LANDMARK PAPERS IN INTERNAL MEDICINE

Len,

With thanks for all you have done for annals.

Hal Sox
July 2009

LANDMARK PAPERS IN INTERNAL MEDICINE

THE FIRST 80 YEARS OF ANNALS OF INTERNAL MEDICINE

HAROLD C. SOX, MD, MACP
EDWARD J. HUTH, MD, MACP
EDITORS

ACP PRESS®
American College of Physicians • Philadelphia

Director, Publishing Operations: Linda Drumheller
Editorial Coordinator: Angela Gabella
Cover Design: Lisa Torrieri, ACP Graphic Services
Interior Design: Michael Ripca, ACP Graphic Services

Printed in the United States of America
Printing/binding by Sheridan Books, Inc.
Composition by Wendy Smith, ACP Graphic Services

Library of Congress Cataloging-in-Publication Data

Landmark papers in internal medicine : the first 80 years of Annals of internal medicine / Hal Sox, editor ; Edward J. Huth, editor emeritus.
p. ; cm.
Includes bibliographical references.
ISBN 978-1-934465-07-3
1. Internal medicine—History—Sources. I. Sox, Harold C. II. Huth, Edward J. III. American College of Physicians (2003-)
[DNLM: 1. Annals of internal medicine. 2. Internal Medicine—history. 3. Internal Medicine—trends. 4. History, 20th Century. 5. History, 21st Century. 6. Review Literature as Topic. 7. Serial Publications. WB 115 L257 2009]

RC39.L36 2009
616—dc22

2009006746

09 10 11 12 13 / 10 9 8 7 6 5 4 3 2 1

Editors of

Annals of Medicine / Annals of Clinical Medicine
Annals of Internal Medicine

Frank Smithies, MD
Editor, *Annals of Medicine*, 1920-1921
Supervising Editor, *Annals of Clinical Medicine*, 1922-1924

Aldred S. Warthin, MD
Editor, *Annals of Clinical Medicine*, 1924-1927
Editor, *Annals of Internal Medicine*, 1927-1931

Carl V. Weller, MD
Editor, *Annals of Internal Medicine*, 1931-1933

Maurice C. Pincoffs, MD
Editor, *Annals of Internal Medicine*, 1933-1960

J. Russell Elkinton, MD
Editor, *Annals of Internal Medicine*, 1960-1971

Edward J. Huth, MD
Editor, *Annals of Internal Medicine*, 1971-1990
Interim Editor, *Annals of Internal Medicine*, 1994-1995

Robert H. Fletcher, MD
Co-Editor, *Annals of Internal Medicine*, 1990-1993

Suzanne W. Fletcher, MD
Co-Editor, *Annals of Internal Medicine*, 1990-1993

Frank F. Davidoff, MD
Editor, *Annals of Internal Medicine*, 1995-2001

Harold C. Sox, MD
Editor, *Annals of Internal Medicine*, 2001-2009

Contributors

Robert G. Dluhy, MD
Senior Physician
Department of Endocrinology, Diabetes and Hypertension
Brigham and Women's Hospital
Professor of Medicine
Harvard Medical School
Boston, Massachusetts

Garabed Eknoyan, MD, FACP
Department of Medicine
Baylor College of Medicine
Houston, Texas

Alfred P. Fishman, MD
Senior Associate Dean
University of Pennsylvania School of Medicine
Philadelphia, Pennsylvania

James N. George, MD, FACP
George Lynn Cross Professor
Departments of Medicine, Biostatistics & Epidemiology
University of Oklahoma Health Sciences Center
Oklahoma City, Oklahoma

DuPont Guerry, MD, FACP
Emeritus Professor of Medicine
School of Medicine
University of Pennsylvania
Philadelphia, Pennsylvania

Daniel G. Haller, MD
Professor of Medicine
Abramson Cancer Center
University of Pennsylvania
Philadelphia, Pennsylvania

Edward D. Harris, Jr., MD, MACP, MACR, FRCP (London)
George DeForest Barnett Professor of Medicine Emeritus
Stanford University
Academic Secretary Emeritus to Stanford University
Executive Secretary, Alpha Omega Alpha
Editor, *The Pharos*
Stanford, California

Edward J. Huth, MD, MACP, FRCP (London)
Editor Emeritus, *Annals of Internal Medicine*
Philadelphia, Pennsylvania

Philip R. Lee, MD, MACP
Professor of Social Medicine, Emeritus
Department of Medicine and Senior Advisor,
Philip R Lee Institute for Health Policy Studies
University of California School of Medicine
San Francisco, California

Bennett Lorber, MD, DSc (Hon), MACP
Thomas M. Durant Professor of Medicine
Professor of Microbiology and Immunology
Temple University School of Medicine
Philadelphia, Pennsylvania

Mark E. Silverman, MD, MACP, FRCP, FACC†

Marvin H. Sleisenger, MD, MACP, DSc (Hon)
Professor of Medicine Emeritus
University of California - San Francisco
Distinguished Physician
Department of Veterans Affairs Medical Center
San Francisco, California

Harold C. Sox, MD, MACP
Editor, *Annals of Internal Medicine*
American College of Physicians
Philadelphia, Pennsylvania

Darren Taichman, MD, PhD
Assistant Professor
University of Pennsylvania School of Medicine
Associate Director
Pulmonary Vascular Disease Program
Penn-Presbyterian Medical Center
Philadelphia, Pennsylvania

Arafat Tfayli, MD
Associate Professor of Medicine
Hematology-Oncology Section
Department of Medicine
University of Oklahoma Health Sciences Center
Oklahoma City, Oklahoma

Charles F. Wooley, MD†

†Deceased

Contents

SECTION VII INFECTIOUS DISEASES

SECTION VIII NEPHROLOGY

SECTION IX ONCOLOGY

SECTION X PULMONARY MEDICINE

SECTION XI RHEUMATOLOGY

Introduction

Any editor of a clinical journal is sure to be aware that relatively few papers that he or she accepts for publication will have a major influence on how medicine is practiced by the journal's readers and other physicians of the time. Some will sink into obscurity; others will be shown in following years to have reached erroneous conclusions. But some will have long lives and bear much fruit, influencing clinical practice and research. They will stand out as truly influential and beneficially so—as turning points in practice, as "landmarks".

We, the current editor and a past editor of *Annals of Internal Medicine*, have collected the landmark articles published by the journal since its inception in 1927. The American College of Physicians is publishing this collection because its leaders believe that internists—and the public that they serve—can learn from the intellectual history of a medical discipline. The edifice of current practice stands on foundations that reflect many small advances in knowledge—and a few large ones. We hope that readers will enjoy reading about some of the large steps, as described in the words of the leaders who advanced the science that shapes daily practice.

But in trying to assemble the "landmarks" published by a journal, what can be the evidence that they are, indeed, landmarks? Are the opinions of editors of journals sufficient? Do judgments have to wait for the opinions of future medical historians, inscribed in the monographs that they write years later on the history of cardiology, of oncology, of medical economics? In beginning to assemble this book, we faced these questions and decided on two solutions.

First, we sought evidence on what papers to select from the frequency with which articles in medical journals cited them. Important and influential papers are likely to be cited by authors whose own work builds upon those papers. While an article whose conclusions prove to be in error may be heavily cited for a year or so, citation over many years is usually the mark of an article with enduring value. So, we used the following procedure in making our selections: We sought citation data for papers published in *Annals of Internal Medicine* through most of its years. For these data, we are truly grateful to Eugene Garfield, the founder of *Science Citation Index*, the authoritative documentation of how widely and frequently a paper is cited in journals in the years after its publication. We made a list of about a dozen of the most frequently cited articles in each subspecialty of internal medicine.

Second, we asked an expert in each subspecialty—the section editors for this book—to help us choose from the lists the most important articles for internal medicine. Because we had to keep the collection of "landmark" *Annals* papers to a number readily accommodated in a book of comfortable size, we asked each of them to choose three articles. Thus, the citation rates were simply the starting point for the selection process. In this way, we introduced a substantial element of subjective judgment into the final choice of the articles that had the most influence in each subspecialty. Some of the section editors judged that the ranking of citation rates was not a sufficient criterion for selection and used their judgment in selecting from the list of the most highly cited articles in their subspecialty.

We asked each section editor to comment briefly on the importance of each of their selections, both at the time of publication and subsequently. We are grateful to them for the commentaries that accompany these "landmark" *Annals* papers. We hope you find their commentaries enlightening and indicative of how these papers played their role in the development of today's standards of medical practice.

Harold C. Sox, MD, MACP, Editor, Annals of Internal Medicine
Edward J. Huth, MD, MACP, Editor Emeritus, Annals of Internal Medicine

Section I

General Medicine

The Medical Review Article: State of the Science.

Mulrow CD. Ann Intern Med. 1987;106:485-488.

This article is a landmark in the development of the modern medical journal. Published under the heading The Literature of Medicine, its subject is the review article, characteristically one of the most popular parts of a clinical journal. The author, Cynthia Mulrow, is a rigorously trained internist-clinical epidemiologist. She is now a senior editor of *Annals*. She evaluated the medical review article according to methodological standards designed to identify reviews that readers could rely upon to provide an unbiased description of the truth. Her findings sparked the beginning of a revolution—still in progress—in how authors should summarize clinical evidence.

Mulrow identified 50 articles published in *Annals, Archives of Internal Medicine, JAMA,* and the *New England Journal of Medicine* during 1985-86. She formulated eight explicit criteria for evaluating reviews: Did it state its purpose? Did it describe the literature search? Did it describe criteria for including and excluding articles? Did it assess study quality? Were the data from different studies combined into a summary measure? and so forth. These criteria are very similar to those now used for evaluating systematic reviews and meta-analyses. No review met all eight criteria, one met six criteria; none met fewer than three criteria. The most commonly met criteria were stating the purpose, doing a qualitative synthesis of the articles, and summarizing the results

Mulrow concluded that a review should meet six standards. First, it should try to answer a precisely defined question. Second, the study question should determine the methods for identifying believable research. Third, the extraction of data should adhere to a protocol and should be done by more than one person. Fourth, the synthesis of the evidence should include all high-quality studies, which means that it will often involve thoughtful weighing of contradictory evidence. Fifth, authors should draw conclusions only when they have adhered to the principles that she described. Finally, the review should state the gaps in the evidence and suggest ways to fill them.

Mulrow's article is a blueprint for the modern systematic review, which now forms the basis for the guidelines and practice measures that increasingly shape medical practice. Systematic reviews are not selective; they are comprehensive. Like a research article, the data speak for themselves to any careful reader. The systematic review—together with the peer review system—are the public's best protection against biased interpretation of clinical evidence. And it started with this four-page article.

Chronic fatigiue syndrome: a working case definition.

Holmes GP, Kaplan JE, Gantz NM, Komaroff AI, Schonberger LB, Straus SE, Jones JF, Dubois RE, Cunningham-Rundles C, Pahwa S, Tosato G, Zegans LS, Purtilo DT, Brown N, Schooley RT, Brus I. Ann Intern Med. 1988;108:387-389.

Chronic fatigue syndrome is a mysterious and disabling affliction that strikes suddenly and can persist for years. Articles about it began to appear in medical journals in the early 1980's. At the very beginning, it acquired the name "chronic Epstein-Barr virus syndrome" because many of the patients had elevated levels of antibodies against the Epstein-Barr virus. The main features of the illness as first described were nonspecific. The dominant symptom is severe, persistent fatigue, often accompanied by low grade fever, sore throat, impaired memory, inability to concentrate on tasks, and confusion. Physical examination is usually normal as are diagnostic tests. Early on, researchers began to question the link to Epstein-Barr virus because antibody levels were often normal and because serum levels of antibodies against other viruses were elevated.

The article by Holmes and his colleagues was pivotal in the short history of this illness. After citing the relatively sparse evidence against a specific linkage to Epstein-Barr virus, the authors said that research on this illness needed to consider other possible causes. Therefore, they said, the illness needs a name that is both descriptive and free of etiological implications. They named the illness "chronic fatigue syndrome," and the name has stuck. Of equal importance, they defined criteria for attaching the new name to a patient, viz., a case definition. A case definition is important in the investigation of any disease because it helps to assure that the subjects of research have the disease. For the same reasons, case definitions are especially important in the early steps in studying a newly recognized illness. If researchers use the same case definition, they are probably studying the same illness, and so they can compare their findings with some confidence.

Although the authors' case definition was updated in 1994 (in an article from the Centers for Disease Control by Fukuda K, Straus SE, Hickie I, Sharpe MC, Dobbins JG, Komaroff AL, International Chronic Fatigue Syndrome Study Group. The chronic fatigue syndrome: a comprehensive approach to its definition and study. Ann Intern Med 1994;121:953-959), it remains important to the present day. It has played an important role in research about chronic fatigue syndrome. However, because the basic features of the authors' case definition have remained widely accepted over two decades, we can infer that researchers have not yet identified the cause of the syndrome, despite progress in defining some of its pathophysiologic manifestations. If they had, their findings would likely have been incorporated into the case definition. Although the search for empirical treatment has led to over 30 randomized trials published from 2003 to the present, the cause of chronic fatigue syndrome remains a mystery.

Screening for colorectal cancer in adults at average risk: a summary of the evidence for the U.S. Preventive Services Task Force.

Pignone M, Rich M, Teutsch SM, Berg AO, Lohr KN. Ann Intern Med. 2002;137:132–141.

The College was one of the first professional organizations in the U.S. to develop practice guidelines, which it began to issue in 1980. Members of the first guidelines committee included many luminaries of the early days of evidence-based medicine, including the redoubtable Alvan Feinstein. Ed Huth was the first *Annals* editor to publish practice guidelines, which he did in the mid-1980's. The *Annals* format persists to the present day: an extensive review of the literature paired with a short article describing the recommendations and briefly summarizing the evidence and the reasoning that connects the evidence to the recommendations. Since 2001, *Annals* has expanded its coverage of practice guidelines and their background reviews. It now publishes all of the U.S. Preventive Services Task Force guidelines for adult medicine as well as the guidelines developed by the College's guidelines program, which is now in its 27th year.

This article is typical of practice guidelines published in *Annals*. The topic is screening for colorectal cancer. The authors were from the Evidence-Based Practice Center at the University of North Carolina, which was funded by the federal government to carry out the literature review. The authors performed a systematic search of the literature from 1966 to 2001, doggedly trying to find everything written on the subject. This article describes the details of their search. As reviews have gotten increasingly complex, *Annals* often publishes the evidence tables on-line but not in the print version of the background review, as is the case for the review reprinted here. These tables are a key element in a systematic review because each row in the table contains a concise description of one of the studies: its patient population, intervention, and key findings. The authors rated the quality of the studies according to criteria developed by the Task Force. The Results section describes the accuracy of the various tests, any randomized trials of screening, and the adverse effects of screening, which would include evaluation of patients who had false-positive screening tests. Table 1 summarizes the effectiveness of the various tests, their accuracy, and the quality of the evidence for these two measures. The article concludes that the evidence is not strong enough to single out one test as clearly preferred.

As an authoritative review of a hot topic in medicine, this article received many citations. The recommendations themselves did not depart much from the guidelines developed by the Task Force in 1996. Little evidence exists to document their influence on the practice of medicine. Indeed, 5 years later, in 2008, the evidence has not changed much. We still do not have a randomized trial of screening with optical colonoscopy or CT colonography, tests that remain prohibitively expensive for a population-wide screening program. Tests for fecal occult blood continue to improve, and the sensitivity has risen to 85% for immunochemical tests. So, this excellent review is a snapshot of a gradually evolving field. For all the excellent recent research, we are farther along but still not close to solid answers. Such is the rhythm of clinical investigation.

THE LITERATURE OF MEDICINE

The Medical Review Article: State of the Science

CYNTHIA D. MULROW, M.D., M.Sc.; San Antonio, Texas

Fifty reviews published during June 1985 to June 1986 in four major medical journals were assessed in a study of the methods of current review articles. Assessments were based on eight explicit criteria adapted from published guidelines for information syntheses. Of the 50 articles, 17 satisfied three of the eight criteria; 32 satisfied four or five criteria; and 1 satisfied six criteria. Most reviews had clearly specified purposes (*n* = 40) and conclusions (*n* = 37). Only one had clearly specified methods of identifying, selecting, and validating included information. Qualitative synthesis was often used to integrate information included in the review (*n* = 43); quantitative synthesis was rarely used (*n* = 3). Future research directives were mentioned in 21. These results indicate that current medical reviews do not routinely use scientific methods to identify, assess, and synthesize information. The methods used in this systematic assessment of reviews are proposed to improve the quality of future review articles.

GOOD REVIEW articles are precious commodities. In this era of a plentiful and burgeoning medical literature, the individual's capacity to read and absorb information has not changed. Reduction of large quantities of information into palatable pieces is essential for digestion.

Adequate refinement of information calls for critical exploration, evaluation, and synthesis. The accomplished reviewer must tediously sift and sort data sources, systematically appraise data quality, and thoughtfully integrate essential data into a unified whole. Such reviewers must synthesize data in a cogent and illuminating way, not just shuffle documents (1).

Unfortunately medical reviews are often subjective, scientifically unsound, and inefficient (2). Strategies for identifying and selecting information are rarely defined. Collected information is reviewed haphazardly with little attention to systematic assessment of quality. Under such circumstances, cogent summarization is an arduous, if not insurmountable, task. The purpose of this article is twofold: to describe the methods of recently published review articles, and to demonstrate a systematic method for preparing review articles.

Methods

Of the 117 journals indexed in the *Abridged Index Medicus,* the four peer-reviewed American medical journals with circulations of greater than 50 000 were identified (3). Articles classified as review or progress articles published in these journals during June 1985 to June 1986 were selected. For *Annals of Internal Medicine* and *Archives of Internal Medicine,* 10 (4-13) and 17 (14-30) review articles, respectively, were identified; for *The Journal of the American Medical Association,* 4 (31-34) state of the art/review articles were identified; and for *The New England Journal of Medicine,* 19 (35-53) medical progress articles were identified. A single assessment was done on reviews published in two parts (54-57).

All reviews were assessed with eight explicit criteria adapted from published guidelines for information syntheses (2, 58, 59): Was the specific purpose of the review stated? Were sources and methods of the citation search identified? Were explicit guidelines provided that determined the material included in and excluded from the review? Was a methodologic validity assessment of material in the review performed? Was the information systematically integrated with explication of data limitations and inconsistencies? Was the information integrated and weighted or pooled metrically? Was a summary of pertinent findings provided? Were specific directives for new research initiatives proposed? Each criterion was categorized as specified, unclear, or not specified.

Results

Assessments of the methods of the 50 review articles are presented in Table 1. No single review clearly specified all eight criteria. One met six criteria; 32 met four or five criteria; and the remaining 17 met three criteria. Most reviews were written by more than 1 author (range, 1 to 12), and the average number of references cited was 100 (range, 18 to 381).

SPECIFIED PURPOSE

The purpose of the review was stated in 40 articles. These purposes were often broad and exhaustive. For example, some reviews addressed multiple aspects of different diseases, such as epidemiology, natural history, physical manifestations, pathogenesis, diagnosis, therapy, and prevention (38, 42). Other reviews had narrower purposes and addressed only treatment (15, 21, 22, 24), pathogenesis (35, 49, 52), clinical presentation (36), or prevention (30). In 10 reviews, no clearly defined purpose was found. Although 1 of these failed to state any purpose whatsoever (44), most were nebulously defined reviews of "current concepts," "aspects of disease," or "lessons derived from 15 years of studies" (23, 45, 51).

Clearly stated purposes are important for several reasons. They give the reader a frame of reference for deciding whether to read further. Specific purposes help determine strategies to select information. For example, reviews concerning therapeutic efficacy might be limited to data from controlled clinical trials; reviews specifically

▶ From the Division of General Internal Medicine, Department of Medicine, University of Texas Health Science Center at San Antonio; San Antonio, Texas.

Table 1. Assessments of Methods Used in Fifty Current Medical Reviews, June 1985 to June 1986

	Specified	Unclear	Not Specified
	←	n	→
Purpose	40	1	9
Data identification	1	2	47
Data selection	1	0	49
Validity assessment	1	1	48
Qualitative synthesis	43	0	7
Quantitative synthesis	3	1	46
Summary	37	12	1
Future directives	21	4	25

addressing natural history might emphasize data from inception cohort studies; and reviews addressing etiology might include data from case-control studies. Finally, the specific purpose of the review can determine appropriate methods of information assessment. Questions concerning where and in whom a particular diagnostic test, intervention, or prevention strategy works might require careful assessment of population and setting. Questions concerning optimal timing of a diagnostic test, intervention, or prevention strategy might concentrate on the actual methods of the test or intervention.

DATA IDENTIFICATION AND SELECTION

The source of the information reviewed was clearly identified in only one review (22), which described a computer-assisted search of English-language articles on MEDLINE. Two reviews (8, 33) stated that published reports had been reviewed but did not specify search processes or time periods. Selection procedures that determined which specific studies to include in the review were provided only by Zarrabi and Rosner (30).

Most reviewers left to conjecture whether included data were identified from automated databases, expert consensus, textbooks, present contents of reference files, or personal-favorite selections. Most also failed to report whether included data were selected on the basis of predetermined criteria, such as particular study designs or population characteristics. As a result, it was impossible to determine whether reviewed material represented information available on a given subject. Selection biases, where authors preferentially cite data that support their opinions, could not be evaluated. Moreover, it was difficult to evaluate whether relevant material had been excluded. This judgment required either considerable personal knowledge of the reviewed topic or considerable faith in the objectivity of the reviewers.

VALIDITY ASSESSMENT

A standardized methodologic assessment of data was used in only one review (22). This article had three authors; whether the assessment ratings represented a consensus or one author's view was not reported. No other review appraised validity in a systematic manner.

Systematic assessment of quality or validity determines, on the basis of a critical examination of the methods used to produce the findings, what conclusions are justifiable. Appraisal of research designs, implementations, and analyses is required. Because authors of most reviews failed to appraise systematically the information regarding population, program, or setting characteristics, judgments on generalizability of the information were limited. Failure to examine details of study design (such as diagnostic and measurement techniques; disease, exposure, and outcome definitions; and intervention and analytic approaches) left the quality of data included open to question.

DATA SYNTHESIS

Although some reviewers (4, 10, 21, 23, 25, 34, 42) merely listed findings, most ($n = 43$) provided some degree of qualitative integration by mentioning limitations and inconsistencies in existing data. Although this qualitative synthesis was often scant and haphazard, three reviews (15, 33, 52) exemplified the value of critically integrating prima-facie conflicting evidence. Hussey (15) elucidated differences in published reports concerning a therapeutic intervention by exploring the differences in study populations, intervention approaches, and outcome measures. Valuable insights about the generalizability of findings were gained: benefits of the therapy were limited to particular populations and settings. Brewster (33) showed that systematic errors in research implementation, such as selection and reporting biases, explained much of the variance in reports on the prevalence of a particular health problem. Clouse and Comp (52) carefully related current knowledge of a pathophysiologic mechanism to differences in laboratory techniques and limitations of measurement methods.

In contrast, synthesis involving quantitative methods was provided in only three reviews. Brewster (33) compared prevalence information among eight studies by converting data to a common numerator and denominator. Houston (24) combined data from four studies involving a drug therapy to determine average response rates, average magnitudes of response, and average times to response. Sakata and colleagues (8) pooled results of several studies to characterize the clinical features of a particular patient group. In these reviews, quantitative methods were used to provide a common unit of comparison and to identify average effects or average characteristics. Other advantages of quantitative techniques, such as identification of interactions and identification of small effects not readily detectable by individual small studies, were not used.

SUMMARIES AND FUTURE DIRECTIVES

Approximately 75% of reviews summarized pertinent findings in remarks in either the initial abstract or the final paragraphs. Although these summaries were helpful in compressing review results into an easily manageable form, they required cautious interpretations. Some resembled "bottom-line" remarks based on "armchair" reviewing techniques; conclusions were not always supported by valid review processes.

Directives for future studies were proposed in only 21 reviews. Specific research recommendations promoted identification of the most promising areas for future research and discouraged duplicative and wasteful efforts. These reviews efficiently enhanced attainment of knowledge by suggesting to the designer of the 100th study what had been learned from the first 99.

Conclusions

This article presents a systematic review method and has shown that current medical reviews do not routinely use such systematic methods to identify, assess, and synthesize information. Although purposes (often broad) were stated in most reviews, the sources and selection methods of reviewed data were rarely defined. Standardized methodologic criteria for assessing the validity of the data were not used. Synthesis of data was weighted toward occasional and informal qualitative critiques with little use of quantitative methods. Summaries were made without showing careful reviewing techniques, and future research directives were often neglected. Although some reviews provided useful overviews of topics, their methods were not replicable and their conclusions might not be valid.

To improve the scope, impact, and quality of reviews, several steps are needed. First, a well-conceived review always answers a question. This question should be made clear at the beginning of the review (60). It should be precisely formulated, rather than broad or ill defined.

Second, efficient strategies for identifying relevant material of substantive quality and excluding irrelevant or poor-quality material are needed. Generally, computer searches of the literature cross-checked with references from other review articles can be used to identify pertinent literature. Experts in the area to be reviewed can be used to verify that all pertinent citations have been identified, but these persons should not serve as the sole source of information. Explicit guidelines for determining what data to include in the review should be stated. These guidelines should coincide with the purpose of the review. In fact, the precise definition of the review's purpose may determine whether characteristics such as study designs, study populations, disease definitions, or time frames should be used as criteria for selecting information for the review.

Third, to manage large quantities of data objectively and effectively, standardized methods of appraising information should be included in more review processes. This involves appraisal of research designs, implementations, and analyses. Standardized appraisal forms addressing these issues can be used by reviewers to optimize uniform assessment of data. To avoid single-reviewer biases, data assessments may be consensus ranked by more than one reviewer. Experts from different areas, such as appropriate specialists, statisticians, and research methodologists, can be used both to help develop the standardized appraisal forms and to rank data.

Fourth, final synthesis of information should involve systematic rather than selective integration. Data regarded as scientifically unsound on the basis of the standardized appraisal should be discarded. Other data can sometimes be assigned a weight or relative value based on its quality as determined by the standardized appraisal (61). Insights gained from careful explorations of divergent findings in scientifically valid data sets should be sought, and limitations of data sets identified. More reviewers should consider quantitative synthesis techniques to complement and supplement their qualitative techniques. Quantitative methods can be used to provide a common unit of comparison between studies and to combine data from several studies. These methods can be used to evaluate generalizability, consistency, interactions, and small effects that are not readily recognizable from individual studies.

Fifth, conclusions are justified only when the aforementioned processes of collecting, analyzing, and integrating information are systematically and thoughtfully applied. The conclusions should be succinct and logically ordered summarizations of data. If the appraisal and synthesis of data involves weighting of evidence according to some type of quality assessment, the conclusions too should reflect the relative weighting.

Finally, reviewers should capitalize on their intensive efforts by clearly identifying gaps in present knowledge and suggesting future initiatives. Unsolved issues and problems can be delineated, and appropriate methods for addressing these issues can be suggested. In this way, the reader finishes the review with a view of what is not known about the subject as well as what is known (60).

By using these systematic methods of exploration, evaluation, and synthesis, the good reviewer can accomplish the task of advancing scientific knowledge.

ACKNOWLEDGMENTS: The author thanks Drs. A. Diehl, R. Bauer, J. Pugh, R. Velez, and P. Mullen for their assistance with this manuscript.

Grant support: by a Teaching and Research Scholar Award from the American College of Physicians.

▶ Requests for reprints should be addressed to Cynthia D. Mulrow, M.D., M.Sc.; Ambulatory Care (11C), Audie Murphy Veterans Administration Hospital, 7400 Merton Minter Drive; San Antonio, TX 78284.

References

1. PRESIDENT'S SCIENCE ADVISORY COMMITTEE. *Science, Government, and Information: The Responsibilities of the Technical Community and the Government in the Transfer of Information.* Washington, D.C.: Government Printing Office; 1963.
2. LIGHT RJ, PILLEMAR DB. *Summing Up: the Science of Reviewing Research.* Cambridge, Massachusetts: Harvard University Press; 1984.
3. *Ulrich's International Periodicals Directory.* 24th ed. New York: R.R. Bowker Co.; 1985.
4. SCHAFER AI. The hypercoagulable states. *Ann Intern Med.* 1985;**102:**814-28.
5. GALE RP, FOON KA. Chronic lymphocytic leukemia: recent advances in biology and treatment. *Ann Intern Med.* 1985;**103:**101-20.
6. PACKER M. Vasodilator therapy for primary pulmonary hypertension: limitations and hazards. *Ann Intern Med.* 1985;**103:**258-70.
7. AUSUBEL K, FURMAN S. The pacemaker syndrome. *Ann Intern Med.* 1985;**103:**420-9.
8. SAKATA S, NAKAMURA S, MIURA K. Autoantibodies against thyroid hormones or iodothyronine: implications in diagnosis, thyroid function, treatment, and pathogenesis. *Ann Intern Med.* 1985;**103:**579-89.
9. BASS E. Cardiopulmonary arrest: pathophysiology and neurologic complications. *Ann Intern Med.* 1985;**103**(6 pt 1):920-7.
10. GRAHAM DY, SMITH JL. Aspirin and the stomach. *Ann Intern Med.* 1986;**104:**390-8.
11. PASULKA PS, BISTRIAN BR, BENOTTI DN, BLACKBURN GL. The risks of surgery in obese patients. *Ann Intern Med.* 1986;**104:**540-6.
12. MELTZER RS, VISSER CA, FUSTER V. Intracardiac thrombi and systemic embolization. *Ann Intern Med.* 1986;**104:**689-98.
13. MARTON KI, GEAN AD. The spinal tap: a new look at an old test. *Ann Intern Med.* 1986;**104:**840-8.
14. BURCH WM. Cushing's disease: a review. *Ann Intern Med.* 1985;**145:**1106-11.

15. Hussey KP. Vasopressin therapy for upper gastrointestinal tract hemorrhage: has its efficacy been proven? *Arch Intern Med.* 1985;**145:**1263-7.
16. Horowitz M, Collins PJ, Shearman DJC. Disorders of gastric emptying in humans and the use of radionuclide techniques. *Arch Intern Med.* 1985;**145:**1467-72.
17. Tobin MJ. Use of bronchodilator aerosols. *Arch Intern Med.* 1985;**145:**1659-63.
18. Barish CF, Wu WC, Castell DO. Respiratory complications of gastroesophageal reflux. *Arch Intern Med.* 1985;**145:**1882-8.
19. Shively B, Goldschlager N. Progress in cardiac pacing: part I. *Arch Intern Med.* 1985;**145:**2103-6.
20. Houston MC. Sodium and hypertension: a review. *Arch Intern Med.* 1986;**145:**179-85.
21. Hoshino PK, Gaasch WH. When to intervene in chronic aortic regurgitation. *Arch Intern Med.* 1986;**146:**349-52.
22. Levine MN, Sackett DL, Bush H. Heroin vs morphine for cancer pain? *Arch Intern Med.* 1986;**146:**353-6.
23. Peterson CE, Kwaan HC. Current concepts of warfarin therapy. *Arch Intern Med.* 1986;**146:**581-4.
24. Houston MC. Treatment of hypertensive emergencies and urgencies with oral clonidine loading and titration: a review. *Arch Intern Med.* 1986;**146:**586-9.
25. Levin ME, Rigg LA, Marshall RE. Pregnancy and diabetes: team approach. *Arch Intern Med.* 1986;**146:**758-67.
26. Mallette LE, Eichhorn F. Effects of lithium carbonate on human calcium metabolism. *Arch Intern Med.* 1986;**146:**770-6.
27. Fulkerson WJ, Coleman RE, Ravin CE, Saltzman HA. Diagnosis of pulmonary embolism. *Arch Intern Med.* 1986;**146:**961-7.
28. Park GD, Spector R, Goldberg MJ, Johnson GF. Expanded role of charcoal therapy in the poisoned and overdosed patient. *Arch Intern Med.* 1986;**146:**969-73.
29. Chan WC, Winton EF, Waldmann TA. Lymphocytosis of large granular lymphocytes. *Arch Intern Med.* 1986;**146:**1201-3.
30. Zarrabi MH, Rosner F. Rarity of failure of penicillin prophylaxis to prevent postsplenectomy sepsis. *Arch Intern Med.* 1986;**146:**1207-8.
31. Schuckit MA. Genetics and the risk for alcoholism. *JAMA.* 1985;**254:**2614-7.
32. Stone KM, Grimes DA, Magder LS. Primary prevention of sexually transmitted diseases: a primer for clinicians. *JAMA.* 1986;**255:**1763-6.
33. Brewster JM. Prevalence of alcohol and other drug problems among physicians. *JAMA.* 1986;**255:**1913-20.
34. Morrison RG. Medical and public health aspects of boxing. *JAMA.* 1986;**255:**2475-80.
35. Britigan BE, Cohen MS, Sparling PF. Gonococcal infection: a model of molecular pathogenesis. *N Engl J Med.* 1985;**312:**1683-94.
36. Huston TP, Puffer JC, Rodney WM. The athletic heart syndrome. *N Engl J Med.* 1985;**313:**24-32.
37. Foley KM. The treatment of cancer pain. *N Engl J Med.* 1985;**313:**84-95.
38. Herzog DB, Copeland PM. Eating disorders. *N Engl J Med.* 1985;**313:**295-303.
39. Rojeski MT, Gharib H. Nodular thyroid disease: evaluation and management. *N Engl J Med.* 1985;**313:**428-36.
40. Fielding JE. Smoking: health effects and control (part 1). *N Engl J Med.* 1985;**313:**491-8.
41. Fraser CL, Arieff AI. Hepatic encephalopathy. *N Engl J Med.* 1985;**313:**865-73.
42. Elliot DL, Tolle SW, Goldberg L, Miller JB. Pet-associated illness. *N Engl J Med.* 1985;**313:**985-95.
43. Lemon SM. Type A viral hepatitis. New developments in an old disease. *N Engl J Med.* 1985;**313:**1059-67.
44. Demling RH. Burns. *N Engl J Med.* 1985;**313:**1389-98.
45. Goorin AM, Abelson HT, Frei E III. Osteosarcoma: fifteen years later. *N Engl J Med.* 1985;**313:**1637-43.
46. DeBusk RF, Blomqvist CG, Kouchoukos NT, et al. Identification and treatment of low-risk patients after acute myocardial infarction and corconary-artery bypass graft surgery. *N Engl J Med.* 1986;**314:**161-6.
47. Benatar SR. Fatal asthma. *N Engl J Med.* 1986;**314:**423-9.
48. Colucci WS, Wright RF, Braunwald E. New positive inotropic agents in the treatment of congestive heart failure: mechanisms of action and recent clinical developments: 1. *N Engl J Med.* 1986;**314:**290-9.
49. Ross R. The pathogenesis of atherosclerosis—an update. *N Engl J Med.* 1986;**314:**488-500.
50. Corey L, Spear PG. Infections with herpes simplex viruses. (part 1). *N Engl J Med.* 1986;**314:**686-91.
51. Katzman R. Alzheimer's disease. *N Engl J Med.* 1986;**314:**964-73.
52. Clouse LH, Comp PC. The regulation of hemostasis: the protein C system. *N Engl J Med.* 1986;**314:**1298-304.
53. Riggs BL, Melton LJ III. Involutional osteoporosis. *N Engl J Med.* 1986;**314:**1676-86.
54. Shively B, Goldschlager N. Progress in cardiac pacing: part II. *Arch Intern Med.* 1985;**145:**2238-44.
55. Fielding JE. Smoking: health effects and control (part 2). *N Engl J Med.* 1985;**313:**555-61.
56. Colucci WS, Wright RF, Braunwald E. New positive inotropic agents in the treatment of congestive heart failure: mechanisms of action and recent clinical developments: 2. *N Engl J Med.* 1986;**314:**349-58.
57. Corey L, Spear PG. Infections with herpes simplex viruses (part 2). *N Engl J Med.* 1986;**314:**749-57.
58. *Policy Research Incorporated Literature Review Validation Procedures Manual.* Baltimore: Policy Research Inc.: 1979.
59. Mullen PD, Ramirez G. Information synthesis and meta-analysis. In: *Advances in Health Education and Promotion.* Vol. 2. Greenwich, Connecticut: Jai Press; 1986.
60. Huth EJ. *How to Write and Publish Papers in the Medical Sciences.* Philadelphia: ISI Press; 1982:64.
61. Morgan PP. Review articles: 2. The literature jungle. *Can Med Assoc J.* 1986;**134:**98-9.

Chronic Fatigue Syndrome: A Working Case Definition

GARY P. HOLMES, M.D.; JONATHAN E. KAPLAN, M.D.; NELSON M. GANTZ, M.D.; ANTHONY L. KOMAROFF, M.D.; LAWRENCE B. SCHONBERGER, M.D.; STEPHEN E. STRAUS, M.D.; JAMES F. JONES, M.D.; RICHARD E. DUBOIS, M.D.; CHARLOTTE CUNNINGHAM-RUNDLES, M.D.; SAVITA PAHWA, M.D.; GIOVANNA TOSATO, M.D.; LEONARD S. ZEGANS, M.D.; DAVID T. PURTILO, M.D.; NATHANIEL BROWN, M.D.; ROBERT T. SCHOOLEY, M.D.; and IRENA BRUS, M.D.; Atlanta, Georgia; Worcester and Boston, Massachusetts; Bethesda, Maryland; Denver, Colorado; New York and Manhasset, New York; San Francisco, California; and Omaha, Nebraska

The chronic Epstein-Barr virus syndrome is a poorly defined symptom complex characterized primarily by chronic or recurrent debilitating fatigue and various combinations of other symptoms, including sore throat, lymph node pain and tenderness, headache, myalgia, and arthralgias. Although the syndrome has received recent attention, and has been diagnosed in many patients, the chronic Epstein-Barr virus syndrome has not been defined consistently. Despite the name of the syndrome, both the diagnostic value of Epstein-Barr virus serologic tests and the proposed causal relationship between Epstein-Barr virus infection and patients who have been diagnosed with the chronic Epstein-Barr virus syndrome remain doubtful. We propose a new name for the chronic Epstein-Barr virus syndrome—the chronic fatigue syndrome—that more accurately describes this symptom complex as a syndrome of unknown cause characterized primarily by chronic fatigue. We also present a working definition for the chronic fatigue syndrome designed to improve the comparability and reproducibility of clinical research and epidemiologic studies, and to provide a rational basis for evaluating patients who have chronic fatigue of undetermined cause.

[**MeSH Terms: axilla; chronic disease; depression; Epstein-Barr virus; fatigue; fever; lymph nodes; memory disorders; neck; pharyngitis.** Other indexing terms: chronic Epstein-Barr virus syndrome; chronic fatigue syndrome; sore throat]

THE CHRONIC EPSTEIN-BARR virus syndrome, also known as chronic mononucleosis or chronic mononucleosis-like syndrome, is a syndrome of unknown cause that has been the subject of interest in both medical and popular literature, particularly since 1985. As it was described (1-4) in four groups of patients, the syndrome consists of a combination of nonspecific symptoms—severe fatigue, weakness, malaise, subjective fever, sore throat, painful lymph nodes, decreased memory, confusion, depression, decreased ability to concentrate on tasks, and various other complaints—with a remarkable absence of objective physical or laboratory abnormalities. The syndrome was linked in these and other reports to Epstein-Barr virus, because many, but not all, of the patients had Epstein-Barr virus antibody profiles that suggested reactivation of latent infection.

Reference laboratories soon began to advertise Epstein-Barr virus serologic tests for use in the diagnosis of the chronic Epstein-Barr virus syndrome (5). Although reliable data are not available, indications are that the syndrome has been diagnosed commonly by physicians, often on the basis of poorly defined diagnostic criteria. Since late 1985, the Division of Viral Diseases, Centers for Disease Control, has responded to several thousand telephone and mail requests for information about the chronic Epstein-Barr virus syndrome, both from physicians and from patients in whom the syndrome has been diagnosed. Judging from the inquiries received, many physicians appear to have based their diagnoses on little more than the presence of detectable serum Epstein-Barr virus antibody titers.

More recent studies (6, 7) have cast doubt on the diagnostic value of positive Epstein-Barr virus serologic results and on the proposed relationship between Epstein-Barr virus infection and patients who have been diagnosed with the chronic Epstein-Barr virus syndrome. Although some statistically significant associations between positive Epstein-Barr virus serologic tests and illnesses diagnosed as the chronic Epstein-Barr virus syndrome were identified in one study using age-, sex-, and race-matched controls (6), the serologic associations between the syndrome and cytomegalovirus, herpes simplex virus types 1 and 2, and measles virus were as strong as or stronger than the association with Epstein-Barr virus. Epstein-Barr virus serologic results in this study were also found to be poorly reproducible, both within and among laboratories, leading to the conclusion that the results of these tests are not directly comparable unless they have been done in parallel.

With the apparent lack of correlation between serum Epstein-Barr virus titers and the presence of chronic fatigue symptoms, it is premature to focus research and diagnostic efforts on Epstein-Barr virus alone. Many public health officials and clinicians are concerned that a di-

▶ From the Division of Viral Diseases, Centers for Disease Control, Atlanta, Georgia; Department of Medicine, University of Massachusetts Medical School, Worcester, Massachusetts; Department of Medicine, Brigham and Women's Hospital, Boston, Massachusetts; Laboratory of Clinical Investigation, National Institutes of Health, Bethesda, Maryland; Department of Pediatrics, National Jewish Center for Immunology and Respiratory Medicine, Denver, Colorado; Atlanta Medical Associates, Atlanta, Georgia; Department of Medicine, Mount Sinai Medical Center, New York, New York; Department of Pediatrics, North Shore University Hospital, Manhasset, New York; Division of Biochemistry and Biophysics, Food and Drug Administration, Bethesda, Maryland; Department of Psychiatry, University of San Francisco School of Medicine, San Francisco, California; Department of Pathology and Microbiology, University of Nebraska Medical Center, Omaha, Nebraska; Department of Medicine, Massachusetts General Hospital, Boston, Massachusetts; and Department of Medicine, Beth Israel Medical Center, New York, New York.

agnosis of the chronic Epstein-Barr virus syndrome may not be appropriate for persons with chronic fatigue who have positive Epstein-Barr virus serologic tests, and that definable occult diseases may actually be the cause of symptoms such as fatigue, weakness, and fever. It is also inappropriate to use a name for the syndrome that implies a specific causal agent. We, therefore, propose a new name—the chronic fatigue syndrome—that describes the most striking clinical characteristic of the chronic Epstein-Barr virus syndrome without implying a causal relationship with Epstein-Barr virus.

Because of the nonspecific nature of the symptoms and the lack of a diagnostic test, researchers have had difficulty devising a case definition for the chronic Epstein-Barr virus syndrome. When definitions have been described, they have differed greatly among the various published studies, making direct comparisons of the study results difficult. We have organized an informal working group of public health epidemiologists, academic researchers, and clinicians, to develop a consensus on the salient clinical characteristics of the chronic Epstein-Barr virus syndrome and to devise a definition for the chronic fatigue syndrome that will be the basis for conducting future epidemiologic and clinical studies. Because the syndrome has no diagnostic test, the definition at present is based on signs and symptoms only. This definition is intentionally restrictive, to maximize the chances that research studies will detect significant associations if such associations truly exist. It identifies persons whose illnesses are most compatible with a possibly unique clinical entity; persons who may have less severe forms of the syndrome or who have less characteristic clinical features may be excluded by the new definition.

The chronic fatigue syndrome is currently an operational concept designed for research purposes that physicians must recognize not necessarily as a single disease but as a syndrome—a complex of potentially related symptoms that tend to occur together—that may have several causes. Periodic reconsideration of conditions such as those listed under major criteria, part 2, should be standard practice in the long-term follow-up of these patients.

Case Definition for The Chronic Fatigue Syndrome

A case of the chronic fatigue syndrome must fulfill major criteria 1 and 2, and the following minor criteria: 6 or more of the 11 symptom criteria and 2 or more of the 3 physical criteria; or 8 or more of the 11 symptom criteria.

MAJOR CRITERIA

1. New onset of persistent or relapsing, debilitating fatigue or easy fatigability in a person who has no previous history of similar symptoms, that does not resolve with bedrest, and that is severe enough to reduce or impair average daily activity below 50% of the patient's premorbid activity level for a period of at least 6 months.

2. Other clinical conditions that may produce similar symptoms must be excluded by thorough evaluation, based on history, physical examination, and appropriate laboratory findings. These conditions include malignancy; autoimmune disease; localized infection (such as occult abscess); chronic or subacute bacterial disease (such as endocarditis, Lyme disease, or tuberculosis), fungal disease (such as histoplasmosis, blastomycosis, or coccidioidomycosis), and parasitic disease (such as toxoplasmosis, amebiasis, giardiasis, or helminthic infestation); disease related to human immunodeficiency virus (HIV) infection; chronic psychiatric disease, either newly diagnosed or by history (such as endogenous depression; hysterical personality disorder; anxiety neurosis; schizophrenia; or chronic use of major tranquilizers, lithium, or antidepressive medications); chronic inflammatory disease (such as sarcoidosis, Wegener granulomatosis, or chronic hepatitis); neuromuscular disease (such as multiple sclerosis or myasthenia gravis); endocrine disease (such as hypothyroidism, Addison disease, Cushing syndrome, or diabetes mellitus); drug dependency or abuse (such as alcohol, controlled prescription drugs, or illicit drugs); side effects of a chronic medication or other toxic agent (such as a chemical solvent, pesticide, or heavy metal); or other known or defined chronic pulmonary, cardiac, gastrointestinal, hepatic, renal, or hematologic disease.

Specific laboratory tests or clinical measurements are not required to satisfy the definition of the chronic fatigue syndrome, but the recommended evaluation includes serial weight measurements (weight change of more than 10% in the absence of dieting suggests other diagnoses); serial morning and afternoon temperature measurements; complete blood count and differential; serum electrolytes; glucose; creatinine, blood urea nitrogen; calcium, phosphorus; total bilirubin, alkaline phosphatase, serum aspartate aminotransferase, serum alanine aminotransferase; creatine phosphokinase or aldolase; urinalysis; posteroanterior and lateral chest roentgenograms; detailed personal and family psychiatric history; erythrocyte sedimentation rate; antinuclear antibody; thyroid-stimulating hormone level; HIV antibody measurement; and intermediate-strength purified protein derivative (PPD) skin test with controls.

If any of the results from these tests are abnormal, the physician should search for other conditions that may cause such a result. If no such conditions are detected by a reasonable evaluation, this criterion is satisfied.

MINOR CRITERIA

Symptom Criteria

To fulfill a symptom criterion, a symptom must have begun at or after the time of onset of increased fatigability, and must have persisted or recurred over a period of at least 6 months (individual symptoms may or may not have occurred simultaneously). Symptoms include:

1. Mild fever—oral temperature between 37.5° C and 38.6° C, if measured by the patient—or chills. (Note: oral temperatures of greater than 38.6° C are less compatible with chronic fatigue syndrome and should prompt studies for other causes of illness.)

2. Sore throat.

3. Painful lymph nodes in the anterior or posterior cervical or axillary distribution.

4. Unexplained generalized muscle weakness.

5. Muscle discomfort or myalgia.

6. Prolonged (24 hours or greater) generalized fatigue after levels of exercise that would have been easily tolerated in the patient's premorbid state.

7. Generalized headaches (of a type, severity, or pattern that is different from headaches the patient may have had in the premorbid state).

8. Migratory arthralgia without joint swelling or redness.

9. Neuropsychologic complaints (one or more of the following: photophobia, transient visual scotomata, forgetfulness, excessive irritability, confusion, difficulty thinking, inability to concentrate, depression).

10. Sleep disturbance (hypersomnia or insomnia).

11. Description of the main symptom complex as initially developing over a few hours to a few days (this is not a true symptom, but may be considered as equivalent to the above symptoms in meeting the requirements of the case definition).

Physical Criteria

Physical criteria must be documented by a physician on at least two occasions, at least 1 month apart.

1. Low-grade fever—oral temperature between 37.6° C and 38.6° C, or rectal temperature between 37.8° C and 38.8° C. (*See* note under Symptom Criterion 1.)

2. Nonexudative pharyngitis.

3. Palpable or tender anterior or posterior cervical or axillary lymph nodes. (Note: lymph nodes greater than 2 cm in diameter suggest other causes. Further evaluation is warranted.)

ACKNOWLEDGMENTS: The authors thank Mrs. Josephine M. Lister for manuscript preparation.

▶ Requests for reprints should be addressed to Gary P. Holmes, M.D.; Division of Viral Diseases, Center for Infectious Diseases, Centers for Disease Control; Atlanta, GA 30333.

References

1. Tobi M, Morag A, Ravid Z, et al. Prolonged atypical illness associated with serological evidence of persistent Epstein-Barr virus infection. *Lancet.* 1982;**1:**61-4.
2. DuBois RE, Seeley JK, Brus I, et al. Chronic mononucleosis syndrome. *South Med J.* 1984;**77:**1376-82.
3. Jones JF, Ray CG, Minnich LL, et al. Evidence for active Epstein-Barr virus infection in patients with persistent, unexplained illnesses: elevated anti-early antigen antibodies. *Ann Intern Med.* 1985;**102:**1-7.
4. Straus SE, Tosato G, Armstrong G, et al. Persisting illness and fatigue in adults with evidence of Epstein-Barr virus infection. *Ann Intern Med.* 1985;**102:**7-16.
5. Merlin TL. Chronic mononucleosis: pitfalls in the laboratory diagnosis. *Hum Pathol.* 1986;**17:**2-8.
6. Holmes GP, Kaplan JE, Stewart JA, Hunt B, Pinsky PF, Schonberger LB. A cluster of patients with a chronic mononucleosis-like syndrome: is Epstein-Barr virus the cause? *JAMA.* 1987;**257:**2297-2302.
7. Buchwald D, Sullivan JL, Komaroff AL. Frequency of "chronic active Epstein-Barr virus infection" in a general medical practice. *JAMA.* 1987;**257:**2303-7.

Screening for Colorectal Cancer in Adults at Average Risk: A Summary of the Evidence for the U.S. Preventive Services Task Force

Michael Pignone, MD, MPH; Melissa Rich, MD; Steven M. Teutsch, MD, MPH; Alfred O. Berg, MD, MPH; and Kathleen N. Lohr, PhD

Purpose: **To assess the effectiveness of different colorectal cancer screening tests for adults at average risk.**

Data Sources: **Recent systematic reviews; *Guide to Clinical Preventive Services*, 2nd edition; and focused searches of MEDLINE from 1966 through September 2001. The authors also conducted hand searches, reviewed bibliographies, and consulted context experts to ensure completeness.**

Study Selection: **When available, the most recent high-quality systematic review was used to identify relevant articles. This review was then supplemented with a MEDLINE search for more recent articles.**

Data Extraction: **One reviewer abstracted information from the final set of studies into evidence tables, and a second reviewer checked the tables for accuracy. Discrepancies were resolved by consensus.**

Data Synthesis: **For average-risk adults older than 50 years of age, evidence from multiple well-conducted randomized trials supported the effectiveness of fecal occult blood testing in reducing colorectal cancer incidence and mortality rates compared with no screening. Data from well-conducted case–control studies supported the effectiveness of sigmoidoscopy and possibly colonoscopy in reducing colon cancer incidence and mortality rates. A nonrandomized, controlled trial examining colorectal cancer mortality rates and randomized trials examining diagnostic yield supported the use of fecal occult blood testing plus sigmoidoscopy. The effectiveness of barium enema is unclear. Data are insufficient to support a definitive determination of the most effective screening strategy.**

Conclusions: **Colorectal cancer screening reduces death from colorectal cancer and can decrease the incidence of disease through removal of adenomatous polyps. Several available screening options seem to be effective, but the single best screening approach cannot be determined because data are insufficient.**

Ann Intern Med. 2002;137:132-141. www.annals.org
For author affiliations, see end of text
See related articles on pp 96-104 and pp 129-131.

The U.S. Preventive Services Task Force (USPSTF) last considered its recommendations regarding colorectal cancer screening in 1996 (1). At that time, the available evidence included one randomized, controlled trial showing that fecal occult blood testing (FOBT) reduced mortality rates (2); a case–control study showing that persons having sigmoidoscopy were less likely to die of colorectal cancer (3); and one nonrandomized, controlled trial of FOBT combined with rigid sigmoidoscopy that suggested some benefit from the two tests together (4). On the basis of this evidence, the USPSTF recommended screening for colorectal cancer with FOBT, sigmoidoscopy, or both (a grade B recommendation) but did not recommend for or against other means of screening (digital rectal examination, double-contrast barium enema, or colonoscopy) because the available evidence was insufficient. (See the companion article in this issue for a description of the USPSTF classification of recommendations.) The Task Force also recommended that FOBT be performed yearly but did not specify an interval for sigmoidoscopy.

Since 1996, important new evidence has emerged regarding the effectiveness of colorectal cancer screening. We performed an updated systematic review to help the USPSTF evaluate new evidence on the effectiveness of different colorectal cancer screening tests as it updated its previous recommendation. We examined the evidence concerning the effectiveness of screening in adults older than 50 years of age who are at average risk for colorectal cancer. The effectiveness, accuracy, and adverse effects of digital rectal examination (with or without a single office-based FOBT), traditional three-card FOBT (hereafter referred to as FOBT), sigmoidoscopy, FOBT with sigmoidoscopy, double-contrast barium enema, and colonoscopy were examined. Other tests or combinations of tests have not been well evaluated and are not discussed here. A more detailed report of our review can be found on the Web site of the U.S. Agency for Healthcare Research and Quality (www.ahrq.gov/clinic/uspstfix.htm) (5). The USPSTF's updated recommendations for colorectal cancer screening recommendations can be found in the companion article in this issue (6).

METHODS

To identify the relevant literature, we used the *Guide to Clinical Preventive Services*, 2nd edition (1); existing systematic reviews; focused MEDLINE literature searches from 1966 through September 2001; and hand searches of key articles. When available, systematic reviews were used to identify older relevant studies. Literature searches were used to identify newer studies. Detailed descriptions of the literature searches can be found in the Appendix (available at www.annals.org).

To identify relevant studies, one reviewer examined the abstracts of the articles identified in the initial search. A second reviewer examined the excluded articles. Disagreements about inclusion were resolved by consensus. Two reviewers examined the full text of the remaining articles to determine final eligibility. We used evidence from randomized, controlled trials or observational studies that measured patient outcomes, particularly changes in colorectal cancer mortality rates and incidence. When such data were not available, we included indirect information on the accuracy of screening tests. Details about study inclusion are available in the Appendix (available at www.annals.org). We rated the quality of the included articles by using the criteria developed by the USPSTF Methods group (7), which are described in the accompanying article in this issue (6). We used the final set of eligible articles to create evidence tables and a draft report. The draft report was extensively peer reviewed by the USPSTF, experts in the field, governmental agencies, and nongovernmental organizations.

Role of the Funding Source

This evidence report was funded through a contract to the Research Triangle Institute–University of North Carolina Evidence-based Practice Center from the Agency for Healthcare Research and Quality. Staff of the funding source contributed to the study design, reviewed draft and final manuscripts, and made editing suggestions.

RESULTS

Our general search identified 719 articles published since 1995 on colorectal cancer screening. We retained 19 of these articles in our final document. Specific searches from 1966 through 2001 for articles about the accuracy of barium enema and complications of screening yielded 621 and 839 articles, respectively. After review, we retained 13 articles about barium enema and 19 articles about complications of screening. We also included 15 articles identified from the previous USPSTF review or from hand searches of other articles. **Table 1** summarizes our findings.

Digital Rectal Examination

Effectiveness

A case–control study from the Kaiser Permanente Medical Care Program in northern California examined the effect of screening with digital rectal examination on death from colorectal cancer (8). The investigators identified patients 45 years of age and older who died of distal rectal cancer between 1971 and 1986 and selected matched controls from the patient membership. They examined medical records to determine whether the patients and controls had undergone screening digital rectal examination within a year of cancer diagnosis. Investigators found no difference between groups after controlling for potential confounders, although the confidence interval was wide (odds ratio, 0.96 [95% CI, 0.56 to 1.7]).

Accuracy

The potential sensitivity of screening digital rectal examination is low; fewer than 10% of cases of colorectal cancer are within reach of the examining finger (28). The specificity of positive results on digital rectal examination has not been examined in outpatients at average risk for colorectal cancer.

In-Office Fecal Occult Blood Testing after Digital Rectal Examination

Effectiveness

No studies have examined the effect of a single in-office FOBT after digital rectal examination on colorectal cancer incidence or mortality rates.

Accuracy

A single in-office FOBT is likely to be less sensitive than the traditional three-card FOBT performed at home because only one sample is taken (9). In a large study from Japan, Yamamoto and Nakama (10) found that the first test card detected only 58% of cancer found after a three-card test. The single in-office FOBT may be less specific than a properly performed three-card FOBT because the in-office test does not allow degradation of the vegetable peroxidases that sometimes produce false-positive results (9). In addition, the potential trauma from the in-office examination itself may also result in lower specificity (9). Two studies of poor to fair quality that used existing data to retrospectively compare the specificity of the single in-office FOBT and the three-card home FOBT (11, 12) found little difference in specificity between the two groups. However, the validity of these studies is limited because neither could ensure that similar patient samples received each test.

Fecal Occult Blood Testing

Effectiveness

In addition to an older randomized trial performed in Minnesota (2), which was available to the USPSTF in 1996, two newer randomized, controlled trials have examined the effectiveness of biennial FOBT for reducing death from colorectal cancer (13, 14). These more recent trials, from the United Kingdom (13) and Denmark (14), found 15% and 18% reductions in mortality rates, respectively, with biennial testing. Neither trial used slides that were rehydrated before development (**Table 2**).

The Minnesota trial compared annual and biennial testing with no screening and rehydrated most test cards (83%). Cumulative colorectal cancer mortality rates after 18 years of follow-up were 33% (CI, 17% to 49%) lower among persons randomly assigned to undergo annual FOBT than in a control group that was not offered screening (absolute rates, 9.5 deaths per 1000 participants vs. 14.1 deaths per 1000 participants; difference, 4.6 deaths per 1000 participants) (2). Biennial screening, which did not show a reduction in mortality rates at 13-year follow-up, produced a 21% (CI, 3% to 38%) reduction in mortality rate at 18 years (15). The 18-year follow-up also showed that the incidence of colorectal cancer decreased by 20% (CI, 10% to 30%) and 17% (CI, 6% to 27%) in the groups screened annually and biennially, respectively, compared with controls (16). Because of differences in hydration, test frequency, duration, and effect size, the results of these trials could not be combined in a meta-analysis.

Table 1. **Characteristics of Screening Tests for Colorectal Cancer***

Screening Strategy for CRC	Effectiveness in Reducing Incidence of and Death from CRC	Evidence Grade†	Ability To Detect Cancer	Evidence Grade†
Digital rectal examination	Case–control study found no difference in mortality rates; OR, 0.96 [0.56–1.7] (8)	Level II—poor	Pathologic data suggest <10% of CRC is within reach of examining finger	
Office FOBT (one card)	Unknown		Only 58% of cancer cases are detected on the first of three cards, suggesting lower sensitivity than three-card testing (10)	Level III—fair
Home FOBT (three cards), unrehydrated	Biennial testing: 2 trials found mortality reductions of 15% [1%–26%] (13) and 18% [1%–32%] (14)	Level I—good	One-time sensitivity 30%–40% Unrehydrated FOBT finds about 25% of cancer cases (9)	
Home FOBT (three cards), rehydrated	Annual testing: 33% [13–50] reduction in mortality (2); 20% [10%–30%] reduction in cancer incidence (16) Biennial testing: 21% [3%–38%] reduction in mortality (15); 17% [6%–27%] reduction in cancer incidence (16)	Level I—good	Single-test accuracy 50% [30%–70%] for cancer, 24% [19%–29%] for advanced neoplasms (17) Over 13 years, rehydrated FOBT finds 50% of cancer cases (2)	Level III—good
Sigmoidoscopy	Small RCT found decreased CRC mortality rates with screening; RR, 0.50 [0.10–2.72] (18) Case–control studies suggest a 59% [31%–75%] reduction in mortality rate within reach of scope (3)	Level I—fair Level II—good	One-time screening detects 68%–78% of advanced neoplasia (17, 20)	Level III—good
Combined FOBT and sigmoidoscopy	Nonrandomized trial found a 43% reduction in mortality rate when FOBT was added to rigid sigmoidoscopy; RR, 0.57 [0.56–1.19] (4)	Level I—fair to poor	One-time screening detects 76% of advanced neoplasia (17) Increased yield when sigmoidoscopy is added to FOBT (21–23)	Level III—good
Double-contrast barium enema	Unknown		Sensitivity of one-time test for cancer or large polyps 48% [24%–67%] (24)	Level III—fair
Colonoscopy	Case–control study found an OR of 0.43 [0.30–0.63] for death from CRC; CRC incidence decreased by 40%–60% (26)	Level II—fair	Sensitivity for large adenomas >90%; sensitivity for cancer probably higher (27)	Level III—good

* CRC = colorectal cancer; FOBT = fecal occult blood test; NA = not applicable (see text); OR = odds ratio; RCT = randomized, controlled trial; RR = relative risk. Numbers in square brackets are 95% CIs; numbers in parentheses are reference numbers.
† Level I = evidence from one or more controlled trials; level II = evidence from cohort or case–control studies; level III = evidence from diagnostic accuracy studies or case series. For each level, the investigators have assigned a quality score based on methods described in reference 7.

Accuracy

A systematic review from 1997 found that the sensitivity of a single unrehydrated FOBT for cancer was approximately 40%; its specificity seems to range from 96% to 98%. Rehydration was found to increase sensitivity to between 50% and 60% but decreased specificity to 90% (9, 29). In a recent study, Lieberman and colleagues (17) found that the sensitivity of rehydrated FOBT for cancer was 50% (CI, 30% to 70%). For advanced neoplasia (cancer and polyps that are large, villous, or dysplastic), sensitivity was 24% (CI, 19% to 29%) and specificity was 94% (CI, 93% to 95%).

In the annual screening arm of the 13-year Minnesota trial, which primarily used rehydrated test cards and had a high initial rate of participation (approximately 90%), 49% of patients who developed colorectal cancer were identified through screening. Thirty-eight percent of all patients had had at least one colonoscopy (2). Biennial screening detected 39% of patients with cancer in the intervention group, and 28% of patients required colonoscopy. Compared with the Minnesota trial, the two European trials were population-based, lasted 8 to 10 years, used only biennial testing, and had lower participation rates (60% to 70% of patients completed the first screening). Screening detected 27% of patients in the intervention group who developed colorectal cancer, and only 5% of patients had colonoscopy (13, 14).

Adverse Effects

Fecal occult blood testing itself has few adverse effects, but false-positive results lead to further tests, such as colonoscopy, during which adverse effects may occur. The specific adverse effects of colonoscopy are described later in this review. Theoretically, a previously negative result on FOBT could falsely reassure patients and lead to delayed response to the development of colorectal symptoms if cancer were to develop, but this concern has not been evaluated empirically.

Sigmoidoscopy

Effectiveness

Thiis-Evensen and coworkers (18) performed a small randomized trial of sigmoidoscopy screening in Norway. In 1983, 799 men and women who were 50 to 59 years of age and were drawn from a population registry were randomly assigned to receive screening flexible sigmoidoscopy (400 patients) or no screening (399 patients). Eighty-one percent of those offered flexible sigmoidoscopy accepted.

Table 1—Continued

Chance of False-Positive Results	Evidence Grade†	Adverse Effects	Evidence Grade†
Unknown		No direct adverse effects known	
Little difference compared with three-card testing (11, 12)	Level III—poor	No direct adverse effects known	
Single-test specificity 96%–98% 5%–10% of patients will require colonoscopy over 10 years of biennial testing (9)	Level III—good	No direct adverse effects known	
Single–test specificity 90% Over 10 to 13 years, 38% of patients tested annually and 28% tested biennially with rehydrated FOBT required colonoscopy (2)	Level III—good	Inconvenience, adverse events resulting from follow-up tests after positive results	
NA		Perforation rate for diagnostic examinations <1 in 10 000; bleeding in 2.5% of patients after diagnostic studies, 5.5% after procedures with polypectomy (19)	Level III—good
NA		Sum of adverse effects from each test alone	
One-time specificity, 85% [82%–88%] (24)	Level III—fair	Perforation rate 1 in 25 000 in a study with screening and symptomatic patients (25)	Level III—poor
NA		Diagnostic procedures: perforation rate 1 in 2000 Polypectomy: perforation rate 1 in 500–1000; bleeding rate 1 in 100–500; mortality rate 1 in 20 000 (5)	Level III—fair to good

All patients found to have polyps on sigmoidoscopy underwent immediate diagnostic colonoscopy and had surveillance examinations 2 and 6 years later. Over the 13 years of the trial, two cases of colorectal cancer were diagnosed in the intervention group and 10 were diagnosed in the control group (relative risk for colorectal cancer, 0.2 [CI, 0.03 to 0.95]). One person who was assigned to the intervention group but never had sigmoidoscopy died of colorectal cancer, as did three controls (relative risk, 0.50 [CI, 0.10 to 2.72]). Overall mortality rate was higher in the intervention group than in the control group (14% vs. 9%; relative risk, 1.57 [CI, 1.03 to 2.40]), mostly because of an excess of cardiovascular deaths. No clear relationship emerged between excess deaths and any procedure-related complications.

Two ongoing randomized trials using flexible sigmoidoscopy will report their initial results within 5 years. One trial in the United Kingdom is examining the effect of screening with sigmoidoscopy once per lifetime (19), and a second trial in the United States is examining sigmoidoscopy screening every 5 years in patients who are assumed to be receiving FOBT as part of usual care (30).

Two older, well-designed case–control studies that provide other important information on the effectiveness of sigmoidoscopy screening were available to the USPSTF in 1996. Using data from the Kaiser Permanente Medical Care Program in northern California, Selby and associates (3) found that rigid sigmoidoscopy had been performed in 9% of persons who died of colorectal cancer occurring within 20 cm of the anus and in 24% of persons who did not die of cancer occurring within 20 cm of the anus. The adjusted odds ratio of 0.41 (CI, 0.25 to 0.69) suggested that sigmoidoscopy screening reduced the risk for death by 59% for cancer within reach of the rigid sigmoidoscope.

The investigators noted that the adjusted odds ratio was 0.96 for proximal colon cancer that was beyond the reach of the sigmoidoscope (3). This finding added support to the hypothesis that the reduced risk for death from cancer within reach of the rigid sigmoidoscope could be attributed to screening rather than to confounding factors. The risk reduction associated with sigmoidoscopy screening did not diminish during the first 9 to 10 years after the test was performed. The study by Selby and associates mostly used rigid sigmoidoscopes. However, in another case–control study supporting the effectiveness of sigmoidoscopy, 75% of the examinations were performed with a flexible instrument (31).

Accuracy

Two recent studies have examined the sensitivity of screening sigmoidoscopy for cancer or advanced adenomas

Table 2. **Trials of Fecal Occult Blood Testing**

Trial Characteristics	Trial (Reference)		
	Minnesota (2)	**United Kingdom (13)**	**Denmark (14)**
Frequency of testing	Annual and biennial	Biennial	Biennial
Participants, *n*	>45 000 men and women	>150 000 men and women	>60 000 men and women
Age, *y*	50–80	45–74	45–74
Duration of follow-up, *y*	18 (annual and biennial)	8	10
Hydration of slides	Yes (83%)	No	No
Participation rate, %*	90 (annual and biennial)	60	67
Patients requiring colonoscopy, %	38 (annual); 28 (biennial)	5	5
Positive predictive value, %	1.9 (annual); 2.7 (biennial)†	10–12	8–18
Relative risk reduction for death from colorectal cancer [95% CI], %	33 [17–49] (annual); 21 [3–38] (biennial)	15 [1–26]	18 [1–32]
Absolute risk reduction for death from colorectal cancer per 1000 participants	4.6 (annual); 2.9 (biennial)	0.8	1.4

* Participation was defined as completion of at least one test.
† Mostly rehydrated slides (83%).

in healthy patients, using colonoscopy as the criterion standard. They found that sigmoidoscopy would identify 70% to 80% of patients with advanced adenomas or cancer (17, 20). Sigmoidoscopy can produce false-positive results by detecting hyperplastic polyps that do not have malignant potential or adenomatous polyps that are unlikely to become malignant during the patient's lifetime. Because studies of diagnostic accuracy cannot measure whether small or large adenomas that are identified and removed would have become cancer, it is not possible to classify such findings in terms of accuracy in detecting cancer. In practice, most investigators consider all adenomas to be "true positives" regardless of whether they would ever progress to cancer. Comparison of the specificity of sigmoidoscopy with that of nonendoscopic screening methods, such as FOBT and barium enema, is therefore difficult.

Adverse Effects

Estimates of bowel perforations from sigmoidoscopy have generally been in the range of 1 to 2 or fewer per 10 000 examinations, particularly since the introduction of the flexible sigmoidoscope (32). Atkin and colleagues (19) recently reported initial results from a trial of sigmoidoscopy screening in which experienced endoscopists performed sigmoidoscopy in 1235 asymptomatic adults 55 to 64 years of age. Two hundred eighty-eight patients had polyps removed during the examination. Adverse effects, including pain, anxiety, or any degree of bleeding, were assessed by a written questionnaire immediately after the test and by a mailed questionnaire 3 months later. Of all patients, 3.2% (40 of 1235) reported bleeding, 16 of 288 (5.5%) after polypectomy and 24 of 947 (2.5%) after diagnostic studies. One patient required hospital admission, and no patients required a transfusion. Fourteen percent of patients reported moderate pain, and 0.4% reported severe pain. More than 25% of patients reported gas or flatus. No perforations were reported, but one patient died of peritonitis after a complicated open surgical procedure to remove a severely dysplastic adenoma. A recent study of endoscopic complications from the Mayo Clinic in Arizona identified two perforations in 49 501 sigmoidoscopy procedures (33).

Fecal Occult Blood Test and Sigmoidoscopy

Effectiveness

Currently, no randomized trials that examine death from colorectal cancer as an end point have compared FOBT alone or sigmoidoscopy alone with a strategy of performing both tests. In 1992, Winawer and coworkers (4) conducted a nonrandomized trial of more than 12 000 first-time attendees at a preventive health clinic in New York. This trial was available to the USPSTF in 1996. The control group received rigid sigmoidoscopy at the first visit, and all study participants were invited to return for annual reexamination with rigid sigmoidoscopy. Patients in the intervention group received rigid sigmoidoscopy and were also asked to complete Hemoccult (Beckman Coulter, Fullerton, California) FOBT cards. Patients who had adenomas larger than 3 mm on sigmoidoscopy or who had positive results on FOBT underwent full colonic examination with barium enema and colonoscopy. The control group received rigid sigmoidoscopy at the first visit, and participants were invited to return for annual reexamination. Few patients continued to participate after the first examination (20% had FOBT at year 2, 15% at year 3). Incidence of colorectal cancer and death were assessed over a 9-year period, and follow-up data were available for 97% of patients.

Demographic and clinical data suggest that the groups were comparable, despite the absence of randomization. More cases of colorectal cancer were detected on initial examination in intervention patients than in control patients (4.5 per 1000 participants vs. 2.5 per 1000 participants). Incidence rates (cancer detected after the initial examination) were similar between groups (0.9 per 1000 person-years in each group). Incidence of death from colorectal cancer was 0.36 per 1000 patient-years in the intervention group and 0.63 per 1000 patient-years among controls (relative risk, 0.56 [CI, 0.25 to 1.19]).

Fecal occult blood testing combined with rigid sigmoidoscopy seems to increase the yield of initial screening and may reduce mortality rates. Because rigid sigmoidoscopy is no longer used for screening, the generalizability of these results to the use of FOBT plus flexible sigmoidoscopy is unclear. Whether the incremental yield of combined screening will change after additional rounds of testing also remains uncertain.

Accuracy

Recent randomized trials from Europe examined the additional diagnostic yield of performing sigmoidoscopy plus FOBT at one point in time for patients who were not already part of an ongoing screening program (21–23). In each study, adding sigmoidoscopy to FOBT increased the identification of significant adenomas or cancer by a factor of two or more. Adding FOBT to sigmoidoscopy did not seem to identify any additional significant lesions. Winawer and coworkers (4), however, found an increased yield from adding FOBT to rigid sigmoidoscopy. In each study, data were limited to a single round of testing. The additional yield of this strategy may be lower after the first round of testing, but the impact of this strategy on mortality rates has not been fully evaluated.

Adverse Effects

The adverse effects of FOBT plus sigmoidoscopy are equal to the adverse effects of each test alone.

Double-Contrast Barium Enema

Effectiveness

We identified no published studies that examined the effectiveness of double-contrast barium enema in reducing incidence of or death from colorectal cancer. Several studies have examined the accuracy of double-contrast barium enema for diagnosing colorectal cancer or adenomatous polyps (24, 34–43). Most are of methodologically poor quality, however, because they examined patients with symptoms or did not prospectively collect blinded data.

The National Polyp Study is a randomized trial of different intervals of surveillance after polypectomy (examinations at 1 and 3 years vs. at 3 years only). In a substudy of this trial, Winawer and colleagues (24) compared the accuracy of double-contrast barium enema with that of colonoscopy. The sensitivity of double-contrast barium enema was 32% (CI, 25% to 39%) for polyps smaller than 0.5 cm; 53% (CI, 40% to 66%) for polyps 0.6 to 1 cm; and 48% (CI, 24% to 67%) for polyps larger than 1 cm, including two cases of cancerous polyps. Results of double-contrast barium enema were positive in 83 of 470 patients in whom colonoscopy detected no polyps (specificity, 85% [CI, 82% to 88%]).

Winawer and colleagues (24) examined patients who previously had colonoscopy and removal of all polyps. Their results, therefore, may have limited generalizability for screening because screening largely involves persons who have not had recent colonoscopic examination and polypectomy and therefore may be more likely to have large polyps or tumors. However, the low sensitivity for large polyps and tumors reported by Winawer and colleagues is cause for concern and may limit the potential effectiveness of screening with double-contrast barium enema.

Adverse Effects

The estimated risk for perforation during barium enema is low. Kewenter and Brevinge (44) found that no perforations or other complications occurred among 1987 screening patients undergoing barium enema as part of a screening work-up. Blakeborough and associates (25) surveyed radiologists in the United Kingdom about complications of barium enema during a 3-year period (1992 through 1994). All examinations were included, regardless of the indication for the procedure. Important complications of any type occurred in 1 in 10 000 examinations. Perforation occurred in 1 of 25 000 examinations, and death occurred in 1 in 55 000 examinations, although it is not clear whether all deaths were procedure related.

Colonoscopy

Effectiveness

The ability of colonoscopy to prevent colorectal cancer or death has not been measured in a screening trial. The National Polyp Study estimated that 76% to 90% of cancer could be prevented by regular colonoscopic surveillance examinations, based on comparison with historic controls (45). However, these results should be interpreted with caution. The comparison groups were not from the same underlying population, which could introduce bias. In addition, all trial participants had polyps detected and removed, limiting generalizability of the results to the average screening population.

Müller and Sonnenberg (26), in a case–control study at Veterans Affairs hospitals, found that patients with a diagnosis of colorectal cancer were less likely to have had previous colonoscopy. The odds ratios for disease incidence were 0.47 (CI, 0.37 to 0.58) for colon cancer and 0.61 (CI, 0.48 to 0.77) for rectal cancer. For death from colorectal cancer, the odds ratio was also lower for patients with previous colonoscopy (odds ratio, 0.43 [CI, 0.30 to 0.63]).

Accuracy

Because colonoscopy is commonly used as the criterion standard examination, it is difficult to calculate its sensitivity. Using tandem colonoscopic examinations, Rex and colleagues (27) found single-test sensitivity to be 90% for large adenomas and 75% for small adenomas (<1 cm); sensitivity for cancer probably exceeds 90%.

Recent identification of flat lesions that can be missed on regular colonoscopy suggests that some histologic variants do not progress through the typical adenoma–carcinoma development sequence and thus may not be easily detectable in the precancerous phase (46). If flat lesions account for 10% of all adenomas, sensitivity of all endoscopic screening methods may be lower than previously thought.

The specificity of colonoscopy with biopsy is generally reported to be 99% or 100%, but this assumes that all detected adenomas represent true-positive results. As with sigmoidoscopy, most detected adenomas, especially small adenomas, will never develop into cancer. If detection of an adenoma that will not become cancer is considered a false-positive result that subjects a patient to risk without benefit, then the actual specificity of colonoscopy would be much lower.

Adverse Effects

Colonoscopy, which uses sedation and requires skilled support personnel, is more expensive and has a higher risk for procedural complications than other screening tests, particularly when polypectomy is performed. Use of conscious sedation adds the risk for complications attributable to the sedative agent. In our systematic review of studies examining the principal complications of colonoscopy (5), we focused on hemorrhage and perforation but noted the less frequent complications of death, infections, sedation-related events, and chemical colitis. Two recent studies examined the incidence of complications from colonoscopy performed in screening populations. Lieberman and associates (17), in a study in patients in Veterans Affairs medical centers, found that 10 of 3121 patients (0.3%) had major complications during or immediately after the procedures. Of these 10 patients, 6 had bleeding that required hospitalization and 1 each had a stroke, myocardial infarction, Fournier gangrene, and thrombophlebitis. Three other patients died within 1 month, probably of causes unrelated to the procedure. In a study of employees of a large corporation, Imperiale and coworkers (20) found that among 1994 persons 50 years of age and older who underwent colonoscopy, 1 (0.05%) had a perforation that did not require surgery and 3 (0.15%) had bleeding that required emergency department visits but not admission or surgery.

Apart from these two screening studies, most of the studies examining colonoscopy complications are retrospective reviews of endoscopy records from U.S. university hospitals that recorded only immediate complications and included a mixture of screening and diagnostic procedures (17, 20, 33, 47–61). A prospective study that also included a patient questionnaire administered 10 days after the procedure identified several additional important complications that occurred outside the hospital, suggesting that hospital record review alone may underestimate actual complication rates (47).

Despite these limitations, these studies provide a useful approximation of the complication rates that can be expected from colonoscopy. For diagnostic procedures, perforation rates were low (0.029% to 0.61%). Bleeding was not reported in enough studies to generate an estimate of its frequency. For therapeutic procedures, complication rates were higher (perforations, 0.07% to 0.72%; bleeding, 0.2% to 2.67%). Deaths occurred infrequently; reported rates ranged from 1 in 30 000 persons to 1 in 3000 persons. Mortality rates were higher in studies that included older patients and more symptomatic patients. The rate of screening-related death may be on the lower end of this range; one cost-effectiveness analysis estimated it to be 1 per 20 000 patients (29). Other clinically relevant complications were reported too infrequently and measured too inconsistently to allow accurate estimation of their true incidence.

DISCUSSION

Our systematic review supports the effectiveness of screening as a means of reducing death from colorectal cancer. For biennial FOBT, three high-quality randomized, controlled trials have shown disease-specific reductions in mortality rate of 15% to 21% over 8 to 13 years. Annual FOBT with rehydrated slides seems to be more effective in reducing mortality rates (33% in one trial). Case–control studies have shown that sigmoidoscopy and possibly colonoscopy are also associated with decreased death from colorectal cancer. The combined strategy of FOBT and sigmoidoscopy was supported by one nonrandomized trial that showed a borderline statistically significant reduction in mortality rates (43%) when FOBT was added to rigid sigmoidoscopy (4). This strategy was also supported by indirect evidence showing increased yield with both tests compared with FOBT alone. Double-contrast barium enema has not been studied as extensively as other screening methods; further data are required in screening populations.

Although strong direct and indirect evidence supports colorectal cancer screening, no trials have directly compared different screening strategies by using colorectal cancer incidence or mortality rates as the end point of interest. Some groups believe that recent evidence showing the superior single-test accuracy of colonoscopy proves its broader superiority and have recommended it as the procedure of choice for screening. However, these analyses have not always considered differences in yield over time, complications, and real-world performance, which may not always favor colonoscopy (62, 63). One solution to these problems would be to perform a trial of colonoscopy, but such a trial would be expensive, particularly if colonoscopy were compared with other screening methods rather than with no screening, and would require many years of follow-up. In the face of good general evidence supporting screening but uncertainty about the most effective screening method, providers and patients may benefit from discussing pros and cons and from incorporating patients' preferences into decisions about how to screen (64).

Several areas of colorectal cancer screening and prevention warrant additional research. There is a critical need to learn more about adherence to screening among informed patients. Furthermore, we need better data on the real-world complication rates of colonoscopic screening and polypectomy, including whether complications become more or less likely as procedure volume increases. Double-contrast barium enema should be studied in a screening population. The accuracy of novel screening techniques, including virtual colonoscopy and genetic stool tests (or other novel noninvasive tests), should be evaluated in screening populations.

Additional means of prevention, including chemopreventive agents (such as nonsteroidal anti-inflammatory drugs, calcium, or estrogen), also warrant further study. Behavioral factors, including physical activity, dietary fat intake, dietary fiber intake, and fruit and vegetable consumption, seem to be related to colorectal cancer incidence. Further research would clarify whether these relationships are causal or the result of uncontrolled confounding.

Despite its apparent effectiveness, colorectal cancer screening is currently underused by age-eligible adults because of patient-, provider-, and system-specific barriers (65). Effective colon cancer screening requires ongoing efforts to ensure test ordering and adherence. Screening with FOBT, for example, may require offering annual testing to 500 to 1000 people for 10 years to prevent one death from colorectal cancer (2). Although this level of effort may seem inefficient or low in yield, the potential benefit is large and the costs per person are small. To achieve high rates of screening in real-world settings rather than in trials, which focused strictly on one aspect of preventive care, colorectal cancer screening must be integrated with other care needs, including other preventive services.

Several strategies have been shown to be effective in raising screening rates in primary care settings over the short term, including reminder systems, patient decision aids, and special screening clinics (66). Further research is needed to determine whether such systems can maintain their effect over time and to identify novel means of reaching persons at risk who currently are not served or are underserved by the existing health care system.

APPENDIX: SEARCH STRATEGIES

To update the evidence on screening for colorectal cancer, we performed three separate literature searches using MEDLINE: one general update from January 1995 to December 2001 and two focused searches for evidence related to barium enema and complications of screening that used search dates from 1966 through December 2001. All searches were limited to "human" subjects.

For the general search, we combined the MeSH headings "colorectal neoplasms" or "occult blood" or "sigmoidoscopy" or "colonoscopy" with the term *mass screening*. This search produced 719 results, 19 of which we retained in the final document. To identify articles on the use of barium enema, we combined the exploded MeSH terms "colorectal neoplasms" and "barium sulfate" and "enema," which yielded 621 results. We retained 13 articles in our final data set. For studies about the complications of screening, we combined the exploded MeSH terms "colonoscopy/ae [adverse effects] and sigmoidoscopy/ae [adverse effects]," "intestinal perforation," "intraoperative complications," "postoperative complications," or "gastrointestinal hemorrhage," with a search combining the test names and the keyword "complications." Our search yielded 839 articles, 16 of which we retained. In addition to these searches, we used peer review and hand searching of the bibliographies of included articles and other systematic reviews, as well as articles from the 1996 document. This yielded an additional 15 references for our final document.

Appendix Table. **Eligibility Criteria***

Test	Type of Studies Included
Digital rectal examination	Diagnostic accuracy studies, observational studies
FOBT	RCTs
Sigmoidoscopy	RCTs, observational studies
FOBT plus sigmoidoscopy	Controlled trials, observational studies, diagnostic accuracy studies
Barium enema	Diagnostic accuracy studies
Colonoscopy	Observational studies, diagnostic accuracy studies
Adverse effects (any test)	Case series, observational studies, RCTs

* FOBT = fecal occult blood test; RCT = randomized, controlled trial.

We developed eligibility criteria to guide decisions about inclusion of articles. In general, we sought to identify and include the highest quality evidence available. The Appendix Table shows the criteria for each specific topic.

From University of North Carolina, Chapel Hill, and Research Triangle Institute, Research Triangle Park, North Carolina; Merck & Co., Inc., West Point, Pennsylvania; and University of Washington, Seattle, Washington.

Disclaimer: The authors of this article are responsible for its contents, including any clinical or treatment recommendations. No statement in this article should be construed as an official position of the U.S. Agency for Healthcare Research and Quality, the U.S. Department of Health and Human Services, or Merck & Co., Inc.

Acknowledgments: The authors thank David Atkins, MD, MPH, Agency for Healthcare Research and Quality, and Eve Shapiro, managing editor of the U.S. Preventive Services Task Force (under contract to the Agency for Healthcare Research and Quality). They also thank the staff of the Research Triangle Institute–University of North Carolina Evidence-based Practice Center; Sonya Sutton, BSPH, Sheila White, and Loraine Monroe, Research Triangle Institute; and Carol Krasnov, University of North Carolina at Chapel Hill Cecil G. Sheps Center for Health Services Research.

Grant Support: This study was developed by the Research Triangle Institute–University of North Carolina Evidence-based Practice Center under contract to the Agency for Healthcare Research and Quality (contract no. 290-97-0011), Rockville, Maryland.

Requests for Reprints: Reprints are available from the AHRQ Web site at www.preventiveservices.ahrq.gov and in print through the AHRQ Publications Clearinghouse (800-358-9295).

Current author addresses are available at www.annals.org.

Current Author Addresses: Dr. Pignone: University of North Carolina at Chapel Hill, Department of Medicine and Cecil Sheps Center for Health Services Research, 5039 Old Clinic Building, CB #7110, Chapel Hill, NC 27599.
Dr. Teutsch: Merck & Co., Inc., 770 Sumneytown Pike, West Point, PA WP399-169.
Dr. Rich: University of North Carolina at Chapel Hill, 724 Burnett Womack, CB 7080, Chapel Hill, NC 27599.
Dr. Berg: University of Washington, Department of Family Medicine, C-408 Health Sciences, Box 356390, Seattle, WA 98195.
Dr. Lohr: Research Triangle Institute, 3040 Cornwallis Road, Research Triangle Park, NC 27709-2194.

References

1. Guide to Clinical Preventive Services. 2nd ed. U.S. Preventive Services Task Force. Alexandria, VA: International Medical Publishing; 1996.
2. **Mandel JS, Bond JH, Church TR, Snover DC, Bradley GM, Schuman LM, et al.** Reducing mortality from colorectal cancer by screening for fecal occult blood. Minnesota Colon Cancer Control Study. N Engl J Med. 1993;328:1365-71. [PMID: 8474513]
3. **Selby JV, Friedman GD, Quesenberry CP Jr, Weiss NS.** A case-control study of screening sigmoidoscopy and mortality from colorectal cancer. N Engl J Med. 1992;326:653-7. [PMID: 1736103]
4. **Winawer SJ, Flehinger BJ, Schottenfeld D, Miller DG.** Screening for colorectal cancer with fecal occult blood testing and sigmoidoscopy. J Natl Cancer Inst. 1993;85:1311-8. [PMID: 8340943]
5. **Pignone MP, Rich M, Teutsch SM, Berg AO, Lohr KN.** Screening for Colorectal Cancer in Adults. Systematic Evidence Review No. 7. AHRQ publication no. 02-S003. Rockville, MD: Agency for Healthcare Research and Quality; 2002.
6. Screening for colorectal cancer: recommendations and rationale. U.S. Preventive Services Task Force. Ann Intern Med. 2002;137:129-131.
7. **Harris RP, Helfand M, Woolf SH, Lohr KN, Mulrow CD, Teutsch SM, et al.** Current methods of the US Preventive Services Task Force: a review of the process. Am J Prev Med. 2001;20:21-35. [PMID: 11306229]
8. **Herrinton LJ, Selby JV, Friedman GD, Quesenberry CP, Weiss NS.** Case-control study of digital-rectal screening in relation to mortality from cancer of the distal rectum. Am J Epidemiol. 1995;142:961-4. [PMID: 7572977]
9. **Ransohoff DF, Lang CA.** Screening for colorectal cancer with the fecal occult blood test: a background paper. American College of Physicians. Ann Intern Med. 1997;126:811-22. [PMID: 9148658]
10. **Yamamoto M, Nakama H.** Cost-effectiveness analysis of immunochemical occult blood screening for colorectal cancer among three fecal sampling methods. Hepatogastroenterology. 2000;47:396-9. [PMID: 10791199]
11. **Eisner MS, Lewis JH.** Diagnostic yield of a positive fecal occult blood test found on digital rectal examination. Does the finger count? Arch Intern Med. 1991;151:2180-4. [PMID: 1953220]
12. **Bini EJ, Rajapaksa RC, Weinshel EH.** The findings and impact of nonrehydrated guaiac examination of the rectum (FINGER) study: a comparison of 2 methods of screening for colorectal cancer in asymptomatic average-risk patients. Arch Intern Med. 1999;159:2022-6. [PMID: 10510987]
13. **Hardcastle JD, Chamberlain JO, Robinson MH, Moss SM, Amar SS, Balfour TW, et al.** Randomised controlled trial of faecal-occult-blood screening for colorectal cancer. Lancet. 1996;348:1472-7. [PMID: 8942775]
14. **Kronborg O, Fenger C, Olsen J, Jørgensen OD, Søndergaard O.** Randomised study of screening for colorectal cancer with faecal-occult-blood test. Lancet. 1996;348:1467-71. [PMID: 8942774]
15. **Mandel JS, Church TR, Ederer F, Bond JH.** Colorectal cancer mortality: effectiveness of biennial screening for fecal occult blood. J Natl Cancer Inst. 1999;91:434-7. [PMID: 10070942]
16. **Mandel JS, Church TR, Bond JH, Ederer F, Geisser MS, Mongin SJ, et al.** The effect of fecal occult-blood screening on the incidence of colorectal cancer. N Engl J Med. 2000;343:1603-7. [PMID: 11096167]
17. **Lieberman DA, Weiss DG, Bond JH, Ahnen DJ, Garewal H, Chejfec G.** Use of colonoscopy to screen asymptomatic adults for colorectal cancer. Veterans Affairs Cooperative Study Group 380. N Engl J Med. 2000;343:162-8. [PMID: 10900274]
18. **Thiis-Evensen E, Hoff GS, Sauar J, Langmark F, Majak BM, Vatn MH.** Population-based surveillance by colonoscopy: effect on the incidence of colorectal cancer. Telemark Polyp Study I. Scand J Gastroenterol. 1999;34:414-20. [PMID: 10365903]
19. **Atkin WS, Hart A, Edwards R, McIntyre P, Aubrey R, Wardle J, et al.** Uptake, yield of neoplasia, and adverse effects of flexible sigmoidoscopy screening. Gut. 1998;42:560-5. [PMID: 9616321]
20. **Imperiale TF, Wagner DR, Lin CY, Larkin GN, Rogge JD, Ransohoff DF.** Risk of advanced proximal neoplasms in asymptomatic adults according to the distal colorectal findings. N Engl J Med. 2000;343:169-74. [PMID: 10900275]
21. **Verne JE, Aubrey R, Love SB, Talbot IC, Northover JM.** Population based randomized study of uptake and yield of screening by flexible sigmoidoscopy compared with screening by faecal occult blood testing. BMJ. 1998;317:182-5. [PMID: 9665902]
22. **Berry DP, Clarke P, Hardcastle JD, Vellacott KD.** Randomized trial of the addition of flexible sigmoidoscopy to faecal occult blood testing for colorectal neoplasia population screening. Br J Surg. 1997;84:1274-6. [PMID: 9313712]
23. **Rasmussen M, Kronborg O, Fenger C, Jørgensen OD.** Possible advantages and drawbacks of adding flexible sigmoidoscopy to hemoccult-II in screening for colorectal cancer. A randomized study. Scand J Gastroenterol. 1999;34:73-8. [PMID: 10048736]
24. **Winawer SJ, Stewart ET, Zauber AG, Bond JH, Ansel H, Waye JD, et al.** A comparison of colonoscopy and double-contrast barium enema for surveillance after polypectomy. National Polyp Study Work Group. N Engl J Med. 2000; 342:1766-72. [PMID: 10852998]
25. **Blakeborough A, Sheridan MB, Chapman AH.** Complications of barium enema examinations: a survey of UK Consultant Radiologists 1992 to 1994. Clin Radiol. 1997;52:142-8. [PMID: 9043049]
26. **Müller AD, Sonnenberg A.** Protection by endoscopy against death from colorectal cancer. A case-control study among veterans. Arch Intern Med. 1995; 155:1741-8. [PMID: 7654107]
27. **Rex DK, Cutler CS, Lemmel GT, Rahmani EY, Clark DW, Helper DJ, et al.** Colonoscopic miss rates of adenomas determined by back-to-back colonoscopies. Gastroenterology. 1997;112:24-8. [PMID: 8978338]
28. **Winawer SJ, Fletcher RH, Miller L, Godlee F, Stolar MH, Mulrow CD, et al.** Colorectal cancer screening: clinical guidelines and rationale. Gastroenterology. 1997;112:594-642. [PMID: 9024315]
29. **Wagner J, Tunis S, Brown M, Ching A, Almeida R.** Cost-effectiveness of colorectal cancer screening in average-risk adults. In: Young G, Rozen P, Levin B, eds. Prevention and Early Detection of Colorectal Cancer. London: Saunders; 1996:321-56.
30. **Kramer BS, Gohagan J, Prorok PC, Smart C.** A National Cancer Institute sponsored screening trial for prostatic, lung, colorectal, and ovarian cancers. Cancer. 1993;71:589-93. [PMID: 8420681]
31. **Newcomb PA, Norfleet RG, Storer BE, Surawicz TS, Marcus PM.** Screening sigmoidoscopy and colorectal cancer mortality. J Natl Cancer Inst. 1992;84: 1572-5. [PMID: 1404450]
32. **Nelson RL, Abcarian H, Prasad ML.** Iatrogenic perforation of the colon and rectum. Dis Colon Rectum. 1982;25:305-8. [PMID: 7083975]
33. **Anderson ML, Pasha TM, Leighton JA.** Endoscopic perforation of the

colon: lessons from a 10-year study. Am J Gastroenterol. 2000;95:3418-22. [PMID: 11151871]

34. **Ott DJ, Scharling ES, Chen YM, Wu WC, Gelfand DW.** Barium enema examination: sensitivity in detecting colonic polyps and carcinomas. South Med J. 1989;82:197-200. [PMID: 2644698]

35. **Rex DK, Rahmani EY, Haseman JH, Lemmel GT, Kaster S, Buckley JS.** Relative sensitivity of colonoscopy and barium enema for detection of colorectal cancer in clinical practice. Gastroenterology. 1997;112:17-23. [PMID: 8978337]

36. **Johnson CD, Carlson HC, Taylor WF, Weiland LP.** Barium enemas of carcinoma of the colon: sensitivity of double- and single-contrast studies. AJR Am J Roentgenol. 1983;140:1143-9. [PMID: 6602483]

37. **Bloomfield JA.** Reliability of barium enema in detecting colonic neoplasia. Med J Aust. 1981;1:631-3. [PMID: 7254054]

38. **Teefey SA, Carlson HC.** The fluoroscopic barium enema in colonic polyp detection. AJR Am J Roentgenol. 1983;141:1279-81. [PMID: 6606327]

39. **Brady AP, Stevenson GW, Stevenson I.** Colorectal cancer overlooked at barium enema examination and colonoscopy: a continuing perceptual problem. Radiology. 1994;192:373-8. [PMID: 8029400]

40. **Strøm E, Larsen JL.** Colon cancer at barium enema examination and colonoscopy: a study from the county of Hordaland, Norway. Radiology. 1999; 211:211-4. [PMID: 10189473]

41. **Brekkan A, Kjartansson O, Tulinius H, Sigvaldason H.** Diagnostic sensitivity of X-ray examination of the large bowel in colorectal cancer. Gastrointest Radiol. 1983;8:363-5. [PMID: 6642154]

42. **Glick S, Wagner JL, Johnson CD.** Cost-effectiveness of double-contrast barium enema in screening for colorectal cancer. AJR Am J Roentgenol. 1998; 170:629-36. [PMID: 9490943]

43. **Myllylä V, Päivänsalo M, Laitinen S.** Sensitivity of single and double contrast barium enema in the detection of colorectal carcinoma. ROFO Fortschr Geb Rontgenstr Nuklearmed. 1984;140:393-7. [PMID: 6425161]

44. **Kewenter J, Brevinge H.** Endoscopic and surgical complications of work-up in screening for colorectal cancer. Dis Colon Rectum. 1996;39:676-80. [PMID: 8646956]

45. **Winawer SJ, Zauber AG, Ho MN, O'Brien MJ, Gottlieb LS, Sternberg SS, et al.** Prevention of colorectal cancer by colonoscopic polypectomy. The National Polyp Study Workgroup. N Engl J Med. 1993;329:1977-81. [PMID: 8247072]

46. **Rembacken BJ, Fujii T, Cairns A, Dixon MF, Yoshida S, Chalmers DM, et al.** Flat and depressed colonic neoplasms: a prospective study of 1000 colonoscopies in the UK. Lancet. 2000;355:1211-4. [PMID: 10770302]

47. **Newcomer MK, Shaw MJ, Williams DM, Jowell PS.** Unplanned work absence following outpatient colonoscopy. J Clin Gastroenterol. 1999;29:76-8. [PMID: 10405238]

48. **Eckardt VF, Kanzler G, Schmitt T, Eckardt AJ, Bernhard G.** Complications and adverse effects of colonoscopy with selective sedation. Gastrointest Endosc. 1999;49:560-65. [PMID: 10228252]

49. **Zubarik R, Fleischer DE, Mastropietro C, Lopez J, Carroll J, Benjamin S, et al.** Prospective analysis of complications 30 days after outpatient colonoscopy. Gastrointest Endosc. 1999;50:322-8. [PMID: 10462650]

50. **Wexner SD, Forde KA, Sellers G, Geron N, Lopes A, Weiss EG, et al.** How well can surgeons perform colonoscopy?. Surg Endosc. 1998;12:1410-4. [PMID: 9822468]

51. **Farley DR, Bannon MP, Zietlow SP, Pemberton JH, Ilstrup DM, Larson DR.** Management of colonoscopic perforations. Mayo Clin Proc. 1997;72:729-33. [PMID: 9276600]

52. **Foliente RL, Chang AC, Youssef AI, Ford LJ, Condon SC, Chen YK.** Endoscopic cecal perforation: mechanisms of injury. Am J Gastroenterol. 1996; 91:705-8. [PMID: 8677933]

53. **Gibbs DH, Opelka FG, Beck DE, Hicks TC, Timmcke AE, Gathright JB Jr.** Postpolypectomy colonic hemorrhage. Dis Colon Rectum. 1996;39:806-10. [PMID: 8674375]

54. **Ure T, Dehghan K, Vernava AM 3rd, Longo WE, Andrus CA, Daniel GL.** Colonoscopy in the elderly. Low risk, high yield. Surg Endosc. 1995;9:505-8. [PMID: 7676371]

55. **Lo AY, Beaton HL.** Selective management of colonoscopic perforations. J Am Coll Surg. 1994;179:333-7. [PMID: 8069431]

56. **Rosen L, Bub DS, Reed JF 3rd, Nastasee SA.** Hemorrhage following colonoscopic polypectomy. Dis Colon Rectum. 1993;36:1126-31. [PMID: 8253009]

57. **DiPrima RE, Barkin JS, Blinder M, Goldberg RI, Phillips RS.** Age as a risk factor in colonoscopy: fact versus fiction. Am J Gastroenterol. 1988;83:123-5. [PMID: 3341334]

58. **Nivatvongs S.** Complications in colonoscopic polypectomy: lessons to learn from an experience with 1576 polyps. Am Surg. 1988;54:61-3. [PMID: 3341645]

59. **Brynitz S, Kjaergård H, Struckmann J.** Perforations from colonoscopy during diagnosis and treatment of polyps. Ann Chir Gynaecol. 1986;75:142-5. [PMID: 3740781]

60. **Webb WA, McDaniel L, Jones L.** Experience with 1000 colonoscopic polypectomies. Ann Surg. 1985;201:626-32. [PMID: 3873221]

61. **Macrae FA, Tan KG, Williams CB.** Towards safer colonoscopy: a report on the complications of 5000 diagnostic or therapeutic colonoscopies. Gut. 1983; 24:376-83. [PMID: 6601604]

62. **Rex DK, Johnson DA, Lieberman DA, Burt RW, Sonnenberg A.** Colorectal cancer prevention 2000: screening recommendations of the American College of Gastroenterology. American College of Gastroenterology. Am J Gastroenterol. 2000;95:868-77. [PMID: 10763931]

63. **Podolsky DK.** Going the distance—the case for true colorectal-cancer screening [Editorial]. N Engl J Med. 2000;343:207-8. [PMID: 10900282]

64. **Woolf SH.** The best screening test for colorectal cancer—a personal choice [Editorial]. N Engl J Med. 2000;343:1641-3. [PMID: 11096175]

65. **Vernon SW.** Participation in colorectal cancer screening: a review. J Natl Cancer Inst. 1997;89:1406-22. [PMID: 9326910]

66. **Balas EA, Weingarten S, Garb CT, Blumenthal D, Boren SA, Brown GD.** Improving preventive care by prompting physicians. Arch Intern Med. 2000;160: 301-8. [PMID: 10668831]

Section II

Health Policy

Human Experimentation: Declaration of Helsinki.

World Medical Association. Ann Intern Med. 1966;65:367-368.

The Declaration of Helsinki remains "a statement of ethical principles to provide guidance to physicians and other participants in medical research involving human subjects" (1). The American College of Physicians and six other major medical societies endorsed the Declaration in 1966. *Annals* Editor J. Russell Elkinton summarized its basic principles (2): "1) the experiment must have adequate scientific background and experimental design, and the experimenter must be adequately trained in his medical and scientific discipline, 2) the human subject, be he [or she] patient or normal subject, must be fully informed to the best of his ability to understand and must freely consent; 3) the risk to the life or health of the patient must be commensurate with the foreseeable gain in new knowledge" He also noted that "These moral and ethical principles are easy to understand and to accept; it is their implementation that is difficult" (2). Forty years after Elkinton wrote these words, they remain at the heart of the matter.

The Declaration of Helsinki is regarded as the cornerstone document in the ethics of human experimentation research because of its influence on national and regional legislation and regulations (3). It has undergone five revisions and two clarifications (4). The first major revision in 1975 introduced the concept of research oversight by an independent committee (5). Additional changes included clarification of informed consent, the primacy of duty to the individual over that to society, and publication of research results. The changes made between 1975 and 2000 were relatively minor; thus, the 1975 version provided guidance for 25 years.

Various developments in the United States, including revelations about gross ethical violations in research (2) and the establishment of the National Commission for the Protection of Human Subjects (1974–1978) (5), have come to have greater influence on policies. than the Declaration. The principles developed by the Commission became the basis for the The Common Rule, which mandates official ethical review of research protocols by an institutional review board and freely given informed consent of research participants for all federally funded research (6). Many federal policies after the 1975 revision of the Declaration of Helsinki were developed independent of the Declaration (7).

The fifth revision of the Declaration of Helsinki, issued in October, 2000, did not reach consensus, and many contentious issues remain. Lurie and Wolfe (7) revealed that trials of zidovudine to prevent HIV transmission from mother to infant in Africa and Thailand used placebo. Brennan (8) reviewed the growth of research by for-profit organizations, the conduct of research in poor countries, and the greater emphasis on utilitarianism with a de-emphasis on the protection of individual research participants. These matters remain critical and provide the context for the next review of the Declaration at the 2008 World Medical Association meeting in Seoul, Korea. As in 1964, the researcher's moral commitment to the research subject and the protection of the research subject's rights remain the crux of the Declaration and discussions about its revision.

References

1. **World Medical Association.** Declaration of Helsinki. Ethical Principles for Medical Research Involving Human Subjects. Edinburgh, Scotland, October 2000. In: Emanuel EJ, Crouch RA, Arras JD, Moreno J, Grady C, eds. Ethical and Regulatory Aspects of Clinical Research. Baltimore: John Hopkins University Press; 2003:30-31.
2. **Elkinton JR.** The experimental use of human beings. Ann Intern Med. 1966;65:372.
3. **Declaration of Helsinki.** Accessed at len.wikipedia.org/wiki/Declaration ofHelsinki.
4. **World Medical Association.** Declaration of Helsinki. Ethical Principles for Medical Research Involving Human Subjects. Edinburgh, Scotland, October 2000. In: Emanuel EJ, Crouch RA, Arras JD, Moreno J, Grady C, eds. Ethical and Regulatory Aspects of Clinical Research. Baltimore: John Hopkins University Press; 2003:30. Also available at www.wma.net/e/policy/b3.htm.
5. Jonsen AR. The Birth of Bioethics. New York: Oxford University Press; 2003:431.
6. **U.S.** Department of Health and Human Services, National Institutes of Health, and Office for Human Research Protection. The Common Rule, Title 45 (Public Welfare) Code of Federal Regulation, Part 46 (Protection of Human Subjects), subparts A–D. revised November 13, 2001; effective December 13, 2001. Washington, DC: U.S. Department of Health and Human Services; 2001.
7. **Lurie P, Wolfe SM.** Unethical trials of interventions to reduce perinatal transmission of the human immunodeficiency virus in developing countries. N Engl J Med. 1997;337:853-856.
8. **Brennan TA.** Proposed revisions to the Declaration of Helsinki—will they weaken the ethical principles underlying human research? N Engl J Med. 1999;341:527-531.

The implications of regional variations in Medicare spending. Part 2: health outcomes and satisfaction with care.

Fisher ES, Wennberg DE, Stukel TA, Gottlieb DJ, Lucas FL, Pinder EL. Ann Intern Med. 2003;138:288-298.

Thanks to the work of Elliot Fisher and David Wennberg and their colleagues, one of the critical issues relating to the costs of medical care in the United States has been clarified and the role of physicians better understood. These investigators analyzed many years of Medicare data and revealed the variations in resources used to treat patients with the same diagnosis in different U.S. regions, states, and hospitals. This article examined the outcomes and satisfaction of care associated with variations in resource use.

Antos and Rivlin (1) further describe Elliott and colleagues' three most important findings. First, resource use per capita varies greatly. As Wennberg and associates (2) noted in 2003, per capita spending in traditional Medicare (parts A and B) was $5,278 for beneficiaries living in the Portland, Oregon, hospital referral region (HRR); $5,661 for those in the Seattle, Washington HHR; $10,752 for those in the Los Angeles HRR; and $11,350 for those in the Miami, Florida HRR. Second, variation in resource use is sensitive to the supply of hospital beds and specialists (the more beds and the more specialists, the greater the use of services and the higher the costs). Finally, more intensive and aggressive treatment styles and expenditures do not result in better outcomes. As Shine (3) has noted, "[c]osts varied primarily by the number of consultations, tests and hospitalization days rather than by the evidence based services required. If anything the mortality rates were somewhat greater in high cost areas." Patients in high-cost HRRs were more likely to see multiple medical subspecialists, and those in lower-cost HRRs were more likely to see family practitioners.

Policymakers in Washington, D.C., have been unable to deal with this issue effectively (4), in part because the fee-for-service payment system used by Medicare rewards more care, not better outcomes. Recently, Wennberg, et al (2) suggested that the pay-for-performance agenda can be applied to reduce waste and improve outcomes. The Medicare Payment Advisory Commission (5), Wilensky (6), Antos and Rivlin (1), Enthoven (7), the Committee for Economic Development (8), and Halverson (9) have proposed broader approaches to the issues of cost, quality, and access. In my view, Bodenheimer (10-12) and Bodenheimer and Fernandez (the paper reprinted herein) list very constructive actions that physicians can take to deal with high and rising health costs.

Fisher and colleagues' work has shed light on the problem of the high cost of medical care, the regional variation in resource use and costs, and the role of physicians in affecting these factors. However, solutions remains elusive.

References

1. **Antos JR, Rivlin AM.** Strategies for slowing the growth of health spending. In: Rivlin AM, Antos JR, eds. Registering Fiscal Sanity 2007. The Health Spending Challenge. Washington, DC: Brookings Institute Press; 2007:35-36.
2. **Wennberg JE, Fisher ES, Skinner JS, Bronner KK.** Extending the P4P agenda, part 2: how Medicare can reduce waste and improve the care of the chronically ill. Health Aff (Millwood). 2007;26:1575-1585.
3. **Shine KI.** Geographical variations in Medicare spending [Editorial]. Ann Intern Med. 2003;138:347-8.
4. **U.S.** Government Accountability Office. Report to Congressional Committees. Medicare Physician Payments. Concern about Spending Target System Prompt Interest in Considering Reforms. Washington, DC: Government Accountability Office; October 2004:68.
5. **Medicare Payment Advisory Commission.** MedPAC Data Book 2006: Healthcare Spending and the Medicare Program. Section 1: National Health Care and Medicare Spending. June 2006. Accessed at www.medpac.900/publications/congressional_reports/Jun06DataBooksec.pdf.
6. **Wilensky GR.** The challenge of Medicare. In: Rivlin AM, Antos JR, eds. Registering Fiscal Sanity 2007. The Health Spending Challenge. Washington, DC: Brookings Institute Press; 2007:81-103.
7. **Enthoven AC.** Open the markets and level the playing field. In: Enthoven AC, Tollen LA, eds. Toward a 21st Century Health Care System: The Contributions and Promise of Pre-Paid Group Practice. San Francisco: Jossey-Bass; 2004:227-245.
8. **Committee for Economic Development.** Quality, Affordable Health Care for All. Moving Beyond the Employer-Based Health Insurance System. Washington, DC: Committee for Economic Development; 2007:117.
9. **Halverson G.** Health Care Reform Now. A Presentation for Change. San Francisco: Jossey-Bass; 2007:361.
10. **Bodenheimer T.** High and rising health care costs. Part 1: seeking an explanation. Ann Intern Med. 2005;142:847-54.
11. **Bodenheimer T.** High and rising health care costs. Part 2: technologic innovation. Ann Intern Med. 2005;142:932-937.
12. **Bodenheimer T.** High and rising health care costs. Part 3: the role of health care providers. Ann Intern Med. 2005;142:996-1002.

High and Rising Health Care Costs. Part 4: Can costs be controlled while preserving quality?

Bodenheimer T, Fernandez A. Ann Intern Med. 2005;143:26-31.

The cost of health care is a complex issue that is too rarely approached with objectivity and thoroughness. In the final article in a four-part series on the high and rising costs of health care, Thomas Bodenheimer and Alicia Fernandez focus on actions that physicians can take to deal with the problem of rising health care costs, with substantial benefit to patients. Bodenheimer and Fernandez describe six strategies:

1. Reducing use of hospital and emergency departments by high-cost patients.

2. Disease management programs, including Edward Wagner's Chronic Care Model.

3. Reducing medical errors, which would result in dollar savings as well as quality improvements. Bodenheimer and Fernandez cite computerized physician order entry for inpatients as a strategy to reduce medical errors. Physician leadership and participation are critical for this strategy to work effectively.

4. Strengthening primary care, which can both improve quality and reduce costs. The March 2007 agreement on a set of joint principles on the patient-centered medical home by the American Academy of Pediatrics, American Academy of Family Physicians, American College of Physicians, and American Osteopathic Association (1) should be a significant impetus to efforts to strengthen primary care. The recently established Patient-Centered Primary Care Collaborative has a membership of more than 330,000 physicians and medical students and encompasses businesses that employ more 50 million workers and influential health care organizations; this collaborative will add a powerful voice to the discussions on primary care and policies that are needed to strengthen primary care.

5. Reducing inappropriate care. Most agree that reduction of inappropriate care is necessary but find hard to reach agreement on a viable strategy to accomplish it, because it is difficult to measure appropriate care. As Bodenheimer and Fernandez note, "Shared decision making, in which educated and active patients are involved in treatment decisions, may be the best remedy for costly inappropriate care" They cite several examples of strategies that have incurred significant cost savings without adverse outcomes. This approach is very much part of the patient-centered medical home.

6. Diffusion of technology assessment, which is discussed in more depth in the second part of the four-part series (2).

For those who believe, as I do, that current health care costs are too high and their continued increase presents a serious problem for individuals and families seeking health care, health insurance companies, physicians, employers, taxpayers, and the uninsured, Bodenheimer and Fernandez provide a refreshing examination of what physicians can do to improve quality while helping to control costs. Their message is a critically important one for physicians, deserving both their attention and action.

References

1. **American Academy of Family Physicians, American Academy of Pediatrics, American College of Physicians, American Osteopathic Association.** Joint principles of the patient-centered medical home. Available at www.acponline.org/hpp/approve_jp.pdf.
2. **Bodenheimer T.** High and rising health care costs. Part 2: technologic innovation. Ann Intern Med. 2005;142:932-937.

SPECIAL ARTICLE

Human Experimentation: Declaration of Helsinki

The rapid expansion in recent years of the experimental study of human patients and normal subjects has led to great concern on the part of both the medical profession and the public that the rights of such individuals be adequately protected. During the past 2 years representatives of certain national medical organizations that are particularly interested in clinical investigation and in the care of the patients have been meeting to consider whether a new code of ethics or set of guidelines should be drawn up to cover this field of medical activity. In February of this year (1966) this ad hoc *committee decided to recommend to their parent organizations that, instead of drawing up a set of detailed rules of procedure, they endorse general principles already embodied in the code of ethics adopted by the World Medical Association in Helsinki in 1964. This code is known as the* Declaration of Helsinki.

Such endorsement has now been made. It is the hope that conscientious physicians and medical investigators everywhere will find the principles of the Declaration *helpful in guiding their activities towards the human beings who are entrusted to them. It also is hoped that the* Declaration *will be useful to those in authority in hospitals, medical schools, and other institutions where humans are serving as experimental subjects, in the implementation of their specific regulation of this important activity.*

Herewith is reproduced the Declaration of Helsinki, *followed by the statement of endorsement and the list of the endorsers; editorial comment on the subject of human experimentation also appears in this issue of the* ANNALS.—Ed.

DECLARATION OF HELSINKI

It is the mission of the doctor to safeguard the health of the people. His knowledge and conscience are dedicated to the fulfillment of this mission.

The Declaration of Geneva of the World Medical Association binds the doctor with the words, "The health of my patient will be my first consideration"; and the International Code of Medical Ethics which declares that "Any act or advice which could weaken physical or mental resistance of a human being may be used only in his interest."

Because it is essential that the results of laboratory experiments be applied to human beings to further scientific knowledge and to help suffering humanity, the World Medical Association has prepared the following recommendations as a guide to each doctor in clinical research. It must be stressed that the standards as drafted are only a guide to physicians all over the world. Doctors are not relieved from criminal, civil, and ethical responsibilities under the laws of their own countries.

In the field of clinical research a fundamental distinction must be recognized between clinical research in which the aim is essentially therapeutic for a patient, and clinical research the essential object of which is purely scientific and without therapeutic value to the person subjected to the research.

I. BASIC PRINCIPLES

1. Clinical research must conform to the moral and scientific principles that justify medical research, and should be based on laboratory and animal experiments or other scientifically established facts.

2. Clinical research should be conducted only by scientifically qualified persons and under the supervision of a qualified medical man.

3. Clinical research cannot legitimately be carried out unless the importance of the objective is in proportion to the inherent risk to the subject.

4. Every clinical research project should

Requests for reprints should be addressed to the Editor, ANNALS OF INTERNAL MEDICINE, 4200 Pine St., Philadelphia, Pa. 19104.

be preceded by careful assessment of inherent risks in comparison to foreseeable benefits to the subject or to others.

5. Special caution should be exercised by the doctor in performing clinical research in which the personality of the subject is liable to be altered by drugs or experimental procedure.

II. CLINICAL RESEARCH COMBINED WITH PROFESSIONAL CARE

1. In the treatment of the sick person the doctor must be free to use a new therapeutic measure if in his judgment it offers hope of saving life, re-establishing health, or alleviating suffering.

If at all possible, consistent with patient psychology, the doctor should obtain the patient's freely given consent after the patient has been given a full explanation. In case of legal incapacity consent should also be procured from the legal guardian; in case of physical incapacity the permission of the legal guardian replaces that of the patient.

2. The doctor can combine clinical research with professional care, the objective being the acquisition of new medical knowledge, only to the extent that clinical research is justified by its therapeutic value for the patient.

III. NON-THERAPEUTIC CLINICAL RESEARCH

1. In the purely scientific application of clinical research carried out on a human being it is the duty of the doctor to remain the protector of the life and health of that person on whom clinical research is being carried out.

2. The nature, the purpose, and the risk of clinical research must be explained to the subject by the doctor.

3a. Clinical research on a human being cannot be undertaken without his free consent, after he has been fully informed; if he is legally incompetent the consent of the legal guardian should be procured.

3b. The subject of clinical research should be in such a mental, physical, and legal state as to be able to exercise fully his power of choice.

3c. Consent should as a rule be obtained in writing. However, the responsibility for clinical research always remains with the research worker; it never falls on the subject, even after consent is obtained.

4a. The investigator must respect the right of each individual to safeguard his personal integrity, especially if the subject is in a dependent relationship to the investigator.

4b. At any time during the course of clinical research the subject or his guardian should be free to withdraw permission for research to be continued. The investigator or the investigating team should discontinue the research if in his or their judgment it may, if continued, be harmful to the individual.

Endorsement of the Declaration of Helsinki By Medical Bodies in the United States

We the undersigned medical organizations endorse the ethical principles set forth in the Declaration of Helsinki by the World Medical Association concerning human experimentation. These principles supplement the principles of medical ethics to which American physicians already subscribe.

American Academy of Pediatrics
American College of Physicians
American College of Surgeons
American Federation for Clinical Research
American Medical Association
American Society for Clinical Investigation
Central Society for Clinical Research
Society for Pediatric Research

The Implications of Regional Variations in Medicare Spending. Part 2: Health Outcomes and Satisfaction with Care

Elliott S. Fisher, MD, MPH; David E. Wennberg, MD, MPH; Thérèse A. Stukel, PhD; Daniel J. Gottlieb, MS; F.L. Lucas, PhD; and Étoile L. Pinder, MS

Background: The health implications of regional differences in Medicare spending are unknown.

Objective: To determine whether regions with higher Medicare spending achieve better survival, functional status, or satisfaction with care.

Design: Cohort study.

Setting: National study of Medicare beneficiaries.

Patients: Patients hospitalized between 1993 and 1995 for hip fracture (n = 614 503), colorectal cancer (n = 195 429), or acute myocardial infarction (n = 159 393) and a representative sample (n = 18 190) drawn from the Medicare Current Beneficiary Survey (MCBS) (1992–1995).

Exposure Measurement: End-of-life spending reflects the component of regional variation in Medicare spending that is unrelated to regional differences in illness. Each cohort member's exposure to different levels of spending was therefore defined by the level of end-of-life spending in his or her hospital referral region of residence (n = 306).

Outcome Measurements: 5-year mortality rate (all four cohorts), change in functional status (MCBS cohort), and satisfaction (MCBS cohort).

Results: Cohort members were similar in baseline health status, but those in regions with higher end-of-life spending received 60% more care. Each 10% increase in regional end-of-life spending was associated with the following relative risks for death: hip fracture cohort, 1.003 (95% CI, 0.999 to 1.006); colorectal cancer cohort, 1.012 (CI, 1.004 to 1.019); acute myocardial infarction cohort, 1.007 (CI, 1.001 to 1.014); and MCBS cohort, 1.01 (CI, 0.99 to 1.03). There were no differences in the rate of decline in functional status across spending levels and no consistent differences in satisfaction.

Conclusions: Medicare enrollees in higher-spending regions receive more care than those in lower-spending regions but do not have better health outcomes or satisfaction with care. Efforts to reduce spending should proceed with caution, but policies to better manage further spending growth are warranted.

Ann Intern Med. 2003;138:288-298. www.annals.org
For author affiliations, see end of text.
See related article on pp 273-287 and editorial comments on pp 347-348, 348-349, and 350-351.

The inexorable growth of health care spending in the United States is widely believed to be due to the greater use of advanced technology of clear-cut benefit (1). Policymakers argue (and the public assumes) that any constraints on growth are likely to be harmful (1, 2). Studies of regional variations in spending and medical practice, however, call these assumptions into question. Earlier research has indicated that the nearly twofold differences in Medicare spending observed across U.S. regions are not due to differences in the prices paid for medical services (3, 4) or to differences in health or socioeconomic status (3, 5, 6). Recent research, some of which is presented in Part 1 of our study, indicates that regional variations in average per capita Medicare spending are not due to more frequent performance of major surgery (7, 8) and that regions with higher per capita spending are no more likely to provide higher-quality care, whether defined in terms of specific evidence-based services or in terms of greater access to basic health care (7, 8). The additional utilization in high-spending regions is largely devoted to discretionary services that have previously been demonstrated to be associated with the local supply of physicians and hospital resources (5, 6). These include the frequency and type of evaluation and management services provided by physicians, the use of specialist consultations, the frequency of diagnostic tests and minor procedures, and the likelihood of treating patients with chronic disease in the inpatient or intensive care unit setting.

Whether the specialist-oriented, more inpatient-based practice observed in high-spending regions offers important health benefits, however, is unknown. Although recent studies have found no benefit in terms of mortality (5, 9, 10), they had limited ability to adjust for possible case-mix differences, inadequate individual-level clinical detail, and limited outcome measures. Our study was designed to address these concerns. In Part 1, we reported on the relationship between regional differences in spending and the content of care, quality of care, and access to care provided to four cohorts of Medicare beneficiaries. In this article, Part 2, we describe associations between increased spending and mortality, functional status, and satisfaction with care.

Methods

Design Overview

As described in greater detail in Part 1, we carried out a cohort study in four parallel populations using a "natural randomization" approach (11). In this approach, one or more exposure variables allow assignment of patients into "treatment groups" (different levels of average spending), as would a randomized trial. Because some of the regional differences in Medicare spending are due to differences in illness levels (enrollees in Louisiana are sicker than those in

Colorado) and price (Medicare pays more for the same service in New York than in Iowa), we could not use Medicare spending itself as the exposure. We therefore assigned U.S. hospital referral regions (HRRs), and thus the cohort members residing within them, to different exposure levels using a measure that reflects the component of regional variation in Medicare spending due to physician practice rather than regional differences in illness or price—the End-of-Life Expenditure Index (EOL-EI). Because regional differences in end-of-life spending are unrelated to underlying illness levels, it is reasonable to consider residence in HRRs with differing levels of end-of-life spending as a random event. The index was calculated as spending on hospital and physician services provided to a reference cohort distinct from the study cohorts: Medicare enrollees in their last 6 months of life. In the current paper, we also present several analyses with an alternative exposure measure, the Acute Care Expenditure Index (AC-EI), to decrease concern about possible residual confounding.

We confirmed that the exposures used to assign the HRRs achieved the goals of "natural randomization": 1) Study samples assigned to different levels of the exposure (the EOL-EI) were similar in baseline health status, and 2) the actual quantity of services delivered to the individuals within the study samples nevertheless differed substantially across exposure levels and was highly correlated with average per capita Medicare spending in the HRRs. We followed the cohorts for up to 5 years after their initial hospitalizations and compared the processes of care (Part 1) and health outcomes (Part 2) across HRRs assigned to different exposure levels.

Context

Per capita Medicare spending varies considerably from region to region. The effect of greater Medicare spending on mortality, functional status, and satisfaction is not known.

Contribution

Using end-of-life care spending as an indicator of Medicare spending, the researchers categorized geographic regions into five quintiles of spending and examined costs and outcomes of care for hip fracture, colorectal cancer, and acute myocardial infarction. Residents of high-spending regions received 60% more care but did not have lower mortality rates, better functional status, or higher satisfaction.

Implications

Medicare beneficiaries who live in higher Medicare spending regions do not necessarily have better health outcomes or satisfaction with health care than those in lower-spending regions.

–The Editors

Study Cohorts

The four study cohorts are described in detail in Part 1. Briefly, we studied fee-for-service Medicare enrollees, ages 65 to 99 years, who were eligible for Medicare Parts A and B. The acute myocardial infarction (MI) cohort was drawn from patients included in the Cooperative Cardiovascular Project, who had index hospitalizations between February 1994 and November 1995. The hip fracture and colorectal cancer cohorts were identified based on an incident hospitalization between 1993 and 1995. The general population sample included participants in the Medicare Current Beneficiary Survey (MCBS) who had initial interviews between 1991 and 1996 (for the survival analysis) or between 1992 and 1995 (for the other analyses) (see Appendix, section C, available at www.annals.org).

Each cohort member was placed in a spending group according to the EOL-EI (as defined in detail in Part 1) in their HRR of residence at the time of the index hospitalization (chronic disease cohorts), or initial interview (MCBS cohort). Characteristics of the study cohorts were ascertained from a variety of sources, as described in detail in Part 1, including Medicare administrative files and claims (all four cohorts), chart reviews (acute MI cohort), in-person interview (MCBS cohort), U.S Census data (attributes of ZIP code of residence, such as income, for the three chronic disease cohorts), and American Hospital Association data (to characterize hospitals).

Assignment to Exposure Levels

As we summarized here and described in detail in Part 1, we used two approaches to determine cohort members' exposure to different levels of Medicare spending in their HRR of residence. Previous research has shown that the dramatic differences in end-of-life treatment across U.S. regions are highly predictive of differences in total spending (8, 12) but are not due to differences in case mix or patient preferences (13). Our primary measure of exposure was the EOL-EI, which was calculated as age-sex-race–adjusted spending (measured with standardized national prices) on hospital and physician services provided to Medicare enrollees who were in their last 6 months of life in each of the 306 U.S. HRRs in mid-1994 to 1997, excluding any members of the study cohorts (Appendix, Section E, available at www.annals.org.) We also repeated the major analyses with an alternative exposure measure, the AC-EI, which was based on differences across HRRs in risk-adjusted spending during an acute illness episode (Appendix, Section F, available at www.annals.org). Both measures were highly predictive of average age-sex-race–adjusted Medicare spending at the HRR level ($r = 0.81$ for the EOL-EI and 0.79 for the AC-EI in the acute MI cohort) and, as was shown in Part 1, of the regional differences in utilization experienced by the study cohorts. For many analyses, we grouped HRRs into quintiles of increasing exposure to the expenditure indices.

Statistical Analyses

To assess the aggregate impact of any differences in individual attributes on average baseline risk for death across regions of increasing EOL-EI, we used logistic regression to determine each individual's predicted 1-year risk for death as a function of his or her baseline characteristics. The models had modest to excellent predictive ability (c-statistics were 0.61 for the colorectal cancer cohort, 0.68 for the hip fracture cohort, 0.77 for the acute MI cohort, and 0.82 for the MCBS cohort). We used these models to determine the average predicted risk for death across quintiles of Medicare expenditure indices.

Mortality Analyses

The association between the HRR-level expenditure index and survival was assessed by using Cox proportional hazards regression models (14), with the expenditure index measured both as a categorical variable (in which each HRR was assigned to a quintile of Medicare spending based on the EOL-EI) and a continuous variable (using the value of the EOL-EI in the HRR of residence as the exposure). The survival models included independent variables to adjust for patient characteristics, hospital characteristics, and attributes of the HRR. Model fit was assessed by using methods for Cox model residuals to examine overall model fit, to test proportional hazards assumptions, and to identify influential observations. The main survival models underpredicted mortality in the first 6 months, possibly because of short-term complications that could not be adequately predicted with the available data; however, the models provided excellent prediction of 1-year mortality rates for each cohort.

The models are presented in **Appendix Tables 6** through **9** (available at www.annals.org). To test whether the overall findings were consistent across subgroups of each cohort, we ran survival models stratified on all major variables. To test whether the findings were sensitive to our choice of the EOL-EI as our primary exposure, we repeated the analyses using the AC-EI. These sensitivity analyses are described in detail in the Appendix, Section F (available at www.annals.org).

Patients in the same hospital are likely to be treated similarly, so their outcomes may not be statistically independent. We adjusted for within-hospital clustering by using overdispersed survival models, clustering by hospital (14). Model fit was assessed by carefully examining the data to identify HRRs that influenced estimates, predicted values, and likelihood ratio tests. Two moderately influential HRRs, Manhattan, New York, and Miami, Florida, were identified, both of which had relatively lower mortality rates and higher spending than predicted. Excluding these regions would have resulted in hazard ratios greater than those we report for quintile 5 (in the categorical model) and overall (in the continuous models). Analyses, however, are presented with these two HRRs included. We used the STCOX routine of Stata 6.0 (Stata Corp., College Station, Texas) to perform survival analyses in the three chronic disease cohorts. For the analyses of the MCBS cohort, we used SUDAAN (Research Triangle Institute, Research Triangle Park, North Carolina) to account for sampling weights and the two-stage design (15).

Change in Functional Status

We used the Health Activities and Limitations Index (HALex) as the primary dependent variable in our longitudinal analyses of changes in functional status (16, 17). The HALex was developed by the National Center for Health Statistics as a composite health status measure that can be calculated by using the responses to the National Health Interview Survey. For our longitudinal analyses, we assigned a HALex score of 0 to respondents who died. Loss to follow-up in these analyses occurred when patients failed to answer enough questions to allow a calculation of the score, did not participate in the survey, or entered a nursing home. Loss to follow-up was as follows: quintile 1, 7.8%; quintile 2, 8.9%; quintile 3, 8.4%; quintile 4, 9.6%; and quintile 5, 13.4%.

The effect of HRR spending on HALex score was modeled by using generalized estimating equation methods for the analysis of continuous longitudinal data (18). The dependent variable was the respondent's annual HALex score for up to 3 years. Each model controlled for individual attributes (**Appendix Table 10**, available at www.annals.org) and included a variable for the time since the initial survey (0, 1, 2, or 3 years). Two sets of models were run, one including indicator variables for quintile of spending, the other including spending as a continuous variable. The principal hypothesis, that increased spending in the HRR of residence would be associated with a slower decline in health status, was tested through the interaction between the EOL-EI of the HRR and the length of time since the initial survey. Different model specifications were tested, both including and excluding interaction terms between time and the other control variables. All analyses yielded similar results for the tests of the principal hypothesis. The models are presented in **Appendix Table 10**, available at www.annals.org. We used the longitudinal sampling weight from the final interview for each respondent and then normalized across all cohort members so that the sum of the weights was equal to the total number in the cohort. The numbers of study participants reported incorporate these weights and are rounded to the nearest integer.

Satisfaction with Care

This analysis was restricted to respondents with at least one physician visit in the previous year. The MCBS interview includes 20 questions on satisfaction with care. Eight items rate the general satisfaction with care received from physicians or hospitals within the past year, while 12 questions are asked only of respondents with a usual physician

Table 1. **Crude and Predicted Mortality Rates in Study Cohorts according to Level of Medicare Spending in Hospital Referral Region of Residence***

Variable	Quintile of EOL-EI					Test for Trend†
	1 (Lowest)	2	3	4	5 (Highest)	
	←——— % ———→					
Hip fracture cohort						
Observed 30-day mortality rate	7.8	7.2	6.9	6.9	6.6	↓
Observed 1-year mortality rate	24.4	23.9	23.9	24.3	24.2	>0.05
Predicted 1-year mortality rate	24.5	24.1	24.1	24.1	23.9	↓
Colorectal cancer cohort						
Observed 30-day mortality rate	4.5	4.6	4.8	4.8	4.4	>0.05
Observed 1-year mortality rate	20.6	20.7	21.7	21.1	20.9	>0.05
Predicted 1-year mortality rate	21.1	20.8	21.2	20.8	20.9	>0.05
Acute MI cohort						
Observed 30-day mortality rate	18.5	18.4	19.2	18.2	18.5	>0.05
Observed 1-year mortality rate	30.7	31.3	32.6	31.6	33.3	↑
Predicted 1-year mortality rate	31.2	31.5	31.8	32.0	33.2	↑
MCBS cohort						
Observed 30-day mortality rate	0.2	0.4	0.4	0.3	0.2	>0.05
Observed 1-year mortality rate	4.6	4.8	5.0	5.1	5.3	>0.05
Predicted 1-year mortality rate	4.9	5.1	5.3	5.0	5.1	>0.05

* Crude mortality rates were based on 30-day and 1-year follow-up for all cohort members with no censoring (follow-up for mortality was complete at 1 year for all). Predicted mortality rates were based on logistic regression equations that included individual- and ZIP code–level variables only. EOL-EI = End-of-Life Expenditure Index; MCBS = Medicare Current Beneficiary Survey; MI = myocardial infarction.
† Arrows show the direction of any statistically significant association ($P \leq 0.05$) between the mortality rate and regional EOL-EI differences. An arrow pointing upward indicates that as spending increases across regions, the mortality rate increases. A P value greater than 0.05 was considered not significant.

(93% of the study sample) and focus on that physician's quality. Following the approach of others (19), we created two summary scores of general satisfaction with care (global quality and accessibility) and three summary scores focused on satisfaction with a usual physician (technical skills, interpersonal manner, and information-giving). To test for significant associations between the expenditure index and each summary scale, we used linear regression with each of the five summary scores as the dependent variable and the exposure measured as the HRR-level EOL-EI. The models controlled for age, sex, race, health status, and major U.S. region of residence (n = 9). We also compared satisfaction scores on these scales across quintiles of spending. The analysis of satisfaction was based on respondents' first interview.

RESULTS

Patient Characteristics

Tables 1 through 4 in Part 1 present selected characteristics of each study cohort grouped into quintiles according to EOL-EI level in their HRRs of residence. Because the sample sizes are large, many small differences for the chronic disease cohorts were statistically significant. Notable differences were found in racial composition (more black persons in higher-expenditure HRRs) and income (higher-expenditure HRRs had more beneficiaries in the highest and lowest income categories). Smaller differences across quintiles were apparent in age, sex, comorbid conditions, and cancer stage. For the acute MI cohort, patients in the highest quintiles had a higher prevalence of non–Q-wave infarctions and congestive heart failure but a lower prevalence of creatine kinase levels greater than 1000 IU/L. For the MCBS cohort, residents of HRRs in the quintiles with higher EOL-EIs were more likely to report being in fair or poor health but were less likely to live in a facility.

Crude 30-day and 1-year mortality rates and average predicted 1-year mortality rates for each cohort are shown in **Table 1**. For the hip fracture cohort, average predicted mortality rates at 1 year were slightly but significantly lower in HRRs with a higher EOL-EI. In the acute MI cohort, however, average predicted mortality rates at 1 year were higher in HRRs with a higher expenditure index. No significant differences were found in predicted mortality across HRRs with differing expenditure indices for the colorectal cancer or MCBS cohorts. These findings reveal no consistent trend toward greater illness burden in HRRs with a higher expenditure index. Observed mortality tended to be lower than predicted in the lowest quintile and equal to or higher than predicted in the highest quintile.

Mortality

Figure 1 presents the relative risk for death over 5 years for residents of HRRs in EOL-EI quintiles 2, 3, 4, and 5 (the higher quintiles) compared with residents of HRRs in the lowest quintile. In each cohort, an increase in EOL-EI was associated with a small increase in the risk for death. We repeated these analyses using the HRR-specific EOL-EI as a continuous variable both overall and in specific subgroups (**Figures 2** through **4**). A relative risk

Figure 1. **Adjusted relative risk for death during follow-up across quintiles of Medicare spending.**

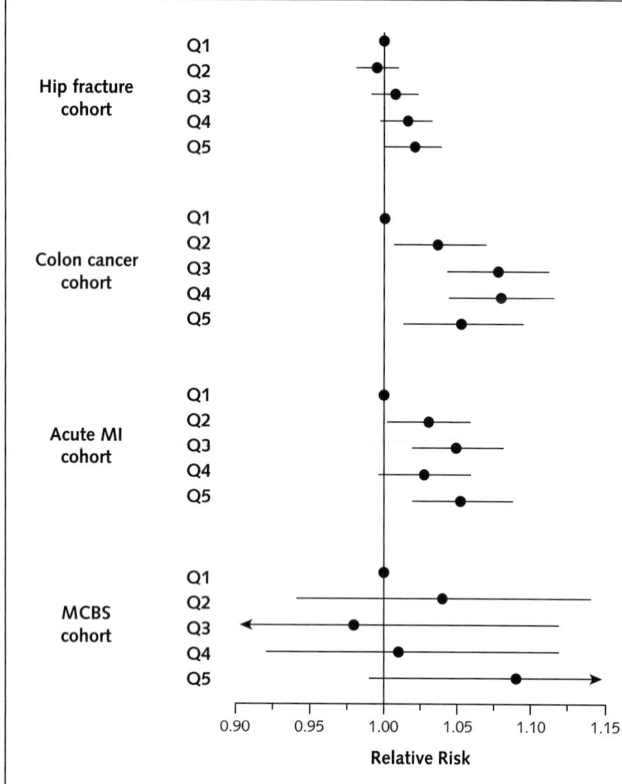

Circles represent adjusted relative risk for death among residents of hospital referral regions in the specified quintile of the End-of-Life Expenditure Index (EOL-EI) compared to the risk for death among residents of hospital referral regions in quintile 1 of the EOL-EI; bars represent 95% CIs. MCBS = Medicare Current Beneficiary Survey; MI = myocardial infarction; Q1 = quintile 1; Q2 = quintile 2; Q3 = quintile 3; Q4 = quintile 4; Q5 = quintile 5.

greater than 1 indicated that residence in an HRR with a higher EOL-EI (higher expenditures) was associated with increased mortality. For every 10% increase in the EOL-EI, the relative risk for death over 5 years was as follows: hip fracture cohort, 1.003 (CI, 0.999 to 1.006); colorectal cancer cohort, 1.012 (CI, 1.004 to 1.019); acute MI cohort, 1.007 (CI, 1.001 to 1.014); and MCBS cohort, 1.01 (CI, 0.99 to 1.03). In none of the subgroups examined was a higher expenditure index associated with a statistically significantly lower mortality rate.

We repeated the mortality analyses using the alternate approach: assigning HRRs to different exposure levels based on the AC-EI. Residents of higher-spending HRRs, according to the AC-EI, had relatively similar baseline health status (**Appendix Table 17**, available at www.annals.org) and yet received substantially more care (**Appendix Table 18**, available at www.annals.org). The results of the mortality analyses are summarized in **Table 2**. For the hip fracture cohort, higher AC-EIs were associated with a small decrease in mortality rates. For all of the other cohorts, mortality rates did not differ or increased slightly in regions with a higher AC-EI.

Change in Functional Status

The average decline in functional status, as measured by using the HALex score, was about 2 points per year (on a 100-point scale) but did not differ across HRRs grouped according to quintiles of the EOL-EI (**Table 3**). In none of the models examined was an increased expenditure index associated with a statistically significant difference in the average rate of decline in health status (**Appendix Table 10**, available at www.annals.org).

Satisfaction with Care

Figure 5 presents average change in adjusted satisfaction scores across quintiles (compared with quintile 1) for the five summary scales. Each scale ranges from 0 to 100, with higher scores implying greater satisfaction. We found substantial variation in satisfaction with care across the nine major U.S. regions (for example, Northeast and Mid-Atlantic), with satisfaction on each scale averaging over five points higher in the Northeast than in the South, controlling for other factors (data not shown). The differences in satisfaction across EOL-EI quintiles, however, were smaller than these regional differences and did not reveal a consistent pattern of greater satisfaction in HRRs with a higher expenditure index. The overall test for trend across HRRs indicated less global satisfaction with care and more satisfaction with interpersonal aspects of care in higher-spending HRRs. No differences were found across HRRs of differing expenditure indices for the other three measures of satisfaction with care.

Discussion

We conducted a cohort study in four distinct samples of Medicare enrollees, comparing the outcomes of care across 306 U.S. HRRs that differed dramatically in levels of Medicare spending and utilization. The primary exposure variable in this study, the EOL-EI, was intended to measure the component of regional variation in Medicare spending that is unrelated to regional differences in illness or price. The goal was to ensure assignment of HRRs (and the patients within them) to "treatment groups" that were similar in baseline health status but differed in subsequent treatment. The validity of the approach was confirmed by our finding that illness levels in each of the four study cohorts differed little across quintiles but that health care utilization rates and spending (for our four study cohorts) increased steadily and substantially across quintiles. Regardless of the measure used to characterize spending, residents of the highest-spending quintile received about 60% more care than those of the lowest-spending quintile.

As shown in detail in Part 1, these differences in spending were explained almost entirely by greater frequency of physician visits, more frequent use of specialist consultations, more frequent tests and minor procedures,

Figure 2. **Adjusted relative risk for death associated with a 10% increase in Medicare spending overall and among specified subgroups of the hip fracture cohort.**

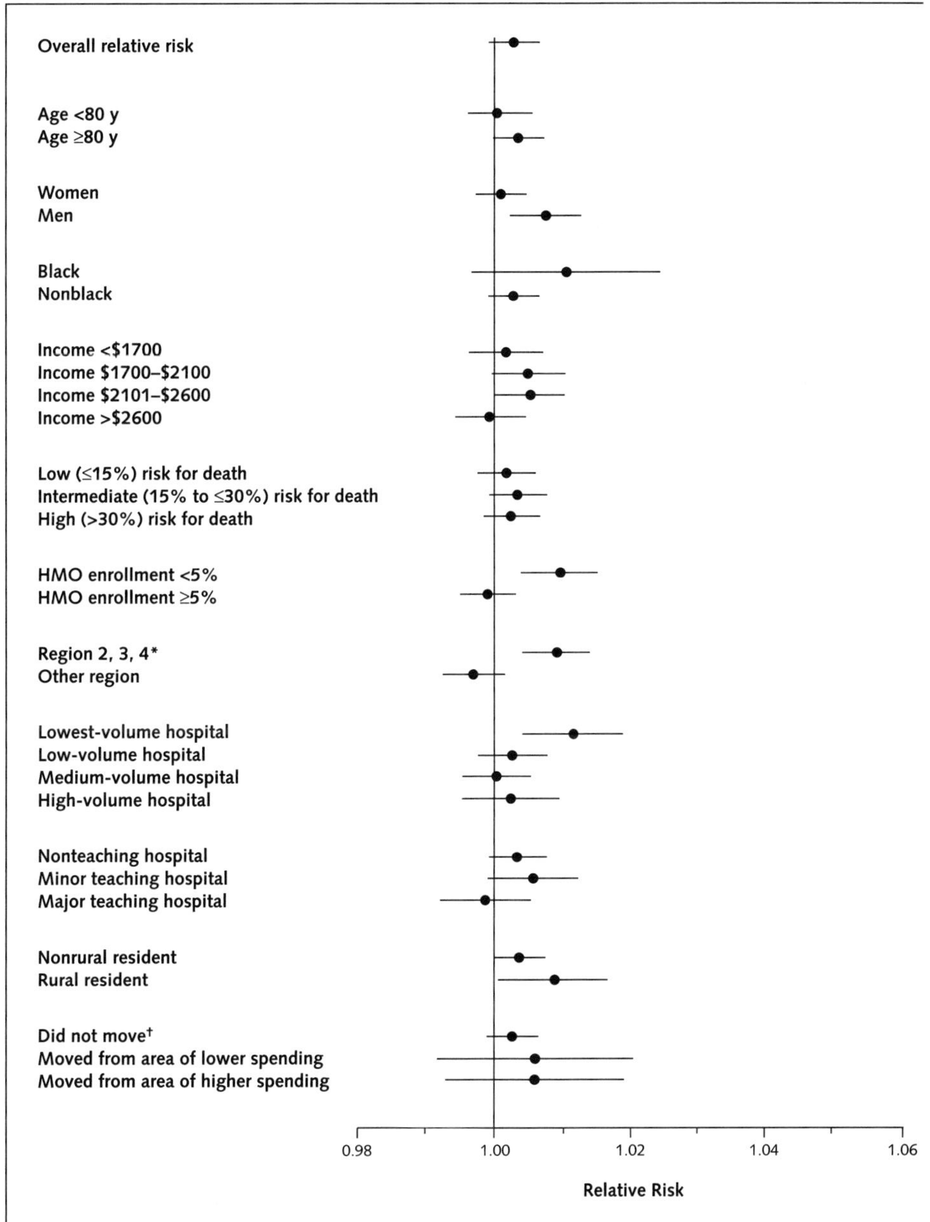

Income figures refer to the average monthly Social Security income of the patients' ZIP codes. Circles represent the adjusted relative risk for death associated with a 10% increase in the End-of-Life Expenditure Index across U.S. hospital referral regions; bars represent 95% CIs for the relative risk. *Mid-Atlantic, South Atlantic, and Great Lakes regions. †Did not change hospital referral region of residence in the 1 to 2 years before index admission. HMO = health maintenance organization.

and greater use of the hospital and intensive care unit in high-spending regions. In this paper, Part 2, we found no evidence to suggest that the pattern of practice observed in higher-spending regions led to improved survival, slower decline in functional status, or improved satisfaction with care.

In Part 1, we discussed the major limitations related to the analyses of utilization. Here we focus primarily on the limitations related to our analysis of health outcomes. First, because of the observational nature of our study, the small increase in mortality rate observed in regions with higher spending levels as assigned by end-of-life spending must be interpreted with caution. It is possible that the higher mortality rates observed in high-spending regions could be caused by the patterns of practice in regions where patients near the end of life are treated more intensively because of either relative overuse of such services as diagnostic tests and hospital-based care (for example, complications of treatment) or lower-quality care (for example, failure to provide such evidence-based services as immunizations).

Figure 3. **Adjusted relative risk for death associated with a 10% increase in Medicare spending overall and among specified subgroups of the colorectal cancer cohort.**

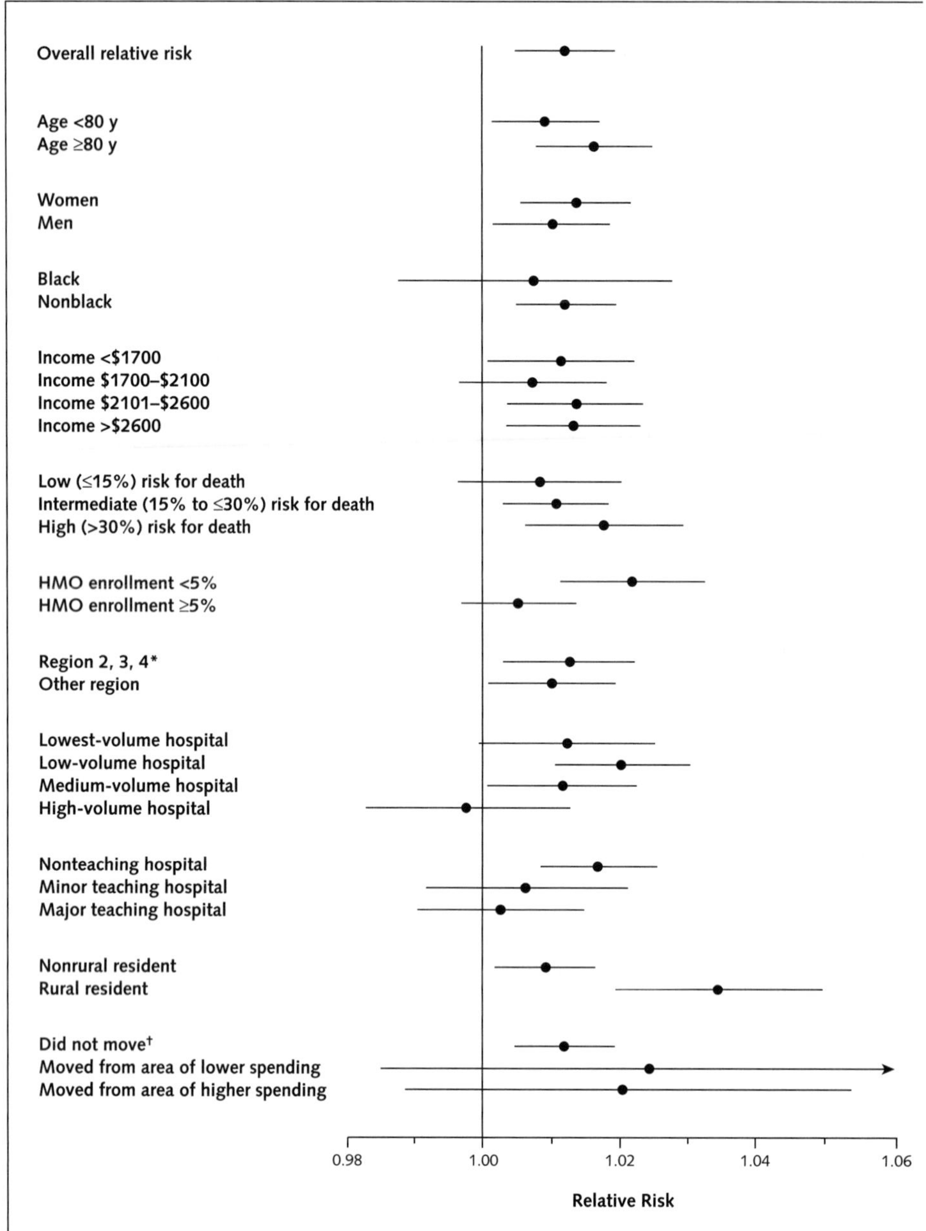

Income figures refer to the average monthly Social Security incomes of the patients' ZIP code. Circles represent the adjusted relative risk for death associated with a 10% increase in the End-of-Life Expenditure Index across U.S. hospital referral regions; bars represent 95% CIs for the relative risk. *Mid-Atlantic, South Atlantic, and Great Lakes regions. †Did not change hospital referral region of residence in the 1 to 2 years before index admission. HMO = health maintenance organization.

On the other hand, it is possible that the increased mortality rate could be explained by unmeasured differences in case mix across regions of differing spending levels. We tried to account for this contingency in our study design (by use of the natural randomization approach) by controlling for numerous patient and regional attributes in our models. The stratified analyses (**Figure 2**) also suggest that unmeasured confounding is unlikely. Any potential confounder would have to operate similarly across all of these strata. Some might argue, for example, that even among similarly ill patients, those who are aware of increased risk might move closer to teaching hospitals or to higher-spending regions (that is, that differences in patterns of migration, with sicker retirees moving to areas where capacity is greatest, explain our findings). That our findings are consistent across patients in teaching and nonteaching hospitals and among patients who had recently moved and those who had not argues against such con-

Figure 4. **Adjusted relative risk for death associated with a 10% increase in Medicare spending overall and among specified subgroups of the acute myocardial infarction (*MI*) cohort.**

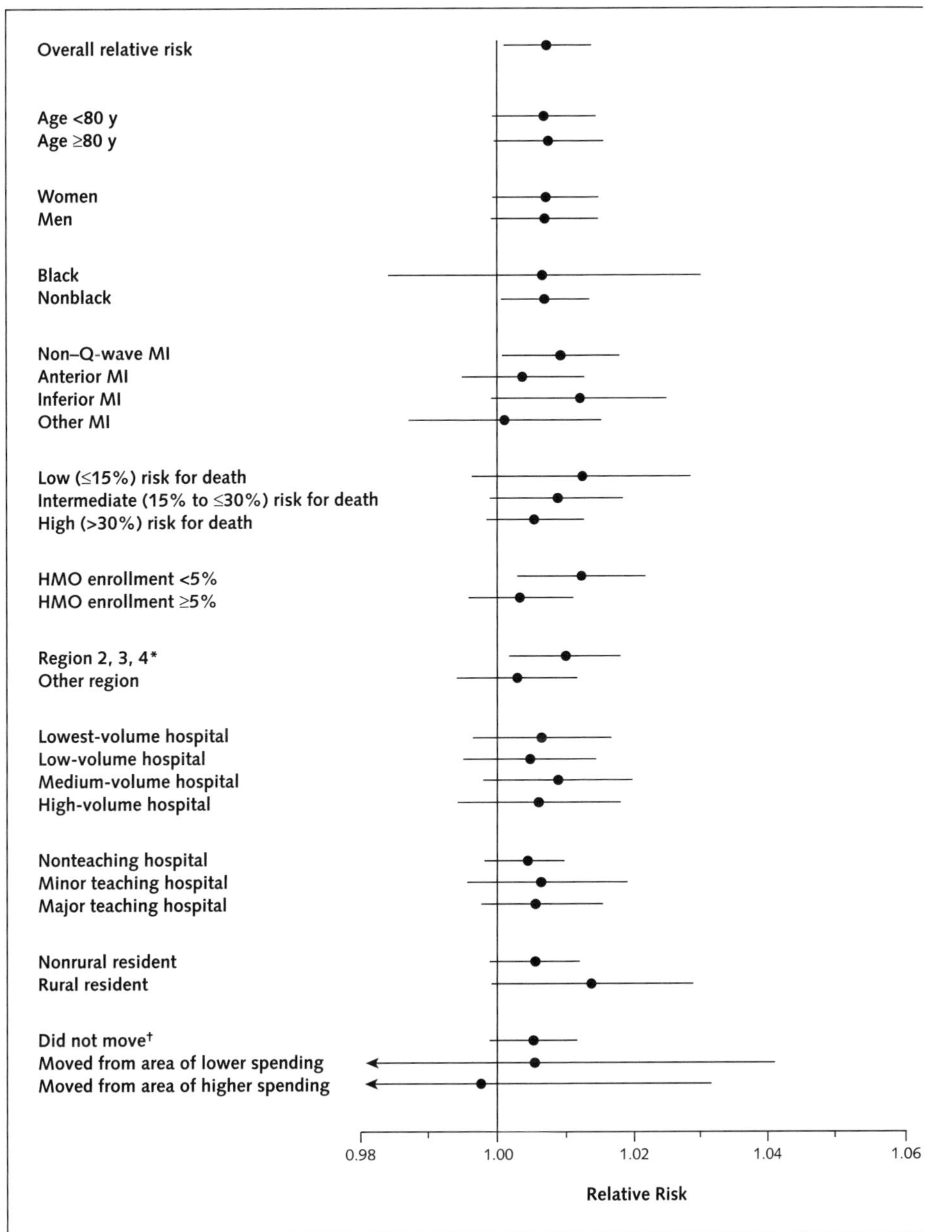

Income figures refer to the average monthly Social Security income of the patients' ZIP codes. Circles represent the adjusted relative risk for death associated with a 10% increase in the End-of-Life Expenditure Index across U.S. hospital referral regions; bars represent 95% CIs for the relative risk. *Mid-Atlantic, South Atlantic, and Great Lakes regions. †Did not change hospital referral region of residence in the 1 to 2 years before index admission. HMO = health maintenance organization.

founding. Nevertheless, the fundamental limitation of observational studies must be acknowledged: We cannot determine whether the small increase in mortality rate is due to the treatment differences (regional differences in practice) or to unmeasured differences in the comparison groups.

Our analyses using the AC-EI provide additional evidence that the regional differences in Medicare spending observed across the United States are unlikely to provide important benefits in terms of improved survival. These findings suggest that even when HRRs are stratified according to differences in how patients are treated during an episode of acute illness, regions that take the more intensive approach to acute care do not achieve better survival. For unmeasured confounding to have led to our findings, the unmeasured confounder would have to be correlated both with end-of-life spending and with regional differences in risk-adjusted acute care spending and would have to predict increased risk for death in all four cohorts. While this possibility must be acknowledged, it appears unlikely.

Table 2. **Adjusted Relative Risk for Death across Quintiles of Medicare Spending and Relative Risk Associated with a 10% Increase in Medicare Spending, as Estimated by Using the Acute Care Expenditure Index (Sensitivity Analysis)***

Cohort	Relative Risk (95% CI)					Continuous Models
	Quintile of AC-EI					
	1 (Lowest)	2	3	4	5 (Highest)	
Hip fracture	1.00 (referent)	1.003 (0.989–1.016)	0.998 (0.984–1.013)	0.993 (0.978–1.009)	0.996 (0.979–1.014)	0.990 (0.983–0.998)
Colorectal cancer	1.00 (referent)	1.024 (0.994–1.055)	1.028 (0.995–1.062)	1.022 (0.987–1.057)	0.995 (0.959–1.032)	1.000 (0.985–1.016)
Acute MI	1.00 (referent)	1.025 (0.999–1.053)	1.029 (1.000–1.058)	1.027 (0.997–1.059)	1.037 (1.004–1.071)	1.009 (0.996–1.023)
MCBS	1.00 (referent)	1.19 (1.04–1.36)	1.16 (0.98–1.37)	1.05 (0.92–1.18)	1.08 (0.95–1.23)	0.99 (0.94–1.05)

* Data were obtained from Cox regression models testing the association between residence in higher-spending hospital referral regions (defined on the basis of the AC-EI) and mortality for up to 5 years. For the quintile models, hospital referral regions were grouped into quintiles of increasing AC-EI levels. For the continuous models, data represent the relative risk for death associated with a 10% increase in the level of the AC-EI in the hospital referral registry of residence. For additional details, see Appendix, Section F, available at www.annals.org. AC-EI = Acute Care Expenditure Index; MCBS = Medicare Current Beneficiary Survey; MI = myocardial infarction.

The consistency of our findings across different measures of the exposure and different study cohorts argues that the increased Medicare spending in high-cost regions provides no important benefits in terms of survival.

A second limitation of this study is that we were able to examine functional outcomes and satisfaction with care only in the general population sample and not in our three high-risk, chronic disease cohorts. Although the quality of care provided to the three chronic disease cohorts appeared no better in higher-spending regions, it remains possible that the increased use of specialists, diagnostic tests, and hospital-based care led to better functional outcomes, quality of life, or satisfaction with care. Further research is warranted to address this possibility.

It is also possible, however, that the increased intensity of treatment provided to severely ill patients could lead to poorer quality of life and less satisfaction. The most striking differences in practice in higher-spending regions are found in the care of patients near the end of life, regardless of whether the definition of a "high-spending" region is based on one of the indices used here or on average per capita Medicare spending (8). Our findings suggest that the more aggressive patterns of practice observed in high-spending regions offer no benefit in terms of their major aim, which is improving survival. In addition, we know of no evidence to suggest that the nearly threefold greater use of invasive life support (intensive care unit utilization, emergency intubation, and feeding tubes) seen in high-spending regions results in improved quality of life or satisfaction with care.

Finally, because our primary exposure variable is ecological, in the sense that residence in a region with higher Medicare spending is a characteristic of patients' environment, some may be concerned that our inferences are suspect because of the "ecological fallacy" (39, 40). The ecological fallacy occurs when one tries to answer a purely individual-level question (for example, Is high saturated fat intake associated with a person's risk for heart disease?) with data derived from groups of people (for example, the average risk for heart disease in a group). The fallacy lies in assuming that an association observed at one level of aggregation (for example, countries) automatically implies the association at a different level (for example, individual patients). It is most likely to occur when both outcomes and predictors of that outcome (including measures of exposure and measures used to adjust for group differences) are ascertained only for the groups and not for individuals. Our research interest was to determine whether a system-level variable—increased Medicare spending in a given region—leads to better care or better outcomes for the average individual Medicare enrollee residing in that region. We chose an ecological (system-level) exposure measure because it is the appropriate exposure measure for this specific research question. In addition, because we were interested in the effects of regional spending on the care of individual patients, our unit of analysis was the patient.

Table 3. **Average Change per Year in Functional Status on Health Activities and Limitation Index among Participants in the Medicare Current Beneficiary Survey according to Medicare Spending in the Hospital Referral Region of Residence***

Variable	Quintile of EOL-EI				
	1 (Lowest)	2	3	4	5 (Highest)
Change in functional status (95% CI)	−1.96 (−2.36 to −1.55)	−2.18 (−2.65 to −1.71)	−2.28 (−2.84 to −1.71)	−1.94 (−2.40 to −1.47)	−1.96 (−2.42 to −1.50)

* Scores on the Health Activities and Limitations Index at follow-up ranged from 0 (death) to 100 (excellent self-assessed health and no limitations). Results controlled for differences in age, sex, race, chronic conditions, residence in a facility, residence in a metropolitan region, whether respondent was bedridden, smoking status, income, education, marital status, and supplemental insurance coverage. EOL-EI = End-of-Life Expenditure Index.

Figure 5. **Satisfaction with care.**

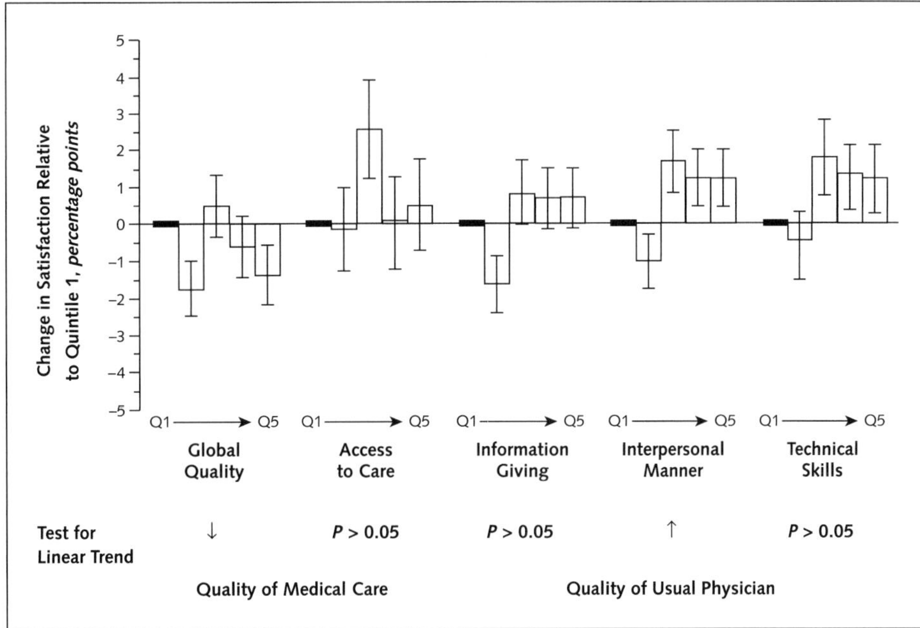

An arrow pointing upward indicates a positive association between increased spending and satisfaction. Bars represents 95% CIs. Q1 = quintile 1; Q5 = quintile 5.

We measured outcomes and variables used to adjust for group differences at the patient level and could therefore control effectively for individual characteristics in the analysis. The ecological fallacy therefore applies neither to our design nor to our analysis. We can legitimately conclude that the average Medicare patient in higher-spending regions (and the average patient in each subgroup examined) receives much more care than those in lower-spending regions and that this additional care is not associated with better access to care, higher-quality care, or better health outcomes.

Previous research on regional variations in utilization and outcomes has been largely ecological in design, examining cross-sectional correlations at the area level between spending and utilization (5) or between spending or utilization and mortality (9, 12, 22). These earlier studies have been criticized for weak designs, inadequate individual-level measures to control for potential differences in case mix, insufficient clinical detail on the process of care to allow inferences on potential causal pathways to be drawn, and limited outcome measures. Our study addressed each of these concerns. We adopted a longitudinal design and obtained extensive baseline data on patients' health and socioeconomic status that allowed us to control for potential differences in need for care. We were also able to characterize in detail patients' access to care, use of services, and quality of care. Finally, we showed that these regional differences in utilization and outcomes were consistently seen in each subgroup of the samples. Black or white, poor or rich, high-risk or low-risk, patients in higher-spending regions received much more care (**Appendix Tables 12 through 14**, available at www.annals.org) but did not have better outcomes.

Our study provides limited guidance on the potential impact of reducing regional disparities in spending or the implementation of policies to constrain the use of these supply-sensitive services. From a clinical perspective, it is important to recognize that our study does not address the question of how the amount of care for an individual patient in a specific case would affect that patient's clinical outcome. What may appear to be relatively low-risk interventions (such as hospitalization or ordering a diagnostic test) may cause harm in some settings, just as failure to provide these or other services (such as bypass surgery in high-risk patients) may cause harm in other settings. From a policy perspective, our study does not tell us definitively that it is possible to reduce Medicare spending within a particular region without affecting patient care or outcomes. Previous research has shown that vulnerable populations may be harmed by reduced access to care (23, 24) or as a consequence of public hospital closures (25). It is not always clear, for example, whether services such as specialist consultations are wasteful or beneficial. The potential adverse impact of reductions in the use of beneficial services and disruptions in current practice patterns underscores the importance of further research on these issues and of the implementation and evaluation of demonstration projects intended to improve quality of care and promote conservative approaches to managing patients with chronic disease (8).

Debates over the need for further growth in medical spending and expansion of the medical workforce are largely based on the assumption that additional services will provide important health benefits to the population served. Our study suggests that this assumption is unwarranted. Our study also underscores the need for research to determine how to safely reduce spending levels. If the United States as a whole could safely achieve spending levels comparable to those of the lowest-spending regions, annual savings of up to 30% of Medicare expenditures could be achieved (3). Such savings could provide the resources to fund important new benefits, such as prescription drugs or expanded Medicare coverage to younger age groups, or to extend the life of the Medicare Trust Fund to better cover the health care needs of future retirees.

From Center for Evaluative Clinical Sciences, Dartmouth Medical School, Hanover, New Hampshire; VA Outcomes Group, White River Junction Veterans Affairs Medical Center, White River Junction, Vermont; and Institute for the Clinical Evaluative Sciences, Toronto, Ontario, Canada.

Disclaimer: The analyses of the Cardiovascular Cooperative Project data were performed under contract number 500-99-NH01, titled "Utilization and Quality Control Peer Review Organization for the State of New Hampshire," sponsored by the Centers for Medicare & Medicare Services (formerly the Health Care Financing Administration), Department of Health and Human Services. The content of this publication does not necessarily reflect the views or policies of the Department of Health and Human Services, nor does mention of trade names, commercial products, or organizations imply endorsement by the U.S. government.

The authors assume full responsibility for the accuracy and completeness of the analyses presented. This article is a direct result of the Health Care Quality Improvement Program initiated by the Centers for Medicare & Medicare Services, which has encouraged identification of quality improvement projects derived from analysis of patterns of care, and therefore required no special funding on the part of this contractor. Ideas and contributions to the author concerning experience with issues presented are welcomed.

The opinions expressed herein are those of the authors alone, and do not necessarily reflect those of the Centers for Medicare & Medicare Services, the Robert Wood Johnson Foundation or the Department of Veterans Affairs.

Grant Support: By the Robert Wood Johnson Foundation, the National Institutes of Health (CA52192), and the National Institute of Aging (1PO1 AG19783-01).

Potential Financial Conflicts of Interest: None disclosed.

Requests for Single Reprints: Elliott S. Fisher, MD, MPH, Strasenburgh Hall, HB 7251, Dartmouth Medical School, Hanover, NH 03755; VA Outcomes Group, White River Junction Veterans Affairs Medical Center, White River Junction, VT 05001; e-mail, elliott.s.fisher@dartmouth.edu.

Current author addresses and author contributions are available at www.annals.org.

References

1. **Cutler DM, McClellan M.** Is technological change in medicine worth it? Health Aff (Millwood). 2001;20:11-29. [PMID: 11558696]

2. **Kleinke JD.** The price of progress: prescription drugs in the health care market. Health Aff (Millwood). 2001;20:43-60. [PMID: 11558720]

3. **Skinner JS, Fisher ES.** Regional disparities in medicare expenditures: an opportunity for reform. National Tax Journal. 1997;50:413-25.

4. **Welch WP, Miller ME, Welch HG, Fisher ES, Wennberg JE.** Geographic variation in expenditures for physicians' services in the United States. N Engl J Med. 1993;328:621-7. [PMID: 8429854]

5. **Fisher ES, Wennberg JE, Stukel TA, Skinner JS, Sharp SM, Freeman JL, et al.** Associations among hospital capacity, utilization, and mortality of US Medicare beneficiaries, controlling for sociodemographic factors. Health Serv Res. 2000;34:1351-62. [PMID: 10654835]

6. **Wennberg JE, Cooper MM.** The Dartmouth Atlas of Health Care 1999. Chicago: American Hospital Publishing; 1999.

7. **Fisher ES, Wennberg DE, Stukel TA, Gottlieb D, Lucas FL, Pinder E.** The health implications of regional variations in Medicare spending. Part 1: Utilization of services and quality of care. Ann Intern Med. 2003;138:273-87.

8. **Wennberg JE, Fisher ES, Skinner J.** Geography and the debate over Medicare reform. Health Aff (Millwood). 13 February 2002. Available at www.healthaffairs.org/WebExclusives/Wennberg_Web_Excl_021302.htm.

9. **Krakauer H, Jacoby I, Millman M, Lukomnik JE.** Physician impact on hospital admission and on mortality rates in the Medicare population. Health Serv Res. 1996;31:191-211. [PMID: 8675439]

10. **Kessler DP, McClellan MB.** Is hospital competition socially wasteful? The Quarterly Journal of Economics. 2000;115:577-616.

11. **McClellan M, McNeil BJ, Newhouse JP.** Does more intensive treatment of acute myocardial infarction in the elderly reduce mortality? Analysis using instrumental variables. JAMA. 1994;272:859-66. [PMID: 8078163]

12. **Skinner JS, Wennberg JE, Fisher ES.** The Efficiency of Medicare. National Bureau of Economic Research Working Papers. Cambridge, MA: National Bureau of Economic Research; 2001.

13. **Pritchard RS, Fisher ES, Teno JM, Sharp SM, Reding DJ, Knaus WA, et al.** Influence of patient preferences and local health system characteristics on the place of death. SUPPORT Investigators. Study to Understand Prognoses and Preferences for Risks and Outcomes of Treatment. J Am Geriatr Soc. 1998;46:1242-50. [PMID: 9777906]

14. **Lin DY.** Cox regression analysis of multivariate failure time data: the marginal approach. Stat Med. 1994;13:2233-47. [PMID: 7846422]

15. **Shah BV, Barnwell BG, Bieler GS.** SUDAAN User's Manual, Release 7.5. Research Triangle Park, NC: Research Triangle Institute; 1997.

16. **Erickson P.** Evaluation of a population-based measure of quality of life: the Health and Activity Limitation Index (HALex). Qual Life Res. 1998;7:101-14. [PMID: 9523491]

17. **Erickson P, Wilson R, Shannon I.** Healthy People Statistical Notes. No. 7. Years of Healthy Life. April 1995. National Center for Health Statistics. Accessed at www.cdc.gov/nchs/data/statnt/statnt07.pdf on 16 December 2003.

18. **Zeger SL, Liang KY.** Longitudinal data analysis for discrete and continuous outcomes. Biometrics. 1986;42:121-30. [PMID: 3719049]

19. **Lee Y, Kasper JD.** Assessment of medical care by elderly people: general satisfaction and physician quality. Health Serv Res. 1998;32:741-58. [PMID: 9460484]

20. **Thorndike EL.** On the fallacy of imputing correlations found for groups to the individuals or smaller groups composing them. American Journal of Psychology. 1939;52:122-4.

21. **Selvin H.** Durkheim's suicide and problems of empirical research. American Journal of Sociology. 1958;63:607-19.

22. **Hadley J.** Medicare spending and mortality rates of the elderly. Inquiry. 1988;25:485-93. [PMID: 2976049]

23. **Lurie N, Ward NB, Shapiro MF, Gallego C, Vaghaiwalla R, Brook RH.** Termination of Medi-Cal benefits. A follow-up study one year later. N Engl J Med. 1986;314:1266-8. [PMID: 3517642]

24. **Lurie N, Ward NB, Shapiro MF, Brook RH.** Termination from Medi-Cal—does it affect health? N Engl J Med. 1984;311:480-4. [PMID: 6379458]

25. **Bindman AB, Keane D, Lurie N.** A public hospital closes. Impact on patients' access to care and health status. JAMA. 1990;264:2899-904. [PMID: 2232084]

High and Rising Health Care Costs. Part 4: Can Costs Be Controlled While Preserving Quality?

Thomas Bodenheimer, MD, and Alicia Fernandez, MD

Several interrelated strategies involving physician leadership and participation have been proposed to contain health care costs while preserving or improving quality. These include programs targeting the 10% of the population that incurs 70% of health care expenditures, disease management programs to prevent costly complications of chronic conditions, efforts to reduce medical errors, the strengthening of primary care practice, decision support tools to avoid inappropriate services, and improved diffusion of technology assessment.

An example of a cost-reducing, quality-enhancing program is post-hospital nurse monitoring and intervention for patients at high risk for repeated hospitalization for congestive heart failure. Disease management programs that target groups with a chronic condition rather than focusing efforts on high-utilizing individuals may be effective in improving quality but may not reduce costs. Error reduction has great potential to improve quality while reducing costs, although the probable cost reduction is a small portion of national health care expenditures. Access to primary care has been shown to correlate with reduced hospital use while preserving quality. Inappropriate care and overuse of new technologies can be reduced through shared decision-making between well-informed physicians and patients. Physicians have a central role to play in fostering these quality-enhancing strategies that can help to slow the growth of health care expenditures.

Ann Intern Med. 2005;143:26-31. **www.annals.org**
For author affiliation, see end of text.

In the first 3 articles, this series on health care costs offered a variety of explanations and remedies for high and rising health care expenditures in the United States (1–3). This final article addresses the question posed at the beginning of the series: Do strategies exist that enable physicians to reduce costs while improving or protecting health care quality?

The first 3 articles discussed various cost-containment methods: making patients more responsible for the costs of their care, encouraging price competition in health care markets, slowing the rate of diffusion of costly new technologies through effective technology assessment programs, reducing the administrative cost burden of the health care system, and counterbalancing the market power of health care providers and suppliers with expenditure caps or global budgets that limit the total amount of money flowing into the health care economy. Most of these approaches are policy initiatives that require the actions of governments or large health insurance plans. Except through political advocacy, physicians cannot readily affect these approaches. Other cost-containment strategies do fall within the purview of physicians' professional work. This article presents quality-preserving cost-control activities that involve physician leadership and cooperation. The strategies discussed overlap with one another; the common theme is the substitution of lower-cost ambulatory care for higher-cost emergency or in-hospital services (**Table**).

Reducing Use of Hospital and Emergency Departments by High-Cost Patients

Physicians are the first to appreciate a fundamental reality: Ten percent of the population accounts for 70% of health care expenditures. Fifty percent of the population—healthy persons—are responsible for only 3% of health care expenditures. These relationships have held steady from 1970 to 1996. In 1996, the healthy 50% incurred an average cost of $122 per person whereas the highest-cost 1% spent $56 000 per person (4). Serious cost control should focus on the high-cost members of the population.

Common diagnoses among the highest-cost 10% are ischemic heart disease (including congestive heart failure), cancer, diabetes, hypertension, pulmonary conditions, mental disorders, and trauma. Moreover, the highest-cost patients have 3 or more comorbid conditions. Particularly for heart disease and cancer, the bulk of expenditures are for inpatient care. Kidney disease and stroke incur the highest average cost per person, but fewer people have these conditions than heart disease, cancer, trauma, mental disorders, and hypertension (5, 6). Almost all high-cost patients utilize inpatient hospital services (7).

High costs result from prolonged hospitalization, brief hospitalization with intensive use of resources, or repeated hospitalization for the same condition. In a study of high-cost patients, repeated hospitalization was considerably more frequent than single prolonged or cost-intensive hospitalization. About 20% of high-cost patients died during the year of the study. Very sick patients, who were kept alive for long periods through multiple clinical interventions, accounted for fewer than 10% of the high-cost patients. Unexpected complications were important factors that elevated patients from low-cost to high-cost status. The study concluded that repeated hospitalizations for the

See also:

Print
Editorial comment. 76

Web-Only
Conversion of table into slide

same illness are an important cause of very high costs (8). A study of hospitalizations for diabetes reached a similar conclusion (9).

Because Medicare data are easy to access and because many high-cost patients are Medicare beneficiaries, analyses of high-cost patients tend to focus on Medicare. Ninety-five percent of Medicare costs are incurred by people with 2 or more chronic conditions; by far, the most expensive Medicare patients in 1999 were elderly persons with 4 or more chronic conditions (10).

If most high-cost patients were near death, the opportunity to reduce spending on those individuals would be limited. However, only one fifth of people in the top 5% of Medicare spending in a given year died by the end of that year. Among Medicare beneficiaries who were consistently high spenders over 5 years (1995 to 1999), 60% were alive at the end of that period (7). Opportunities exist for cost reduction among persistently high-cost patients who are not near death, particularly because a substantial proportion of their costs are inpatient related. To take full advantage of this opportunity, high-cost patients must be identified and interventions made before these patients become high spenders (7). One successful cost-reduction program for high-cost patients is the improved management of congestive heart failure.

Post-Hospital Management of Congestive Heart Failure

Congestive heart failure is the most common indication for hospitalization among older adults (11). In 1995, Rich and colleagues (12) studied a nurse-directed program of patient education with post-hospital telephone calls and home visit follow-up for patients with congestive heart failure. Within 90 days, hospital readmissions decreased markedly and quality of life improved, resulting in a cost reduction of $460 per patient in the intervention group compared with controls (12). Eleven randomized, controlled trials of similar nurse-led post-hospital interventions for congestive heart failure have been published; 7 of 8 trials that reported cost data saved money. Eight of the 11 trials found that readmission rates decreased from 22% to 45% in the intervention group. For the 9 trials in which multidisciplinary follow-up teams were used, the summary risk ratio for readmission for heart failure was 0.77 (95% CI, 0.68 to 0.86), indicating a reduction in readmissions of 23%. Quality outcomes improved or remained the same (11, 13).

Recent publications suggest that these programs are not cost-effective for all patients with congestive heart failure (14, 15). The programs that successfully reduce costs are targeted to high-risk patients, are initiated in the hospital or shortly after discharge, and include postdischarge face-to-face encounters with nurse care managers rather than telephone-only contact (16). Because these programs reduce hospital revenues, hospitals are unlikely to sponsor them. The Medicare program, which realizes the savings, is the logical entity to require or reimburse such programs.

Table. **Thinking about Specific Cost-Reduction Programs**

It is helpful to ask 5 questions about concrete cost-reduction programs in specific institutions.

1. Who benefits from a cost reduction effort: purchaser, insurer, provider, patient, or society?
2. Are financial incentives aligned to promote cost reduction? An organization that earns more money by providing more services is unlikely to engage in cost reduction. Cost-containment programs in globally budgeted institutions, such as Kaiser Permanente or the Veterans Affairs systems, may not generalize to other settings because these institutions have aligned their financial incentives in favor of cost reduction.
3. Is it possible to identify the patients whose health expenditures might be lowered? Ideally, efforts would be made to identify and case-manage patients whose costs are likely to be high in the future.
4. Is the timeline for cost reduction short or long? How does the timeline affect the "business case" for cost-reduction programs? Few health plans will invest in cost-control efforts whose savings will be delayed for 10 or 20 years.
5. Will the cost reduction effort truly protect quality of care?

Other Post-Hospital Programs

The concept of nurse-run post-hospital programs can be extended from patients with congestive heart failure to elderly people with multiple diagnoses. In 1 study, such a program markedly reduced the readmission rate, causing mean total charges to be 63% less for the intervention group than the control group (17).

Forty percent to 50% of patients with chronic obstructive pulmonary disease—another high-cost diagnosis—who are discharged from hospitals are readmitted during the following year. A patient education program with regular follow-up was associated with a 40% reduction in admissions for chronic obstructive pulmonary disease and improved quality of life compared with controls (18).

Fewer hospitalizations could not only reduce costs but also avoid serious illnesses in elderly persons. Many functionally independent elderly persons are no longer independent after hospital discharge. Bed rest rapidly reduces muscle strength and aerobic ventilatory capacity, thereby increasing the risk for falls, confusion, and future dependency. The vertebral bone loss caused by 10 days of bed rest requires 4 months to restore, thereby increasing risk for fracture. The cascade of physiologic decline initiated by a hospitalization may prove irreversible (19).

Physicians are ideally suited to encourage post-hospital interventions for high-utilizing patients with congestive heart failure and other chronic conditions, thereby contributing to cost reduction and quality enhancement.

DISEASE MANAGEMENT PROGRAMS

"Disease management" is a general term for programs that focus on 1 or more chronic illnesses and attempt to improve quality and reduce costs incurred by people with chronic conditions. Post-hospital heart failure interventions are an example. The success of programs such as those targeting high-risk patients with heart failure has helped drive enthusiasm for disease management. Disease management programs may or may not be high-user interventions, depending on whether they target entire groups with chronic conditions or restrict their focus to high-risk patients.

Because care of chronic illness consumes 78% of national health care expenditures (20), the disease management movement has become a growth industry in the United States (21). The premise is that consistent intervention in chronic disease, guided by evidence-based medicine and coordinated care, results in better care, less illness, and lower costs.

Do disease management programs truly cut costs? Some do and some do not. The programs for management of congestive heart failure described earlier reduce expenditures because they target individuals, most of whom are in the top 10% of health care spenders. Programs for children with moderate or severe persistent asthma who have been hospitalized have been shown to save money, whereas similar programs for children with less severe asthma do not reduce costs (22). The cost-saving congestive heart failure and asthma interventions are programs only for high users of health care resources. Disease management vendors who proclaim cost savings often restrict their efforts to high users rather than large groups (23, 24).

Savings are difficult to demonstrate for programs aimed at all patients with chronic conditions of high prevalence (most of whom are not yet high users), particularly conditions whose complications manifest themselves far in the future. A review of diabetes programs involving components of Edward Wagner's Chronic Care Model—planned visit clinics, case management, reminder prompts, and performance feedback reports—found that 7 of 9 studies reported reduced health care use or reduced costs. However, most of these programs were experimental and of short duration, and in some cases costs increased again when the research protocol ended (22). A study of 4 disease management programs (for coronary artery disease, heart failure, diabetes, and asthma) at Kaiser Permanente from 1996 to 2002 found that the programs were associated with substantial quality improvement but not cost savings (25, 26). A recent report from the U.S. Congressional Budget Office also raises questions about the cost-saving promise of disease management (15).

Under most fee-for-service arrangements, the costs of disease management programs may be borne by the provider organization, whereas savings (if they exist) accrue to the insurer. Integrated systems with global budgets (for example, Kaiser Permanente and Veterans Affairs hospitals) both bear the program costs and reap the benefits of reduced use of hospitals and emergency departments. Analyses of "costs to whom" and the related alignment of incentives are an essential part of constructing the elusive business case for chronic disease management (27). In the case of diabetes, effective cost reduction requires identifying which patients will be the high-cost patients of the future and effectively intervening with those patients (7). Although some prediction models for future high-cost patients exist (28), they have not always proven to be reliable (7).

The time frame for return on investment poses challenges to the cost-control potential of disease management programs. If a person with diabetes receives excellent care, thereby delaying the onset of end-organ complications, are costs saved through reductions in myocardial infarctions and end-stage renal disease, or are costs increased because the patient lives longer and incurs more expenditures by virtue of needing medical care for more years? Lubitz and associates (29) compared noninstitutionalized patients in good health at 70 years of age with those in poor health at 70 years of age. People in good health lived longer, thereby incurring more years of medical expenditures; those in poor health had more expenditures per year for fewer years. The data showed that total health expenditures from 70 years of age to death were equal for the 2 groups, suggesting that improved chronic care before 70 years of age neither increases nor reduces health expenditures over the lifetime of the patient (29). A business-case "home run" in diabetes management would be hit by a program that lasts at least 20 years within the organization reaping the cost reductions; is utilized by patients who remain in that organization for at least 20 years; and markedly reduces the rate of myocardial infarctions, strokes, leg amputations, and end-stage renal disease among its participants. Such home runs are rare.

Even though the cost-containment potential of disease management programs is uncertain, these programs aspire to the dual goals of quality improvement and cost containment. Disease management programs initiated by health insurance plans and managed by vendor companies often fail to involve physicians in a central role. In contrast, programs that develop within provider organizations—hospitals; physician groups; and group-model health maintenance organizations, such as Kaiser Permanente, Group Health in Seattle, and HealthPartners in Minnesota—offer important innovations in which physicians can lead and participate.

REDUCING MEDICAL ERRORS

Quality problems are generally categorized as underuse, overuse, and misuse (30). High-user and chronic disease management programs attempt to correct underuse of ambulatory and home-care programs in order to reduce overuse of hospitals and emergency departments. Error reduction is aimed at misuse.

Unexpected complications, often resulting from medical errors, may catapult hospitalized patients from the low-cost to the high-cost category (8). One study estimated savings from eliminating preventable errors during hospitalization as being in the range of $5 billion to $10 billion per year (31). Another estimate placed savings at $17 billion per year (32). These amounts may be small in relation to total health expenditures, but they are substantial.

Solutions to the problem of medical errors involve physician-driven activities that combine cost reduction with quality improvement. One example of an error-reduction intervention is computerized physician order entry for inpatients (33). Physicians have resisted this intervention when it was poorly implemented (34). An alternative would be for all physicians to participate in planning in-hospital computerization so that the innovation is implemented in an effective and physician-friendly manner.

STRENGTHENING PRIMARY CARE

Primary care has the potential to reduce costs while preserving quality. Studies of ambulatory care–sensitive conditions (conditions, such as diabetes or congestive heart failure, for which timely, appropriate diagnosis and treatment may result in reduced hospitalization) have shown that hospitalization rates and expenditures for those conditions are higher in areas with fewer primary care physicians (35) and limited access to primary care (36). Systems that link patients with primary care physicians are associated with reduced hospitalizations for ambulatory care–sensitive conditions (37, 38). Adults 18 to 64 years of age in urban California communities with poorer access to primary care had higher hospitalization rates for 5 ambulatory care–sensitive chronic conditions than did similar patients with better access to primary care (39).

Strengthening primary care may also result in more appropriate use of specialists (40). Schroeder and Sandy (41) have labeled specialty care as "the invisible driver of health care costs." Costs are higher in regions with higher ratios of specialist to generalist physicians (42, 43). Baicker and Chandra (44) showed that states with more specialists have higher per capita Medicare spending, suggesting that this relationship may be driven by the use of more intensive, costly interventions. Although specialists provide higher-quality care for some conditions, the large Medical Outcomes Study showed that primary care physicians, using fewer resources, deliver care similar in quality to that of specialists for such conditions as diabetes and hypertension (45, 46).

Both specialists and primary care physicians can encourage efforts to strengthen primary care structures that may reduce unnecessary hospitalizations while maintaining quality. These efforts may or may not involve an increased number of primary care physicians per capita (depending on the geographic region); more important, they include modes of primary care reimbursement that are adequate and that promote better quality, and redesign of primary care practices to improve the basic management of ambulatory care–sensitive conditions.

REDUCING INAPPROPRIATE CARE

Eliminating inappropriate care is a well-recognized strategy to reduce costs while improving quality. Although appropriateness is difficult to measure (47), well-recognized criteria, which were clinically tested in several cases, have been developed for the appropriateness of various procedures (48).

Examples of inappropriate or possibly inappropriate care abound in the literature (49). Some studies have examined variation in rates of procedures; others may have applied appropriateness criteria to specific cases by using chart audits. More than 20% of patients with cancer receive chemotherapy in the last 3 months of life, and this percentage is similar for patients whose cancer is responsive to chemotherapy and those whose disease is unresponsive (50). Estimates of unnecessary inpatient hospital days have ranged from 25% to 50% (51, 52). A recent analysis of Medicare beneficiaries 65 to 75 years of age found that 15% of coronary artery bypass surgeries were performed for an uncertain indication and 10% were inappropriate; 54% of angioplasties had an uncertain indication and 14% were inappropriate (53). Increasing rates of spinal fusion surgery for conditions for which no evidence of benefit exists—with high rates of reoperation and complications—suggest substantial inappropriate care (54, 55).

Elimination of inappropriate prescriptions could also generate cost savings. In 1 study, 40% of prescriptions written for hypertension did not conform to evidence-based guidelines (56). For elderly patients with hypertension in the United States in 2001, physician noncompliance with guidelines cost about $1.2 billion (56).

As noted in article 3 of this series (3), states and regions featuring high-intensity medical practice with high per capita Medicare costs do not provide better quality of care, as measured by use of various preventive or treatment processes associated with improved outcomes, than do states and regions with more conservative practice patterns (57–59). A major difference between conservative and high-intensity regions is the number of physicians involved in the care of a given patient. High-intensity practice is likely to involve inappropriate and harmful care (60).

Achievement of quality-enhancing cost reduction by reduction of inappropriate care is difficult. It is easier to judge appropriateness after, rather than before, an intervention has been performed. Shared decision making, in which educated and active patients are involved in treatment decisions, may be the best remedy for costly, inappropriate care. In 6 of 7 studies, shared decision making was associated with 21% to 44% reductions in more invasive surgical options—including coronary revascularization, hysterectomy, mastectomy, back surgery, and prostatectomy—without adverse outcomes (61).

High-quality shared decision making requires patients who can engage in discussions as informed partners, which in turn requires use of patient decision aids. These are evidence-based tools that allow physicians to accurately inform patients of available options and their consequences. These tools are not widely utilized at present (61). For chronic illnesses, such as diabetes, shared decision making is associated with better health-related behaviors and improved clinical outcomes (62, 63). Physicians can seek to minimize inappropriate care by using decision aids that bring evidence-based knowledge to the point of care and by engaging patients in shared decision making.

DIFFUSION OF TECHNOLOGY ASSESSMENT

Article 2 in this series reviewed the evidence that new technologies are adopted more rapidly in the United States compared with other developed nations, thereby increasing their use and cost (2). Although novel technologies may benefit patient care, high rates of use of these technologies could represent inappropriate care. Technology assessment—the process of determining which technologies are clinically indicated for which patients (64)—is an important tool to assist physicians in limiting inappropriate use of medical advances. The results of technology assessment can be incorporated into patient decision aids and used when engaging patients in shared decision making.

CONCLUSION

The 4-part series that concludes with this article explains that the high and rising health care expenditures in the United States are caused by a variety of factors. The most important of these are the market power of physicians, hospitals, and pharmaceutical companies, which has enabled these providers and suppliers to garner high prices for their services and products, and the rapid diffusion of high-cost innovative technologies.

Several measures may contain rising health care costs. Among these are encouragement of competition among providers and health insurance plans, linking of provider payment to health technology assessment so that new technologies are not utilized inappropriately, placing of controls on prices of services and products or on the quantities of services provided, and institution of expenditure caps or global budgets that limit the total amount of money flowing into the health system.

Most of these cost-containment measures do not connect closely with physician practice. They are instituted, strengthened, weakened, or discontinued by governments or large health insurance plans. However, several approaches to high and rising health care costs are directly tied to daily medical practice. It is these physician-connected strategies—which may help to control health care expenditures while protecting quality—that have been the topic of this final article.

We believe that high and rising costs are a serious menace to the future of our health care system. As expenditures rise, Medicare, Medicaid, and private insurers reduce coverage; costs are shifted to individuals, thereby reducing access to needed care for some. Most of us, as physicians, have experienced how rising costs can create difficulties in caring for our patients: For example, the growing cost of prescription drugs, which are frequently not covered by insurance, has often restricted our therapeutic choices for elderly patients. Escalating patient responsibility for payment in an environment of rising prices will further restrict physicians' diagnostic and treatment options for the sizable proportion of patients with limited financial means. If cost increases are not moderated, our satisfaction at being able to offer patients beneficial clinical innovations may give way to frustration, as our patients become unable to afford those same innovations.

From the University of California, San Francisco, San Francisco, California.

Potential Financial Conflicts of Interest: None disclosed.

Requests for Single Reprints: Thomas Bodenheimer, MD, Department of Family and Community Medicine, University of California, San Francisco, Building 80-83, San Francisco General Hospital, 1001 Potrero Avenue, San Francisco, CA 94110; e-mail, tbodenheimer@medsch.ucsf.edu.

Current author addresses are available at www.annals.org.

References

1. **Bodenheimer T.** High and rising health care costs. Part 1: seeking an explanation. Ann Intern Med. 2005;142:847-54.
2. **Bodenheimer T.** High and rising health care costs. Part 2: technologic innovation. Ann Intern Med. 2005;142:932-7.
3. **Bodenheimer T.** High and rising health care costs. Part 3: the role of health care providers. Ann Intern Med. 2005;142:996-1002.
4. **Berk ML, Monheit AC.** The concentration of health care expenditures, revisited. Health Aff (Millwood). 2001;20:9-18. [PMID: 11260963]
5. **Cohen JW, Krauss NA.** Spending and service use among people with the fifteen most costly medical conditions, 1997. Health Aff (Millwood). 2003;22:129-38. [PMID: 12674416]
6. **Thorpe KE, Florence CS, Joski P.** Which medical conditions account for the rise in health care spending? Health Affairs. Web Exclusive. 25 August 2004. W-4-437-445. Accessed at http://content.healthaffairs.org/cgi/content/full/hlthaff.w4.437/DC1 on 24 November 2004.
7. **Lieberman SM, Lee J, Anderson T, Crippen DL.** Reducing the growth of Medicare spending: geographic versus patient-based strategies. Health Affairs. Web Exclusive. 10 December 2003. W3-603-613. Accessed at http://content.healthaffairs.org/cgi/content/full/hlthaff.w3.603v1/DC1 on 24 November 2004.
8. **Zook CJ, Moore FD.** High-cost users of medical care. N Engl J Med. 1980;302:996-1002. [PMID: 6767975]
9. **Jiang HJ, Stryer D, Friedman B, Andrews R.** Multiple hospitalizations for patients with diabetes. Diabetes Care. 2003;26:1421-6. [PMID: 12716799]
10. **Wolff JL, Starfield B, Anderson G.** Prevalence, expenditures, and complications of multiple chronic conditions in the elderly. Arch Intern Med. 2002;162:2269-76. [PMID: 12418941]
11. **Rich MW.** Heart failure disease management programs: efficacy and limitations [Editorial]. Am J Med. 2001;110:410-2. [PMID: 11286961]
12. **Rich MW, Beckham V, Wittenberg C, Leven CL, Freedland KE, Carney RM.** A multidisciplinary intervention to prevent the readmission of elderly patients with congestive heart failure. N Engl J Med. 1995;333:1190-5. [PMID: 7565975]
13. **McAlister FA, Lawson FM, Teo KK, Armstrong PW.** A systematic review of randomized trials of disease management programs in heart failure. Am J Med. 2001;110:378-84. [PMID: 11286953]
14. **DeBusk RF, Miller NH, Parker KM, Bandura A, Kraemer HC, Cher DJ, et al.** Care management for low-risk patients with heart failure: a randomized, controlled trial. Ann Intern Med. 2004;141:606-13. [PMID: 15492340]
15. Congressional Budget Office. An Analysis of the Literature on Disease Management Programs, October 13, 2004. Accessed at www.cbo.gov on 29 November 2004.
16. **Wagner EH.** Deconstructing heart failure disease management [Editorial].

Ann Intern Med. 2004;141:644-6. [PMID: 15492346]
17. **Naylor M, Brooten D, Jones R, Lavizzo-Mourey R, Mezey M, Pauly M.** Comprehensive discharge planning for the hospitalized elderly. A randomized clinical trial. Ann Intern Med. 1994;120:999-1006. [PMID: 8185149]
18. **Bourbeau J, Julien M, Maltais F, Rouleau M, Beaupre A, Begin R, et al.** Reduction of hospital utilization in patients with chronic obstructive pulmonary disease: a disease-specific self-management intervention. Arch Intern Med. 2003; 163:585-91. [PMID: 12622605]
19. **Creditor MC.** Hazards of hospitalization of the elderly. Ann Intern Med. 1993;118:219-23. [PMID: 8417639]
20. **Anderson G, Horvath J.** Chronic Conditions: Making the Case for Ongoing Care. Baltimore: Johns Hopkins Univ Pr; 2002.
21. **Bodenheimer T.** Disease management—promises and pitfalls. N Engl J Med. 1999;340:1202-5. [PMID: 10202174]
22. **Bodenheimer T, Wagner EH, Grumbach K.** Improving primary care for patients with chronic illness: the chronic care model, Part 2. JAMA. 2002;288: 1909-14. [PMID: 12377092]
23. **Villagra VG, Ahmed T.** Effectiveness of a disease management program for patients with diabetes. Health Aff (Millwood). 2004;23:255-66. [PMID: 15318587]
24. **Fetterolf D, Wennberg D, Devries A.** Estimating the return on investment in disease management programs using a pre-post analysis. Dis Manag. 2004;7: 5-23. [PMID: 15035830]
25. **Fireman B, Bartlett J, Selby J.** Can disease management reduce health care costs by improving quality? Health Aff (Millwood). 2004;23:63-75. [PMID: 15584100]
26. **Crosson FJ, Madvig P.** Does population management of chronic disease lead to lower costs of care? Health Aff (Millwood). 2004;23:76-8. [PMID: 15537587]
27. **Leatherman S, Berwick D, Iles D, Lewin LS, Davidoff F, Nolan T, et al.** The business case for quality: case studies and an analysis. Health Aff (Millwood). 2003;22:17-30. [PMID: 12674405]
28. **Dove HG, Duncan I, Robb A.** A prediction model for targeting low-cost, high-risk members of managed care organizations. Am J Manag Care. 2003;9: 381-9. [PMID: 12744300]
29. **Lubitz J, Cai L, Kramarow E, Lentzner H.** Health, life expectancy, and health care spending among the elderly. N Engl J Med. 2003;349:1048-55. [PMID: 12968089]
30. **Institute of Medicine.** Crossing the Quality Chasm: A New Health System for the 21st Century. Washington, DC: National Academy Pr; 2001.
31. **Zhan C, Miller MR.** Excess length of stay, charges, and mortality attributable to medical injuries during hospitalization. JAMA. 2003;290:1868-74. [PMID: 14532315]
32. Medical Errors: The Scope of the Problem. Fact Sheet. Rockville, MD: Agency for Healthcare Research and Quality; 2000. Publication no. AHRQ 00-P037. Accessed at www.ahrq.gov/qual/errback.htm on 7 December 2004.
33. **Bates DW, Leape LL, Cullen DJ, Laird N, Petersen LA, Teich JM, et al.** Effect of computerized physician order entry and a team intervention on prevention of serious medication errors. JAMA. 1998;280:1311-6. [PMID: 9794308]
34. Cedars-Sinai Medical Center suspends use of computerized physician order entry system. Los Angeles Times. 22 January 2003:B.1.
35. **Parchman ML, Culler S.** Primary care physicians and avoidable hospitalizations. J Fam Pract. 1994;39:123-8. [PMID: 8057062]
36. **Basu J, Friedman B, Burstin H.** Managed care and preventable hospitalization among Medicaid adults. Health Serv Res. 2004;39:489-510. [PMID: 15149475]
37. **Zhan C, Miller MR, Wong H, Meyer GS.** The effects of HMO penetration on preventable hospitalizations. Health Serv Res. 2004;39:345-61. [PMID: 15032958]
38. **Backus L, Moron M, Bacchetti P, Baker LC, Bindman AB.** Effect of managed care on preventable hospitalization rates in California. Med Care. 2002;40: 315-24. [PMID: 12021687]
39. **Bindman AB, Grumbach K, Osmond D, Komaromy M, Vranizan K, Lurie N, et al.** Preventable hospitalizations and access to health care. JAMA. 1995;274: 305-11. [PMID: 7609259]
40. **Franks P, Clancy CM, Nutting PA.** Gatekeeping revisited—protecting patients from overtreatment. N Engl J Med. 1992;327:424-9. [PMID: 1625720]
41. **Schroeder SA, Sandy LG.** Specialty distribution of U.S. physicians—the invisible driver of health care costs [Editorial]. N Engl J Med. 1993;328:961-3. [PMID: 8446146]
42. **Starfield B.** Primary Care. New York: Oxford Univ Pr; 1998.
43. **Welch WP, Miller ME, Welch HG, Fisher ES, Wennberg JE.** Geographic variation in expenditures for physicians' services in the United States. N Engl J Med. 1993;328:621-7. [PMID: 8429854]
44. **Baicker K, Chandra A.** Medicare spending, the physician workforce, and beneficiaries' quality of care. Health Affairs. Web Exclusive. 7 April 2004. Accessed at http://content.healthaffairs.org/cgi/content/full/hlthaff.w4.184v1/DC1 on 24 November 2004.
45. **Greenfield S, Rogers W, Mangotich M, Carney MF, Tarlov AR.** Outcomes of patients with hypertension and non-insulin dependent diabetes mellitus treated by different systems and specialties. Results from the medical outcomes study. JAMA. 1995;274:1436-44. [PMID: 7474189]
46. **Greenfield S, Nelson EC, Zubkoff M, Manning W, Rogers W, Kravitz RL, et al.** Variations in resource utilization among medical specialties and systems of care. Results from the medical outcomes study. JAMA. 1992;267:1624-30. [PMID: 1542172]
47. **Naylor CD.** What is appropriate care? [Editorial] N Engl J Med. 1998;338: 1918-20. [PMID: 9637815]
48. **Shekelle PG.** Are appropriateness criteria ready for use in clinical practice? [Editorial] N Engl J Med. 2001;344:677-8. [PMID: 11228286]
49. **Leape LL.** Unnecessary surgery. Annu Rev Public Health. 1992;13:363-83. [PMID: 1599594]
50. **Emanuel EJ, Young-Xu Y, Levinsky NG, Gazelle G, Saynina O, Ash AS.** Chemotherapy use among Medicare beneficiaries at the end of life. Ann Intern Med. 2003;138:639-43. [PMID: 12693886]
51. **Brook RH.** Practice guidelines and practicing medicine. Are they compatible? JAMA. 1989;262:3027-30. [PMID: 2810647]
52. **Axene DV, Doyle RL, van der Burch D.** Analysis of Medically Unnecessary Inpatient Services. New York: Milliman & Robertson; 1997.
53. **Schneider EC, Leape LL, Weissman JS, Piana RN, Gatsonis C, Epstein AM.** Racial differences in cardiac revascularization rates: does "overuse" explain higher rates among white patients? Ann Intern Med. 2001;135:328-37. [PMID: 11529696]
54. **Deyo RA, Nachemson A, Mirza SK.** Spinal-fusion surgery—the case for restraint. N Engl J Med. 2004;350:722-6. [PMID: 14960750]
55. **Deyo RA.** Cascade effects of medical technology. Annu Rev Public Health. 2002;23:23-44. [PMID: 11910053]
56. **Fischer MA, Avorn J.** Economic implications of evidence-based prescribing for hypertension: can better care cost less? JAMA. 2004;291:1850-6. [PMID: 15100203]
57. **Fisher ES, Wennberg DE, Stukel TA, Gottlieb DJ, Lucas FL, Pinder EL.** The implications of regional variations in Medicare spending. Part 1: the content, quality, and accessibility of care. Ann Intern Med. 2003;138:273-87. [PMID: 12585825]
58. **Fisher ES, Wennberg DE, Stukel TA, Gottlieb DJ, Lucas FL, Pinder EL.** The implications of regional variations in Medicare spending. Part 2: health outcomes and satisfaction with care. Ann Intern Med. 2003;138:288-98. [PMID: 12585826]
59. **Medicare Payment Advisory Commission.** Variation and Innovation in Medicare. June 2003. Accessed at www.medpac.gov/publications on 25 January 2005.
60. **Fisher ES.** Medical care—is more always better? [Editorial] N Engl J Med. 2003;349:1665-7. [PMID: 14573739]
61. **O'Connor AM, Llewellyn-Thomas HA, Floor AB.** Modifying unwarranted variations in health care: shared decision making using patient decision aids. Health Affairs. Web Exclusive. 7 October 2004. VAR-63-72. Accessed at http://content.healthaffairs.org/cgi/content/full/hlthaff.var.63/DC2 on 24 November 2004.
62. **O'Brien MK, Petrie K, Raeburn J.** Adherence to medication regimens: updating a complex medical issue. Med Care Rev. 1992;49:435-54. [PMID: 10123082]
63. **Heisler M, Bouknight RR, Hayward RA, Smith DM, Kerr EA.** The relative importance of physician communication, participatory decision making, and patient understanding in diabetes self-management. J Gen Intern Med. 2002;17: 243-52. [PMID: 11972720]
64. **Banta D.** The development of health technology assessment. Health Policy. 2003;63:121-32. [PMID: 12543525]

Section III

Cardiology

Aortic stenosis with special reference to angina pectoris and syncope.

Contratto AW, Levine SA. Ann Intern Med. 1937;10:1636-1653.

In the 19th century, use of the stethoscope dominated the cardiac examination, and systolic murmurs were of great interest and debate. New technology introduced at the beginning of the 20th century—chest radiography, cardiac fluoroscopy, and electrocardiography—marked a turning point that would advance cardiovascular diagnosis. Samuel A. Levine, a master clinician with a special interest in auscultation, was a central figure in this time of transition. Levine brought his passion for collection and analysis of clinical data to the task of clarifying diagnostic precision. In this 1937 article, Contratto and Levine discuss the clinical features of 180 patients with a definite diagnosis of aortic stenosis based on three criteria: a systolic thrill at the base of the heart, calcification of the aortic valve on fluoroscopy, and postmortem findings. Thirty-two percent of the patients had a history of rheumatic fever or chorea. Forty-one patients described "definite" angina pectoris, 21 had syncope, and 16 had with significant dizziness. The most diagnostic finding was a basal grade 3 or louder systolic murmur and thrill. The aortic second sound was generally diminished or absent, and a plateau arterial pulse was characteristic. Of 32 patients who had cardiac fluoroscopy, 26 had calcification of the aortic valve; Contratto and Levine considered this finding to be the most accurate single indicator of aortic stenosis. Electrocardiographic studies demonstrated bundle-branch block in 14 patients and atrioventricular block in 3. In general, the patients had a long natural history before the onset of symptoms or complications. Among 95 documented deaths, 44 were due to congestive heart failure, 15 to subacute bacterial endocarditis, and 15 to sudden unexpected death; the average age at death among these patients was 51 years, 36 years, and 45 years, respectively.

Contratto and Levine's study improved precision in the clinical diagnosis and understanding of the natural history of aortic valvular stenosis in an era when catheterization and surgery were not yet available. They emphasized the significance of angina pectoris, syncope, and sudden death, and their use of technology marked a sea change in cardiac diagnosis, with routine use of chest radiography to determine cardiomegaly and fluoroscopy to detect aortic valvular calcification. Electrocardiographic evidence of bundle-branch block and atrioventricular block raised new questions about significance of signs, mechanisms, and pathogenesis. The study stands out as a prototype for reporting the presentation of specific cardiovascular entities and is a transition piece in the diagnosis and understanding of aortic valvular cardiac disease.

Since then, the patient history has remained the most important determinant of the timing of surgery; survival rates plummet when congestive heart failure, syncope, and angina are present. An abnormal carotid pulse, grade 4 or greater systolic murmur, and diminished second heart sound are closely correlated with peak systolic gradients of 75 mm or more and aortic valve areas less than 1.0 cm^2. Rheumatic fever is a rare cause of aortic stenosis in industrialized countries; the usual cause is a calcified tricuspid or bicuspid valve. Recent pathogenic studies implicate an underlying atherosclerotic process, driven by the usual risk factors.

Studies on experimental hypertension. V. The pathogenesis of experimental hypertension due to renal ischemia.

Goldblatt H. Ann Intern Med. 1937;11:69-103.

In 1836, Richard Bright in London observed an association between kidney disease and cardiac hypertrophy. By 1898, Robert Tigerstedt at the Karolinska Institute had discovered a pressor compound in the rabbit renal vein that increased blood pressure when injected. He called this substance "renin" and conjectured that cardiac hypertrophy occurred in response to this vasoactive substance. Studies to determine a renal origin of essential hypertension followed but were unsuccessful until 1934, when Harry Goldblatt, a pathologist at Case Western Reserve University in Cleveland, masterminded the solution. Goldblatt postulated that essential hypertension was due to renal ischemia: "If the arteriolar disease of the kidney be responsible for the origin of hypertension then the more likely mechanism of its action is persistent reduction of blood flow to the functioning elements of this organ." Using a silver clip, he found that partial, bilateral constriction of the main renal arteries—the Goldblatt technique—produced a significant rise in blood pressure that abated after the clip was removed. The more severe the constriction, the greater the renal ischemia. An "effective substance" (not further elucidated) was found in the renal vein, and additional evidence indicated that the adrenal cortex played a role. In 1937, *Annals of Internal Medicine* published Goldblatt's carefully analyzed review of his evidence and all previous work stating his conclusions and showing why essential hypertension could not be due to a nervous reflex, constriction of the splenic or femoral vessels, bilateral nephrectomy, or occlusion of the renal veins. Subsequent studies led by Bernardo Houssay in Buenos Aires and Irvine Page in Indianapolis (1937–1941) revealed that Goldblatt's "effective substance" functioned indirectly as a proteolytic enzyme, which was finally called "rennin."

The renin–angiotensin–aldosterone system (RAS), as it became known in 1960, begins with the juxtaglomerular apparatus of the kidney releasing renin in response to a decrease in blood pressure, sodium, or blood volume. Renin, acting on angiotensinogen formed in the liver, cleaves it to produce angiotensin I. Angiotensin-converting enzyme (ACE) then processes angiotensin I to form angiotensin II, a potent, direct vasopressor which also stimulates aldosterone secretion to retain salt and water. The net effect is to elevate blood pressure; renin production is then suppressed. Many organs have since been shown to have their own RAS system that maintains their homeostasis.

Because hypertension is found in 26% of adults globally and is a leading cause of stroke, myocardial infarction, and kidney failure, its control is a major concern. Surprisingly, despite the central importance of the RAS feedback loop in blood pressure control, only 20% of hypertensive patients have elevated renin levels; 30% have low renin levels, and 50% have normal levels. Nevertheless, ACE inhibitors and angiotensin-receptor blockers have become first-line treatments for hypertension and heart failure.

Factors of risk in the development of coronary heart disease—six-year follow-up experience. The Framingham Study.

Kannel WB, Dawber TR, Kagan A, Revotskie N, Stokes J 3rd.
Ann Intern Med. 1961;55:33-50.

The Framingham Heart Study, a longitudinal study of 5209 men and women 30 to 62 years of age living in Framingham, Massachusetts, was initiated in 1948 by the National Heart, Lung, and Blood Institute. The purpose of the study was to check whether certain risk factors—blood pressure, cholesterol levels, and the electrocardiographic pattern of left ventricular hypertrophy—influenced the "proneness to the development of [coronary heart disease] CHD." In 1961, the group reported their 6-year experience in *Annals of Internal Medicine*. Key findings from this landmark study, which has been ongoing for more than 58 years and is internationally recognized as one of the most important epidemiologic studies of the 20th century, include the following: At least one risk factor was present in 40% of the study group; CHD (angina pectoris, infarction, sudden death) manifested differently in men and women; silent infarction and sudden death occurred without prior symptoms; a previously recognized influence of hypertension and higher cholesterol levels was confirmed; left ventricular hypertrophy was associated with CHD; multiple risk factors augmented the consequences; and the incidence of CHD was strikingly low when no risk factors were present.

The Framingham investigators have since issued more than 1200 reports that have greatly influenced our understanding of CHD. They have shown the importance of both systolic and diastolic hypertension, high levels of low-density lipoprotein, low levels of high-density lipoprotein, cigarette smoking, diabetes, obesity, psychosocial factors, menopause, and physical inactivity. The Framingham Offspring Study, begun in 1972, has shown the influence of heritable risk factors.

Since the 1961 report, the basic concept of atherosclerosis has changed dramatically. Instead of a primary role played by lipids imbibed by the arterial wall, the fundamental theory is that an inflammatory disorder interferes with endothelial homeostasis. The various risk factors drive the process beginning early in life; nevertheless, high cholesterol levels remain a basic requirement.

The Framingham investigators cautiously commented, "Whether or not the correction of these abnormalities once they are discovered will favorably alter the risk of development of disease, while reasonable to contemplate and perhaps attempt, remains to be demonstrated." Since the 1960s, the age-adjusted death rate from cardiovascular disease has decreased by 60% in the United States, and life expectancy has increased by 5 years. A recent analysis has attributed 44% of the decline in coronary mortality to risk factor reduction.

AN ARTICLE CONTRIBUTED TO AN ANNIVERSARY VOLUME IN HONOR OF DOCTOR JOSEPH HERSEY PRATT

AORTIC STENOSIS WITH SPECIAL REFERENCE TO ANGINA PECTORIS AND SYNCOPE *

By A. W. Contratto, M.D., and Samuel A. Levine, M.D., F.A.C.P.,
Boston, Massachusetts

Introduction

The accuracy of diagnosis, the interpretation of physical findings and the etiology, frequency and symptomatology of aortic stenosis have been matters of considerable controversy in recent years. About 30 years ago the diagnosis was often made on the basis of a systolic murmur over the aortic area without any other confirmatory evidence. It became particularly clear during the great war that this was entirely insufficient evidence to warrant the diagnosis, when in some army camps and in the hands of some boards that were examining recruits, large numbers of cases of aortic stenosis were being reported. Such cases were subsequently regarded as having neuro-circulatory asthenia, showing a basal systolic murmur frequently found in this condition. The result of this experience led to the view that still prevails in the minds of many, that aortic stenosis is rare. It will be clear from this study that the pendulum has swung much too far in this direction, and that many clinical aspects of aortic stenosis need reconsideration and reappraisal. Certainly it can be stated at the outset that aortic stenosis is a fairly common lesion, and that basal systolic murmurs cannot be dismissed lightly.

The purpose of this study is to review some of the clinical features of aortic stenosis that might help in diagnosis, and especially to discuss two complications to which attention has recently been called, i.e. the occurrence of syncope and angina pectoris.

Although there are numerous isolated references to aortic stenosis in the older literature briefly reviewed by Marvin [1] and Margolies,[2] it is only in the last decade that the importance of this lesion has been stressed. Cabot [3] in 1926 reported 28 autopsied cases. He called attention to the greater frequency of aortic stenosis in the male sex, the absence of evidence of aortic regurgitation in approximately half of the cases, and the occurrence of the disease predominantly in individuals past 40 years of age. Willius [4] studied 96 cases, and stressed the fact that anginal pain was a common occurrence in 21 per cent of his cases. Forty-six per cent also gave a clear cut history of rheumatic fever. Margolies [2] emphasized the frequency of calcification of the valve in aortic stenosis but regarded the process in the most part as

* Received for publication March 17, 1937.
From the medical clinic of the Peter Bent Brigham Hospital, Boston.

sclerotic in nature. Christian[5] reported 57 cases that came to autopsy, 21 of which had calcification of the aortic valve. He also predicted that the calcification could be visualized by the roentgen-ray. McGinn and White[6] reviewed 123 cases of aortic stenosis that came to autopsy and 113 that were examined clinically. Only one-third of the cases that came to autopsy were accurately diagnosed during life. A definite history of rheumatic fever was obtained in 23 per cent of the autopsied group and 46 per cent of the clinical series. Faintness, dizziness or actual syncope were fairly common complaints, occurring in 22 per cent of the cases. Nineteen per cent had angina pectoris. Nine of the patients in their series died suddenly.

Marvin and Sullivan[1] reported 11 cases of aortic stenosis that died suddenly and presented the view that syncope and sudden death in cases of aortic stenosis may be due to a hypersensitive carotid sinus. Boas[7] discussed 19 cases, four of which had angina pectoris, and believed that the angina pectoris was due to the narrowing of the aortic valve. LaPlace[8] reported a series of cases of aortic valve disease and found that the degree of aortic regurgitation as measured by the diastolic pressure had no relationship to the presence of angina pectoris.

Material in This Study

In the selection of material for this review only those cases were included that could be regarded as having definite evidence of aortic stenosis. The three main criteria were the presence of a systolic thrill at the base of the heart, the detection of calcification in the aortic valve on fluoroscopic examination and the postmortem findings. All cases that had definite evidence of organic involvement of the mitral valve were excluded in order to study the features of aortic stenosis per se, eliminating any complicating events that the presence of mitral valve disease might entail. For this purpose all the clinical and pathological data in the records of the Peter Bent Brigham Hospital, from the year 1913 to 1935 inclusive, were analyzed together with the cases seen by one of us in private consultation practice. This comprised a group of 180 definite cases of aortic stenosis.

Etiological Considerations

It has been and still is often difficult to establish a conclusive relationship between an early rheumatic infection and a subsequent valvular lesion. There is no indisputable and constant pathological finding which determines the rheumatic nature of any cardiac abnormality. The presence of Aschoff nodules in the heart, although very distinctive, is often wanting, even when there is every reason to believe that the lesion is rheumatic. An early rheumatic infection may have taken on one of the many bizarre forms so that the proper diagnosis never was made. Even when the correct diagnosis was made the patient and his family may not have been informed of it. When a great many years elapse, as often happens, before cardiac embarrassment develops, the early diagnosis may readily be forgotten. Finally a positive past history of a rheumatic infection and the presence of a valve lesion is not necessarily proof that the former is the cause of the latter. One is therefore left with opinions rather than with proof.

If specific diseases from a clinical point of view are rarely if ever associated with the subsequent development of stenosis of the aortic valve, it is reasonable to eliminate them entirely from our discussion of causation. In this group may be included pneumonia, typhoid fever, syphilis, and many other specific infections. It may be mentioned at this point that we did not find a single instance in which aortic stenosis could have been due to syphilis, notwithstanding the great frequency with which this disease produces aortic insufficiency and aortitis. It is not certain, however, how often nonspecific infections of a mild degree such as the "common cold," influenza or sore throat were the etiological cause of cases included in this study.

The great frequency of calcification of the aortic cusps naturally led to the belief in the past that in many instances it was purely arteriosclerotic. This opinion seemed to be further validated, in many instances, by the absence of any previous history of rheumatism or of any other significant infections. In refutation one might offer the evidence that is found in the mitral valve. Here stenosis occurs and is frequently accompanied by marked calcification, even in comparatively young people in whom very few would deny the rheumatic etiology. This often occurs when there is no available history of previous rheumatism. In fact it is a common experience to find calcification developing in any old and prolonged inflammatory process like tuberculosis, syphilis, parasitic cysts and other conditions. From the above considerations it follows that a particular lesion of the heart may be regarded as rheumatic in origin if an early history of rheumatic fever, chorea, or other stigmata of rheumatic disease are present in a large percentage of the cases, and if there is no other predominating etiological cause. It is well to recall that in a large series of cases of mitral stenosis, which all regard as almost invariably due to rheumatism, a history of this early infection can only be obtained in slightly more than 50 per cent of the cases. If a similar incidence can be found in relation to any other valve lesion it is equally logical to assume that rheumatic fever is the etiological factor.

In this series of 180 cases there was a definite history of rheumatic fever or chorea in 57 instances (31.7 per cent). The figures for the two sexes were approximately the same. The interval between the first rheumatic infection and the time these patients were first examined averaged 23.3 years for the females and 28.9 years for the males. The extremes were quite wide, from a few years to 60 years. This is considerably longer than similar figures would be for cases of mitral stenosis. In addition there were 23 in which the history was questionable. By this is meant that there was a history of previous "rheumatism," sciatica, growing pains, nosebleeds, etc., or that a heart murmur developed after an early acute infection. If these are included the total incidence would be 44.4 per cent. This corresponds fairly closely to the observations of Willius [4] who found a history of rheumatic fever in 46 per cent of 96 cases of aortic stenosis. It is a somewhat lower figure than the 50 per cent that is generally found in cases of mitral stenosis. The difference in the two groups can readily be explained by the fact that aortic cases when detected are on the average 10 years older than those with mitral disease, the latter coming to a physician earlier in their course because of troublesome symptoms of congestive failure. The result is that the aortic cases have more frequently forgotten their early infections or these infections have occurred in an era when rheumatic fever was not so well understood.

From the above discussion it would seem logical to conclude that rheumatic fever is the most frequent and most important cause of aortic stenosis. Furthermore, we are of the opinion that arteriosclerosis and calcification are secondary manifestations superimposed on lesions due to rheumatic fever or to some other early nonspecific apparently mild infection.

Age and Sex

The age distribution in this group of 180 cases of pure aortic stenosis ranged from 13 to 81 years, with an average of 52.5 years. There were 108 males and 72 females, i.e. 60 per cent and 40 per cent respectively. The average age of the males was 53.6 years and of the females 51.4 years. There was no significant difference in the distribution of the two sexes in the various decades (figure 1) although the largest number occurred in

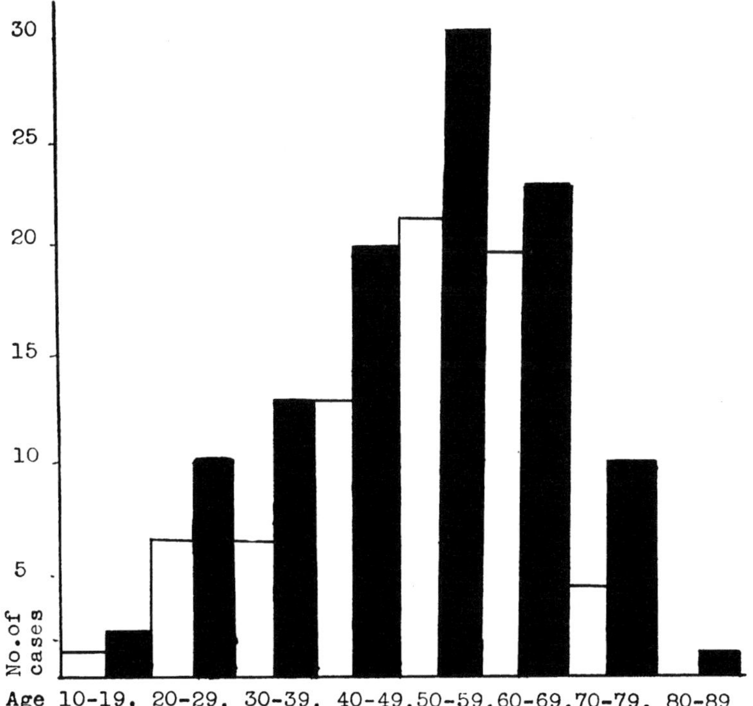

Fig. 1. Number of cases of aortic stenosis in various decades. ■ males; □ females.

the sixth decade. The incidence in the fifth and seventh decades was considerable. The number of females in this series was considerably greater than that reported by Margolies [2] or Willius,[4] but more closely approximated that given by McGinn and White.[6] The preponderance of males may possibly be explained by the greater frequency of chorea as the rheumatic manifestation in the female sex and by the fact that chorea rarely is responsible for subsequent aortic involvement.

Blood Pressure Considerations

The average blood pressure of 147 cases of aortic stenosis, in which readings were available, was 145 mm. of mercury systolic and 84 mm. diastolic. The range varied from a highest systolic reading of 260 mm. and a highest diastolic of 156 mm., to a lowest systolic of 80 mm. and a lowest diastolic of 10 mm. That hypertension was common is shown by the fact that there were 17 with systolic readings over 200 mm. and 22 with a diastolic over 110 mm. The average pressures for the 85 males was 138 mm. systolic and 79 mm. diastolic; that of the 62 females was 153 mm. systolic and 81 mm. diastolic (figures 2 and 3). This tendency for the females to have a higher blood pressure is in accord with findings obtained in a comparative study of the two sexes in relation to other forms of heart disease, such as mitral stenosis or angina pectoris.

There are two factors in addition to the stenosis of the aortic valve, which have some bearing on the blood pressure level. Insofar as there might be an accompanying aortic insufficiency there will be a tendency for the systolic pressure to be somewhat elevated and the diastolic to be depressed. Such effects are commonly observed in pure aortic insufficiency. The other factor is the one generally called essential hypertension, or that associated with an aging process. This will tend to show higher pressure readings in the older group. The common occurrence of hypertension in many types of cardiac disease makes one suspect that the intrinsic lesions of the heart may in some reflex fashion be partly responsible for hypertension. Another possibility is that the original etiological factor, namely rheumatic infection, may not only have been the cause of the valvular lesion but also may have produced changes in the peripheral vessels which eventually led to hypertension. The study of individual cases of aortic stenosis gives one the impression that when no other mechanisms are involved the systolic pressure is likely to be low and the diastolic slightly elevated, resulting in a small pulse pressure. Notwithstanding this, all ranges of systolic and diastolic levels from very low to very high may occur.

Physical Findings

Among the physical findings in cases of aortic stenosis there are some that are more peculiarly diagnostic of the anatomical lesion, and there are others less characteristic because of their common occurrence in a variety of other conditions. A systolic thrill in the aortic area, roentgen-ray evi-

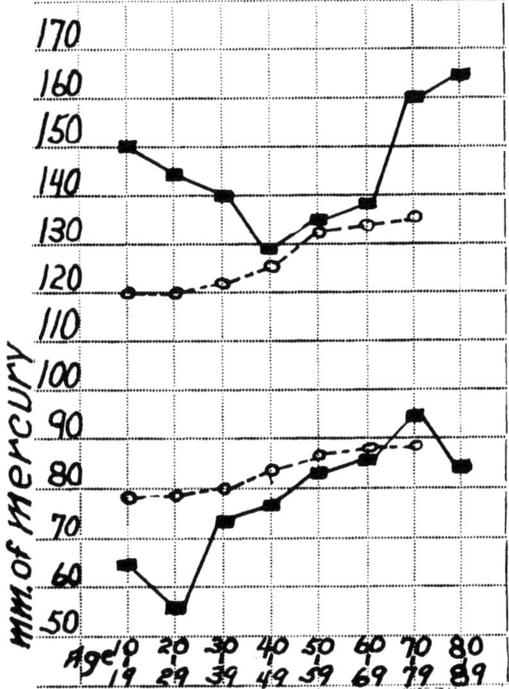

FIG. 2. Average blood pressure readings of cases of aortic stenosis (solid squares), as compared to normal individuals (circles). Male group.

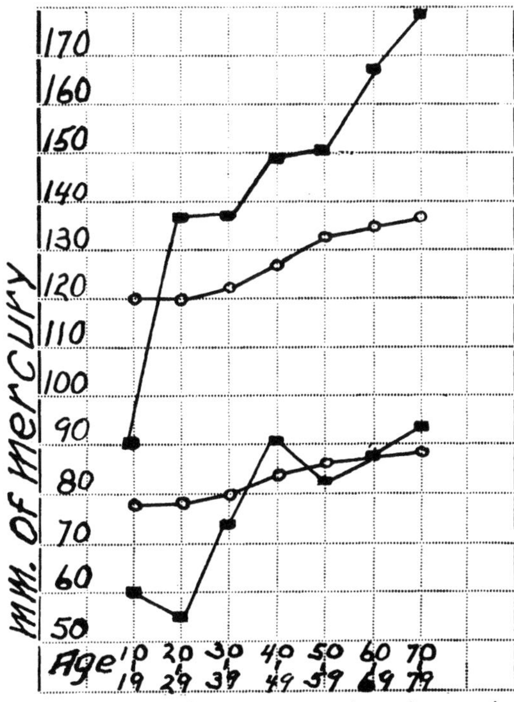

FIG. 3. Average blood pressure readings of cases of aortic stenosis (solid squares), as compared to normal individuals (circles). Female group.

dence of calcification of the aortic valve, a loud systolic murmur at the aortic area and a plateau pulse belong to the former group. Cardiac enlargement and an apical systolic murmur belong to the latter.

Cardiac hypertrophy is practically invariable in well marked aortic stenosis. In most cases this can be readily made out on physical examination, although during the early stages the percussion outlines do not always extend very much beyond normal limits. Marked dilation of the chambers such as occurs in mitral stenosis is not present as a rule, and therefore the cardiac silhouette is likely to be smaller, although the heart weight is greater in aortic stenosis than in mitral stenosis. In a previous study [9] it was found that the average weight of the heart in cases of aortic stenosis was 669 grams while in cases of mitral stenosis it was 474 grams. The great difference is due to the marked hypertrophy of the left ventricle of the former. When the left border of dullness does not extend much beyond the nipple line the finding of a forceful apical impulse will often indicate that there is considerable hypertrophy of the left ventricle. This type of impulse, which lifts the finger slowly and remains lifted for an instant before it recedes, is quite unlike the short snapping impulse that is found in mitral stenosis.

An apical systolic murmur is a quite common finding but one that is difficult to appraise. It can be partly due to a transmission of a loud basal bruit, and to some extent it may result from an accompanying mitral insufficiency, either relative or structural in nature. Its presence or absence does not aid in establishing or eliminating the diagnosis of aortic stenosis.

The most constant physical finding is a loud basal systolic murmur best heard at the second right interspace, or over the midsternum. This murmur is often harsh in quality but we feel that its intensity is of greater importance than its quality. In fact one may say that faint murmurs are rarely harsh. When the loudness of murmurs was graded from I to VI [10] as was done in many of the cases studied here, with rare exceptions the basal bruit was found to be of grade III intensity or louder. Often the apical murmur was just as loud as the basal and occasionally it was louder. There are other conditions in which loud systolic murmurs are heard at the base of the heart such as hypertension, congenital heart disease, anemia and hyperthyroidism. If these can be eliminated from consideration a loud aortic systolic murmur must always bring up the possibility of aortic stenosis. The direction of propagation of this murmur has been of no great aid in diagnosis. When loud it often could be heard throughout the chest, even in the right axilla. The importance of its transmission to the vessels of the neck has been exaggerated for this is due mainly to its intensity and to the proximity of its point of origin. There are occasional instances when the state of the circulation is so feeble that the murmur is quite faint and may only regain its loud and more characteristic intensity when the heart improves. It is in such cases particularly that roentgen-ray examination may be very valuable.

A blowing diastolic murmur heard in the second right interspace or along the left sternal border is a common, but by no means invariable finding in aortic stenosis. Stenosis of either the aortic or mitral valve frequently occurs without any auscultatory evidence of regurgitation. There are many instances of well marked mitral stenosis that show no systolic murmur whatever, and likewise many cases of aortic stenosis that have no diastolic murmur. In fact, of these 180 cases there were 87 in which no diastolic murmur was heard. To be sure this group excluded all cases with free aortic insufficiency, for this study was confined to well marked stenosis of the valve. In trying to elicit the aortic diastolic murmur, the fainter ones may be overlooked unless auscultation is carried out carefully, both in the recumbent and upright positions and during held expiration.

The most diagnostic physical finding is a systolic thrill. This is generally best felt at the aortic area but is occasionally present over the upper or midsternum and rarely to the left of the manubrium. A systolic impact must not be confused with a true purr that has duration, for when the latter is really felt and congenital heart disease can be ruled out a diagnosis of aortic stenosis is almost certain. There will be very rare exceptions when a loud basal systolic murmur and a definite systolic thrill will be found and yet stenosis will be absent. The explanation of such findings is still obscure. The difficulty is that in less than one half of the cases will a thrill be palpable.

In only 21 of the 51 instances in this series that came to autopsy was a thrill found. Possibly in some, more careful palpation might have been more successful. In others terminal cardiac weakness may have been the cause of the absence of this sign. The thrill is often overlooked because palpation is not carried out or because when a thrill is faint it may be detectable only in certain positions. It may be necessary to have the patient sit up or lean forward or even hold a deep expiration while the base of the heart is palpated.

No careful analysis was made of the frequency of an absent aortic second sound, or the reliability of this sign in the diagnosis of aortic stenosis. We are certain, however, that in some of the cases a clear second sound was heard in the second right interspace, although in many it was either diminished or absent. In according importance to the character of the second sounds at the base one should remember that the sound heard over the aortic or the pulmonary area is not necessarily made by the corresponding valve. In some obvious cases of hypertension the second sound is louder over the pulmonary than over the aortic area, although aortic pressure is considerably higher than pulmonary pressure. Likewise in some cases of aortic stenosis a second sound heard to the right of the manubrium may be partly a transmission from the pulmonary snap. In general it may therefore be said that the aortic second sound in these cases occasionally is present, though generally diminished or absent.

A plateau form of peripheral pulse has long been regarded as a characteristic of aortic stenosis. The frequency with which this peculiarity of the pulse is observed is diminished by the difficulty of its recognition and also by the fact that its typical form is commonly altered in the presence of an accompanying aortic insufficiency or hypertension. However, there are instances in which careful attention to the quality of the radial pulse may supply valuable supportive evidence.

A peculiarity of the pulse less generally appreciated is that the rate not infrequently is slow. This was quite well known to the clinicians of former times for Fothergill [11] in discussing aortic obstruction states, "the pulse is usually slow and steady." There are very few conditions apart from aortic stenosis in which the rate of the heart may be so slow in the presence of severe congestive heart failure, and where the slowing cannot be accounted for by a digitalis effect or heart block. This peculiarity on several occasions has been the first clue in reaching the correct diagnosis. The rhythm of the heart, unlike that observed in mitral stenosis, is generally regular. Of the 180 instances in this study auricular fibrillation was present in only 11 cases. Four of these were examined post mortem and none showed mitral stenosis. Factors such as age, sex, blood pressure and previous rheumatic infection were no different in the fibrillators than in those with regular rhythm.

Electrocardiographic Observations

In 82 cases electrocardiographic studies were made. Our findings concerning conduction disturbances were similar to those recently reported.[7] There were 14 instances of defective intraventricular conduction, including seven with typical bundle branch block. Three of the above 14 showed appreciable delay in the P–R interval and one had complete heart block. There were two additional cases of complete heart block. Conduction defects seemed to be more common in the cases of aortic stenosis that had angina pectoris than in those that did not have this complication. Eleven of the 82 cases had auricular fibrillation. Some of the others had extrasystoles of ventricular or nodal origin. It is significant that we did not have a single instance of right axis deviation in the entire series. If such a change in the electrical axis is found in aortic stenosis it should lead one to suspect an additional mitral stenosis. The main conclusion from the electrocardiographic studies is that defects in conduction are commonly associated with aortic stenosis.

Roentgen-Ray Findings and Calcification of the Aortic Valve

In the past there have been no distinctive roentgen-ray findings that characterized aortic stenosis. The boot shaped heart denoting a hypertrophied left ventricle, although common in aortic stenosis is also frequently present in pure aortic insufficiency and in some cases of hypertensive heart disease with left ventricular hypertrophy. Recently, however, the detection of calcification in the aortic valve by fluoroscopic examination [12] has been of tremendous diagnostic value. This has invariably been indicative of a significant degree of stenosis of the valve. Inasmuch as this technic has been developed in the past several years, only 32 of the more recent cases of this series were fluoroscoped. Among these there were 26 instances in which this examination positively identified calcification of the aortic valve. Two of the remaining six were examined post mortem; one showed calcification, the other did not. It is evident that aortic stenosis may be present for a long period of time before calcification occurs in the leaflets. Such cases will necessarily be negative on fluoroscopy, and others may be missed because of the thickness of the chest wall or the faintness of the shadow. It also follows that calcification will be found more readily in the long standing cases. This is well borne out by the following figures. The average age of the group showing calcification was 60.3 years while that of the negative group was 42.6 years. The youngest of the positive cases was 45 years old, although younger individuals not included in this study have shown calcification of the valves by roentgen-ray. The value of roentgenographic examination is readily appreciated by the fact that in one half of the 26 cases, no aortic systolic thrill could be felt. In some of these the roentgen-ray was the only means of establishing the diagnosis. At present it may be stated that the roentgenological finding of calcification of the aortic valve is the most accurate single evidence of aortic stenosis, but that calcification may not be detectable during the early years of the production of this lesion.

The Occurrence of Angina Pectoris

Little mention was made in the older writings concerning the association of angina pectoris with aortic stenosis. Mackenzie [13] stated that, "there may be symptoms of angina pectoris but these are due to associated changes in the heart muscle." Recently more attention has been paid to this relationship.[6, 7, 14] The more recent teaching has been that although angina pectoris is commonly associated with aortic valvular disease it is due to insufficiency of the valve rather than to stenosis. The explanation that is offered for this association is that coronary flow takes place during diastole and that with the low diastolic pressure that accompanies aortic insufficiency there is inadequate flow through the coronary system with resultant relative myocardial anoxemia. This explanation is open to some doubt for there are those who believe that the main flow through the heart occurs during systole.[15] Apart from the theoretical controversy there are certain clinical experiences which make one doubt the accepted importance of aortic regurgitation in the production of anginal pain.

Free aortic insufficiency, syphilitic in origin, is rarely associated with angina except in those cases in which the coronary orifices are narrowed. Furthermore, as will be seen from the following data, angina occurs quite commonly in aortic stenosis without any clinical evidence of insufficiency of the valve. The following explanation was kindly suggested to us by Dr. Tinsley R. Harrison: " The two important points about angina and aortic stenosis seem to be (1) that there is no evidence of anything which can decrease the circulation to the heart in these cases and (2) that in such patients there is much less relationship of the pain to exercise than in ordinary coronary angina. As regards the first point, while in cases without aortic stenosis one almost always finds at autopsy either coronary arteriosclerosis, luetic narrowing of a coronary orifice, or a well marked aortic insufficiency with a low diastolic pressure during life (the latter producing angina by causing interference with the blood supply to the heart during diastole), in persons with aortic stenosis typical anginal seizures may occur in the absence of any of these factors, the aortic insufficiency either not being present at all or in many cases of such mild degree as to cause no lowering of the diastolic pressure. In such cases the pathological evidence does not point toward a diminution in coronary flow and the enlarged coronary arteries suggest that the flow during life was actually greater than normal. However, this does not mean that the mechanism of angina is any different in such cases from that occurring in other patients. The coronary flow has to be looked at not per se but from the standpoint of its relationship to the need for blood; the latter of course depends on the oxygen consumption of the heart, which in turn depends largely on the work done by the heart. The latter depends on three factors—the amount of blood expelled per unit of time, the pressure against which this blood is expelled, and the energy expended in imparting velocity to this blood. As regards the output of blood, the only case which we studied had a normal cardiac output. However, the pressure within the ventricle during systole is probably enormously increased and this of course tends to increase the cardiac work. Furthermore, while the velocity factor is, under certain conditions, a relatively small fraction of the cardiac work, it may become the greatest factor in aortic stenosis, where with a markedly narrowed orifice the rate of flow must be enormously greater during systole. It is possible and indeed quite likely that the velocity factor is more than 50 per cent of the cardiac work in a case of marked aortic stenosis. Therefore, even though the coronary flow increases, say three-fold, it is quite likely that the cardiac work may be increased four-fold, and this would of course tend to produce angina through the usual mechanism of myocardial anoxemia.

" As regards the second point; in the young patients with aortic stenosis we do not have pipe-stem coronaries but normal vessels which are capable of opening and closing. The attacks which come on at rest may very well be due to slight vasomotor changes in the caliber of the coronaries. Suppose that the arteries are wide open and are just able to transmit enough blood to prevent angina. Then even a very slight diminution in caliber could cause an attack. This is quite different from a normal person, where the arteries have large reserve and different from a person with extensive coronary sclerosis where one can't imagine any opening and closing of the pipe-stem vessels."

Another explanation depends on the likeness of the aorta and coronary system to the common water faucet suction pump. The water flowing through the larger orifice causes a suction on the smaller orifice which enters it at right angles. The amount of suction is somewhat dependent upon the velocity of flow through the larger orifice. It seems reasonable to assume that in the normal heart with "paper thin" aortic valves, during systole these leaflets are fairly close to the coronary ostia preventing any such suction action. In cases of aortic stenosis with rigid, calcified immovable aortic valves, and markedly increased velocity of the blood flow, it is possible that this suction action may even draw blood out of the coronary arteries and lead to relative myocardial ischemia.

It was significant but by no means surprising that as many as 41 of the 180 cases, or 22.7 per cent had definite angina pectoris. (There were 28 additional questionable cases.) Of these 41 cases 22 were male and 19 were female; the average age of the former was 49 years (youngest 13 and oldest 64) and of the latter 59 years (youngest 25 and oldest 74). There was one case in the second decade, two in the third, three in the fourth, seven in the fifth, and the remaining 28 in the later decades. The average blood pressures for the two sexes in these cases were 136 mm. systolic and 80 mm. diastolic in the males, and 154 mm. systolic and 85 mm. diastolic in the females. These figures were similar to the blood pressure readings of the cases of aortic stenosis in general, but somewhat lower than those found in angina pectoris, unassociated with aortic stenosis.[16] It follows that hypertension is not a factor in the causation of angina associated with aortic stenosis.

The frequent absence of aortic insufficiency in this group with angina pectoris is indicated by the fact that in 19 of the 41 instances, no diastolic murmur was heard. This signifies that not only is pure aortic stenosis a common occurrence but that a concomitant angina is frequently present without an accompanying regurgitation.

To further validate this point of view 31 consecutive cases of free aortic insufficiency were studied. Only four were found to have angina pectoris and they were all luetic. Very likely the coronary orifices were involved in these. The average age of the 31 cases was 41.6 years and nine of them were over 50 years of age. The blood pressure readings in this group were typical of free aortic insufficiency, the average readings being systolic 154 mm. and diastolic 32 mm. In 15 instances a definite past history of rheumatic fever was obtained but the lesion had not progressed to detectable clinical aortic stenosis. The comparative rarity of angina in these cases of aortic insufficiency is in striking contrast to its frequency when the aortic valve is stenosed.

Inasmuch as the diagnosis of angina pectoris can only be made by a proper appraisal of the symptoms and because the subjective complaints that lead to this diagnosis are often mild and may be over-shadowed by the more distressing breathlessness, the diagnosis is often overlooked. In many cases one has to initiate a direct inquiry into the possibility of any ill feeling in the chest on hurrying in the street, because the patient often will not spontaneously mention it. We feel that this type of careful questioning was responsible for the large number of cases of angina detected in this study. The importance of eliciting these symptoms lies in the fact that the frequency of angina throws some light on the prevalence of sudden unexpected death in aortic stenosis. Whenever the diagnosis of angina pectoris is correctly made one infers that that patient is subject to such a fatal outcome. It is interesting that of the 80 cases in which the type of death was known, nine dropped dead suddenly. In five of these nine cases a diagnosis of angina pectoris had already been made. We believe that in some of the others that died suddenly a diagnosis of angina pectoris could have been made if we had had the opportunity of inquiring carefully into the history.

One experience that we had bears directly on this point. A man of 50 entered the hospital complaining of increasing breathlessness. He showed the typical signs of aortic stenosis and marked congestive failure, and was studied most carefully by many physicians including ourselves. He improved on medical treatment and returned about one year later with recurrent failure. On this second admission a clear cut history was elicited by direct questioning of anginal distress, that antedated the first admission. It had been entirely overlooked by all members of the staff. After he had again recovered a fair degree of compensation and while feeling quite comfortable, he died instantly. If a proper history had not by chance been obtained he would have been classified in that vague group of cases of sudden death from aortic stenosis. Sudden death of this type can occur even in the very young who have aortic stenosis and angina pectoris, as was the case in a boy of 15 in whom both of these diagnoses were made, who dropped dead while going to school.

The duration of life in cases of aortic stenosis after the development of angina pectoris is not very different from what is found in ordinary angina. In the 19 patients of this present series who were known to have died, the duration of life after anginal pain first occurred was 3.3 years. Of 10 who were known to be still alive the duration was 5.5 years. The cases varied considerably and were too few in number to permit drawing any clear cut conclusions, but we have the general impression that the young rheumatic aortic case with anginal pain may carry on many years, although typical sudden fatality may occur at any time.

Syncope

The occurrence of syncope in aortic stenosis was lost sight of until a few years ago. This was recently discussed by McGinn and White [6] and in greater detail by Marvin and Sullivan.[1] Knowledge of the rôle that the carotid sinus may play in the production of syncope,[17] naturally led to the suspicion that this same mechanism might account for the dizziness and fainting attacks that occur in aortic stenosis. With this in mind an investigation was carried out to test the irritability of the carotid sinus in some of these cases. In 19 a test for carotid sinus irritability was performed on each side and in none were positive results obtained for syncope, or dizziness was not produced.* Among these were two with a clear cut history of syncopal attacks. From this it seems unlikely that carotid sinus irritability can be a common occurrence in aortic stenosis or that it will explain, in the majority of cases, either the dizziness and fainting, or the sudden death. The possible rôle of the carotid sinus cannot be dismissed entirely, however, and further investigation is necessary. It is possible that reflex inhibition of the heart from a sensitive carotid sinus may be the cause of sudden death in rare instances. A more likely cause of sudden death is the same mechanism that prevails in ordinary angina. This assumption is particularly applicable in those cases in which the diagnosis of angina pectoris can be made. One may even postulate that some of the others die suddenly in their first attack of angina.

An attempt was made to detect clinical features which were characteristic of cases showing syncope or dizziness. There were 21 instances of true syncope and an additional 16 had significant dizziness without syncope. The average age of those with true syncope was five years greater among the males and 10 years greater among the females than the general averages. Despite their more advanced years those with syncope tended to have a somewhat lower blood pressure. Although these two differences were not great they may have some bearing on the production of the cerebral symptoms since both age and lower blood pressure may predispose to cerebral anoxemia.

Type of Death

Ninety-five of 180 cases studied were known to have died. Of these 18 died of unknown cause, 44 died of congestive heart failure, 15 of subacute bacterial endocarditis, four of coronary thrombosis, two of cerebral accidents, two of pneumonia and one of Adams-Stokes disease. The remaining nine died suddenly and unexpectedly. There were some differences in age between these various groups. Although the average age at death of all the fatal cases was 51.3 years, the group with subacute bacterial endocarditis died at an average age of 36 years. Those that died suddenly had an average age of 45 years. The three most common types of death are congestive failure, subacute bacterial endocarditis and angina pectoris.

It is of some interest to analyze the duration of the more important subjective symptoms and objective findings in the group of fatal cases. Such an analysis gives one a guide as to the prognosis when particular

* Since this study was completed two cases of aortic stenosis were seen without any previous history of syncope or dizziness that showed definite positive reactions to carotid sinus stimulation.

features develop in the progress of the disease. Palpitation of the heart was an early complaint and the average duration of life after its onset was eight years. Dyspnea on the other hand came much later, as the average length of life after its first occurrence was only 23 months. The average period of survival after edema was 9.3 months and after appearance of syncope 9.1 months. Syncopal attacks that occurred early in life, 15 years or so before the patient was seen, were disregarded as they were considered to be unrelated to the disease. The duration of life after congestive râles were found in the lungs and definite pitting edema of the legs occurred was 6.3 and 4.3 months, respectively. In many of these cases the features just enumerated may have been present for some time before they were first noted, but in general it may be said that life expectancy is quite short once clear cut heart failure has developed.

Diagnostic Considerations

The more important diagnostic findings in aortic stenosis are a loud systolic murmur at the base of the heart, a basal systolic thrill, a plateau pulse and calcification of the aortic valve on fluoroscopic examination. The presence of a true thrill or calcification by roentgen-ray are quite reliable diagnostically. The other two features are not as trustworthy. This explains the difficulty in diagnosis and the fact that the majority of cases are overlooked. It is obvious that a fair degree of stenosis must exist for years before all the above criteria will be apparent. The early stages of the process must therefore be diagnosed on data that have been regarded in the past as inadequate. In a previous publication [10] attention has been called to the importance of interpreting the presence of a systolic murmur as a possible early sign of aortic stenosis. In fact it was found that during the early stages a moderately loud systolic murmur that eventually proves to be due to aortic stenosis could be somewhat louder at the apex of the heart or the mid-precordium than in the aortic area. Also some cases regarded as having benign or insignificant systolic murmurs eventually prove to have aortic stenosis. With this in mind an analysis was made of 16 cases seen by one of us over the course of years, that eventually proved to have definite aortic stenosis but that had previously been misdiagnosed. Four of these were thought to have had mitral insufficiency, four aortic insufficiency, one a normal heart with a benign systolic murmur, six hypertensive heart disease and one chronic myocarditis. In none of these was a systolic thrill present at first, but in all either a systolic thrill or calcification of aortic valve or both developed. In conclusion it may be emphasized that loud basal systolic murmurs, especially in the absence of hypertension, must lead one to suspect the presence of aortic stenosis and make one search all the more diligently for other more convincing evidence.

Postmortem Findings

The main pathological finding that was investigated in this group of cases was the condition of the coronary arteries. The question naturally arises whether angina pectoris which accompanies aortic stenosis is due to atheromatous changes in the coronary arteries similar to those seen in patients without aortic stenosis or to the valvular lesion itself. The frequent occurrence of pathological changes in the coronary system in older people makes it necessary to appraise this problem in the younger group.

There were nine cases in this study with angina pectoris that were examined post mortem. Six were over and three were under 50 years of age. Two of the older group, aged 71 and 66, merely showed minimal changes in the coronary arteries without any narrowing of the vessels or infarction of the heart muscle. One case, aged 52, showed moderate sclerosis with narrowing of the coronary arteries and no myocardial infarction. Another, aged 66, had marked sclerosis and narrowing of the vessels with several small old infarctions. There was one, aged 62, that showed typical coronary thrombosis with infarction of the ventricle. The last one of this group, aged 52, had syphilitic aortitis, almost completely occluding both coronary orifices. Two of the younger cases, aged 46 and 25, had perfectly normal coronary arteries and the third, aged 46, showed moderate coronary changes without narrowing of the vessels. None of the last three had any old or recent infarctions of the ventricle. The complete absence of any alterations in the coronary system in two of the younger cases and the occurrence of only minimal alteration in some of the others, we consider as adequate proof that the anginal attacks were due to some other cause. It is more logical to regard this other factor as the actual valvular lesion. How this burden may be conducive to anginal attacks has previously been discussed.

Another pathological finding of interest is the localization of the calcification to the aortic valve and the ring. The deposits did not extend up to the mouth of the coronary vessels, which were distinctly free and open. In fact many cases of aortic stenosis, even in the older group, were comparatively free of atheromatous changes in the wall of the aorta itself.

Summary

1. A study was made of 180 cases of aortic stenosis, unassociated with any other significant valve disease, 53 of which were examined post mortem.

2. Evidence was presented to indicate that the etiology in most instances was a previous rheumatic infection. It was thought that some early ill defined infections may have been the cause in a few cases.

3. It was found that although the male sex predominates, the ratio was not more than three to two. The largest number occurred in the sixth decade.

4. The average blood pressure of the males was 138 mm. of mercury systolic and 79 mm. diastolic, and for the females 153 mm. systolic and

81 mm. diastolic. The range of these readings, however, varied from very low to very high systolic and diastolic levels.

5. The most distinctive physical findings in aortic stenosis were a loud basal systolic murmur, a systolic thrill near the aortic area, and the detection of calcification of the valve on fluoroscopic examination. In about one half of the cases no aortic diastolic murmur was audible.

6. Disturbances in conduction such as bundle branch block and auriculo ventricular block were quite common.

7. Twenty-six of 32 cases that were examined showed calcification of the valve fluoroscopically.

8. Angina pectoris was found to be quite common, occurring in 22.7 per cent of the cases. There is reason to believe that many cases are overlooked because of inadequate histories. An explanation of the possible mechanism of angina in these cases, not dependent upon coronary sclerosis was suggested.

9. There were 21 instances of syncope in this series. In four of these and 15 other cases the sensitivity of the carotid sinus was tested and found normal. It was found that sudden death occurred particularly in those with an anginal history, and that the carotid sinus was an unlikely cause of such eventuality.

10. The three most common types of death were congestive heart failure, subacute bacterial endocarditis, and sudden death. Once major symptoms developed in this group the average life expectancy was short.

11. Although the finding of a basal systolic thrill or calcification on roentgen-ray examination are very reliable evidences of aortic stenosis, the diagnosis in many cases and especially during the early stages, will have to depend upon the intelligent appraisal of a moderately loud basal systolic murmur.

12. A study of the postmortem material showed that the calcification is limited to the valve and does not involve the coronary orifices. The finding of normal coronary vessels in two of the young patients who had angina, and the presence of only minimal atheroma in the vessels of some of the others that had angina strongly suggest that the deformity of the valve itself is in some way responsible for this complication.

BIBLIOGRAPHY

1. Marvin, H. M., and Sullivan, A. G.: Clinical observations upon syncope and sudden death in aortic stenosis, Am. Heart Jr., 1935, x, 705.
2. Margolies, H. M., Ziellessen, F. O., and Barnes, A. R.: Calcareous aortic valvular disease, Am. Heart Jr., 1930–31, vi, 349.
3. Cabot, R. C.: Facts on the heart, 1926, W. B. Saunders Company, Philadelphia.
4. Willius, T. A.: A clinical study of aortic stenosis, Proc. Staff Meet. Mayo Clinic, 1927, ii, 123.
5. Christian, H. A.: Aortic stenosis with calcification of the cusps, Jr. Am. Med. Assoc., 1931, xcvii, 158.

6. McGinn, S., and White, P. D.: Clinical observations in aortic stenosis, Am. Jr. Med. Sci., 1934, clxxxviii, 1.
7. Boas, E. P.: Aortic stenosis, angina pectoris and heart block as symptoms of calcareous stenosis, Am. Jr. Med. Sci., 1935, cxc, 376–383.
8. LaPlace, L. B.: Aortic valve diseases, relationship of angina pectoris, Am. Heart Jr., 1933, viii, 810–820.
9. Laws, C. H., and Levine, S. A.: Clinical notes on rheumatic heart disease with special reference to the cause of death, Am. Jr. Med. Sci., 1933, clxxxvi, 833.
10. Levine, S. A.: The systolic murmur; its clinical significance, Jr. Am. Med. Assoc., 1933, ci, 436–438.
11. Fothergill: The heart and its diseases, 1879, J. Millner, p. 162.
12. Sosman, M. C., and Wosika, P. H.: Calcification in aortic and mitral valves with a report of 23 cases, Am. Jr. Roent. and Radium Therapy, 1933, xxx, 3.
13. Mackenzie, J.: Diseases of the heart, Third edition, 1918, p. 339.
14. Levine, S. A.: Clinical heart disease, 1936, W. B. Saunders, Philadelphia.
15. Hochrein, M., and Keller, C. J.: Beiträge zur Blutzirkulation im klienen Kreislauf; über die Beeinflussung der mittleren Durchblutung der Lunge durch pharmakologische Mittel, Arch. f. exper. Path. u. Pharmak., 1932, clxiv, 529–564.
16. Eppinger, E. C., and Levine, S. A.: Angina pectoris, some clinical considerations with special reference to prognosis, Arch. Int. Med., 1934, liii, 120–130.
17. Weiss, S., and Baker, J. P.: The carotid sinus reflex in health and disease, Medicine, 1933, xii, 297.

STUDIES ON EXPERIMENTAL HYPERTENSION

V. THE PATHOGENESIS OF EXPERIMENTAL HYPERTENSION DUE TO RENAL ISCHEMIA *

By Harry Goldblatt, M.D., C.M., *Cleveland, Ohio*

The production of persistent hypertension in dogs and monkeys has been reported in previous communications.[1-4] This was accomplished by constricting the main renal arteries by means of a special silver clamp devised for the purpose. In some of the dogs hypertension of severe degree has now existed for more than five years. The type of hypertension produced by this method depends upon the degree of constriction of the renal arteries. When the constriction is not very great, there is little or no disturbance of renal function accompanying the hypertension and it resembles benign hypertension in man. When the constriction is very severe, there is often accompanying damage of renal function which may also be severe. Such animals may die in uremia so that in this respect the hypertension resembles malignant hypertension in man. Constriction of splenic and of femoral vessels had no effect on blood pressure.[2] This is in keeping with the negative results obtained by Longcope and McClintock [5] from constriction of the superior mesenteric artery. These findings have been confirmed for the dog by other investigators.[6-18] The present report deals with experiments designed to determine the mechanism whereby the reduction of blood flow to the functioning components of the kidney, that is, renal ischemia, induces the development of hypertension.

That some pathological change in the kidney may be the cause of some forms of cardiovascular disease in man has been suspected on the basis of clinical observations and pathological findings from the time of Bright.[19, 20] That a pathological change in the kidney may initiate hypertension in man, especially the type that is associated with so-called diffuse vascular disease, has been recognized by some investigators for more than 50 years, since the existence of hypertension was first recognized. This view is still upheld by some, like Fahr,[21] who, on teleological grounds, regards the hypertension as compensatory to the reduced blood flow through the kidney, and by Volhard,[22a, 22b] on the basis of a humoral mechanism of renal origin, for at least the so-called malignant type of hypertension. It is opposed by others, like Kylin,[23, 24] who does not admit a primary renal origin even for the hypertension that accompanies glomerulonephritis. The mechanism whereby the kidneys produce their effect is still regarded as unsolved even by those who

* Presented by invitation, before the American College of Physicians in St. Louis, Mo., April 20, 1937.
From the Institute of Pathology, Western Reserve University, Cleveland, Ohio.
These studies were supported by the Beaumont-Richman-Kohn Fund.

consider that these organs can play a primary part in the origin of hypertension.

Many experiments have been performed to determine whether the kidneys can be the primary site of origin of hypertension in animals.

A Summary of Other Experiments Designed to Determine the Possible Renal Origin of Hypertension

Bilateral nephrectomy.

Mosler,[25] (1912). Used rabbits. Insignificant elevation of blood pressure.

Backmann,[26] (1916). Used cats. No elevation of blood pressure.

Cash,[27] (1926). Used dogs. No elevation of blood pressure.

Hartwich,[28] (1930). Used dogs. No elevation of blood pressure.

Harrison, Blalock and Mason,[11] (1936). Used dogs. No elevation of blood pressure in 16 out of 18 dogs.

Reduction of the amount of functioning renal tissue.

Grawitz and Israel,[29] (1879). Used rabbits. Slight hypertrophy of heart, interpreted by the authors as due to hypertension.

Pässler and Heineke,[30] (1905). Used dogs. Slight elevation of blood pressure.

Backmann,[26] (1916). Used cats. Slight elevation of blood pressure.

Allen and collaborators,[31, 32, 33] (1923). Used dogs. Slight temporary elevation of blood pressure.

Mark,[41a, 41b] (1925, 1928). Used dogs. Slight elevation of blood pressure.

Anderson,[34] (1926). Used rabbits. No elevation of blood pressure.

Friedman and Wachsmuth,[35] (1930). Used dogs. No elevation of blood pressure.

Chanutin and Ferris,[36] (1932). Used rats. Great elevation of blood pressure.

Rytand, D. A. and Dock, W.,[37] (1935). Used rats. Great elevation of blood pressure.

Reduction of amount of renal substance by coagulation necrosis due to ligation of branches of renal arteries.

Janeway,[38, 39] (1908), assisted by Carrel.[40] Used dogs. Slight elevation of blood pressure.

Mark,[41b] (1928). Used dogs. No elevation of blood pressure.

Reduction of amount of renal substance by partial renal excision and unilateral nephrectomy combined with coagulation necrosis of part of the remaining kidney by ligation of branches of renal artery.

Cash,[42] (1924). Used dogs. Slight to moderate temporary elevation of blood pressure.

Mark and Giesendorfer,[43] (1930). Used dogs. Moderate temporary elevation of blood pressure.

Ferris and Heynes,[44] (1931). Used dogs. Slight temporary elevation of blood pressure.

Destruction of renal substance by irradiation of kidneys with roentgen-rays.

Hartman, Bolliger and Doub,[45] (1929). Used dogs. Moderate elevation of blood pressure.

Page,[6] (1935). Used dogs. Moderate elevation of blood pressure.

Renal infarction due to multiple emboli.

Senator,[46] (1911). Used cats. Injected liquid paraffin into renal arteries. No rise of blood pressure.

Cash,[42] (1924). Used dogs. Injected insoluble Berlin blue. No elevation of blood pressure.

Apfelbach and Jensen,[47] (1931). Used dogs. Injected particles of charcoal into renal arteries. No elevation of blood pressure.

Occlusion of one main renal artery or its branches.

Friedman and Wachsmuth,[35] (1930). Used dogs. Slight temporary elevation of blood pressure.

Occlusion of both main renal arteries.

Katzenstein,[48] (1905). Used rabbits and dogs. No rise of blood pressure.

Cash,[27] (1926). Used dogs. Moderate to severe elevation of blood pressure.

Occlusion (permanent or temporary) of renal arteries, veins and ureters.

Cash,[27] (1926). Permanent occlusion. Used dogs. No elevation of blood pressure.

Loesch,[49] (1933). Intermittent brief occlusion, every 2 or 3 days. Used dogs. Moderate persistent elevation of blood pressure.

Passive hyperemia (constriction of renal vein) of one kidney.

Pedersen,[50] (1927), and Bell and Pedersen,[51] (1930). Used dogs. Moderate temporary elevation of blood pressure.

Menendez,[52] (1933). Used dogs. Slight temporary elevation of blood pressure in some; none in others.

Compression of kidneys by oncometer.

Alwens,[53] (1909). Used cats. Acute experiments. Slight elevation of blood pressure.

Permanent obstruction of ureters.

Hartwich,[28] (1930). Used dogs. Moderate elevation of blood pressure.

Harrison, Mason, Resnik and Rainey,[54] (1936). Used dogs. Moderate elevation of blood pressure.

Temporary obstruction of one ureter followed by release of obstruction and excision of other kidney.

Rautenberg,[55] (1912). Used rabbits. Moderate elevation of blood pressure.

Effect of nephrotoxic substances.

Dominguez,[56] (1928). Used rabbits. Injected uranium salts. Nc elevation of blood pressure except in one animal that developed severe arterial and arteriolar sclerosis, especially in the kidneys.

Arnott and Kellar,[57, 58] (1935, 1936). Used rabbits. Injected sodium oxalate. Moderate elevation of blood pressure.

Scarff and McGeorge,[59] (1937). Used rabbits. Injected sodium oxalate. No elevation of blood pressure.

In the earlier investigations summarized above the hypertension that was observed was usually slight and lasted from only a few hours to several days. Some of the later investigators also reported the development of hypertension of slight or moderate degree and of short duration while others succeeded in producing moderate or severe hypertension of longer duration. Under practically every heading contradictory reports occur. These differences are partly due to the various methods, including cardiac hypertrophy, used for determining the existence of hypertension, the various types of animal employed and the slight changes of blood pressure which were regarded as significant by some and not by others. For some of the opposite results there is no obvious explanation. While the results of these experiments do indicate that various pathological changes in the kidneys can, in some way, play a primary part in initiating some degree of hypertension in animals, yet by none of these methods was a condition produced in the kidney which is comparable to that of the kidney in human hypertension that is associated with arteriolar disease. To reproduce a state resembling the condition of the kidney in arteriolar disease, any method must effect a decreased flow of blood to the functioning elements of this organ. Loesch [49] approximated this condition by completely occluding the circulation to and from the kidneys, and probably the ureter, for a short while, every two or three days, by clamping the entire pedicle of explanted kidneys. However, there is no good reason for believing that such intermittent occlusion of the arterial blood supply to the kidneys as well as complete interference with the return of venous blood from the kidneys reproduces the functional effects of arteriolar disease in the kidney. If the arteriolar disease of the kidney be responsible for the origin of hypertension then the more likely mechanism of its action is persistent reduction of blood flow to the functioning elements of this organ. The only method which would reproduce this exactly is one that would result in functional or organic narrowing of the arterioles of the kidney. No one has yet succeeded in producing either generalized arteriolar sclerosis or arteriolar sclerosis limited to the kidneys. The closest approach, therefore, to the functional effects of arteriolar disease on the kidneys has been accomplished by reducing the calibre of the main renal arteries alone,[1-4] with resultant renal ischemia, due to persistent reduction of blood flow into the organs. It was considered possible, therefore, that an elucidation of the mechanism of development of this type of experimental hypertension might make some contribution to our knowledge of the pathogenesis of the hypertension in man that is associated with arteriolar sclerosis and consequent ischemia of the kidneys. This is to be regarded as a preliminary communication on this part of the subject.

Experiments

The following experiments were performed for the purpose of elucidating the mechanism of hypertension due to renal ischemia.

Release or Removal of the Clamp. In six dogs, one or both clamps were released or removed some time after hypertension due to renal ischemia had

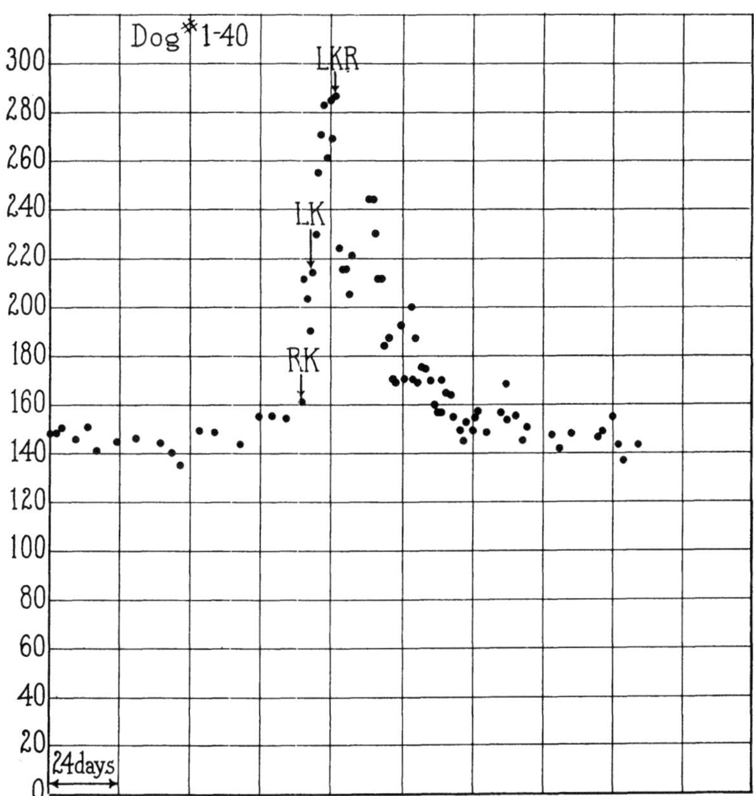

Figure 1. Dog 1–40. Female. 13.4 Kg.

● = Systolic blood pressure, van Leersum carotid loop method. RK = Right main renal artery severely constricted. LK = Left main renal artery severely constricted. LKR = Left clamp completely released but left on the artery.

The blood pressure, which had risen to a very high level after the constriction of the second renal artery, fell to normal in about one month after the release of the clamp on this artery.

been established. Quite promptly, but after a variable period, the blood pressure in these animals returned to the original level. In Dog 1–40 (figure 1), release of one clamp was followed by a rather slow fall of the blood pressure to the original level. In this animal there was no impairment of renal function. In Dog 2–67 (figure 2), after unilateral nephrectomy (LN), severe constriction of the main artery of the remaining kidney (RK_1) resulted in severe hypertension and severe impairment of renal function. When the clamp was released, (RKR_1) blood pressure and renal function promptly returned to normal. Reconstriction of the artery (RK_2) again resulted in hypertension and uremia. Slight release of the constriction (RKR_2) relieved the uremia but the blood pressure remained slightly elevated.

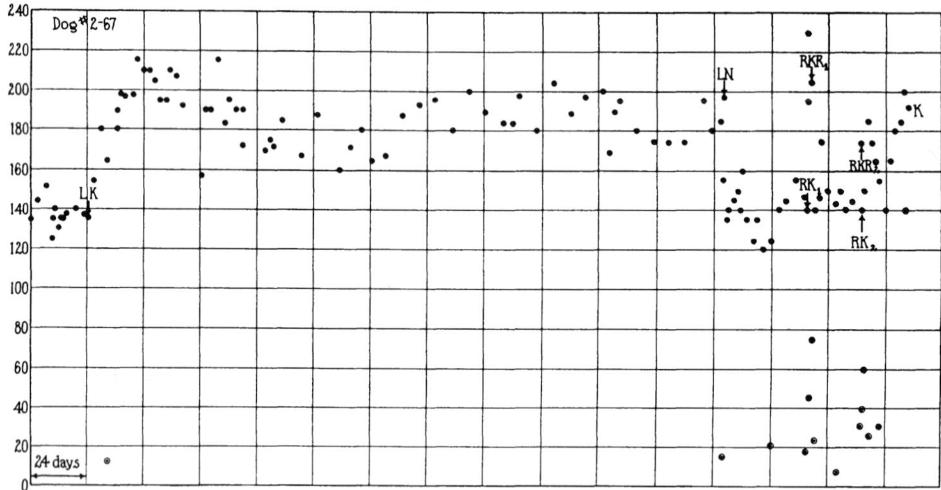

FIGURE 2. Dog 2–67. Female. 13.6 Kg.

● = Mean blood pressure, mm. Hg; ⊙ = blood urea mg. per 100 c.c. plasma. LK = Left main renal artery severely constricted. The blood pressure became greatly elevated. During about ten months after this the blood pressure remained elevated but gradually fell to a moderately elevated level. LN = The ischemic left kidney was excised and the blood pressure promptly fell to the normal level. RK_1 = The right main renal artery was severely constricted. The blood pressure became elevated and uremia developed. RKR_1 = The clamp on the right main renal artery was released. The blood pressure, blood urea, creatinine and non-protein nitrogen promptly returned to normal. RK_2 = The right main renal artery again constricted. Elevated blood pressure and uremia again resulted. RKR_2 = The right main renal artery partly released. Blood pressure dropped temporarily, then rose again and remained elevated. The animal developed severe uremia. K = Killed.

Removal of the Ischemic Kidney During the Period of Hypertension Following the Constriction of One Main Renal Artery. It was shown in the original communications[1,2] that hypertension of some degree follows the constriction of the main renal artery of only one kidney but that after a variable period the blood pressure tends to return to the original level. In some dogs the blood pressure remains elevated for a considerable period following unilateral renal ischemia. In one dog, 2–67 (figure 2), the mean blood pressure remained at a higher level than normal for about nine months following the constriction of the main renal artery of only one kidney. During this period there was no impairment of renal function. After the removal of this kidney (LN) the blood pressure promptly fell to the normal level. Severe constriction of the main renal artery of the remaining kidney

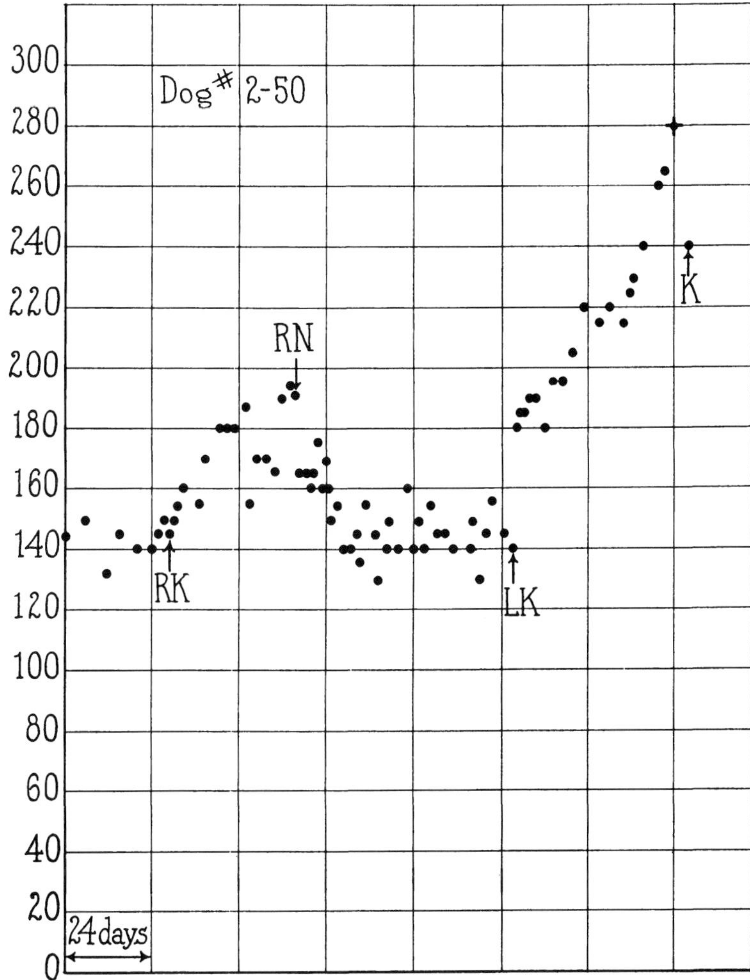

FIGURE 3. Dog 2–50. Female. 17.8 Kg.

● = Mean blood pressure, mm. Hg. RK = Right main renal artery moderately constricted. RN = Right nephrectomy at a time when the mean blood pressure was elevated resulted in its prompt return to normal. LK = Severe constriction of main renal artery of left kidney. This was followed by very high elevation of mean blood pressure. + = The mean blood pressure at this time was more than 300 mm. Hg. K = Killed.

(RK_1) resulted in reëlevation of mean blood pressure and impairment of renal function. In two other dogs also, at the height of elevation of blood pressure, after moderate to severe constriction of the main renal artery of one kidney, this ischemic kidney was excised. Dog 2–50 (figure 3), illustrates what happened in these animals. As in the case of Dog 2–67 (figure 2), removal of the ischemic kidney (RN) was followed by a prompt return of the mean blood pressure to the original level. Constriction of the main renal artery of the remaining kidney (LK) was followed by a prompt re-elevation of blood pressure which persisted. The results of these experiments indicate the importance of ischemia as the pathologic change and the kidney as the primary site of origin of this type of hypertension.

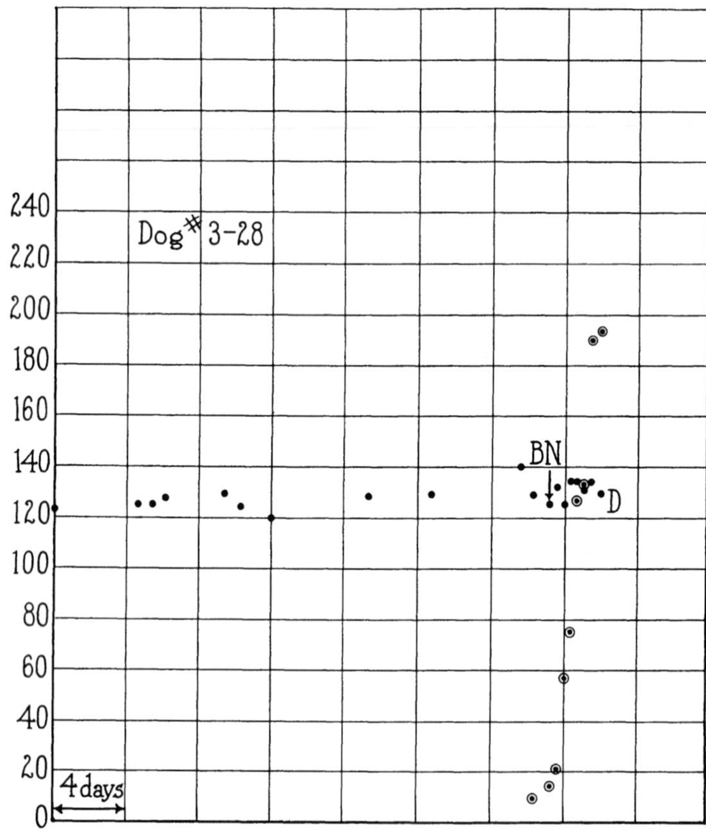

FIGURE 4. Dog 3–28. Male. 16.6 Kg.
● = Mean blood pressure, mm. Hg. ⊙ = Blood urea nitrogen mg. per 100 c.c. plasma. BN = Bilateral nephrectomy. The blood pressure did not become elevated. D = Died.

Bilateral Nephrectomy. If uremia alone were the cause of hypertension, then the removal of both kidneys, which is always followed by the development of uremia, should also, invariably, be followed by the development of hypertension.

In five dogs, both kidneys were removed. In three, bilateral nephrectomy was performed at one time and in two, the nephrectomies were separated by an interval of a week or longer. Most of the animals appeared in good condition for about 48 hours following the operation. All the animals died in uremia but the blood pressure did not rise during the period of survival which varied from two to five days. Figure 4, Dog 3–28, illustrates one of these experiments. This finding is in keeping with the results obtained by other investigators.[11, 25, 26, 27, 28]

Occlusion of the Main Renal Artery of Both Kidneys. It might be considered that occlusion of both main renal arteries would be equal to, and give the same results, as bilateral nephrectomy. This is not the case. In

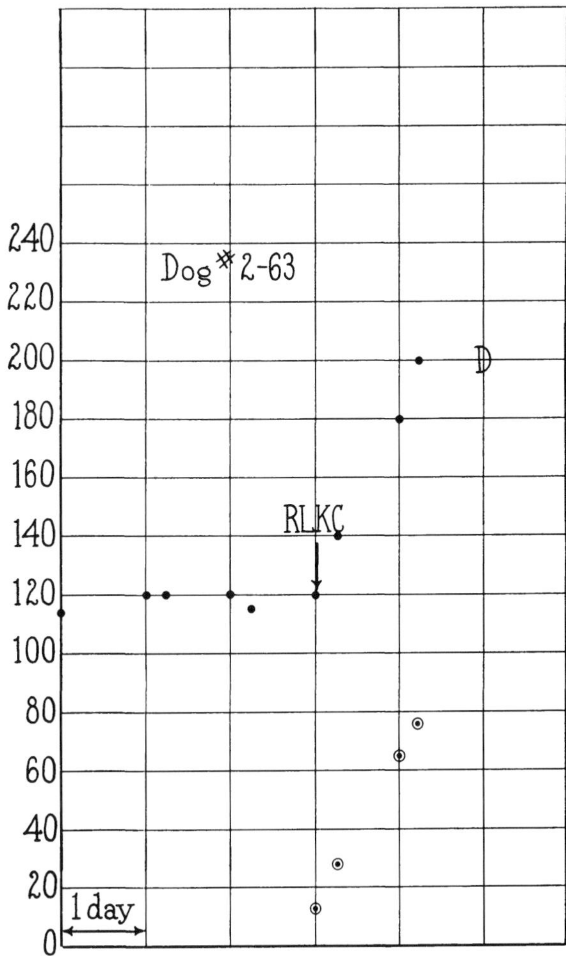

FIGURE 5. Dog 2–63. Female. 16.2 Kg.
● = Mean blood pressure, mm. Hg. ⊙ = Blood urea, mg. per 100 c.c. of plasma. RLKC = Both main renal arteries occluded. The blood pressure rose to quite a high level. D = The animal died in uremia.

four dogs the main renal artery of both kidneys was clamped completely at one operation and in two dogs the occlusion of the second artery was carried out after an interval of a week or longer. The complete occlusion of one main renal artery was not followed by either uremia or a significant elevation of blood pressure. In all four animals, however, simultaneous occlusion of the main renal artery of both kidneys was followed by the development of severe uremia and slight or moderate elevation of the blood pressure. The degree of hypertension in the animals with both renal arteries occluded was not as great as in dogs with both main renal arteries only moderately or

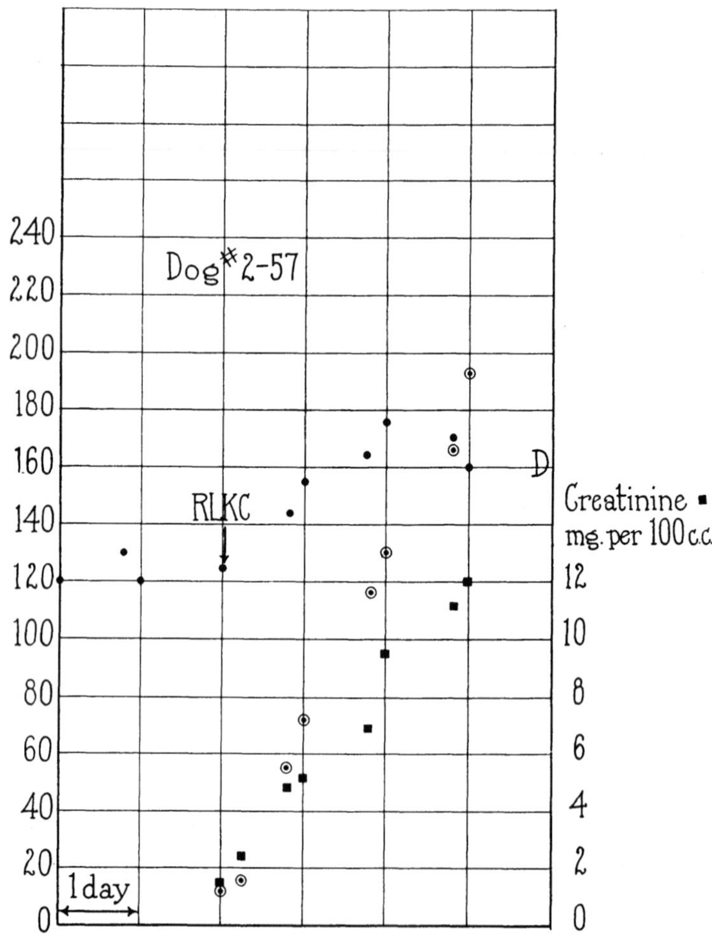

FIGURE 6. Dog 2–57. Female. 18.4 Kg.
● = Mean blood pressure, mm. Hg. ⊙ = Blood urea, mg. per 100 c.c. of plasma. ■ = Blood creatinine mg. per 100 c.c. of plasma. RLKC = Right and left main renal arteries occluded. The blood pressure showed a moderate elevation following the occlusion of the arteries. D = The animal died in uremia.

severely constricted.[2] The period of survival was about the same as that of the bilaterally nephrectomized animals. In the animals with both main renal arteries occluded, as in those bilaterally nephrectomized, the shock of the operation was evidently not great and for about 48 hours they seemed in excellent condition. Both groups survived about the same period and all developed severe uremia, yet the animals with both arteries occluded did show a significant elevation of blood pressure which is illustrated for three of the dogs in figures 5, 6 and 7, while the nephrectomized animals failed to show a rise of blood pressure. In Dog 2–65, as a control, all of the arteries to the spleen were tied off completely (figure 7), some time before

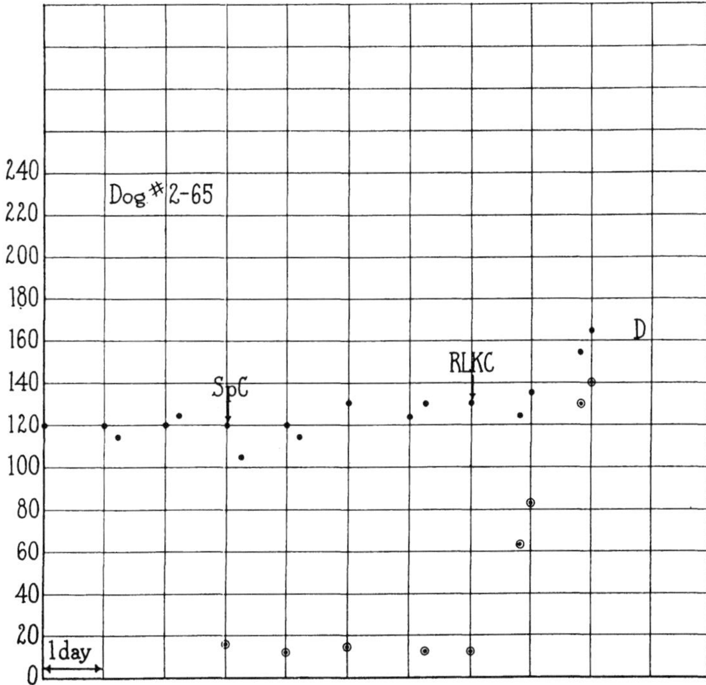

FIGURE 7. Dog 2–65. Female. 15.2 Kg.

● = Mean blood pressure, mm. Hg. ⊙ = Blood urea nitrogen mg. per 100 c.c. of plasma. SpC = Splenic arteries occluded. There was no significant rise of blood pressure after this procedure. RLKC = Right and left main renal arteries occluded. After this there was a moderate elevation of blood pressure. D = The animal died in uremia.

the renal arteries were occluded. The occlusion of the splenic vessels was not followed by a significant elevation of mean blood pressure. When both main renal arteries were occluded (RLKC) (figure 7), the blood pressure became slightly elevated, severe uremia developed and the animal died.

That a dog can survive for a long time the occlusion of both main renal arteries, provided the occlusion is not accomplished abruptly, has been well shown by four animals, in which the occlusion was accomplished in two or more stages. One dog has proved this very strikingly. At the second clamping of both main renal arteries, carried out successively about one year after the initial partial constriction, both main renal arteries were occluded. This animal survived the complete occlusion of both main renal arteries for four years. Hypertension of severe degree persisted during the entire period and renal function, as shown by urea clearance, was only slightly affected. At autopsy, one kidney was very small and the other only moderately reduced in size. No accessory arteries were found except those that entered the kidney through the capsule. Other experiments of this kind, to be reported later, are being carried out to determine the exact source and extent of the supply of blood to such kidneys.

Discussion

As in the case of partial constriction of both main renal arteries,[2] the hypertension which follows occlusion of both main renal arteries can be explained by a possible nervous reflex from the kidney by way of the central nervous system to the peripheral vasomotor apparatus or by some humoral mechanism, or by a combination of both mechanisms.

That hypertension due to occlusion of both renal arteries is not due to a nervous reflex from the kidney is indicated by the fact that in some of these animals the renal pedicle was carefully denervated before the clamp was applied. It has also been shown by other investigators,[6, 10] and we have confirmed this, that renal denervation does not interfere with the development of experimental hypertension due to partial constriction of the main renal arteries. Section of the splanchnic nerves in the thorax, combined with excision of the lower four thoracic sympathetic ganglia, does not interfere with the development of hypertension or permanently reduce the hypertension produced by renal ischemia.[3] In an investigation soon to be published in collaboration with Dr. W. B. Wartman, it will be shown that section of the anterior nerve roots, from the sixth dorsal to the second lumbar inclusive, also does not interfere with the development of hypertension or permanently reduce the hypertension produced by renal ischemia. Finally, Freeman and Page [60] have shown that total sympathectomy does not interfere with the development of hypertension due to bilateral renal ischemia. These results are not to be interpreted as evidence or proof that the surgical procedures being practised on human beings with hypertension are not justifiable and that no improvement is to be expected from these procedures. What they do show is that in experimental hypertension, due to the permanent renal ischemia effected by the clamps, section or excision of various portions of the nervous system controlling a large part of the vasomotor mechanism of the abdominal organs, does not result in prevention or reduction of this type of experimental hypertension. These experiments serve to emphasize the importance of the reduction of the circulation to the functioning components of the kidney rather than a primary effect on the general vasomotor mechanism of the abdomen as the cause of this type of hypertension. This is in keeping with the views of Prinzmetal and Wilson [61] and of Pickering [62] about the secondary part played by the vasomotor mechanism in human hypertension. In man it is at least possible that as a result of some or all of the surgical procedures being practised on the nervous system for the cure of hypertension, actual improvement of the circulation to the functioning components of the kidney may occur. Dilatation of renal arterioles without fixed organic changes in their walls might occur in some cases, as a result of these procedures. Since, in man, there is frequently no narrowing of the large renal vessels to interfere with the flow of blood into the kidney, it is at least conceivable that improved circulation to the functioning components of the kidney may follow as a result of dilatation of arterioles. This improvement of renal circulation could then account for the fall of blood pressure which has been observed in about the same rather small percentage of cases treated by the various surgical procedures on the nervous system. This view is in agreement with that of Peet [69] on the mode of action of resection of the splanchnic nerves in lowering the blood pressure in human beings with hypertension. It is not, however, the view that is generally accepted by those who have been performing operations on the nervous system for the cure of hypertension in man.[63-75] They prefer to regard the improvement following section or excision of the nerves as due to the elimination of their control over the corresponding portion of the vasomotor mechanism. The same improvement of the circulation cannot happen, or can happen to only a very limited degree, as the result of increased dilatation of the arterioles in the experimental kidney, as long as the main renal artery remains constricted by the clamp. These observations do minimize the importance of the effect of the vasoconstrictor mechanism in the abdomen in hypertension due to renal ischemia, because the removal of this mechanism by the various surgical procedures does not prevent or cure the hypertension as long as the clamps remain applied and the blood flow to the functioning components of the kidneys remains unimproved.

If the mechanism whereby constriction of the main renal arteries produces its effect on blood pressure be humoral and of renal origin then, in the case of the hypertension which also follows occlusion of both main renal arteries, it must be assumed that the natural accessory circulation through the capsule which may become more prominent in these circumstances, is sufficient to wash some hypothetical " effective substance " into the systemic circulation through the main renal veins. The term " effective substance " will be used in this paper to avoid commitment to the existence of a direct pressor substance rather than one which acts indirectly to produce the pressor effect. The effective substance, for example, might act synergistically with a known pressor hormone from an endocrine organ, such as the hypophysis or adrenal. It is also possible for the hypothetical effective substance from the kidney to act by sensitizing the contractile elements of the arterioles to the action of the pressor hormone, or the reverse may be the case. The effective substance might also produce its effect by neutralizing or reducing the amount of a hypothetical depressor substance circulating in the blood. That there may be an effective substance from the kidney is indicated by reports of the pressor effect of extract of ischemic kidneys from dogs with experimental hypertension,[11, 13, 17] and of arteriosclerotic kidneys [13] from human beings with hypertension. However, the results of such investigations should be interpreted with caution because a pressor effect has also been obtained with extracts of normal kidneys [118, 119] and with extracts of various

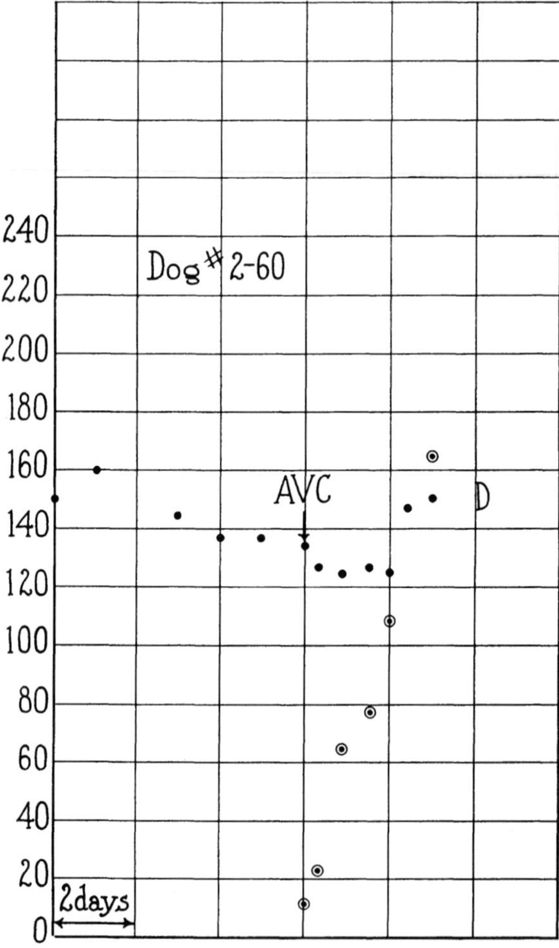

FIGURE 8. Dog 2–60. Male. 16.6 Kg.
● = Mean blood pressure mm. Hg. ⊙ = Blood urea nitrogen mg. 100 c.c. plasma. AVC = Both main renal arteries and veins occluded. The blood pressure did not become elevated. D = Died.

other normal organs.[120] The existence of a pressor substance in the systemic or renal vein blood of animals with hypertension due to renal ischemia has not been demonstrated [12] and no greater quantity of pressor substance than the normal has been found [12] in the extract of plasma of dogs with this type of experimental hypertension. It has not been proved that the systemic blood, spinal fluid, or urine of human beings with hypertension of any type invariably contains a pressor substance. Many reports of the finding of a pressor substance [76-104] and of the failure to find a pressor substance [105-117] have been published. A discussion of these results would serve no useful purpose here. The pitfalls of such investigations were well shown by O'Connor.[126] The burden of the proof still rests with those who claim the

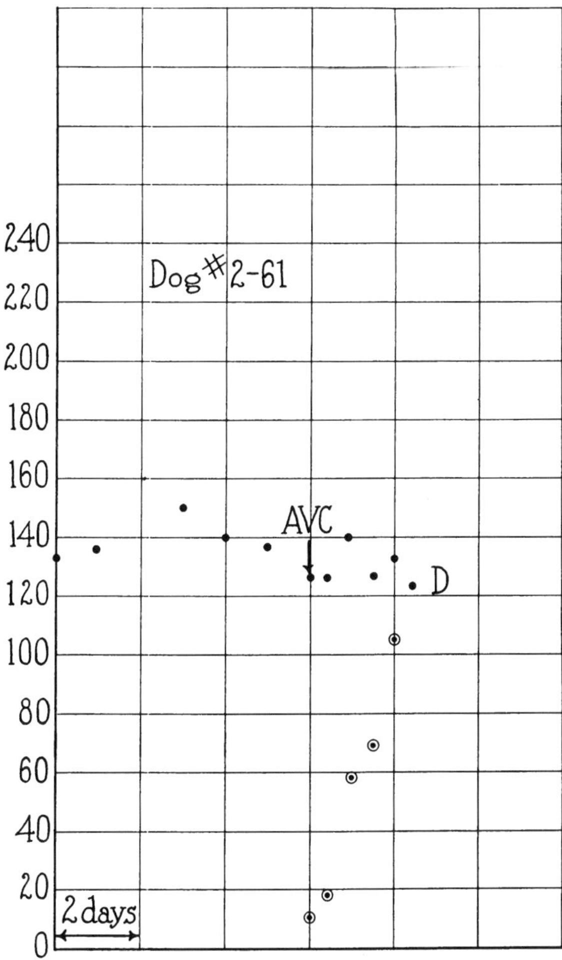

FIGURE 9. Dog 2-61. Female. 14.8 Kg.
● = Mean blood pressure mm. Hg. ⊙ = Blood urea nitrogen mg. per 100 c.c. plasma. AVC = Both main renal arteries and veins occluded. The blood pressure did not become elevated. D = Died.

invariable presence of an unusual amount of a known pressor hormone or of a new kind of pressor substance in pure or extracted blood, spinal fluid or urine of human beings with hypertension, especially the so-called benign or essential type. The experiments which follow are part of an investigation that is being carried out to determine the part played by a possible humoral mechanism in the pathogenesis of hypertension due to renal ischemia.

Constriction or Occlusion of Both Main Renal Arteries with Simultaneous Occlusion of Both Main Renal Veins. One obvious but indirect way of testing for a possible humoral mechanism originating in the kidney is to constrict or occlude the main renal arteries, procedures which are now known to produce hypertension, and, at the same time, to occlude the main

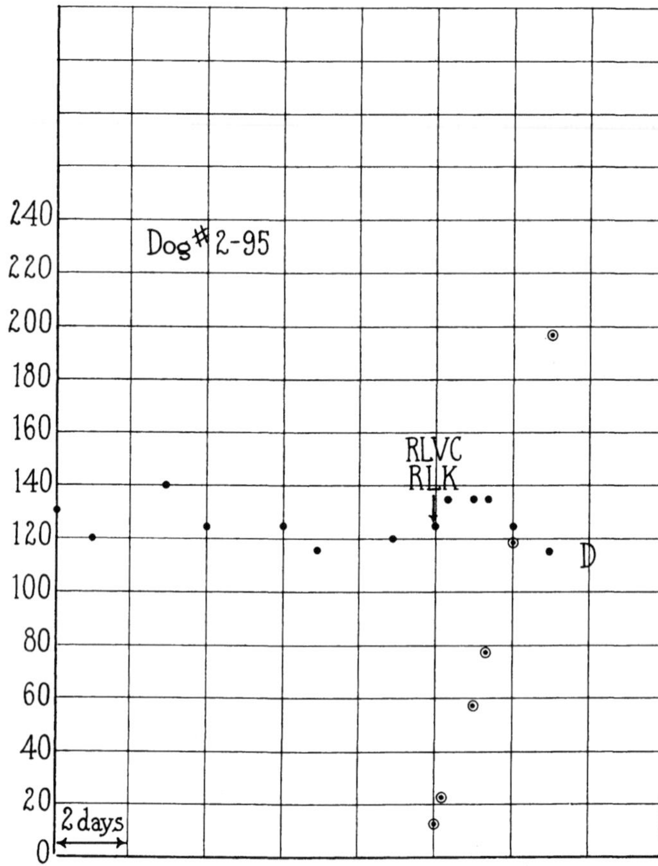

FIGURE 10. Dog 2-95. Female. 16.4 Kg.
● = Mean blood pressure, mm. Hg. ⊙ = Blood urea nitrogen mg. per 100 c.c. RLVC = Both main renal veins occluded. RLK = Both main renal arteries severely constricted. The animal died in uremia but the blood pressure did not become significantly elevated.

renal veins in order to prevent the hypothetical effective substance from leaving the kidneys. Failure of development of hypertension would be evidence in favor of a humoral mechanism originating in the kidney as the cause of the hypertension.

In two dogs (2-60 and 2-61) the main renal arteries and veins of both kidneys were occluded at one time. The blood pressure and some of the chemical changes in the blood of these dogs are illustrated in figures 8 and 9. Both developed severe uremia but no rise of blood pressure occurred during the short period of survival. These results are in keeping with those of Cash [27] who found that no elevation of blood pressure occurred in dogs after the permanent occlusion of both main renal arteries, veins and ureters.

In two dogs (2–51 and 2–95) the main renal veins were occluded and the main renal arteries were only severely constricted. The animals developed severe uremia but no elevation of blood pressure occurred during the short period of survival. Figure 10 illustrates the blood pressure and chemical changes in the blood of one of these animals, Dog 2–95.

Since it has been shown that the permanent constriction or occlusion of the main renal arteries alone is followed by a definite rise of blood pressure, these results may be interpreted as indicating the probable interference with the entrance of the hypothetical effective substance into the systemic circulation by way of the renal veins.

The Part Played by Endocrine Organs in the Origin of Hypertension Due to Renal Ischemia

As part of the study of the humoral mechanism, an attempt has been made to investigate the part played by the endocrine organs that are known to produce a vaso-pressor hormone.

Hypophysis. Page [7] has shown that in dogs, hypophysectomy does not prevent the development of experimental hypertension due to renal ischemia, but that it does reduce the blood pressure in some animals with this type of hypertension. The significance of these contradictory findings cannot be evaluated at the present time. More experiments of this kind should be performed. The effect on this type of hypertension of removal of the various portions of the pituitary body have not yet been investigated.

Adrenals. In a previous communication [2] an experiment on Dog No. 8–9 was described in which excision of the right adrenal, the destruction of the medulla of the left adrenal, denervation of this adrenal and section of the left splanchnic nerves in the abdomen did not prevent the development of hypertension after the renal arteries were moderately constricted. The only conclusion that can be drawn from this experiment is that hypertension can develop in the absence of the medulla of both adrenal glands, as a consequence of renal ischemia, and that the presence of the medulla of the adrenal is not necessary for the development of this type of hypertension. Since then other experiments have been performed which were designed to determine the part which the cortex of the adrenal gland may play in the development of experimental hypertension due to renal ischemia. This is in the nature of a preliminary communication on this subject. The study is being continued and full details, including chemical studies, will be published later in collaboration with Dr. R. F. Hanzal. Up to the present time the following experiments have been performed.

Bilateral Adrenalectomy, without Supportive or Substitution Therapy, and Renal Ischemia. In this group of animals no supportive (sodium chloride and sodium bicarbonate or sodium citrate by mouth) or substitution (intra-venous cortical extract *) therapy was given after the removal of both adrenals.

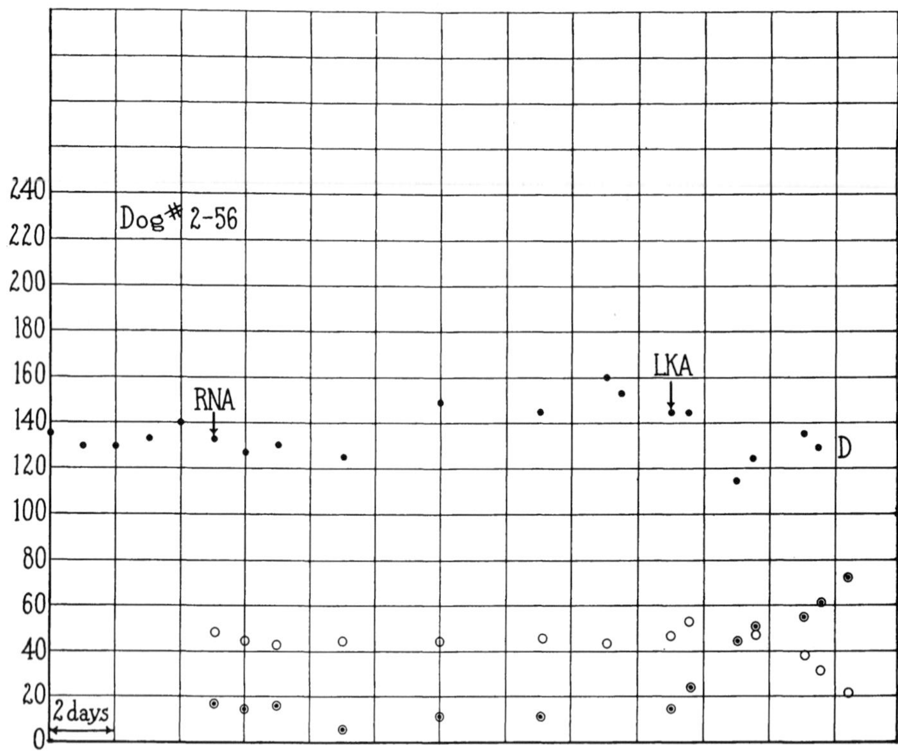

FIGURE 11. Dog 2–56. Female. 23.2 Kg.

● = Mean blood pressure, mm. Hg. ⊙ = Blood urea nitrogen mg. per 100 c.c. of plasma. ○ = CO_2 combining power, volumes per 100 c.c. RNA = Right adrenalectomy and right nephrectomy. If anything, a slight elevation of blood pressure occurred after these procedures. LKA = Left adrenalectomy and left main renal artery severely constricted. The animal developed uremia and the blood pressure fell. D = The animal died in uremia.

In three dogs, both main renal arteries were permanently constricted at the time of the second adrenalectomy. In two of these (2–56 and 2–62) the first adrenalectomy preceded the second by about two weeks, but in one animal the adrenalectomy and the constriction of both main renal arteries were carried out at the same time (Dog 3–22). The blood pressure did not become elevated in any of these animals, but the period of survival was short. (Figure 11.)

* The cortical extract used in these experiments was Eschatin which was generously supplied by Parke, Davis and Co.

In one dog (2–64, figure 12) one adrenal was first removed and the main artery of the kidney on this side was constricted 12 days later. The blood pressure rose significantly, showing the responsiveness of the blood pressure of this animal. At the height of elevation of the blood pressure, the second adrenal was excised and the main renal artery of the corresponding side was permanently constricted. Instead of rising to a higher level, or at least remaining elevated, the blood pressure soon fell to a level below the previous normal for this animal and it died in 11 days of acute adrenal insufficiency.

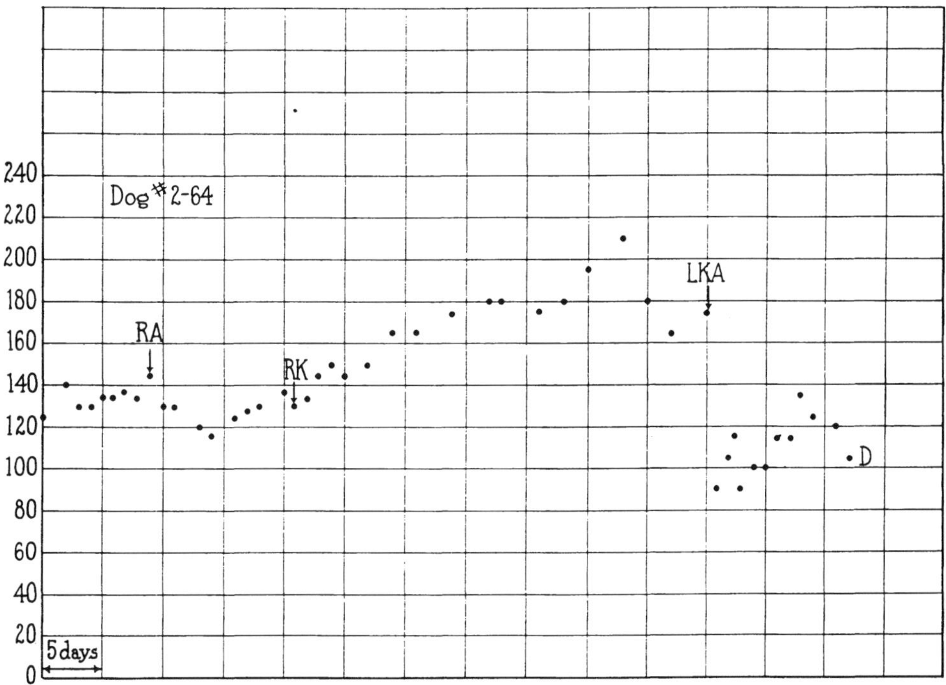

FIGURE 12. Dog 2–64. Female. 18.8 Kg.

● = Mean blood pressure, mm. Hg. RA = Right adrenalectomy. RK = Right main renal artery severely constricted. The blood pressure became significantly elevated. LKA = Left adrenalectomy and left main renal artery moderately constricted. The blood pressure fell to below normal level and the animal died of acute adrenal insufficiency. D = Died.

The results of these experiments show that bilateral adrenalectomy, without supportive or substitution therapy, interferes with the development and maintenance of hypertension which usually follows the production of renal ischemia.

Bilateral Adrenalectomy with Supportive Treatment and Renal Ischemia. It has been shown that the life of bilaterally adrenalectomized animals can be prolonged by the administration of sodium chloride [121-124] or sodium chloride and sodium bicarbonate or sodium citrate.[125]

In one dog (2–89, figure 13), the constriction of the main renal artery was carried out on the same side and at the same time as the first adrenalectomy. After this the blood pressure became significantly elevated, which demonstrated the responsiveness of the blood pressure of this animal to the effect of renal ischemia. At the end of four weeks, while the blood pressure was still elevated, the second adrenal was removed and the main artery of the kidney on the same side was constricted. Supportive treatment in the form of sodium chloride alone was given by stomach tube during the first 10 days and then sodium bicarbonate was added. After the second adrenalectomy and constriction of both main renal arteries, instead of rising to a higher level, the blood pressure gradually fell to a level below the normal for this animal and death occurred in 19 days.

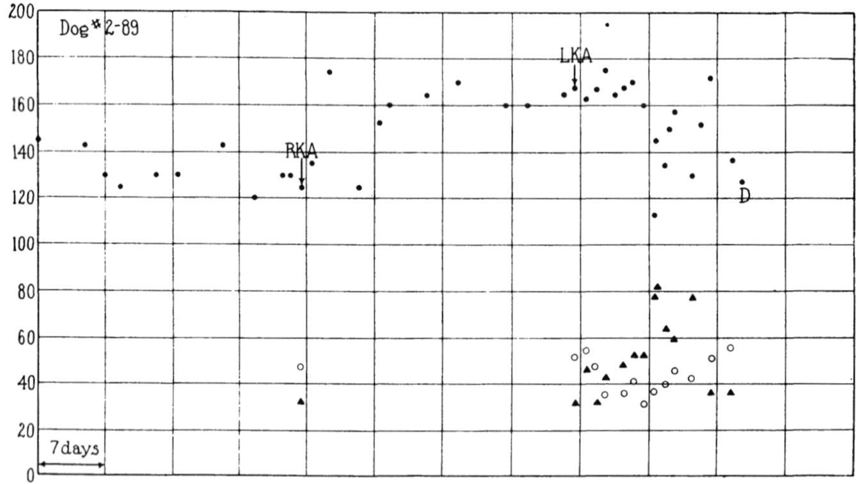

FIGURE 13. Dog 2–89. Male. 17.6 Kg.

● = Mean blood pressure, mm. Hg. ○ = CO_2 combining power, volumes per 100 c.c. plasma. ▲ = Non-protein nitrogen mg. per 100 c.c. plasma. RKA = Right adrenalectomy and right main renal artery moderately constricted. After this the blood pressure showed a moderate elevation. LKA = Left adrenalectomy and left main renal artery moderately constricted. From the time of the second adrenalectomy this animal received sodium chloride (0.75 gm. per kg. of body weight) by stomach tube for 9 days and from then on received in addition sodium bicarbonate (0.25 gm. per kg. of body weight). There was no greater elevation of blood pressure following the clamping of the second renal artery and the blood pressure gradually fell to below the original level. D = The animal died of acute adrenal insufficiency.

In another dog (2–81) the constriction of both main renal arteries was carried out at the same time as the bilateral adrenalectomy. This was followed by the administration of supportive treatment in the form of sodium chloride and sodium citrate by mouth. The animal survived 15 days but the blood pressure did not become elevated during that period. It fell gradually to a low level and the animal died of acute adrenal insufficiency.

The most convincing proof that in bilaterally adrenalectomized animals supportive treatment alone is not sufficient to permit elevation of blood pressure or maintenance of elevated blood pressure due to renal ischemia was furnished by four dogs 2–77, 2–87, 2–88 and 3–08 (figures 14 to 17). These animals received both supportive and substitution therapy after the second adrenalectomy but after a varying length of time the administration of cortical extract was discontinued for varying periods. As a result, some of the animals received only supportive treatment in the form of sodium chloride and sodium bicarbonate or sodium citrate by stomach tube for as long as six weeks. In some of these animals the blood pressure remained at the normal or elevated level for a while, but invariably the blood pressure fell to a lower level and rose again to the normal level or higher only when the administration of cortical extract was resumed. These results show that bilateral adrenalectomy, even if followed by supportive treatment, interferes with the development and maintenance of the hypertension which is usually produced by renal ischemia.

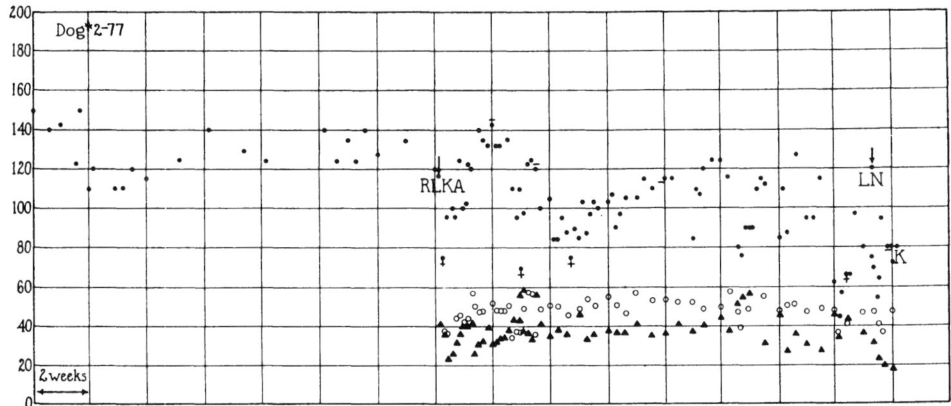

FIGURE 14. Dog 2–77. Female. 11.4 Kg.

● = Mean blood pressure, mm. Hg. ▲ = Non-protein nitrogen, mg. per 100 c.c. ○ = CO_2 combining power, volumes per 100 c.c. RLKA = Bilateral adrenalectomy and both main renal arteries moderately constricted. LN = Left nephrectomy. + = Intravenous adrenal cortical extract begun. — = Adrenal cortical extract discontinued. During the entire period following the bilateral adrenalectomy the animal received by stomach tube, in two equal doses (9:00 a.m. and 4:00 p.m.) a total of 0.75 gm. per kg. of body weight of sodium chloride and 0.25 gm. per kg. of body weight of sodium bicarbonate. At no time during the four months of survival did the animal show elevated blood pressure. Several times, when cortical extract was discontinued, the blood pressure fell to very low levels. K = Killed.

Bilateral Adrenalectomy with Supportive and Substitution Treatment and Renal Ischemia. In Dog 2–77, both adrenals were excised and at the same time both main renal arteries were permanently constricted (RLKA, figure 14). During the entire four months of survival following these operations the animal received supportive treatment daily in the form of sodium chloride and sodium bicarbonate by stomach tube and intermittent substitution treatment in the form of intravenous cortical extract. Immediately after the operation the administration of adrenal cortical extract was begun (+, figure 14). At intervals, for varying periods, the administration of cortical extract was discontinued. The blood pressure remained at about the normal level during the periods when the cortical extract was also being administered. When the cortical extract was discontinued (—, figure 14) the mean blood pressure gradually fell to a low level. When the administration of cortical extract was resumed, the blood pressure rose again but never above the normal level. This was repeated several times with the same result. At no time was the pressure in this animal above normal.

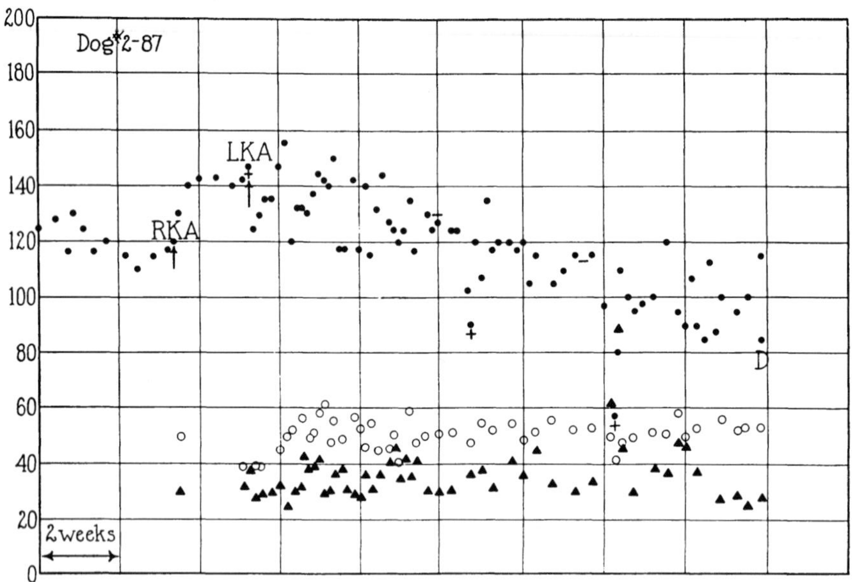

FIGURE 15. Dog 2–87. Female. 12.8 Kg.
● = Mean blood pressure, mm. Hg. ○ = CO_2 combining power, volumes per 100 c.c. ▲ = Non-protein nitrogen, mg. per 100 c.c. + = Intravenous adrenal cortical extract begun. — = Intravenous adrenal cortical extract discontinued.

Sodium chloride (0.75 mg. per kg. of body weight) and sodium bicarbonate (0.25 gm. per kg. body weight) were given during the entire period following the second adrenalectomy. RKA = Right adrenalectomy and right main renal artery moderately constricted. The blood pressure rose moderately. LKA = Left adrenalectomy and left main renal artery severely constricted. From this time the blood pressure gradually fell to a low level despite the supportive and substitution therapy. D = Died.

In dog 2–87 (figure 15) unilateral adrenalectomy and constriction of the main renal artery on the same side were first carried out. After this first operation no supportive or substitution therapy was given. Definite though slight elevation of blood pressure followed this procedure, which demonstrated the responsiveness of the blood pressure of this animal to renal ischemia. After the second adrenalectomy and constriction of the corresponding main renal artery, both of which were performed at the same time, about two weeks after the first adrenalectomy, supportive and substitution treatment were begun. The blood pressure remained elevated for a while but it did not rise to a higher level and, despite the treatment, gradually fell to below the previous normal.

In two dogs (2–88 and 3–08), one adrenal and the kidney on the same side were first removed. After an interval, the second adrenal was removed and the main artery of the only remaining kidney was constricted. During the entire period after the second adrenalectomy, these animals were given supportive treatment in the form of sodium chloride and sodium citrate by stomach tube. Immediately after the second adrenalectomy the administration of intravenous adrenal cortical extract was also begun. At intervals, for varying periods, the administration of cortical extract was

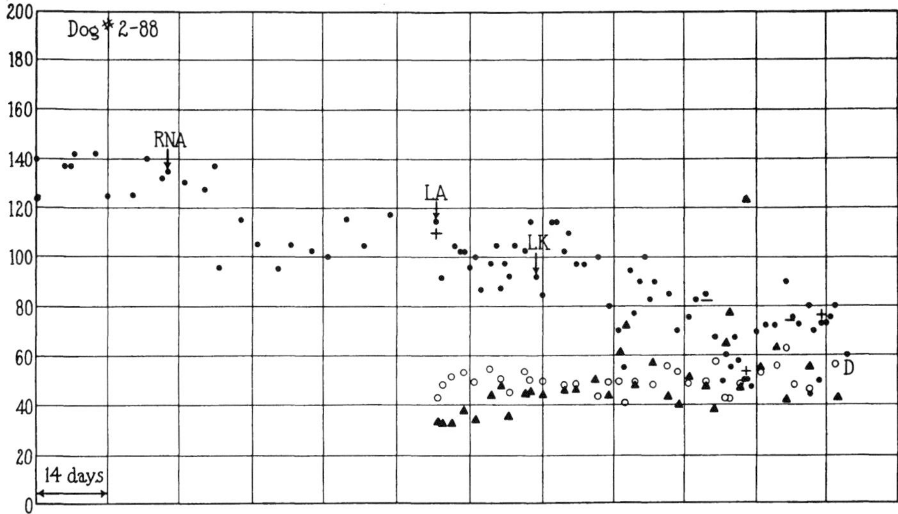

FIGURE 16. Dog 2–88. Female. 16.8 Kg.

● = Mean blood pressure, mm. Hg. ▲ = Blood non-protein nitrogen mg. per 100 c.c. of plasma. ○ = CO_2 combining power of blood, volumes per 100 c.c. of plasma. RNA = Right nephrectomy and adrenalectomy. LA = Left adrenalectomy. LK = Left main renal artery moderately constricted. + = Intravenous adrenal cortical extract begun. — = Intravenous adrenal cortical extract discontinued.

After the left main artery was constricted (LK) the blood pressure gradually fell to a very low level despite the intravenous adrenal cortical extract which was given for long periods at a time and the sodium chloride and sodium citrate which were given by stomach tube twice daily during the entire period following the second adrenalectomy. D = Died.

discontinued. In dog 2–88 (figure 16), the main artery of the only remaining kidney was constricted about two weeks after the second adrenalectomy. There was no elevation of mean blood pressure following this procedure but instead the blood pressure fell gradually to a low level despite supportive and substitution therapy. When the cortical extract was discontinued, the blood pressure fell to even a lower level. The animal survived the second adrenalectomy about 12 weeks. During the intervals when cortical extract was discontinued, the mean blood pressure fell to unusually low levels and rose again, but not even to the original level, when cortical extract was resumed. In the other dog, 3–08 (figure 17), the constriction of the main artery of the remaining kidney was carried out at the time of the second adrenalectomy. Definite elevation of mean blood pressure followed for a period of about one month. During this entire time intravenous adrenal cortical extract was given daily in addition to the salt and

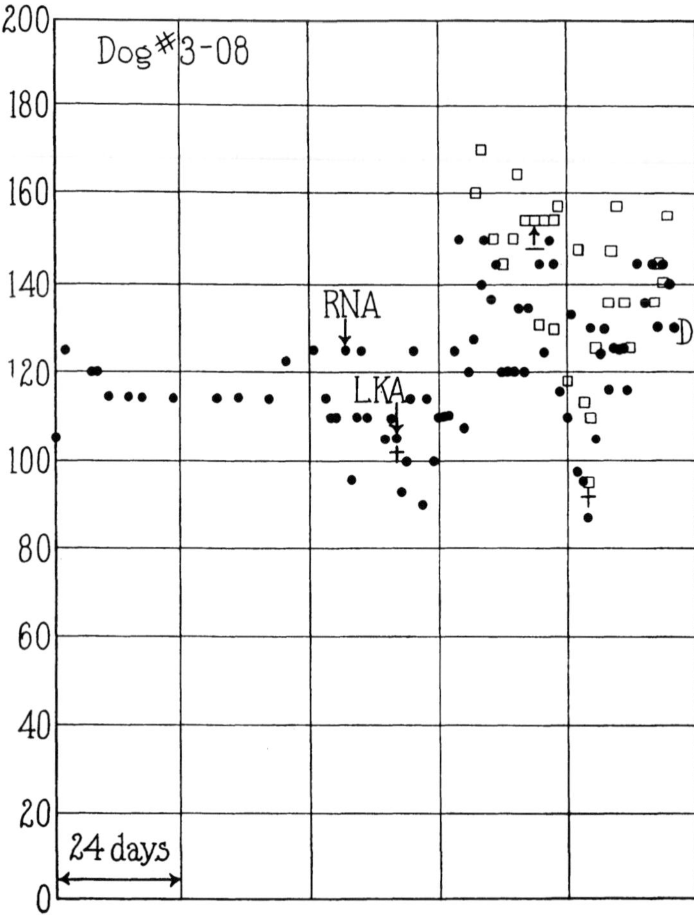

FIGURE 17. Dog 3–08. Female. 9.0 Kg.

● = Mean blood pressure, mm. Hg. Determinations made in a.m. □ = Mean blood pressure, mm. Hg. Determinations made in p.m. 5 hours after the administration of the morning dose of cortical extract, sodium chloride and sodium citrate. RNA = Right adrenalectomy and right nephrectomy. LKA = Left adrenalectomy and left main renal artery severely constricted. + = Intravenous cortical extract begun. — = Intravenous cortical extract discontinued.

Sodium chloride and sodium citrate by stomach tube were given daily during the entire period after the second adrenalectomy.

The blood pressure became moderately elevated and remained elevated for one month during which the dog received substitution as well as supportive treatment. Whenever the intravenous cortical extract was discontinued (—) the blood pressure gradually fell to a level below normal. When cortical extract was begun again (+) the blood pressure gradually rose but did not reach the previous hypertensive level. D = Died of pneumonia.

sodium citrate by stomach tube. When the cortical extract was discontinued at the end of one month, the blood pressure gradually fell to a lower level. When the administration of cortical extract was resumed the blood pressure again became slightly elevated. The animal was accidentally exposed to cold and died of pneumonia.

Up to the present time, definite elevation of blood pressure due to renal ischemia has occurred in one other bilaterally adrenalectomized animal (Dog 2–96) that received substitution and supportive treatment. This animal survived the second adrenalectomy only 19 days. After the constriction of one main renal artery, which was performed eight days after the second adrenalectomy, there was a definite elevation of the blood pressure. Six days later, while the blood pressure was still elevated the main artery of the other kidney was constricted but the animal died the next day.

These results show that, even in the absence of both adrenals, provided adequate substitution and supportive treatment are given, some dogs do develop a significant but not great elevation of blood pressure due to renal ischemia. Without substitution treatment such animals do not develop or maintain hypertension due to renal ischemia.

Renal Ischemia in Dogs with No Adrenal Medulla and Only a Small Remnant of Adrenal Cortex. Additional evidence that adrenal cortical hormone is necessary for the development of hypertension due to renal ischemia is provided by the following experiments.

In one dog (3–12, figure 18) approximately three-fifths of one adrenal was excised and the medulla of the remaining portion removed by means of a curette. At this operation the kidney on the same side was removed. At the second operation, carried out 19 days later, the other adrenal was excised, and the main artery of the only remaining kidney was constricted. In a second dog (3–16, figure 19) exactly the same procedure was carried out but this animal was left with about three-fifths of the cortex alone of one adrenal. There was an interval of 33 days between the two adrenal operations. For a few days following the removal of the second adrenal and constriction of the main renal artery of the only kidney, both dogs received supportive treatment in the form of sodium chloride and sodium citrate by stomach tube. No adrenal cortical extract was given at any time. The blood pressure rose promptly following the production of renal ischemia. Even when the supportive treatment was discontinued, the blood pressure remained elevated and, in 3–16 rose to even a higher level.

These results are interpreted as indicating the preservation of the function of the small portion of adrenal cortex which was left. In both animals, without the aid of supportive or substitution treatment, this small remnant of cortex was sufficient to permit elevation of blood pressure due to renal ischemia. This is additional evidence in support of the view that the hormone of the cortex of the adrenal gland in some way plays a part in the pathogenesis of hypertension due to renal ischemia. More experiments are being performed in order to elucidate the manner in which this hormone, itself not a vasopressor substance, helps to bring about the pressor effect which follows the production of renal ischemia.

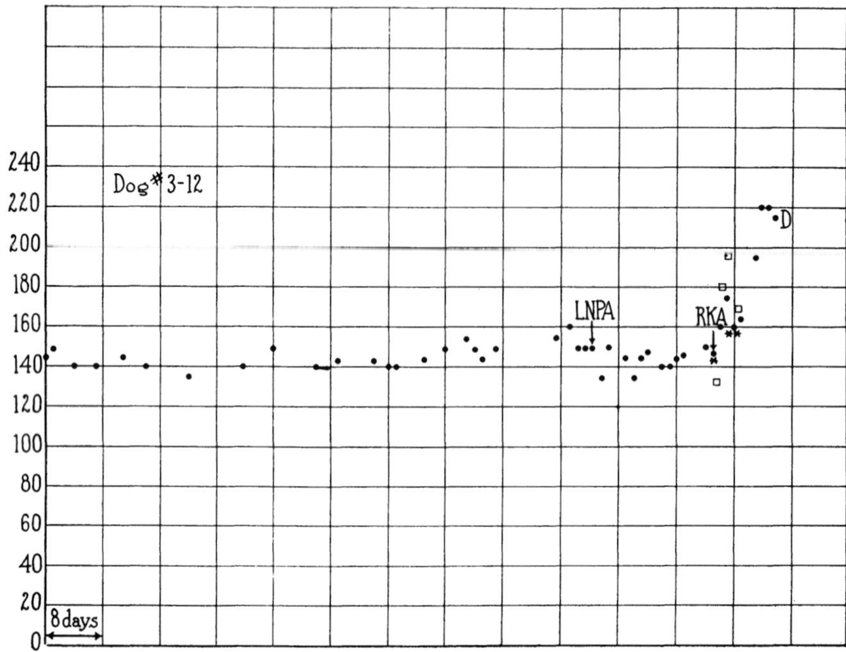

FIGURE 18. Dog 3–12. Female. 11.4 Kg.

● = Mean blood pressure, mm. Hg. LNPA = Left nephrectomy and partial adrenalectomy. The medulla was destroyed. About two-fifths of the cortex was left. RKA = Right adrenalectomy and right main renal artery severely constricted. * = Sodium chloride (0.75 gm. per kg. of body weight) and sodium citrate (0.25 gm. per kg. of body weight) were given by stomach tube from this time on. ** = Sodium chloride and sodium citrate discontinued. No cortical extract was given at any time. The blood pressure rose moderately following the constriction of the renal artery and remained elevated when supportive treatment was discontinued. D = Died.

SUMMARY

The results of the experiments that have been performed up to the present time on the pathogenesis of hypertension due to renal ischemia indicate that the mechanism of the development of this type of hypertension is primarily a humoral one of renal origin.

The failure of the various surgical procedures carried out on the nervous system to affect this type of experimental hypertension is evidently due to the persistence of the renal ischemia which cannot be altered by these procedures as long as the clamps remain applied. These experiments do not in any way controvert the results that have been obtained by the same procedures in the treatment of hypertension in man. They do emphasize, however, the importance of the reduced blood flow to the functioning components of the kidney as the primary cause of this type of experimental hypertension and perhaps of human hypertension that is associated with arteriolar disease of the kidneys. Since the reduced blood flow in the human kidney is frequently due to narrowing of the arterioles alone, without narrowing of the large arteries, improvement of the circulation

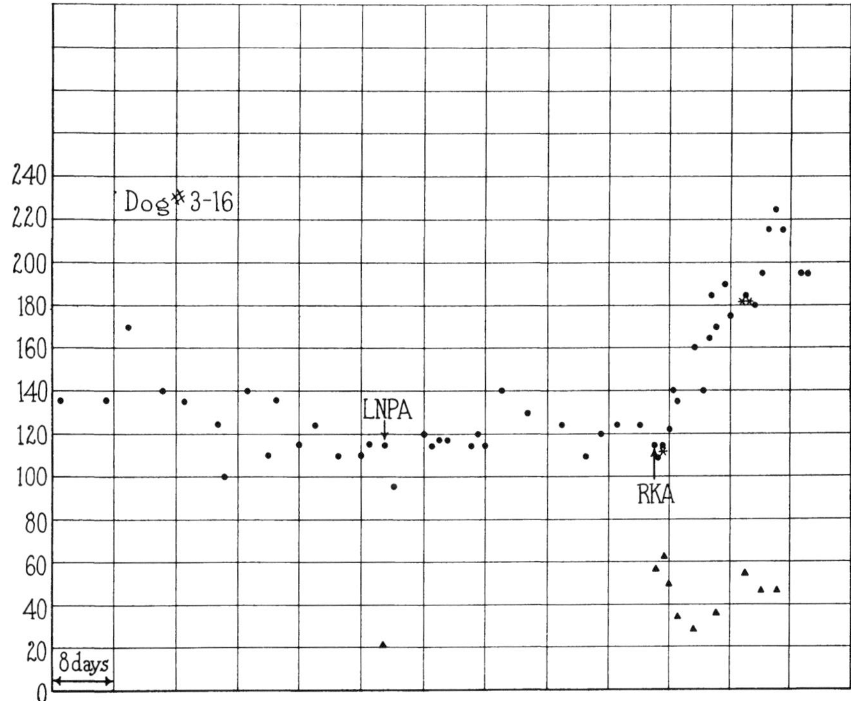

FIGURE 19. Dog 3–16. Female. 14.0 Kg.

● = Mean blood pressure, mm. Hg. ▲ = Non-protein nitrogen, mg. per 100 c.c. plasma. LNPA = Left nephrectomy and partial adrenalectomy. The medulla was destroyed. About two-fifths of the cortex was left. RKA = Right adrenalectomy and right main renal artery severely constricted. * = Sodium chloride (0.75 gm. per kg. of body weight) and sodium citrate (0.25 gm. per kg. of body weight) were given by stomach tube from this time on. ** = Sodium chloride and sodium citrate discontinued. No cortical extract was given at any time. The blood pressure rose moderately following the constriction of the renal artery and remained elevated when supportive treatment was discontinued. The animal is still living.

may result from these procedures on the nervous system due to relaxation of the arterioles in which the organic changes are not fixed. The beneficial effects reported in about the same percentage of cases of hypertension by surgeons using various procedures affecting the vasomotor nervous mechanism in the abdomen may therefore all be due to one cause, the improvement of the circulation through the kidney and not, as has been suggested by some, to the effect on the vasomotor mechanism of a large part of the vascular bed in the abdomen. The latter view has no support in these experiments. Whether or not improved circulation through the kidney is responsible for the effect should be put to the test by a large series of renal denervations alone in cases of human hypertension. If improvement of the circulation through the kidneys be the common basis of improvement as a result of all of the various surgical procedures that have been carried out, then denervation of the kidneys alone, if it can be accomplished, should give improvement in about the same small percentage of cases of hypertension.

The view that in the pathogenesis of hypertension due to renal ischemia a humoral mechanism involving a hypothetical effective substance of renal origin plays a part of primary importance is based almost entirely upon indirect evidence. Bilateral nephrectomy is not followed by hypertension, yet varying degrees of constriction and even complete occlusion of both main renal arteries are followed by hypertension. This difference is attributed to the absence of a hypothetical effective renal substance when the kidneys are absent. Even when both renal arteries are occluded, the hypothetical effective substance can still be formed and washed into the renal veins by the accessory circulation through the capsule. The constriction or occlusion of both main renal arteries, when accompanied by occlusion of the main renal veins, is not followed by the development of hypertension. This is interpreted as being due to interference with the entrance of the hypothetical effective substance into the circulation. Release of the constriction of the renal arteries, by unscrewing or removing the clamps, causes a prompt return of the blood pressure to normal. The release of the clamp on the main renal artery of only one of two ischemic kidneys is also followed by return of the blood pressure to normal, but it takes longer for the blood pressure to reach the normal than when both clamps are released. This is in keeping with the finding that the clamping of one main renal artery causes only a temporary rise of blood pressure for a varying period. Excision of the ischemic kidney at the height of the hypertension which follows constriction of one main renal artery is also followed by prompt return of the blood pressure to normal. These experiments indicate that if one or two normal kidneys could be transplanted into an animal with hypertension due to renal ischemia, the blood pressure would return to normal because the source of the effective renal substance would be eliminated. Such a study is being carried out at the present time in collaboration with Doctor J. R. Kahn and Doctor W. B. Wartman. Up to the present time the only direct evidence suggestive of the existence of an effective substance has been the demonstration by other investigators [11, 13] of an increased amount of pressor substance in ischemic kidneys as compared with normal ones.

Various experiments that have been carried out on the effect of complete adrenalectomy, with and without supportive and substitution therapy, and the effect of a small remnant of adrenal cortex only on the prevention or maintenance of hypertension due to renal ischemia, indicate that the medulla plays no part, but that the cortex of the adrenal gland may play an important part in the mechanism of development of this type of hypertension

Complete bilateral adrenalectomy, without supportive or substitution therapy, interfered with the development of this type of hypertension. Even with supportive treatment, but without substitution therapy, the animals failed to develop or to maintain hypertension due to renal ischemia. In several bilaterally adrenalectomized animals, however, moderate hypertension did develop when adequate supportive and substitution therapy was given. Because of this and because an amount of cortex close to the minimum requisite for survival and even the absence of both adrenals, if supplemented by the administration of cortical extract, still permitted the development of hypertension due to renal ischemia, the rationale of partial adrenalectomy which has been proposed and practised [127-133] for the treatment of hypertension is questionable to say the least, except in cases of suprarenal tumor [134-140] with hypertension in which the improvement results from the removal of the tumor in the adrenal.

The exact way in which the adrenal cortical hormone acts in conjunction with the hypothetical effective renal substance in the development and maintenance of hypertension due to renal ischemia has not been elucidated. Although the cortical hormone is not by itself a vasopressor substance, yet it may prepare the arteriolar musculature for the action of the hypothetical effective renal substance, or the reverse may be the case. The two may even combine before exerting their synergistic effect on the arteriolar musculature or they may act in conjunction with other hormones. These various possibilities are now being investigated.

Conclusions

Persistent hypertension has been produced in animals (dog and monkey) by constricting the main renal arteries, which reduces the blood flow to the functioning components of the kidneys (renal ischemia).

Hypertension without or with disturbance of renal function, resembling in this respect the benign and malignant types, respectively, in man, can be produced by varying the degree of constriction of the renal arteries.

The results of various experiments indicate that this type of experimental hypertension is due primarily to a humoral and not to a nervous mechanism initiated by the ischemia of the kidneys.

The nature of the effective substance responsible for inducing the hypertension has not yet been elucidated.

The present indication is that the adrenal cortical hormone plays a part in conjunction with the hypothetical effective substance of renal origin in the pathogenesis of hypertension due to constriction of the main renal arteries.

BIBLIOGRAPHY

1. Goldblatt, H., Lynch, J., Hanzal, R. F., and Summerville, W. W.: Experimental hypertension due to renal ischemia, Bull. Acad. of Medicine of Clev., 1932, xvi, 6. Preliminary report before the experimental section of the Academy of Medicine of Cleveland, Nov. 11, 1932.

2. Goldblatt, H., Lynch, J., Hanzal, R. F., and Summerville, W. W.: Studies on experimental hypertension. (1) The production of persistent elevation of systolic blood pressure by means of renal ischemia, Jr. Exper. Med., 1934, lix, 347.
3. Goldblatt, H., Gross, J., and Hanzal, R. F.: Studies on experimental hypertension. II. The effect of resection of splanchnic nerves on experimental renal hypertension, Jr. Exper. Med., 1937, lxv, 233.
4. Goldblatt, H.: Studies on experimental hypertension. III. The production of persistent hypertension in monkeys (macaque) by renal ischemia, Jr. Exper. Med., 1937, lxv, 671.
5. Longcope, W. T., and McClintock, A. T.: The effect of permanent constriction of the splanchnic arteries and the association of cardiac hypertrophy with arteriosclerosis, Arch. Int. Med., 1910, vi, 439.
6. Page, I. H.: Relationship of extrinsic renal nerves to origin of experimental hypertension, Am. Jr. Physiol., 1935, cxii, 166.
7. Page, I. H., and Sweet, J. E.: Extirpation of pituitary gland on arterial blood pressure of dogs with experimental hypertension, Proc. Soc. Exper. Biol. and Med., 1936, xxxiv, 260.
8. Elaut, L.: Hypertension artérielle chronique chez le chien par ischémie rénale, Compt. rend. Soc. de biol., 1936, cxxii, 126.
9. Wood, J. E., Jr., and Cash, J. R.: Experimental hypertension observations on sustained elevation of systolic and diastolic blood pressure in dogs, Jr. Clin. Invest., 1936, xv, 543.
10. Collins, D. A.: Hypertension from constriction of the arteries of denervated kidneys, Am. Jr. Physiol., 1936, cxvi, 616.
11. Harrison, T. R., Blalock, A., and Mason, M. F.: Effects on blood pressure of injection of kidney extracts of dogs with renal hypertension, Proc. Soc. Exper. Biol. and Med., 1936, xxxv, 38.
12. Page, I. H.: Vaso-pressor action of extracts of plasma of normal dogs and dogs with experimentally produced hypertension, Proc. Soc. Exper. Biol. and Med., 1936, xxxv, 112.
13. Prinzmetal, M., and Friedman, B.: Pressor effects of kidney extracts from patients and dogs with hypertension, Proc. Soc. Exper. Biol. and Med., 1936, xxxv, 122.
14. Bouckaert, J. J., Elaut, L., and Heymans, C.: Vasomotor carotid sinus reflexes in experimental hypertension produced by renal ischemia, Jr. Physiol., 1936, lxxxix, 3P.
15. Govaerts, P., and Dicker, E.: Mise en Évidence de Propriétés hypertensives dans le liquide céphalo-rachidien et dans le sang de néphritiques hypertendus, Bull. Acad. Roy. Méd., Belgium, VIe Serie, 1936, i, 131.
16. Dicker, E.: Existence de substances hypertensives dans le sang du chien pendant la compression permanente des artères rénaux, Compt. rend. Soc. biol., 1936, cxxii, 476.
17. Govaerts, P., and Dicker, E.: Production intrarénale de substances hypertensives par ligature ou pincement de l'artère rénal, Compt. rend. Soc. biol., 1936, cxxii, 809.
18. Collins, D. A., and Hoffbauer, F. W.: Effect of transfusion of blood from dogs with experimental renal hypertension into normal dogs, Proc. Soc. Exper. Biol. and Med., 1937, xxxv, 538.
19. Bright, R.: Cases and observations illustrative of renal disease accompanied with the secretion of albuminous urine, Guy's Hosp. Rep., 1836, i, 338.
20. Bright, R.: Tabular view of the morbid appearances in 100 cases connected with albuminous urine, Guy's Hosp. Rep., 1836, i, 380.
21. Fahr, Th.: Pathologische Anatomie des Morbus Brightii, Handbuch der speziellen pathologischen Anatomie und Histologie, VI/1 Niere, 156–472.
22*a*. Volhard, F., and Fahr, Th.: Die Brightsche Nierenkrankheit, Verlag von Julius Springer, Berlin, 1914.
22*b*. Volhard, F., and Suter, F.: Nieren und ableitende Harnwege, Handbuch der inneren Medizin, 1931, vi, 2 Teil, Verlag von Julius Springer, Berlin.

23. Kylin, E.: Über Hypertonie und Nierenkrankheit, Zentralbl. f. inn. Med., 1921, xlii, 441.
24. Kylin, E.: On the etiology of essential hypertension, Acta med. Scandinav., 1925, xvi, 282.
25. Mosler, E.: Über Blutdrucksteigerung nach doppelseitiger Nierenexstirpation, Ztschr. f. klin. Med., 1912, lxxiv, 297.
26. Backmann, E. L.: Einige Versuche über das Verhalten des Blutdruckes nach Nierenentfernung und Nierenverkleinerung, Ztschr. f. d. gesammt. exper. Med., 1916, iv, 63.
27. Cash, J. R.: Further studies of arterial hypertension, Proc. Soc. Exper. Biol. and Med., 1926, xxiii, 609.
28. Hartwich, A.: Der Blutdruck bei experimenteller Urämie und partieller Nierenausscheidung, Ztschr. f. d. ges. exp. Med., 1930, lxix, 462.
29. Grawitz, P., and Israel, O.: Experimentelle Untersuchungen über den Zusammenhang zwischen Nierenerkrankung und Herzhypertrophie, Virchow's Arch. f. pathol. Anat., 1879, lxxvii, 315.
30. Pässler, H., and Heineke, D.: Versuche zur Pathologie des Morbus Brightii, Verhandl. d. deutsch. path. Gesell., 1905, ix, 99.
31. Allen, F. M.: Auscultatory estimation of the blood pressure of dogs, Jr. Metab. Res., 1923, iv, 431.
32. Allen, F. M., Scharf, R., and Lundin, H.: Clinical and experimental renal deficiency, Jr. Am. Med. Assoc., 1925, lxxxv, 1698.
33. Lundin, H., and Mark, R.: Feeding of protein to partially nephrectomized animals, Jr. Metab. Res., 1925–1926, vii–viii, 221.
34. Anderson, H.: Experimental renal insufficiency. The effects of high protein diet in the presence of low renal function on the kidneys, aorta and liver; changes in the blood pressure and concentration of blood metabolites, Arch. Int. Med., 1926, xxxvii, 297.
35. Friedman, L., and Wachsmuth, W.: Experimentelle Studien zur Frage der renalen Hypertonie, Arch. f. exper. Path., 1930, cl, 173.
36. Chanutin, A., and Ferris, E. B.: Experimental renal insufficiency produced by partial nephrectomy, Arch. Int. Med., 1932, xlix, 767.
37. Rytand, D. A., and Dock, W.: Experimental concentric and eccentric cardiac hypertrophy in rats, Arch. Int. Med., 1935, lvi, 511.
38. Janeway, T. C.: Note on the blood pressure changes following reduction of the renal arterial circulation, Proc. Soc. Exper. Biol. and Med., 1908–9, vi, 109.
39. Janeway, T. C.: Nephritic hypertension: clinical and experimental studies, Am. Jr. Med. Sci., 1913, cxlv, 625.
40. Carrel, O.: Note on the production of kidney insufficiency by reduction of the arterial circulation of the kidney, Proc. Soc. Exper. Biol. and Med., 1909, vi, 107.
41*a*. Mark, R. E.: Ergebnisse partieller Nierenexstirpation am Tiere, Ztschr. f. exper. Med., 1925, xlvi, 1.
41*b*. Mark, R. E.: Untersuchungen über die Nierenfunction. Ergebnisse partieller Nierenarterienunterbindung am Hunde, Ztschr. f. exper. Med., 1928, lix, 601.
42. Cash, J. R.: A preliminary study of the blood pressure following reduction of renal substance with a note on simultaneous changes in blood chemistry and blood volume, Bull. Johns Hopkins Hosp., 1924, xxxv, 168.
43. Mark, R. E., and Giesendorfer, H.: Untersuchungen über die Nierenfunction: Zur Frage des Zusammenhanges von Nierenmasse Herzhypertrophie und Blutdrucksteigerung, Ztschr. f. d. ges. exper. Med., 1930, lxxiv, 350.
44. Ferris, E. B., and Heynes, J. F.: Indirect blood pressure readings in dogs: description of method and report of results, Jr. Lab. and Clin. Invest., 1931, xvi, 597.
45. Hartman, F. W., Bolliger, A., and Doub, H. P.: Experimental nephritis produced by irradiation, Am. Jr. Med. Sci., 1929, clxxii, 487.

46. SENATOR, H.: Über die Beziehungen des Nierenkreislaufs zum arteriellen Blutdruck und über die Ursachen der Herzhypertrophie bei Nierenkranken, Ztschr. f. klin. Med., 1911, lxxii, 189.
47. APFELBACH, C. W., and JENSEN, C. R.: Experimental renal insufficiency in dogs with special reference to arterial hypertension, Jr. Clin. Invest., 1931, x, 162.
48. KATZENSTEIN, M.: Experimenteller Beitrag zur Erkenntnis der bei Nephritis auftretenden Hypertrophie des linken Herzes, Virchow's Arch. f. path. Anat., 1905, clxxxii, 327.
49. LOESCH, J.: Ein Beitrag zur experimentellen Nephritis und zum arteriellen Hochdruck, Zentralbl. f. inn. Med., 1933, liv, 145, 177.
50. PEDERSEN, A. H.: A method of producing experimental chronic hypertension in the rabbit, Arch. Path., 1927, iii, 912.
51. BELL, E. T., and PEDERSEN, A. H.: The causes of hypertension, ANN. INT. MED., 1930, iv, 227.
52. MENENDEZ, E. B.: Stase veineuse du Rein normal ou énervé et hypertension artérielle, Compt. rend. Soc. de biol., 1933, cxiii, 461.
53. ALWENS, W.: Experimentelle Untersuchungen über die Bedeutung der mechanischen Theorie der nephritischen Blutdrucksteigerung, Deutsch. Arch. f. klin. Med., 1909, xcviii, 137.
54. HARRISON, T. R., MASON, M. F., RESNIK, H., and RAINEY, J.: Changes in blood pressure in relation to experimental renal insufficiency, Trans. Assoc. Am. Phys., 1936, ci, 281.
55. RAUTENBERG, E.: Erzeugung chronischer Nierenkrankungen mit folgender Blutdrucksteigerung und Arteriosklerose, Deutsch. med. Wchnschr., 1910, xxxvi, 51.
56. DOMINGUEZ, R.: Effect on the blood pressure of the rabbit of arteriosclerosis and nephritis caused by uranium, Arch. Path., 1928, v, 577.
57. ARNOTT, W. M., and KELLAR, R. J.: Hypertension associated with experimental oxalate nephritis, British Jr. Exper. Path., 1935, xvi, 265.
58. ARNOTT, W. M., and KELLAR, R. J.: The effect of renal denervation on the blood pressure in experimental renal hypertension, Jr. Path. and Bact., 1936, xlii, 141.
59. SCARFF, R. W., and McGEORGE, M.: Experimental renal lesions and blood pressure in rabbits, British Jr. Exper. Path., 1937, xviii, 59.
60. FREEMAN, N. E., and PAGE, I. H.: Presented before American Heart Assoc. June 7, 1937.
61. PRINZMETAL, M., and WILSON, C.: The nature of the peripheral resistance in arterial hypertension with special reference to the vasomotor system, Jr. Clin. Invest., 1936, xv, 63.
62. PICKERING, G. W.: The peripheral resistance in persistent arterial hypertension, Clin. Sci., 1936, ii, 209.
63. ROWNTREE, L. G., and ADSON, A. W.: Bilateral lumbar sympathetic neurectomy in the treatment of malignant hypertension, Jr. Am. Med. Assoc., 1925, lxxxv, 959.
64. ADSON, A. W., and BROWN, G. E.: Malignant hypertension. Report of a case treated by bilateral section of anterior spinal nerve roots from the sixth thoracic to the second lumbar inclusive, Jr. Am. Med. Assoc., 1934, cii, 1115.
65. CRAIG, W. M., and BROWN, G. E.: Unilateral and bilateral resection of major and minor splanchnic nerves. Its effects in cases of essential hypertension, Arch. Int. Med., 1934, liv, 577.
66. BROWN, G. E.: Sympathectomy for early malignant hypertension, Med. Clin. N. Am., 1934, lxviii, 577.
67. PEET, M. M.: Splanchnic section for hypertension, University Hosp. Bull. Ann Arbor, 1935, i, 17.
68. PAGE, I. H., and HEUER, G. J.: A surgical treatment of essential hypertension, Jr. Clin. Invest., 1935, xiv, 22.

69. Fralick, F. B., and Peet, M. M.: Hypertensive fundus oculi after resection of the splanchnic sympathetic nerves. A preliminary report, Arch. Ophth., 1936, xv, 840.
70. Heuer, G. J.: The surgical treatment of essential hypertension, Ann. Surg., 1936, civ, 771.
71. Crile, G. W.: Comparative anatomy and pathologic physiology of the adrenal-sympathetic complex with relation to the genesis and surgical treatment of essential hypertension, Jr. Mich. State Med. Soc., 1936, xxxv, 694.
72. Crile, G. W.: The surgical treatment of essential hypertension. Report of progress in 106 cases, Cleve. Clinic Quarterly, 1936, iii, 201.
73. Crile, G., and Crile, G., Jr.: Blood pressure changes in essential hypertension after excision of the celiac ganglion and denervation of the aortic plexus, Cleve. Clinic Quarterly, 1936, iii, 268.
74. Crile, G. W.: A critical review of 822 operations on the adrenal sympathetic system with special reference to essential hypertension, Ill. Med. Jr., 1936, lxx, 115.
75. Page, I. H., and Heuer, G. J.: Treatment of essential and malignant hypertension by section of anterior nerve roots, Arch. Int. Med., 1937, lix, 245.
76. Major, R. H.: Relationship between certain products of metabolism and arterial hypertension, Jr. Am. Med. Assoc., 1924, lxxxiii, 81.
77. Hülse, W., and Strauss, H.: Zur Frage der Blutdrucksteigerung. V. Über die Wirkung höherer Eiweisspaltprodukte auf den Blutdruck und ihr Vorkommen im Blute bei hypertonischen Nierenkrankheiten, Ztschr. f. exper. Med., 1924, xxxix, 426.
78. Hülse, W.: Zur Frage der Blutdrucksteigerung. IV. Experimentelle Untersuchungen über sensibilisierende Eigenschaften des Hypertonikerblutes, Ztschr. f. d. ges. exp. Med., Berlin, 1924, xxxix, 413.
79. Gheorghian, I., and Niculescu, Gh.: Recherches expérimentales sur la circulation générale avec le serum des malades hypertoniques, Compt. rend. Soc. biol., 1924, xc, 1163.
80. Major, R. H.: The possible relationship between guanidin and high blood pressure, Am. Jr. Med. Sci., 1925, clxx, 229.
81. Danzer, C. S., Brody, J. G., and Miles, A. L.: On the existence of a pressor substance in the blood of clinical cases of hypertension, Proc. Soc. Exper. Biol. and Med., 1926, xxiii, 454.
82. Danzer, C. S.: Further observations on the pressor substance in the blood of certain hypertensives, Am. Jr. Physiol., 1927, lxxxi, 472.
83. Major, R. H., and Weber, C. J.: The probable presence of increased amounts of guanidine in the blood of patients with arterial hypertension, Bull. Johns Hopkins Hosp., 1927, xl, 85.
84. Kahlson, G., and Werz, R.: Über Nachweis und Vorkommen gefässverengernder Substanzen im menschlichen Blute, Arch. f. exp. Path. u. Pharmak., 1928, cxlviii, 173.
85. Major, R. H.: Blood chemical studies in arterial hypertension, Am. Jr. Med. Sci., 1929, clxxvii, 188.
86. Hülse, W.: Experimentelle Untersuchungen zur Genese des essentiellen Hochdruckes, Arch. f. exper. Path., 1929, cxlvi, 282.
87. Anselmino, K. J., and Hoffmann, F.: Die Übereinstimmungen in den klinischen Symptomen der Nephropathie und Eklampsie der Schwangeren mit den Wirkungen des Hypophysenhinterlappenhormons, Arch. f. Gyn., 1931, cxlvii, 597.
88. Anselmino, K. J., and Hoffmann, F.: Nachweis der antidiuretischen Komponente des Hypophysenhinterlappenhormons und einer Blutdrucksteigernden Substanz im Blute bei Nephropathie und Eklampsie der Schwangeren, Klin. Wchnschr., 1931, x, 1438.
89. Major, R. H.: Chemical factors regulating blood pressure, Am. Jr. Med. Sci., 1932, clxxxiii, 81.
90. Bohn, H.: Untersuchungen zum Mechanismus des blassen Hochdrucks. I. Mitteilung gefässverengernde Stoffe im Blute beim blassen Hochdruck, Ztschr. f. klin. Med., 1932, cxix, 100.

91. Bohn, H.: Weitere Untersuchungen zum Mechanismus des blassen Hochdrucks, Zentralbl. f. inn. Med., 1932, liii, 1593.
92. Anselmino, K. J., Hoffmann, F., and Kennedy, W. P.: The relation of hyperfunction of the posterior lobe of the hypophysis to eclampsia and nephropathy of pregnancy, Edinburgh Med. Jr., 1932, xxxix, 376.
93. Lange, F.: Der Stoffliche Anteil an der Regulation des Kreislaufes und seine Bedeutung für die Hypertonie, Klin. Wchnschr., 1933, xii, 173.
94. Bohn, H., and Hahn, F.: Untersuchungen zum Mechanismus des blassen Hochdrucks. VI. Mitteilung blutdrucksteigernde Stoffe im Harn, insbesondere beim blassen und roten Hochdruck, Ztschr. f. klin. Med., 1933, cxxiii, 558.
95. Marx, H., and Hefke, K.: Untersuchungen zur Pathogenese der Hypertonie, Klin. Wchnschr., 1933, xii, 1318.
96. Scheps, M.: Beitrage zur Ätiologie der essentiellem Hypertonie und Eklampsie, Klin. Wchnschr., 1934, xiii, 1151.
97. Heinsen, H. A., and Wolf, H. J.: Tyramin als blutdrucksteigernde Substanz beim blassen Hochdruck, Klin. Wchnschr., 1934, ii, 1688.
98. Bohn, H., and Coestes, C.: Untersuchungen zum Mechanismus des blassen Hochdrucks. IX. Mitteilung. Pressorische und antidiuretische Stoffe im Harn beim blassen Hochdruck, Ztschr. f. klin. Med., 1934, cxxvi, 593.
99. Weiser, J.: Zum Nachweis von pressorischen Substanzen im Blute bei blassen Hochdruck, Zentralbl. f. inn. Med., 1934, lv, 65.
100. Heinsen, H. A., and Wolf, H. J.: Tyramin als blutdrucksteigernde Substanz beim blassen Hochdruck, Ztschr. f. klin. Med., 1935, cxxviii, 213.
101. Wolf, H. J., and Heinsen, H. A.: Tyramin und Nierendurchblutung, Arch. f. exp. Path. u. Pharmak., 1935, clxxix, 15.
102. Bohn, H., and Schlapp, W.: Untersuchungen zum Mechanismus des blassen Hochdrucks. XIII. Mitteilung. Weitere Erfahrungen über den Nachweis pressorischer Stoffe im Blute beim blassen Hochdruck, Ztschr. f. klin. Med., 1935, cxxvii, 233.
103. Pick, E. P.: Über humorale Uebertagung hohen und niedrigen Blutdrucks, Wien. klin. Wchnschr., 1935, xlviii, 634.
104. Hantschmann, L.: Über vasokonstriktorisch wirksame Stoffe im Blut mit besonderem Hinblick auf das Problem des Hochdrucks, Ztschr. f. exp. Med., 1935, xcvi, 442.
105. Stewart, G. N.: So-called biological tests for adrenalin in blood, with some observations on arterial hypertonus, Jr. Exper. Med., 1911, xiv, 377.
106. Bröking, E., and Trendelenburg, P.: Adrenalinnachweis und Adrenalingehalt des menschlichen Blutes, Deutsch. Arch. f. klin. Med., 1911, ciii, 168.
107. Curtis, F. R., Moncrieff, A. A., and Wright, S.: The supposed presence of a pressor substance in the blood of patients with high blood pressure, Jr. Path. and Bact., 1927, xxx, 55.
108. Turries, J., and Robert, S.: La guanidine du Sang, Presse méd., 1930, xxxviii, 85.
109. Wakerlin, G. E., and Bruner, H. D.: The question of the presence of a pressor substance in the blood in essential hypertension, Arch. Int. Med., 1933, lii, 57.
110. Theobald, G. W.: The alleged relation of hyperfunction of the posterior lobe of the hypophysis to eclampsia and the nephropathy of pregnancy, Clin. Sci., 1933–1934, i, 225.
111. de Wesselow, O. L. V., and Griffith, W. J.: On the question of pressor bodies in the blood of hypertensive subjects, Brit. Jr. Exper. Path., 1934, xv, 45.
112. Hurwitz, D., and Bullock, L. T.: Failure to find pressor and antidiuretic substances in patients with toxemia of pregnancy, Am. Jr. Med. Sci., 1935, clxxxix, 613.
113. Page, I. H.: Pressor substances from the body fluids of man in health and disease, Jr. Exper. Med., 1935, lxi, 67.
114. Aitken, R. S., and Wilson, C.: An attempt to demonstrate a pressor substance in the blood in malignant hypertension, Quart. Jr. Med., 1935, iv, 179.
115. Capps, R. B., Ferris, E. B., Taylor, F. H., and Weiss, S.: Rôle of pressor substances in arterial hypertension, Arch. Int. Med., 1935, lvi, 864.

116. Friedman, B., and Prinzmetal, M.: Vasomotor effects of blood in patients with hypertension, Proc. Soc. Exper. Biol. and Med., 1936, xxxiv, 543.

117. Prinzmetal, M., Friedman, B., and Rosenthal, N.: Nature of peripheral resistance in arterial hypertension, Proc. Soc. Exper. Biol. and Med., 1936, xxxiv, 545.

118. Tigerstedt, R., and Bergman, P. G.: Niere und Kreislauf, Skand. Arch. f. Physiol., 1898, viii, 223.

119. Hessel, G., and Hans, M. H.: Über das Renin, einen körpereigenen kreislaufwirksamen Stoff, Verhandl. deutsch. Ges. inn. Med., 1934, xlvi, 347.

120. Collip, J. B.: A non-specific pressor principle derived from a variety of tissues, Jr. Physiol., 1928, lxvi, 416.

121. Stewart, G. N., and Rogoff, J. M.: Studies on adrenal insufficiency, Proc. Soc. Exper. Biol. and Med., 1925, xxii, 394.

122. Stewart, G. N., and Rogoff, J. M.: Studies on adrenal insufficiency. IV. The influence of intravenous injections of Ringer's solution upon the survival period in adrenalectomized dogs, Am. Jr. Physiol., 1928, lxxxiv, 649.

123. Marine, D., and Baumann, E. J.: Duration of life after suprarenalectomy in cats and attempts to prolong it by injections of solutions containing sodium salts, glucose and glycerol, Am. Jr. Physiol., 1927, lxxxi, 86.

124. Loeb, R. F., Atchley, D. W., Benedict, E. M., and Leland, J.: Electrolyte balance studies in adrenalectomized dogs with particular reference to the secretion of sodium, Jr. Exper. Med., 1933, lvii, 775.

125. Harrop, G. A., Soffer, L. J., Nicholson, W. M., and Strauss, M.: Studies on the suprarenal cortex. IV. The effect of sodium salts in sustaining the supra-renalectomized dog, Jr. Exper. Med., 1935, lxi, 839.

126. O'Connor, J. M.: Über den Adrenalingehalt des Blutes, Arch. f. exp. Path. u. Pharmakol., 1912, lxvii, 195.

127. Galata, G.: Di un caso d'ipertensione climaterica colla surrenectomia unilaterale, Riforma med., 1929, xlv, 1449.

128. Monier-Vinard and Desmarest: Hypertension artérielle permanente et primitive avec paroxysmes hypertensifs démesures. Influence de la rachianesthésie, de la surrénalectomie, de la radiothérapie et de la ponction lombaire, Bull. et mém. Soc. méd. d. hôp. de Paris, 1930, liv, 1084.

129. Piere, G.: Tentativi di cura chirurgica dell' ipertensione arteriosa essenziale, Riforma med., 1932, xlviii, 1173.

130. DeCourcy, J. L., DeCourcy, C., and Thuss, O.: Subtotal bilateral suprarenalectomy for hypersuprarenalism, Jr. Am. Med. Assoc., 1934, cii, 1118.

131. DeCourcy, J. L.: The technique of adrenalectomy and adrenal denervation, Am. Jr. Surg., 1935, xxx, 404.

132. DeCourcy, J. L.: Subtotal bilateral adrenalectomy for the relief of essential hypertension, Jr. Med., 1935, xvi, 244.

133. DeCourcy, J. L.: Surgical treatment of hypertension, Jr. Med., 1936, xvii, 505.

134. Labbé, Tinel and Doumer: Crises solaires et hypertension paroxystique, en rapport avec une tumeur surrénale, Bull. et mém. Soc. méd. d. hôp. de Paris, 1922, xlvi, 982.

135. Oberling, C., and Jung, G.: Paragangliome de la surrénale avec hypertension, Bull. et mém. Soc. méd. d. hôp. de Paris, 1927, li, 366.

136. Pincoffs, M. C.: A case of paroxysmal hypertension associated with suprarenal tumor, Trans. Assoc. Am. Phys., 1929, xliv, 295.

137. Rabin, C. B.: Chromaffin cell tumor of the suprarenal medulla, Arch. Path., 1929, vii, 228.

138. Shipley, A. M.: Paroxysmal hypertension associated with tumor of suprarenal, Ann. Surg., 1929, xc, 742.

139. Wilder, R. M.: Recently discovered endocrine diseases; hyperepinephrinism, hyperinsulinism and hyperparathyroidism, Internat. Clin., 1930, i, 293.

140. Eisenberg, A. A., and Wallerstein, H.: Pheochromocytoma of suprarenal medulla, Arch. Path., 1932, xiv, 818.

Factors of Risk in the Development of Coronary Heart Disease—Six-Year Follow-up Experience

The Framingham Study

William B. Kannel, m.d., Thomas R. Dawber, m.d., f.a.c.p.,
Abraham Kagan, m.d., f.a.c.p., Nicholas Revotskie, m.d.,
and Joseph Stokes, III, m.d.
Framingham, Massachusetts

Increasingly reliable estimates of the prevalence and incidence of coronary heart disease (CHD) emphasize the importance of this disease as a contemporary health hazard. Cardiovascular disease is now the leading cause of death, with coronary heart disease accounting for two-thirds of all heart disease deaths. While advances in the diagnosis and therapeutic management of CHD have been made in the past decade, no important reduction in morbidity and mortality from CHD has occurred. This is apparent in the relatively slight increase in life expectancy at age 40 which has been achieved in the past several decades, while life expectancy at birth has been substantially prolonged.

Because coronary heart disease is often manifested as sudden unexpected death or "silent" infarction and since the immediate mortality in those surviving to enter a hospital is still distressingly high in spite of the best therapeutic efforts, it appears that a preventive program is clearly necessary. Since it has been established that coronary atherosclerosis is present for many years prior to the development of symptomatic CHD, it seems evident that efforts at prevention must begin many years before the appearance of clinical CHD. A knowledge of the epidemiology of the disease is highly desirable if a program of prevention is to be developed. From a study of the characteristics of persons who develop coronary heart disease under observation in comparison with those who remain free of disease it is possible to determine the characteristics of susceptible individuals. This allows the identification of the coronary prone individual many years before the occurrence of clinically recognizable disease.

Multiple interrelated factors have been demonstrated to be associated with increased risk of development of CHD. To date no single essential factor has been identified. However, epidemiologic information has accumulated which now allows the physician to recognize certain characteristics of increased risk in patients he sees in his practice. Some of these characteristics have been convincingly demonstrated, others are still under investigation. More precise identification will undoubtedly be possible in the future.

The present report deals with three characteristics believed to be associated with proneness to the development of CHD: elevated serum cholesterol levels, hypertension, and the electrocardiographic pat-

Received for publication April 19, 1961.

From the Heart Disease Epidemiology Study, Framingham, Mass., and the National Heart Institute, National Institutes of Health, Public Health Service, U. S. Department of Health, Education, and Welfare, Washington, D. C.

Presented at the Forty-second Annual Session, The American College of Physicians, May 8–12, 1961, Bal Harbour, Fla.

Requests for reprints should be addressed to Thomas R. Dawber, M.D., F.A.C.P., Medical Director, Heart Disease Epidemiology Study, 25 Evergreen St., Framingham, Mass.

tern of left ventricular hypertrophy. These characteristics have been demonstrated to be associated qualitatively with the development of CHD in a previous report (1). No precise estimate of the magnitude of the increased risk could be made at that time. The present report represents two more years of observation and allows more detailed analysis of these factors as they affect both men and women. Sufficient data have now been accumulated to permit quantitative estimation of the increase in risk associated with these characteristics singly and in combination.

Because of the apparent need to obtain more epidemiologic data in coronary heart disease, a study was established in Framingham, Massachusetts, during the period 1948 to 1950. The Framingham Study was designed to investigate the incidence of cardiovascular disease and factors related to its development. Details of the organization and first four-year follow-up experience have been previously reported (1–5).

Methods

A description of the town of Framingham, the method of selection of the study population, and the response of selected persons has been previously reported (1, 5, 6). Of the 6,507 persons selected at random, 4,469 persons aged 30 to 59 came in for examination and comprised the sample population. An additional 740 persons who volunteered to cooperate in the Study have also been included. The rationale for including the group of volunteers has been discussed elsewhere (1, 5). While the sample and volunteer groups differ in a number of minor particulars, none of the recorded differences appears to present any difficulties in analysis (5). The incidence of new coronary heart disease in the two groups is very similar. Accordingly, these two groups have been combined.

All subjects have been examined in a clinic set up for the Study. A detailed history and a physical examination were completed by a physician assigned to the Study and the findings were entered on standard forms. If any possibility of the new development of CHD was considered, the opinion of a second physician was obtained. Laboratory studies included chest X ray, electrocardiogram, vital capacity determination, urinalysis, hemoglobin, hematocrit, blood glucose, uric acid, lipoproteins, cholesterol, phospholipid, and other special studies.

Upon completion of each examination a diagnosis was made using uniformly applied criteria as indicated below. An abstract of the findings was sent to the personal physician indicated by the subject. No medical advice was provided to any participant beyond encouragement to visit his physician if the need was indicated.

CRITERIA FOR CORONARY HEART DISEASE

The criteria used for the classification of coronary heart disease in the Framingham Study are based upon those recommended by the New York Heart Association (7).

1. Angina pectoris: Minimal criteria for the diagnosis of angina pectoris consisted of substernal discomfort of brief duration (i.e., two to three minutes), definitely related to exertion or emotional upset, promptly relieved by rest, and seldom if ever occurring during periods of quiet or rest. The diagnosis was made when symptoms were sufficiently clear cut to allow at least two observers to agree readily as to its presence. Because of the subjective nature of this diagnosis, no possible or questionable instances are included in the group designated as having coronary heart disease.

2. Myocardial infarction: This diagnosis was made only in the presence of electrocardiographic changes of infarction.* All

* Recent or acute myocardial infarction was designated when S-T segment elevation was present associated with late inversion of T waves and the occurrence of loss of initial QRS potentials (i.e., development of "pathological" Q waves of four

TABLE 1. Composition of Framingham Study Group

	Total	Men	Women
Random sample	6,507	3,074	3,433
Respondents	4,469	2,024	2,445
Volunteers	740	312	428
Respondents free of CHD*	4,393	1,976	2,417
Volunteers free of CHD	734	307	427
Total free of CHD:			
Framingham Study Group	5,127	2,283	2,844

* Coronary heart disease.

hospital records and electrocardiograms were reviewed by the Study personnel. In cases that lacked a history, the development of an unequivocal pattern of myocardial infarction since the previous electrocardiographic tracing was obtained, was accepted as evidence of an unrecognized myocardial infarction. In addition, for the purpose of the present analysis, instances of prolonged acute coronary insufficiency with associated electrocardiographic abnormality were included in this category.

3. Sudden death: This was considered to be due to CHD when it was documented to have occurred in a matter of minutes and was attributed to no other cause by the physician who completed the death certificate and when no other cause of death was suggested by prior medical history. All death certificates and information available regarding the death of the patient were reviewed by clinic personnel.

Whenever available, autopsy information was utilized only to confirm the clinical diagnosis of CHD. The autopsy rate was not high enough to use post-mortem findings as a basis for diagnosis.

hundredths of a second duration or greater), followed by serial changes of evolution if available.

An old or remote myocardial infarction was considered to be present when there was a pathological Q wave of four hundredths of a second duration or greater, or loss of initial QRS potential (R-wave) in those leads in which this would not be expected to occur. This electrocardiographic diagnosis was also considered when changes from a previous tracing indicated a loss of R wave potential previously present and not otherwise explained. More weight was given to this finding if T wave abnormality was also associated. In all instances electrocardiograms antedating the event were available for comparison, a factor of considerable assistance in evaluating patterns of old myocardial infarction.

COMPOSITION OF STUDY GROUP

Table 1 shows the composition of the population being observed for the development of coronary heart disease. The population at risk of developing CHD consisted of those persons who were free of this disease at the initial examination. Of the 6,507 persons selected for study, 4,469 responded and were examined. Of these, 4,393 were found to be free of CHD and were suitable for follow-up study. Of the 740 volunteers, 734 were free of disease. Thus, a group of 5,127 persons free of CHD on entry to the study could be periodically re-examined for the subsequent development of disease; they constituted the Framingham Study Group.

FOLLOW-UP

Of the original study group it was possible to re-examine 87% at the clinic on the fourth biennial examination or later (Table 2). Another 2.4% are known to have died before their fourth examination was due. For this group the cause of death has been ascertained and in each instance

TABLE 2. Six-Year Follow-Up: Framingham Study Group

	Number	Per Cent
Framingham Study Group	5,127	100.0
Examined at clinic at Exam IV*	4,478	87.3
Not examined at clinic at Exam IV*	649	12.7
Dead before Exam IV*	122	2.4
Alive at Exam IV*	523	10.2
Unknown whether alive or dead	4	0.1

* Fourth biennial examination.

TABLE 3A. Six-Year Incidence of CHD* by Age and Sex

	Framingham Study Group		Sample Respondents		Volunteers	
Age at Entry	New CHD	Population at Risk	New CHD	Population at Risk	New CHD	Population at Risk
Men	125	2,283	106	1,976	19	307
30–34	5	388	4	333	1	55
35–39	11	438	9	388	2	50
40–44	15	420	13	357	2	63
45–49	15	352	14	308	1	44
50–54	27	353	19	301	8	52
55–59	41	262	36	221	5	41
60–62	11	70	11	68	—	2
Women	61	2,844	52	2,417	9	427
30–34	—	453	—	388	—	65
35–39	—	582	—	489	—	93
40–44	3	508	3	433	—	75
45–49	16	446	13	376	3	70
50–54	14	421	10	357	4	64
55–59	24	371	22	313	2	58
60–62	4	63	4	61	—	2

* Coronary heart disease.

documentation has been sought to determine whether coronary heart disease had developed by the time of death. From observation of the population at subsequent examinations at the clinic, routine surveillance of admissions to the local hospitals, and inquiries made of friends and relatives appearing at the clinic for examination it was possible to reach a conclusion about the state of health with respect to CHD for another 10.2%. In many instances the physicians of the community, knowing of our interest in the problem, have advised us of the development of new disease in our subjects. It is considered to be unlikely that a significant number of new events of CHD have been missed in the six years of follow-up.

RESULTS

INCIDENCE AND CLINICAL MANIFESTATION OF HEART DISEASE IN SIX YEARS OF OBSERVATION

The incidence of coronary heart disease (defined above as myocardial infarction, angina pectoris, and sudden death) is shown in Tables 3 A and B. The population at risk for this observation was composed of all subjects found to be free of CHD at entry into the Study. There were 186 men and women free of definite CHD at the first examination who developed the disease in the subsequent six years of observation. This represents an over-all six-year incidence of 36.3 per thousand in the age groups under study. The six-year incidence of coronary heart disease in the men was 54.8 per thousand as compared with 21.4 per thousand in the women. In the younger age group (30 to 44 years) there was an incidence of 1.9 per thousand in women as compared with 24.9 per thousand in men (a thirteenfold difference). In the older age group (45 to 62 at entry into the Study) this sex ratio becomes attenuated to only a twofold difference with an incidence of 90.6 per thousand in men as compared with 44.6 per thousand in women. As indicated in Table 4, 24 of the 88 men who developed myocardial infarction* died suddenly.

* All sudden deaths are considered to be myocardial infarctions.

TABLE 3B. Six-Year Incidence Rate of New CHD by Age and Sex

Age at Entry	Rate per 1,000 Population: Framingham Study Group	Sample Respondents	Volunteers
Men	54.8	53.6	61.9
30–44	24.9	24.1	29.8
45–62	90.6	89.1	100.7
Women	21.4	21.5	21.1
30–44	1.9	2.3	0
45–62	44.6	44.3	46.4

Of these, 15 (62.5%) had no previous evidence of CHD and this constituted the only known manifestation of the disease. Seven of the men who suffered myocardial infarction had no clinical evidence of the event other than the development of characteristic electrocardiographic evidence of infarction, and the disease would have been undetected unless periodic routine electrocardiograms were undertaken in apparently well individuals. Three of 19 women who suffered myocardial infarction manifested the disease as sudden death. All of these occurred as the first reported manifestation of CHD.

There is clearly a difference in the predominant clinical manifestation of coronary heart disease in the sexes (Table 4). The CHD appearing in the women was predominantly angina pectoris without associated myocardial infarction (69%). This is in contrast to the men in whom angina pectoris without associated myocardial infarction constituted only 30% of the coronary heart disease developing in the six years of observation. Among all cases of

TABLE 4. Clinical Manifestations of CHD Developing in Six Years of Follow-Up

Clinical Manifestation	Number: Men	Number: Women	Per Cent: Men	Per Cent: Women
Total CHD	125	61	100.0	100.0
Definite myocardial infarction by history and ECG*	57	14	45.6	23.0
With AP†	32	7		
Without AP†	25	7		
Definite myocardial infarction by ECG only	7	2	5.6	3.3
Sudden death	24	3	19.2	4.9
With pre-existing MI‡	3	—		
With pre-existing AP†	6	—		
Without pre-existing CHD	15	3		
Definite angina pectoris	37	42	29.6	68.8

* Electrocardiogram.
† Angina pectoris.
‡ Myocardial infarction.

TABLE 5. Mean Serum Cholesterol at Initial Examination: Comparison New CHD and Population at Risk

Age at Entry	Number		Mean		Standard Deviation of Population
	New CHD	Population at Risk	New CHD	Population at Risk	
Men					
30–34	5	375	257*	219	45
35–39	11	419	267*	222	42
40–44	14	402	259*	229	46
45–49	14	341	250*	231	37
50–54	27	338	245*	227	40
55–59	41	252	248*	229	43
Women					
40–44	3	480	316*	222	39
45–49	14	423	286*	240	48
50–54	13	403	239	250	46
55–59	24	355	260	258	48

* Significantly elevated (at the 5% level) compared with population at risk.

CHD, myocardial infarction with or without associated angina pectoris occurred as the manifestation of CHD approximately twice as frequently in the male coronary subjects as in the female. The incidence of angina pectoris in subjects with myocardial infarction, however, is about the same in the sexes.

SERUM CHOLESTEROL

The data presented here are based on determinations of serum cholesterol which were made in the Framingham Laboratory by the method of Abell, Levy, Brodie, and Kendall (8). During the period when much of the data was being collected, the laboratory standardized its results by exchange

TABLE 6. Six-Year Incidence of CHD According to Initial Serum Cholesterol Level: Ages 40–59

Serum Cholesterol (mg/100 ml)	New CHD	Population at Risk	Incidence Rate per 1,000 Population	
			Observed	Expected*
Men, 40–59	96†	1,333	72.0	70.6
Less than 210	16	454	35.2‡	69.4
210–244	29	455	63.7	70.8
245 or more	51	424	120.3‡	71.8
Women, 40–59	54†	1,661	32.5	32.7
Less than 210	8	445	18.0	25.2
210–244	16	527	30.4	31.3
245 or more	30	689	43.5	38.7

* Expected rate is calculated by applying age-sex-specific incidence rates (five-year age interval) in the Framingham Study Group to the population in the specified category of sex and cholesterol.

† Total number of new cases of CHD and the population at risk varies in different tabulations since it was not possible to obtain blood specimens on every subject.

‡ Significantly different (at the 5% level) from the expected rate.

TABLE 7A. Mean Systolic and Diastolic Blood Pressures at Initial Exam. Comparison of New CHD and Population at Risk

Age and Sex	Number of Persons		Systolic Blood Pressure			Diastolic Blood Pressure		
			Mean		Standard Deviation,	Mean		Standard Deviation,
	New CHD	Population at Risk	New CHD	Population at Risk	Population	New CHD	Population at Risk	Population
Men								
30–34	5	388	128	131	16	83	83	11
35–39	11	438	144*	132	17	95*	85	12
40–44	15	420	133	135	18	90	87	12
45–49	15	352	144	138	21	93*	88	12
50–54	27	353	148*	140	22	90	89	13
55–59	41	262	162*	145	27	96*	88	15
Women								
40–44	3	508	125	131	20	81	83	12
45–49	16	446	158*	142	24	97*	87	12
50–54	14	421	171*	150	30	96	90	14
55–59	24	371	178*	154	31	100*	91	15

* Significantly elevated (at the 5% level) compared with population at risk.
Note: Blood pressures are available for everyone in the Study Group. This is not true for other measures.

of serum lipids with the four laboratories participating in the Cooperative Lipoprotein Study (9).

Higher mean cholesterol levels were demonstrated among subjects who developed coronary heart disease than in the population at risk (Table 5). This indicates an association between serum cholesterol levels and the subsequent development of CHD. In men, serum cholesterol levels tended to be higher for those who subsequently developed CHD in the six years of observation than in the population at risk. This elevation was most marked for men in the youngest age group and diminished with age. Beyond age 59 there were too few persons in the Study for analysis.

The risk associated with serum cholesterol level was analyzed in men in the broad age group, 40 to 59 years at entry into the Study (Table 6). Separation of the men in the population at risk into three categories according to increasing levels of serum cholesterol yields groups of similar size when dividing points are made at levels of 210 and 245 mg per 100 ml. Analysis of these groups reveals a gradient of risk of developing CHD with increasing levels of serum cholesterol, such that those with serum cholesterols over 244 mg per 100 ml have more than three times the incidence of CHD as do those with cholesterol levels less than 210 mg per 100 ml (Table 6). This cannot be attributed to aging within the group studied since no significant gradient of serum cholesterol with age can be demonstrated in men (Table 5). In evaluating the risk associated with elevation of serum cholesterol levels it is important to recognize that in the Framingham population the reference base for serum cholesterol (i.e., "normal" cholesterol) may be high when compared with some other populations in which lower rates of CHD have been claimed.

Since no new coronary heart disease developed in women less than 40 years of age at entry into the Study, no analysis of the association of serum cholesterol level with the risk of CHD was possible. A significant elevation of mean serum cholesterol is evident for women 40 to 49 years old who de-

TABLE 7B. Mean Systolic and Diastolic Blood Pressures at Initial Exam: Comparison of New CHD and Population at Risk, Framingham Study Group Without Left Ventricular Hypertrophy by Electrocardiogram

Age and Sex	Number of Persons		Systolic Blood Pressure			Diastolic Blood Pressure		
			Mean		Standard Deviation, Population	Mean		Standard Deviation, Population
	New CHD	Population at Risk	New CHD	Population at Risk		New CHD	Population at Risk	
Men								
30–34	4	382	128	131	15	84	82	10
35–39	11	426	144*	132	16	95*	84	11
40–44	14	407	133	135	17	90	87	12
45–49	14	336	140	137	20	91	87	11
50–54	24	337	145	139	21	90	88	13
55–59	31	238	158*	143	25	92*	87	14
Women								
40–44	3	501	125	130	19	81	83	12
45–49	15	439	157*	141	23	96*	87	12
50–54	13	397	164*	147	26	93	90	13
55–59	21	357	173*	152	29	97*	90	15

* Significantly elevated (at the 5% level) compared with population at risk.
Note: Blood pressures are available for everyone in the Study Group. This is not true for other measures.

veloped coronary heart disease but not for women 50 to 59 years old (Table 5). However, a significant (although not striking) gradient of risk with increasing cholesterol levels could be demonstrated for the entire group of women aged 40 to 59 years (Table 6).

BLOOD PRESSURE AND ASSOCIATED CHARACTERISTICS

It was evident on the basis of the four-year follow-up experience that elevation of blood pressure was associated with an increased risk of the development of CHD among men 45 to 62 years of age (1). The occurrence of additional cases of new CHD during two more years of observation permits the analysis of this factor to be extended to younger men and to women.

In Tables 7A and B are shown the mean blood pressures of the population at risk (those free of coronary heart disease at the initial examination) and of those of the group who developed CHD during the six years of observation. Among both men and women aged 45 to 59 years on entry, blood pressures, either systolic or diastolic, were significantly higher in the group who subsequently developed CHD than in the whole population at risk. Outside of this age range, the association of elevated blood pressure levels with CHD is not consistently significant. As indicated in Table 8 progressive degrees of blood pressure elevation were associated with increased risk of the subsequent development of CHD. Hypertension associated with the electrocardiographic pattern of left ventricular hypertrophy (LVH by ECG) was associated with a higher incidence of coronary heart disease than was hypertension alone.

It was not possible on the basis of the data to assign greater importance to the diastolic than to the systolic blood pressure level as a predictor of subsequent coronary heart disease. This can be explained by the high correlation between systolic and diastolic blood pressure. Two other values of blood pressure measurement, pulse pressure and systolic lability, were also considered. Both of these measures varied with the level of systolic pressure and both were higher in the coronary group than in the population as a whole. Elevation of either measure, however, did not contribute independently to the risk of subsequent CHD. As previously noted, the electrocardiographic finding of left ventricular hypertrophy is associated with an unusually high risk of the subsequent development of CHD among men age 40 to 59 years (Table 8). Within six years one-third of the men 40 to 59 years of age with this finding had developed overt CHD, as had one-fifth of these men with "possible" LVH by electrocardiogram. The relative infrequency of CHD among women and among younger men during the six years of observation precluded the demonstration of a comparable association among them, though the data are suggestive for older women.

Several possible explanations for the high incidence of coronary heart disease associated with left ventricular hypertrophy by ECG are suggested. It is possible that the group with this finding includes a sizable proportion with subclinical CHD at entry. This might happen if electrocardiographic evidence of LVH masked evidence of CHD in the ECG or if the electrocardiographic patterns for the two conditions could be confused. It could also happen if, in fact, the LVH pattern was an indicator of CHD. These possibilities led to a preliminary analysis excluding persons with left ventricular hypertrophy by electrocardiogram from the population at risk. The effect of this on the analysis of blood pressure can be judged by com-

TABLE 8. Six-Year Incidence Rate of CHD by Blood Pressure Category and Electrocardiogram of Left Ventricular Hypertrophy: Ages 40 to 59

Sex, Hypertensive Status, ECG Evidence of LVH*	Number of Persons		Incidence Rate per 1,000 Population	
	New CHD	Population at Risk	Observed	Expected
Men, 40 to 59	98	1,387	70.7	70.7
Normotension	23	556	41.4	68.8
Borderline hypertension	38	532	71.4	68.6
Definite hypertension	37	299	123.7	77.8
Definite hypertension and ECG evidence:				
No LVH	27	265	101.9	75.8
Possible LVH	3	15	200.0	78.4
Definite LVH	7	19	368.4	105.1
Women, 40 to 59	57	1,746	32.6	32.6
Normotension	6	704	8.5	26.5
Borderline hypertension	20	647	30.9	35.0
Definite hypertension	31	395	78.5	39.8
Definite hypertension and ECG evidence:				
No LVH	26	357	72.8	40.0
Possible LVH	1	19	52.6	34.6
Definite LVH	4	19	210.5	42.2

* Left ventricular hypertrophy.

Note: Expected rate is calculated by applying the age-sex-specific incidence rates (in five-year age intervals) of the Framingham Study Group to the population in the specified sex-hypertension LVH category.

TABLE 9. Mean Systolic and Diastolic Blood Pressures According to Presence or Absence of ECG Evidence of LVH at Initial Examination: Men Aged 45 to 62

ECG Evidence of LVH	New CHD	No CHD
	Mean Systolic Pressure	
Total	154	140
Definite or possible LVH	171	162
No LVH	149	139
	Mean Diastolic Pressure	
Total	93	87
Definite or possible LVH	100	98
No LVH	91	87
	Number of Men Aged 45–62	
Total	94	943
Definite or possible LVH	18	45
No LVH	76	898

paring the results displayed in Table 7A with those in Table 7B. There is a very slight reduction in the association between CHD and blood pressure when the group having LVH by ECG is excluded from the analysis. In general, the omission of this group from the analysis of the factors related to the development of coronary heart disease under consideration in this paper had only a minor effect.

Another possibility which may explain the association of left ventricular hypertrophy by electrocardiogram with the development of CHD is a strong inter-relationship between the electrocardiographic pattern and hypertension. The electrocardiographic abnormality may well reflect either long standing or sevère degrees of hypertension. Among the men without LVH by ECG, those who developed coronary heart disease had blood pressures which were higher on the average by 10.4 mm systolic and by 3.9 mm diastolic compared with those who did not develop CHD (Table 9). A similar elevation of blood pressure in those who developed CHD is found within the group of men with definite or possible LVH by ECG. This indicates that blood pressure is associated with the risk of developing coronary heart disease independently of the presence or absence of left ventricular hypertrophy by electrocardiogram.

Whether left ventricular hypertrophy by electrocardiogram is associated with the risk of developing coronary heart disease independently of blood pressure levels is not as easily evaluated. Blood pressures are much higher in the small group with LVH by ECG than in those without it, and this in itself should enhance the risk of developing CHD. How much of the excess risk associated with the electrocardiographic finding is accounted for by elevated blood pressure is difficult to judge because of the small number of cases and because of the large sampling variability in incidence rates among men with this electrocardiographic finding. However, reference to Table 10 indicates the effect of left ventricular hypertrophy by electrocardiogram in blood pressure diagnostic categories. It can be seen that at each diagnostic blood pressure category, the presence of LVH by ECG is associated with an excess incidence of coronary heart disease. Left ventricular hypertrophy by ECG appears to make an

TABLE 10. Six-Year Incidence of CHD According to Hypertensive Status and ECG Evidence of LVH at Initial Exam: Men Aged 40 to 59

Hypertension	LVH Present	LVH Absent
	Incidence Rate per 1,000	
None	200.0	38.5
Borderline	120.0	69.0
Definite	294.1	101.9
	New CHD	
None	2	21
Borderline	3	35
Definite	10	27
	Population at Risk	
None	10	546
Borderline	25	507
Definite	34	265

Note: LVH means definite or "possible" left ventricular hypertrophy.

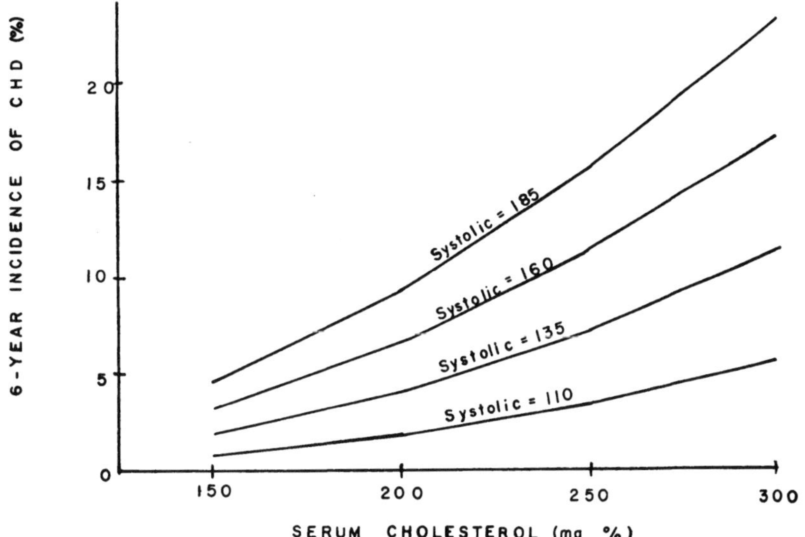

FIGURE 1. Six year incidence of coronary heart disease according to serum cholesterol levels at specified systolic blood pressures (men 45 to 62 years). These curves are based on the following assumptions: (1) The joint distribution of the logarithms of blood pressure value minus 75 and cholesterol value is bi-variate normal within both the coronary heart disease and non-coronary heart disease groups; (2) The variance-covariance matrices in the coronary heart disease and non-coronary heart disease groups are equal (14).

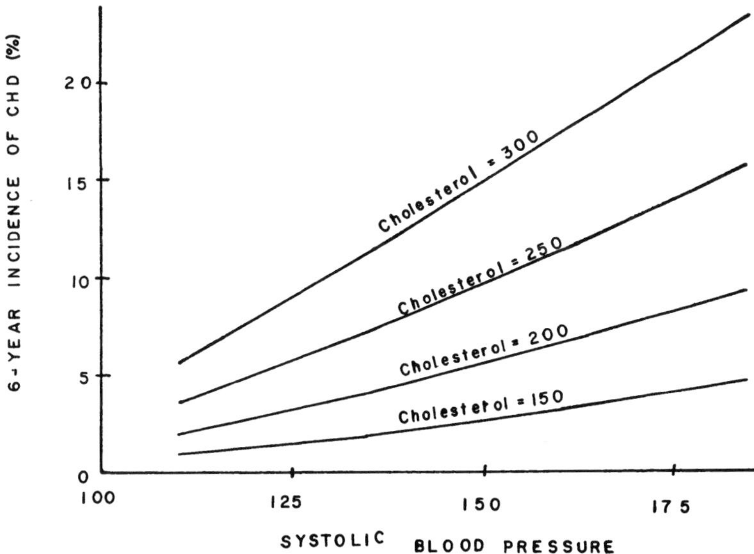

FIGURE 2. Six-year incidence of coronary heart disease according to level of systolic blood pressure at specified serum cholesterol levels (men 45 to 62 years). For explanation, see legends for Figure 1.

TABLE 11. Six-Year Incidence of CHD, According to Combinations of Blood Pressure, Serum Cholesterol, and ECG Evidence of LVH at Initial Exam: Ages 40–59

Sex and Combinations of Blood Pressure, Serum Cholesterol, and ECG Evidence of LVH	Population at Risk		New CHD	Incidence Rate per 1,000 Population	
	Number	Per Cent		Observed	Expected
Men, 40 to 59	1,333	100.0	96	72.0	70.6
Normal* on all three	811	60.8	29	35.8	67.5
Abnormal* on one only	416	31.2	43	103.4	73.6
Blood pressure	186	14.0	17	91.4	76.8
Cholesterol	207	15.5	25	120.8	70.4
LVH	23	1.7	1	43.5	76.4
Abnormal* on two only	98	7.4	20	204.1	81.4
BP and cholesterol	65	4.9	10	153.8	74.1
BP and LVH	25	1.9	6	240.0	87.7
Cholesterol and LVH	8	0.6	4	500.0	121.4
Abnormal* on all three	8	0.6	4	500.0	102.9
Abnormal* on two or three	106	8.0	24	226.4	83.0
Women, 40 to 59	1,661	100.0	54	32.5	32.7
Normal* on all three	888	53.5	15	16.9	27.2
Abnormal* on one only	597	35.9	24	40.2	38.1
Blood pressure	206	12.4	14	68.0	38.0
Cholesterol	382	23.0	10	26.2	38.2
LVH	9	0.5	—	0	37.9
Abnormal* on two only	162	9.8	13	80.2	42.1
BP and cholesterol	134	8.1	10	74.6	43.3
BP and LVH	23	1.4	3	130.4	35.8
Cholesterol and LVH	5	0.3	—	0	39.5
Abnormal* on all three	14	0.8	2	142.9	42.7
Abnormal* on two or three	176	10.6	15	85.2	42.2

* Abnormal blood pressure is defined as definite hypertension, abnormal cholesterol is a serum cholesterol reading of 260 mg/100 ml or higher, and abnormal LVH is a diagnosis of possible or definite LVH on the electrocardiogram. "Normal" means not abnormal; it includes normotension and borderline hypertension, serum cholesterol less than 260 mg/100 ml, no LVH by ECG.

independent contribution to the risk of development of CHD, increasing the risk of development of coronary heart disease two to threefold when blood pressure is held constant. Because of the small numbers it was necessary to examine the broad age group 40 to 59 years in men and hence it is not possible to assess completely the possible effect of age.

INTERACTION OF HYPERTENSION, HYPERCHOLESTEROLEMIA, AND THE ELECTROCARDIOGRAPHIC PATTERN OF LEFT VENTRICULAR HYPERTROPHY

Data already presented indicate that hypertension, hypercholesterolemia, and the electrocardiographic pattern of left ventricular hypertrophy are each associated with an increased risk of the development of CHD in men 40 to 59 years of age. It has been previously shown (1) that there is almost no correlation between serum cholesterol level and diastolic or systolic blood pressure. Left ventricular hypertrophy by ECG is strongly associated with hypertension, and has been shown to contribute to risk of development of CHD (Tables 8 and 9). At each level of blood pressure in hypertensives the presence of LVH is associated with a two to threefold increase in incidence of CHD (Table 10). Consequently each of these characteristics would be expected to contribute to the risk of development of CHD and combinations of these factors could be expected to augment the risk. From Figures 1 and 2 it can be seen that the incidence of CHD does indeed rise progressively with increasing levels of both blood pressure and serum cholesterol and that a combination of these two factors further augments the risk. In Table 11 the six-year incidence of coronary heart disease in persons having various combinations of these three characteristics is given. Men aged 40 to 59 years, normal in all these characteristics, had a six-year incidence of CHD of only 35.8 per thousand. When abnormal with respect to one of these characteristics the risk almost tripled (103.4 per thousand). If abnormal in two of these characteristics the six-year incidence climbs to 204.1 per thousand, approximately doubling the risk associated with abnormality in one characteristic. Abnormality in all three characteristics probably again doubles the incidence, but because of small numbers available and sampling variability, it is not possible to assess this risk reliably. Abnormality of two or more of these risk characteristics is associated with a six-year incidence of 226.4 per thousand. Approximately the same magnitude of compounding of risk associated with these characteristics (hypertension, hypercholesterolemia, and the ECG pattern of left ventricular hypertrophy) is seen in women 40 to 59 years of age. The incidence rates are generally lower, women normal in all three characteristics having an incidence of 16.9 per thousand, rising to 40.2 per thousand when abnormal in only one characteristic, and doubling to 80.2 per thousand when two abnormal characteristics are present. When two or more factors are abnormal, a six-year incidence of 85.2 per thousand is noted.

These risk characteristics are found with some frequency in the population: 39% of men and 46% of women 40 to 59 years of age have at least one of these abnormal characteristics, while 8% of men and 11% of women have two or more of these abnormal characteristics.

Discussion

The rarity of coronary heart disease in the younger female (two per thousand) is in sharp contrast to the incidence of this disease in the male of the same age (25 per thousand) as indicated in Table 3B. This sex differential is greater than the differences in incidence produced by any other factor thus far investigated in this disease. Clearly, any statement regarding the etiology of CHD will have to explain the sex ratio. This also indicates a fruitful area for research into the pathogenetic mechanism of this disease. The gap between the sexes closes after age 45 so that only a twofold difference exists. This strongly suggests, among other things, an endocrine influence related to the menopause.

Not only the incidence, but the clinical manifestation of CHD appeared to differ markedly in the sexes (Table 4). Coronary heart disease in the female is manifested chiefly as angina pectoris. Seventy per cent of all CHD occurring in females exhibited this manifestation. In the male, on the other hand, the disease is manifested chiefly as myocardial infarction or sudden death with only 30% exhibiting angina pectoris alone. The percentage of sudden death in men (19.2%) greatly exceeded that in women (4.9%). Myocardial infarction was approximately twice as frequently exhibited by men. It thus appears that the seriousness of the disease developed in the two sexes as well as the incidence differs markedly.

On the basis of clinical studies it is commonly believed that angina pectoris occurs predominantly in males (10). Data presented in Table 4 indicate that if all cases of angina pectoris occurring in a community are considered, rather than only those presenting themselves for medical care, angina pectoris is as common in the female as in the male. In six years of follow-up of persons initially free of CHD 124 cases of angina pectoris developed. In 79 instances this occurred alone, in 39 instances the angina was associated with myocardial infarction, and in six instances it antedated sudden death. Of the 79 instances of angina pectoris unassociated with myocardial infarction 42 occurred in women (53.2%), while of the 39 cases of angina pectoris associated with myocardial infarction only seven were in women (17.9%). Forty per cent of all angina encountered in the study population occurred in women. Angina pectoris in association with myocardial infarction was more common in men.

It is widely accepted that sudden death (occurring within a matter of minutes) is usually the result of coronary heart disease with or without coronary occlusion (11). This is especially likely if other possible causes such as aortic valvular deformity, pulmonary embolism, and aortic dissection or rupture can be excluded. Examination of the Framingham Study subjects prior to the event and careful evaluation of the circumstances under which the sudden death occurred renders it unlikely, although still possible, that these other etiologies were responsible for the deaths. It is recognized that sudden death may be the only manifestation of CHD (11). It has not been possible up until now, however, to determine how often sudden death occurs as the initial manifestation of CHD. In the six years of observation of men in the Framingham Study group, 24 sudden deaths occurred. Nine (37.5%) of these had pre-existing evidence of coronary heart disease (six had angina pectoris and three had myocardial infarction). Thus 62.5% of all sudden deaths attributed to CHD in men occurred as the initial manifestation of the disease.

TABLE 12. Immediate Mortality Following Initial Myocardial Infarction: Men in Framingham Study Group

	Total	Survived*	Died within Three Weeks
Hospitalized	49	43	6
Not hospitalized	39	19	20†
Total	88	62	26

* Known living up to time of report or died of other causes after two-year survival. All survivals in excess of two months.

† All sudden deaths.

It can be seen from Table 12 that there is a high immediate mortality associated with myocardial infarction. For purposes of this discussion sudden death is classified as myocardial infarction. Of 88 cases of myocardial infarction in men occurring in the six years of observation, 26 (29.5%) died within three weeks of the initial infarction. Indeed, 20 of the 26 (77%) deaths wihin three weeks were sudden, occurring in a matter of minutes.

It is also noteworthy that approximately 45% of those with the initial myocardial infarction never got hospitalized. Of these, one-half never had the opportunity to be hospitalized because of the occurrence of sudden death. Approximately 25% of those not hospitalized had unrecognized infarctions discovered only because of routine electrocardiographic studies on biennial examinations. Thus approximately 70% of the initial infarctions not hospitalized in the community never had the opportunity to be hospitalized in order to receive the benefits of therapeutic medicine. Indeed, the majority of these could not even be seen by a physician prior to their demise. Of the 49 who survived to enter a hospital, six (12.2%) died shortly after admission (only one survived more than ten days). As indicated previously 15 of the 24 (62.5%) sudden deaths which occurred had no prior evidence of coronary heart disease. These data suggest to the authors that in efforts to control CHD, major emphasis must be placed on prevention.

Six years of follow-up experience in the longitudinal prospective study of coronary heart disease in Framingham have confirmed the widely recognized influence of hypertension and hypercholesterolemia on the development of CHD. These factors have been noted in clinical studies to occur in excess in persons with coronary heart disease, and in animal experiments to be associated with the development of atherosclerosis. It is now demonstrated that these factors *precede* the development of overt CHD in humans and are associated with increased risk of the development of CHD. The association of these factors with the subsequent development of coronary heart disease has been independently demonstrated in other longitudinal studies (12, 13). In addition, it is now demonstrated that the electrocardiographic pattern of left ventricular hypertrophy is also associated with increased risk of developing CHD.

It is now possible to assess the magnitude of the increase in risk associated with these characteristics. It can be seen from Table 8, by comparing the ratios of observed to expected incidence rates, that hypertension, as defined, is associated with a 2.6-fold increase in risk of development of CHD in men 40 to 59 years of age and a sixfold increase in women in the same age. This represents a considerable increase in risk. Of interest also is the comparison of risk in the sexes. It is often stated that women tolerate hypertension better than do men. Insofar as the relationship between hypertension and coronary heart disease is concerned, the six-year incidence figures do not support this thesis. If the independent contribution of hypertension to risk is assessed by holding the other factors which contribute to risk constant (i.e., left ventricular hypertrophy by electrocardiogram and elevated serum cholesterol), then, of the three characteristics under consideration, hypertension represents a greater relative increase in risk in women than in men although the absolute incidence of CHD in women never reaches that of men in any category (Table 11). Elevation of serum cholesterol level (i.e., 245 mg per 100 ml or more) is associated with more than a threefold increase in risk in men aged 40 to 59, while in women of the same age a 1.6-fold increase is noted (Table 6). As seen in a comparison of Table 6 and Table 8, and in Table 11, when blood pressure and left ventricular hypertrophy factors are removed from consideration, the independent contribution of cholesterol (at slightly higher levels of 260 mg per 100 ml or greater) to risk in women is further reduced so that cholesterol levels contribute only slightly to the increased risk among women but very significantly among men. Some of the increased risk is undoubtedly attributable to a higher mean age of women with higher cholesterol level, since cholesterol increase with age occurs to a greater extent in women than in men. It thus appears that, in assessing the contribution to risk of developing CHD, of the three factors under consideration, hypertension represents a greater risk factor for women than for men, whereas for serum cholesterol levels the converse is true, cholesterol contributing only slightly to the increased risk among women, but very significantly increasing risk among men.

Combinations of the three risk factors under consideration appear to augment further the risk of subsequent development of coronary heart disease. It has been demonstrated (Figures 1 and 2 and Table 11) that the incidence of coronary heart disease rises progressively as these factors are combined.

There can be no doubt that absence of these characteristics is distinctly advantageous since such persons demonstrate a relatively low risk of developing CHD. Whether or not the correction of these abnormalities once they are discovered will favorably alter the risk of development of disease, while reasonable to contemplate and perhaps attempt, remains to be demonstrated.

As additional longitudinal observations are made, it is hoped that additional risk factors will be determined. This will allow further identification of susceptible individuals and hopefully suggest methods of control.

Summary and Conclusions

A six-year longitudinal study is reported of a stratified random sample of the population of Framingham, Massachusetts, aged 30 to 59 years, covering factors related to the development and clinical manifestations of coronary heart disease. The factors studied include blood pressure, serum cholesterol levels, and certain electrocardiographic abnormalities. Follow-up of the study group free of CHD at the initial examination has been reasonably complete.

One hundred and eighty-six men and women aged 30 to 59 years on entry into the study developed coronary heart disease in the six years of observation, representing an over-all six years' incidence of 36.3 per thousand. In the younger age group, 30 to 44 years, a male to female ratio of 13 to 1 was noted. In the older age group, 45 to 62 years, this sex ratio became attenuated to only a twofold difference.

In addition to incidence, the clinical manifestations of CHD were noted to differ markedly in the sexes. Coronary heart disease in the female was noted to be manifested chiefly as angina pectoris (70%). In the male, the disease was manifested chiefly as myocardial infarction or sudden death, with only 30% exhibiting angina pectoris alone. The incidence rate of sudden death was ten times as common in men (10.5 per 1,000) as in women (1 per 1,000) and the incidence rate of myocardial infarction was five times as high in men. Contrary to general belief, uncomplicated angina pectoris was noted to occur as frequently in women as in men; 53% of all such angina pectoris developing in the population occurred in women. Only angina pectoris in association with myocardial infarction was noted to be more common in men.

It has been noted that 62.5% of all sudden deaths attributed to coronary heart disease in men occurred as the initial manifestation of the disease. A high immediate mortality was noted to be associated with myocardial infarction. Of 88 cases of myocardial infarction in men, 26 (29.5%) died within three weeks of the initial infarction. Of those with initial myocardial infarction 44% were not hospitalized, half of these because of the occurrence of sudden death. Another 23% of those not hospitalized had infarctions that were unrecognized. Thus three of four initial infarctions not hospitalized in the community could not have been hospitalized owing to sudden death or unrecognized infarction. Of those who survived to enter a hospital, 12.2% died shortly after admission.

The well-recognized influence of hypertension and hypercholesterolemia on the development of coronary heart disease is confirmed. It is now demonstrated that these factors precede the development of overt CHD and are associated with increased risk of its development. In addition, it is now demonstrated that the electrocardiographic pattern of left ventricular hypertrophy is also associated with increased risk of developing CHD.

The magnitude of the increase in risk associated with these characteristics has been assessed. Hypertension has been noted to be associated with a 2.6-fold increase in risk in men 40 to 59 years of age and a six-fold increase in women the same age. With respect to the development of coronary heart disease, hypertension was noted to represent a greater risk factor in women than in men, while elevated serum cholesterol levels contributed only slightly to increased risk among women as compared with men. Elevation of serum cholesterol levels (i.e., 245 mg per 100 ml or more) was associated with more than a threefold increase in risk among men aged 40 to 59 years.

A pattern of left ventricular hypertrophy by electrocardiogram was noted to be associated with a two or three-fold increase in risk of development of CHD at given hypertensive blood pressure levels in men. Combinations of these risk factors (hypertension, elevated serum cholesterol level, and left ventricular hypertrophy by electrocardiogram) were noted to augment further the risk of development of CHD. Men 40 to 59 years of age, lacking these three abnormal characteristics, were noted to have a six-year incidence of coronary heart disease of 35.8 per thousand. When all of these characteristics were present the incidence rose to approximately 500 per thousand. These risk characteristics were shown to occur with sufficient frequency in the population to merit concern, 8% of men and 11% of women having two or more of these abnormal characteristics. At least one abnormal characteristic was present in over 40% of the population aged 30 to 59 years.

Summario in Interlingua

Un specimen de 5.127 subjectos de etates de 30 a 59 annos, le quales initialmente esseva libere de morbo cardiac coronari, esseva observate durante sex annos. In le curso de iste intervallo, 125 masculos e 61 feminas disveloppava manifestationes de morbo cardiac coronari. Inter le 34 casos in le gruppo de etates ab 30 ad 44 annos, le proportion mascule a feminin de incidentia esseva 13 a 1. Inter le 152 casos in le gruppo de etates ab 45 ad 62 annos, le proportion mascule a feminin del incidentia esseva approximativemente 2 a 1. Le incidentia de angina de pectore esseva plus o minus equal pro le duo sexos. Tamen, infarcimento myocardial esseva duo vices plus commun in masculos e morte subite dece vices.

In masculos, un alte mortalitate immediate (30%) esseva associate con infarcimento myocardial initial (incluse mortes subite). Quaranta-cinque pro cento de 88 masculos suffrente infarcimento myocardial non esseva hospitalisate, primarimente a causa del facto que morte superveniva subitemente o que le infarcimento myocardial non esseva recognoscite como tal.

Factores de risco esseva evalutate in le gruppo de etates inter 40 e 59 annos. Hypertension (160/95 mm de Hg o plus) esseva associate con un quasi triplice augmento del risco in homines e un sextuple augmento in feminas. Elevation del nivello seral de cholesterol (245 mg per 100 ml o plus) esseva associate con un augmento plus que triplice del risco in masculos, durante que illo contribueva pauco (o nihil del toto) al augmento del risco in feminas. Le configuration electrocardiographic de hypertrophia sinistro-ventricular esseva associate con un augmento duplice o triplice del risco de un disveloppamento de morbo cardiac coronari.

Combinationes del tres characteristicas resultava in un augmento progressive in le risco de disveloppar morbo cardiac coronari, durante que subjectos libere de omne le mentionate anormalitates disveloppava le morbo a un prorata de solmente un medietate de illo del population total de iste studio. Le anormalitates occurreva in le population con un frequentia sufficientemente alte pro meritar nostre sollicitude.

References

1. Dawber, T. R., Moore, F. E., Jr., Mann, G. V.: II. Coronary heart disease in the Framingham Study. *Amer. J. Public Health* 47: 4, 1957.
2. Dawber, T. R., Meadors, G. F., Moore, F. E., Jr.: Epidemiological approaches to heart disease: the Framingham Study. *Amer. J. Public Health* 41: 279, 1951.
3. Dawber, T. R., Moore, F. E.: Longitudinal study of heart disease in Framingham, Massachusetts. An interim report: research in public health. 1951 Annual Conference of the Milbank Memorial Fund. *Milbank Mem. Fund Quart.* 1952.
4. Dawber, T. R., Kannel, W. B.: An epidemiological study of heart disease: the Framingham Study. *Nutr. Rev.* 16: 1, 1958.

5. Gordon, T., Moore, F. E., Jr., Shurtleff, D., Dawber, T. R.: Some methodologic problems in the long-term study of cardiovascular disease: observations on the Framingham Study. *J. Chron. Dis.* 10: 186, 1959.
6. Dawber, T. R., Kannel, W. B., Revotskie, N., Stokes, J., III, Kagan, A., Gordon, T.: Some factors associated with the development of coronary heart disease. Six years' follow-up experience in the Framingham Study. *Amer. J. Public Health* 49: 1349, 195 9.
7. *Nomenclature and Criteria for Diagnosis of Diseases of the Heart and Blood Vessels,* Criteria Committee of the N. Y. Heart Association, 5th Ed., New York, 1953.
8. Abell, L. L., Levy, B. B., Brodie, B. B., Kendall, F. E.: A simplified method for the estimation of total cholesterol in serum and the demonstration of its specificity. *J. Biol. Chem.* 195: 357, 1952.
9. Technical Group, Committee on Lipoproteins and Atherosclerosis of the National Advisory Heart Council: An evaluation of serum lipoproteins and cholesterol measurements as predictors of clinical complications of atherosclerosis: a report of a cooperative study of lipoproteins and atherosclerosis. *Circulation* 14: 691, 1956.
10. Friedberg, C. K.: *Diseases of the Heart,* 2nd Ed., W. B. Saunders Company, Philadelphia, 1956, p. 455.
11. Friedberg, C. K.: *Diseases of the Heart,* 2nd Ed., W. B. Saunders Company, Philadelphia, 1956, pp. 317, 433, 543.
12. Doyle, J. T., Heslin, S. A., Hilleboe, H. E., Formel, P. F., Korns, R. F.: A prospective study of degenerative cardiovascular disease in Albany: report of three years' experience. I. Ischemic heart disease. *Amer. J. Public Health* 47: 25, 1957.
13. Chapman, J. M., Goerke, L. S., Dixon, W., Loveland, D. B., Phillips, E.: The clinical status of a population group in Los Angeles under observation for two to three years. *Amer. J. Public Health* 47: 43, 1957.
14. Cornfield, J., Gordon, T., Smith, W.: Quantal response curves for experimentally uncontrolled variables. *Proceedings of the 32nd Session of the International Statistical Institute, Tokyo, 1960. To be published.*

SECTION IV

ENDOCRINOLOGY

Addison's disease: evaluation of synthetic desoxycorticosterone acetate therapy in 158 patients.

Thorn GW, Dorrance SS, Day E. Ann Intern Med. 1942;16:1053-1096.

In clinical medicine, a defining experience can direct practice. In this article, George Thorn and colleagues evaluated the use of synthetic desoxycorticosterone acetate (DOCA) to treat patients with Addison's disease. I was privileged to inherit one of the patients in Thorn's 1942 report from his practice when he retired. The story of this patient's clinical response to a DOCA pellet implant was riveting. His life was rapidly transformed from a bed-bound existence to a restored sense of well-being, amelioration of anorexia and nausea, and weight gain. The patient was able to return to work; however, he remained mildly symptomatic and continued to experience episodes of acute adrenal insufficiency with sepsis. He was eventually restored to full health when cortisone acetate became available.

Thorn and colleagues described 158 patients treated with DOCA. Sixty-four patients were under direct observation at The Johns Hopkins Hospital, and 94 were treated by physicians elsewhere. The crucial finding was a dramatic reduction in the comparative mortality rate with "specific" (DOCA) therapy compared with historical controls and patients treated with adrenal extract.

The report provides detailed demographic data and dosing schedules for patients treated with daily intramuscular DOCA in sesame oil or with once-yearly subcutaneous pellet implantations. Although DOCA represented a significant advance over treatment with adrenocortical extract, it also posed a therapeutic challenge, since this potent mineralocorticoid was used for its weak glucocorticoid actions. The metabolic studies performed at Johns Hopkins that counseled clinicians on the balance between a DOCA dosage sufficient to ameliorate the symptoms of glucocorticoid deficiency and dietary sodium to avoid such complications as edema and hypertension were an important contribution to clinical practice.

Thorn and colleagues' article heralds the age of clinical research which was to follow, and it stands as an outstanding example of the importance of controlled metabolic studies in the investigation of adrenocortical diseases. It remains a management primer for adrenal insufficiency even in the modern era, in which specific glucocorticoid and mineralocorticoid treatments are available to treat primary adrenal insufficiency. The authors commented that abnormalities in carbohydrate metabolism continued despite DOCA treatment, setting the stage for our current understanding of the different metabolic actions of glucocorticoid and mineralocorticoid hormones. They also recognized that the adrenal cortex participates in the "stress response," noting rapid deterioration of patients into adrenal crisis in the setting of intercurrent infection unless they received DOCA supplementation, and proposed techniques for preparing patients with Addison's disease for surgery.

Primary aldosteronism, a new clinical entity.

Conn JW, Louis LH. Ann Intern Med. 1956;44:1-15.

The early 1950s was the dawn of the era of mineralocorticoid research. Extraordinary clinical investigators, such as Luetscher, Liddle, and Bartter were performing metabolic studies in such disease states as congestive heart failure and cirrhosis, documenting excessive levels of a salt-retaining factor found in human urine. In 1954, Simpson and Tait reported the isolation and structural characterization of aldosterone. Enter Jerome Conn and Lawrence Louis, who described a new clinical entity: primary aldosteronism. Their article was a paradigm of the new science of clinical investigation. Conn and Louis performed extensive metabolic balance studies before, during, and after surgery over 227 days on a single patient. The clinical and biochemical description of this patient—hypertension without edema, muscle weakness, and hypernatremia and hypokalemic alkalosis with alkaline urine—defined this new syndrome. Conn and Louis chose the term "primary aldosteronism" because the patient was ultimately found to have a 4-cm adrenocortical adenoma; that is, the disease originated in the adrenal gland. They used the term "secondary aldosteronism" to describe conditions usually associated with edema, in which they reasoned that a "metabolic event . . . triggers the production of excessive quantities of aldosterone" (subsequently found to be an activated renin–angiotensin system).

Postoperative studies in the patient showed reversal of hypertension and the electrolyte abnormalities. Of note, Conn and Louis observed that compared with preoperative values, "urinary sodium-retaining corticoid" was undetectable on postoperative bioassay. Their speculations in the Comment section of the article pointed researchers into new directions. Conn and Louis guessed that because the remaining contralateral adrenal gland was hypofunctional and anatomically atrophic, the hyperaldosteronism "did suppress something"—but not adrenocorticotropic hormone, since cortisol production was normal.

Conn and Louis wondered about the relationship between the hyperaldosteronism and hypertension. They also predicted that some patients with this syndrome would not have an adenoma at surgery, foreseeing that primary aldosteronism results from bilateral hyperplasia. Conn and Louis surmised that when it became possible to accurately measure urinary aldosterone, a substantial percentage of hypertensive patients would be found to have primary aldosteronism. In fact, screening of hypokalemic–hypertensive patients revealed a low prevalence of this disorder ([1%). Accurate measurements of plasma aldosterone and plasma renin activity in blood as screening tests (the ratio of these two substances) have confirmed Conn and Louis's earlier prediction. Most studies now agree that the prevalence of primary aldosteronism in essential hypertension is approximately 10%.

Our current understanding of the pathophysiology of primary aldosteronism is that aldosterone production is viewed as inappropriate for the level of sodium intake.

Hypertension ensues in this setting, but recent evidence also indicates that long-term exposure to excess aldosterone results in direct cardiovascular damage. Conn and Louis would have enjoyed this recent chapter in the disorder that they so elegantly defined.

Nonenzymatic glycosylation and the pathogenesis of diabetic complications.

Brownlee M, Vlassara H, Cerami A. Ann Intern Med. 1984;101:527-537.

Brownlee and colleagues hypothesized that nonenzymatic glycosylation of a number of substrates, including proteins and nucleic acids, formed the basis of diabetic complications. They proposed an understanding of the biochemical basis of these progressive complications. Two types of nonenzymatic glycosylation were described. One type involved Amadori products, proteins with half-lives of days to weeks; accumulation of these proteins had been extensively studied using human hemoglobin as a model protein. The other type of glycosylation involved long-lived proteins (e.g., collagen, elastin, myelin) that turned over at a much slower rate such. As a result, nonenzymatic glycosylation—which could modify such processes as enzyme activity, binding of regulatory molecules, cross-linking of proteins, and immunogenicity—could alter physiologic processes.

At the time this article was published, there were two opposing schools of thought regarding diabetic complications. One ignored hyperglycemia as causal, invoking other factors; the other proposed that attempts to achieve normoglycemia would provide benefit. Brownlee and colleagues' hypothesis strengthened the role of control of hyperglycemia. They found, in vitro, that "Glucose concentration and incubation time are the most clinically relevant variables affecting the extent of nonenzymatic glycosylation, because only these two variables have counterparts that also differ in vivo." The other variables that affected glycosylation in vitro (pH, temperature, protein concentration, and NH2 microenvironment) were constant in vivo. Brownlee and colleagues concluded that long-term diabetic complications result from nonenzymatic glycosylation due to chronic hyperglycemia. They wisely admonished that current epidemiologic data suggested that for any given level of sustained hyperglycemia, some patients seemed to be at greater risk. Nonetheless, their article provided a rationale for performing studies that compared outcomes in patients with rigorous glycemic control versus usual care—for example, the Diabetes Control and Complications Trial conducted from 1983 to 1993 in 1400 patients with type 1 diabetes who were randomized to standard therapy or intensive control. This trial found that lowering the blood glucose level reduces risk for eye disease by 76%, kidney disease by 50%, and nerve disease by 60%.

It is now acknowledged that normoglycemia is an important clinical goal, and one glycosylated protein (hemoglobin A1c) is an easily measured analyte that helps the clinician and the patient achieve this goal. We also now know that the pathogenesis of diabetic microvascular and macrovascular complications is complex, involving alterations in endothelial function, inflammation, dyslipidemia, and genetic factors. Nevertheless, the Brownlee hypothesis merits acclaim for stimulating clinicians to consider control of hyperglycemia on the basis of a plausible biochemical mechanism of disease.

ANNALS OF
INTERNAL MEDICINE

VOLUME 16 JUNE, 1942 NUMBER 6

ADDISON'S DISEASE: EVALUATION OF SYNTHETIC DESOXYCORTICOSTERONE ACETATE THERAPY IN 158 PATIENTS*

By GEORGE W. THORN, F.A.C.P., SAMUEL S. DORRANCE,† and EMERSON DAY,‡ *Baltimore, Maryland*

INTRODUCTION

THE immediate and favorable response of patients with Addison's disease to synthetic desoxycorticosterone acetate therapy is now well established.[1, 2, 3, 4, 5] The effect which treatment with desoxycorticosterone acetate will have on the life expectancy of patients with Addison's disease cannot be stated at this early date, although our experience indicates that there has been a considerable reduction in mortality rate during the first 18 months of therapy.

The present report summarizes our experience with synthetic desoxycorticosterone acetate therapy during the past three years. In this period 158 patients with classical signs and symptoms of Addison's disease have been treated with the synthetic hormone. Sixty-four patients have been under our direct observation in The Johns Hopkins Hospital, and 94 patients have been treated by physicians elsewhere. The majority of these patients (148) have received subcutaneous implantations of pellets of crystalline hormone * following a carefully conducted assay period in which the optimum daily maintenance dose of hormone was determined by means of a single daily intramuscular injection of hormone in oil (4 to 12 weeks).

* Received for publication April 4, 1942.
From the Chemical Division, Department of Medicine, The Johns Hopkins University and Hospital. This study was aided by a grant from the Committee on Research in Endocrinology, National Research Council.

† Dazian Foundation Fellow in Medicine, Chemical Division, Department of Medicine.
‡ Emanuel Libman Fellow in Medicine, Department of Medicine.

* In all instances we have used standardized sterile pellets of crystalline desoxycorticosterone acetate weighing approximately 125 mg., which were provided through the courtesy of the Ciba Pharmaceutical Products, Inc., Summit, N. J.

In this report data relating to the age and sex of the patients, etiology of the disease, hormone requirement and mortality rate will be presented for the entire group of 158 patients. More detailed observations relating to the course of the disease during treatment, changes in body weight, blood pressure, blood chemistry, electrocardiogram and electroencephalogram will be limited to the group of 64 patients who were directly under our observation

TABLE I

Etiology of Addison's Disease in a Group of 158 Patients Treated with Desoxycorticosterone Acetate

	MALE		FEMALE		TOTAL	
	Total No. of Cases	Non-Tuberculous	Total No. of Cases	Non-Tuberculous	Number of Cases	Non-Tuberculous
Johns Hopkins Hospital	34	80%	30	77%	64	78%
Other Cases	55	37%	39	64%	94	48%
TOTAL	89	53%	69	70%	158	60%

in The Johns Hopkins Hospital. All cases of Addison's disease which have been reported previously by us [1, 2, 5] are included in the present report.

Etiology of the Disease: For convenience the etiological factors responsible for the adrenal cortical insufficiency in this group of patients have been classified as *tuberculous* or *non-tuberculous* (table 1). There appears to be a much lower incidence of tuberculosis of the adrenals in this group (40 per cent on the basis of clinical and laboratory diagnosis; 50 per cent on the basis of the 14 autopsy records) than has been observed previously (table 2). Conybeare and Millis [6] noted an incidence of 76 per cent of tuberculosis

TABLE II

Etiology of Addison's Disease—Postmortem Studies (Patients Treated with Desoxycorticosterone Acetate)

Patient	Age	Sex	Classification (Clinical and Lab. Studies)	Postmortem Findings—Adrenals
J. B.	52	M	Tuberculous	Tuberculosis
M. B.	31	F	Non-Tuberculous	Atrophy
R. B.	45	F	Non-Tuberculous	Atrophy
A. K.	30	F	Non-Tuberculous	Atrophy
J. L.	41	M	Tuberculous	Tuberculosis
A. M.	48	M	Tuberculous	Tuberculosis
G. M.	32	F	Non-Tuberculous	Atrophy
M. M.	27	F	Non-Tuberculous	Atrophy
S. M.	50	M	Tuberculous	Tuberculosis
S. O.	30	M	Tuberculous	Tuberculosis
O. Q.	62	M	Non-Tuberculous	Atrophy
D. R.	27	F	Non-Tuberculous	Atrophy
F. S.	28	M	Tuberculous	Tuberculosis
I. T.	69	F	Tuberculous	Tuberculosis

SUMMARY:

Tuberculous —7
Non-Tuberculous—7

of the adrenals in a series of 29 autopsies and Rowntree and Snell[7] report 84 per cent in a group of 31 cases (autopsy records) of Addison's disease.

Age and Sex: Approximately 80 per cent of the total number of cases in this series occurred in patients 20 to 50 years of age (table 3). The average

TABLE III

Age and Sex of Patients with Addison's Disease Treated with Desoxycorticosterone Acetate

Age	Males	Females	Total
0–10	0	0	0
10–20	7	3	10
20–30	20	12	32
30–40	24	22	46
40–50	26	21	47
50–60	7	9	16
60–70	5	1	6
70–80	0	1	1
TOTAL	89 (56%)	69 (44%)	158

age of the male patients was 37.2 years and the average age of the female patients was 40.0 years, the average for the entire group of 158 patients being 38.4 years. A comparison between the number of patients in this age group and the general population (chart 1) indicates that the apparent in-

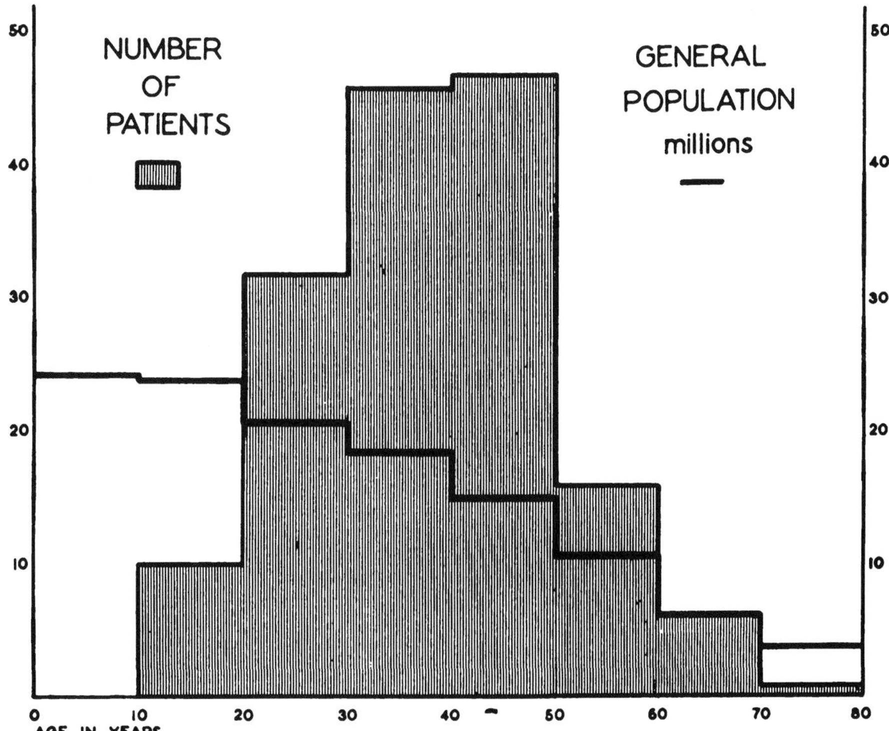

CHART 1. Age of patients with Addison's disease (158 cases).

creased incidence of Addison's disease in this age group is real. Although the number of males predominated (table 3), the difference in incidence between the sexes was not great.

Symptomatology: An analysis of the presenting symptoms in the 64 patients with Addison's disease who were seen in The Johns Hopkins Hospital is recorded in table 4. Weakness, fatigability, increasing pigmentation, anorexia and nausea were present in most instances. Ten patients (16 per cent) noted a definitely increased desire for salt and salty foods. A similar increase in "salt appetite" has been noted in adrenalectomized rats.[8]

TABLE IV
Analysis of Symptoms in 64 Patients with Addison's Disease

	Number	Per Cent
Weakness and fatigability	64	100
Increasing pigmentation	60	94
Anorexia	58	91
Nausea	55	86
Vomiting	48	75
Constipation	21	33
Abdominal pain	20	31
Diarrhea	10	16
Salt craving	10	16
Muscle pain	8	13

Diagnosis: From the group of 64 patients reported from The Johns Hopkins Hospital we have excluded all in whom there was the slightest doubt regarding the diagnosis of Addison's disease. Fifty-eight of the 64 patients had been seen at some time in typical adrenal crisis. The diagnosis in the other four patients was substantiated by careful clinical observations over a period of years. In the 94 patients who were not under our direct care we have relied upon the diagnosis of Addison's disease as established by the attending physician. In most instances these patients have also been seen in adrenal crisis and have, in addition, exhibited the changes characteristic of the syndrome, i.e., increasing pigmentation, hypotension, weakness, weight loss, anorexia and hypochloremia. The diagnosis of Addison's disease was substantiated in each instance in which a postmortem examination was made.

Desoxycorticosterone Acetate Therapy: In most patients treatment with desoxycorticosterone acetate was initiated by administering a daily intramuscular injection of the synthetic hormone in sesame oil (Percorten, Ciba; 1 c.c. contains 5 mg. of hormone) with or without supplementary sodium chloride therapy. The majority of patients required 5 mg. or less of Percorten daily (table 5) with 4 gm. (average) of supplementary sodium chloride medication. Less than 10 per cent of the patients required more than 5 mg. of hormone daily. The initial dose of hormone was usually much greater than the ultimate maintenance dose, since most patients were in rather poor condition at the time synthetic hormone therapy was instituted. As their condition subsequently improved under desoxycorticosterone acetate treatment, the hormone requirement decreased considerably. However, it often required several weeks before the minimum maintenance dose was attained.

Although supplementary sodium chloride therapy was not required in order to obtain successful regulation with the synthetic hormone,[2] it was used in most instances because it greatly reduced the hormone requirement and hence the cost of therapy. For most patients this was a consideration

TABLE V

Daily Maintenance Dose of Desoxycorticosterone Acetate in Sesame Oil of 141* Patients with Addison's Disease

Daily Dose of Hormone mg.	Number of Patients
0–1	0
1–2	53
2–3	20
3–4	8
4–5	48
5–10	8
10+	4
3.8 mg. per day, average	141 patients

* Assays in 17 patients were not standardized sufficiently to warrant inclusion in this table.

which could not be neglected. However, at present, 60 patients are being maintained with pellets of synthetic hormone *without* supplementary sodium chloride therapy. Supplementary sodium chloride therapy was best tolerated when given in the form of *1 gm. enteric coated tablets, at meal time with food,* a total of 3–5 gm. per day being the quantity most frequently used. It is undesirable to administer more than 5 gm. of supplementary sodium chloride therapy daily to most patients, even though well tolerated, since the onset of an acute infection or gastrointestinal disorder is usually accompanied by an inability to take the sodium chloride tablets and hence the patient is suddenly deprived of a large part of his therapy at a time when his need is greatest. A supplement of 3 gm. of sodium chloride daily was always used when patients were being prepared for pellet implantation (vide infra). Sodium chloride therapy in conjunction with desoxycorticosterone acetate treatment is *contraindicated* in patients who are predisposed to edema formation, hypertension or circulatory insufficiency.

The desirability of implanting pellets of crystalline hormone was considered after a patient had been maintained in good condition for a period of one month or more with daily injections of Percorten (crystalline hormone in sesame oil). Pellets were implanted in 148 of the patients in this group (table 6) after careful clinical control had permitted the daily requirement of hormone in oil to be determined accurately (table 5). In most instances it required at least four weeks to determine the optimum maintenance dose of hormone.

Calculation of Pellet Requirement: The number of pellets (Ciba; 125 mg. each) to be implanted was calculated directly from the daily maintenance dose of hormone in oil, injected intramuscularly. One pellet of 125 mg.* was implanted for each 0.5 mg. of hormone so required by daily injection.

TABLE VI

Initial Pellet Requirement of Patients with Addison's Disease

Number of Patients	Average Number of Pellets of Crystalline Desoxycorticosterone Acetate †	Total Quantity of Hormone per Patient (Aver.)
148*	6.4 (Range 2–15)	820 mg. (Range 250–1875)

* 10 patients have been treated with intramuscular injections of hormone in oil (Percorten) only.
† Pellets weighed 125 mg. ± 6 mg.

A small constant quantity of supplementary sodium chloride medication (3 gm. daily) was administered during the period of assay. This provided a balancing mechanism which could be used after pellets were implanted to compensate for any temporary excess of hormone. Thus, in the event that excessive sodium chloride was retained (edema) following pellet implantation it was possible to correct this by discontinuing a part or all of the added sodium chloride medication. If necessary, sodium chloride in the diet could also be restricted. Maintaining the sodium chloride therapy at a low dosage level (3 gm. daily) permitted an appreciable increase in the quantity of supplementary sodium chloride at a later date, should this be desirable. In this way a temporary need for additional therapy might easily be met by increasing the quantity of sodium chloride therapy. This could not have been done had the patient been receiving large doses of sodium chloride.

Pellets, weighing 125 mg. each, provided effective therapy in most patients for a period of at least 12 months. The fact that pellets were no longer providing an adequate supply of hormone was first indicated in most instances by a gradual reduction in blood pressure. Later fatigue, loss of weight and appetite were observed. However, in most instances, as soon as the reduction in blood pressure was noted, without awaiting the further development of symptoms of adrenal insufficiency, the patient was given intramuscular injections of hormone. One injection of 2 to 5 mg. (0.4 to 1.0 c.c.) of Percorten, twice weekly, was adequate for most patients at this

* Standardized pellets of desoxycorticosterone acetate prepared by Ciba Pharmaceutical Products, Inc., Summit, N. J., were used throughout these studies. The rate of absorption of these pellets has been shown to be 0.3 to 0.5 mg. per day per pellet. Pellets prepared in a different manner with a different rate of absorption should not be implanted on the basis of the calculation used in these studies, i.e., 1 pellet of 125 mg. for each 0.5 mg. of hormone required by daily injection.

time. Later daily injections of the hormone were resumed and a new assay was conducted. Three grams of sodium chloride daily were administered during this new assay period. When the maintenance hormone requirement had again been ascertained, and when it was certain that little, if any, of the original pellets remained, new pellets were implanted. *New pellets of desoxycorticosterone were never implanted arbitrarily at the end of one year, on the basis of the original assay* for two reasons: first, patients' hormone requirement often changed considerably after a year of sustained therapy; secondly, in many patients at the end of 12 months, there was still an appreciable quantity of hormone which was being absorbed from the original pellets and which would have led to overdosage if supplemented by a full complement of new pellets. At present 61 of the patients have received two or more implantations (table 7). The average duration of time which

TABLE VII

Number of Implantations of Pellets of Crystalline Desoxycorticosterone Acetate

Number of Implantations	Number of Patients
1	148
2	61
3	12
4	1
Total Number of Implantations	222

elapsed between the first and second implantations was 12.3 months. In most patients supplementary injections of hormone in oil were not required during the first 12 months subsequent to the initial pellet implantation.

Technic of Pellet Implantation: The infrascapular region posteriorly was selected for pellet implantation. Strict asepsis was observed. The operative field was prepared with iodine and alcohol and the site of incision was infiltrated with procaine, 1:200 solution. A transverse incision 2 to 4 cm. in length was made a few centimeters below the inferior spine of the scapula. With blunt dissection a number of small pockets, 2 to 3 cm. in depth were prepared in the subcutaneous tissues. The opening of each pocket was held far enough apart by a nasal dilator to permit pellets to be dropped gently to the bottom of the pocket without the use of force. This was important, for if the opening into the pocket were too small the fragile pellet could easily be crushed by the force used to insert it; furthermore, if the pocket were not deep enough, the pellet might be extruded subsequently through the incision. The wounds were closed with subcuticular stitches of fine black silk. It was possible to insert as many as 10 to 15 pellets through a single incision.[5]

At present 131 of the 132 patients now alive are being treated with pellets of hormone. Of this number 60 are receiving *no supplementary sodium chloride medication* at present. Six patients in addition to desoxycorticosterone acetate treatment are receiving 3 to 6 c.c. daily of adrenal cortex extract (Wilson, Upjohn or Parke, Davis & Co.). Supplementary injections of synthetic hormone in oil (Percorten, Ciba), intravenous administration of saline and glucose solutions and large doses of adrenal cortex extract, 5 to 10 c.c. at 4 to 8 hour intervals have been administered to many of these patients during the course of acute infections or in preparation for operative procedures.

The sublingual administration of desoxycorticosterone acetate in propylene glycol according to the method of Anderson et al.[9] has been tested in five patients with Addison's disease.[10] It was shown that this method was effective, but not efficient (table 8). It appears that administration of hormone sublingually may be useful in the treatment of patients whose hormone requirement is small and who are able to afford the increased quantity of hormone required by this route of administration. Recently we have tested solid tablets of crystalline desoxycorticosterone acetate "Linguets"* for sublingual administration and have found them very much more convenient to administer than the hormone in propylene glycol although the tablets are no more efficient than hormone in propylene glycol administered sublingually. The results obtained on a comparative assay of "Linguets" and Percorten are presented in chart 2. Patients receiving desoxycorticosterone acetate sublingually are not immune from the complications which have been reported in patients treated with intramuscular injections or subcutaneous implants of hormone. In patient M. D. edema readily developed when the dose of hormone, administered in propylene glycol sublingually, was increased above the minimum maintenance dose.

TABLE VIII

Relative Effectiveness of Desoxycorticosterone Acetate Administered Subcutaneously (Pellets), Intramuscularly, and Sublingually

	Equivalents
Subcutaneous implantation of pellets of crystalline hormone	1.2 mg. daily
Intramuscular injection of hormone in oil (once daily)	2.0 mg. daily
Sublingual administration of	
(*a*) Desoxycorticosterone acetate in propylene glycol	6.0–8.0 mg. daily
(*b*) Solid tablets of crystalline hormone in glucose	6.0–8.0 mg. daily

Results of Therapy: The mortality rate for the entire group of 158 patients was 15.4 per cent for a period of 1.7 years of therapy, or an annual mortality rate of 9.2 per cent, per year (table 9). A comparison with earlier reports on the life expectancy of patients with Addison's disease before the

* Tablets ("Linguets") composed of desoxycorticosterone acetate (1, 2, 5 and 10 mg. respectively), lactose, sucrose, talcum and gum arabic for sublingual use were prepared by Ciba Pharmaceutical Products, Inc.

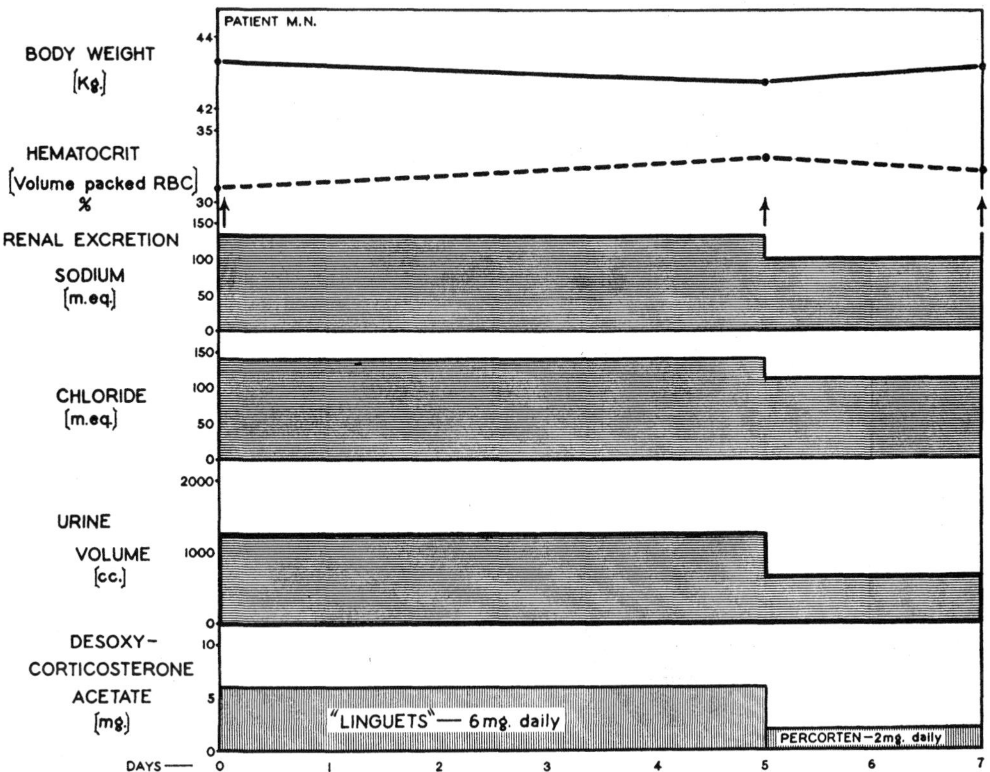

CHART 2. The relative effectiveness of desoxycorticosterone acetate tablets ("linguets") for sublingual use and a single daily injection of synthetic hormone in oil ("percorten").

TABLE IX

Mortality Rate in 158 Patients with Addison's Disease Treated with Desoxycorticosterone Acetate

	Number of Patients	Duration of Therapy	Number of Deaths	Mortality Rate
Johns Hopkins Hospital...	64	1.8 yr.	10	16.0%
Other Cases............	94	1.6 yr.	14	14.9%
TOTAL.............	158	1.7 yr.	24	15.2%

era of specific therapy and during the period of extract and sodium chloride therapy has been made (chart 3). The possible rôle played by added sodium chloride therapy in the present series of cases is controlled by the mortality rate which was observed when combined extract and sodium chloride therapy were employed (44.2 per cent at the end of 1.5 years). In regard to the group treated with adrenal cortex extract it is only fair to state that in all likelihood these patients did not, for the most part, receive adequate hormone therapy. There is no doubt, however, that they received all of the sodium chloride medication which they could tolerate. Thus, the mortality rate for this group more correctly represents the mortality rate for a group of patients who received adequate sodium chloride therapy, but, for the most part, inadequate extract therapy. The reasons for the latter were, and still remain, the high cost of adrenal cortex extract therapy and the necessity for frequent injections of this hormone preparation if the best clinical results are to be obtained.

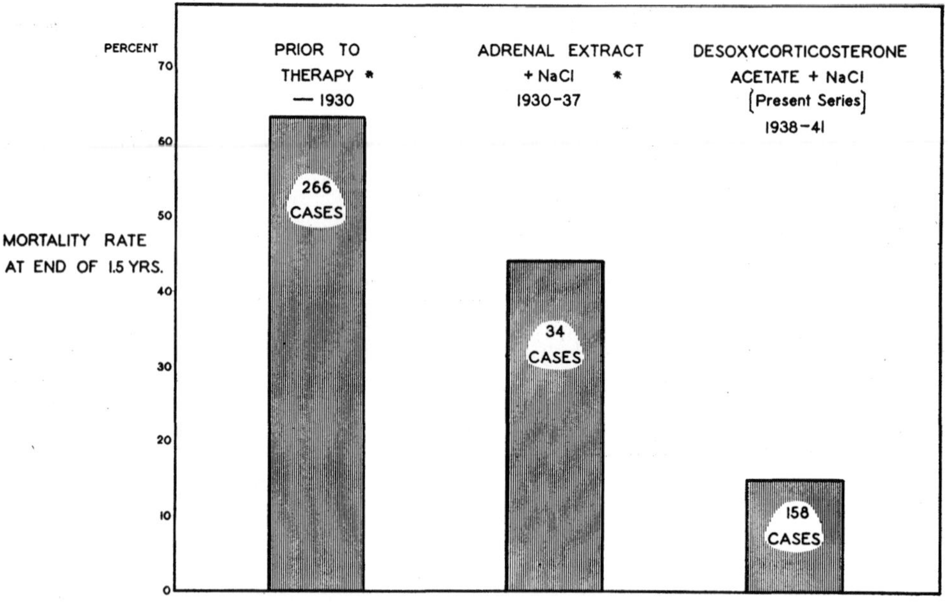

CHART 3. Comparative mortality rates in patients with Addison's disease prior to and subsequent to use of specific therapy.

Not only was the mortality rate greatly reduced in the group of patients treated with desoxycorticosterone acetate but the clinical improvement in the majority of patients was very striking. At this point it may be of interest to quote from Rowntree[7] who stated prior to the use of specific hormone therapy: "Most patients with Addison's disease are invalids throughout the course of the disease. Not more than one patient out of four or five is rehabilitated even to 50 per cent of former working capacity for as long as one year, and not more than one in sixty is rehabilitated to the extent of 75 to 80 per cent of previous working capacity for five years. None of the patients in our series has been completely restored to health and normal strength." In the group of 64 patients studied in the Johns Hopkins Hospital there occurred an average gain of approximately 4 kg. during the 1.7 years of therapy (chart 4). There was also a corresponding rise in blood pressure from an average level of 100 mm. Hg systolic and 66 mm. diastolic prior to therapy to a level of 126 mm. Hg systolic and 76 mm. diastolic at present.

Statistical analysis of these data indicates that the changes in all instances are significant.* The factor for difference between means is 4.9 in respect to the values for body weight, 6.3 for systolic blood pressure values, and 6.5 for diastolic pressure values.

A total of 31 of the 64 patients in our group improved so markedly during desoxycorticosterone acetate treatment that they were fully rehabilitated

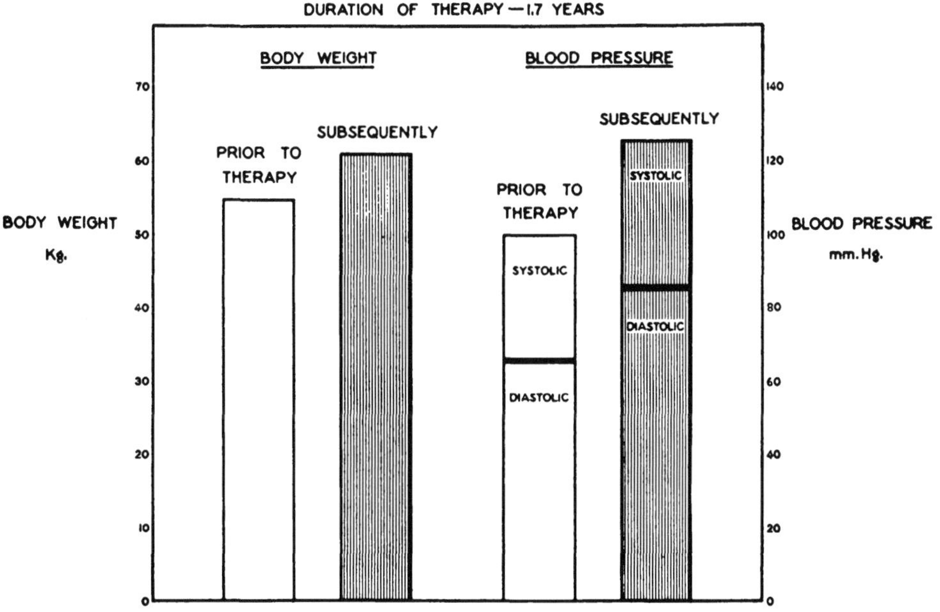

CHART 4. Effect of desoxycorticosterone acetate therapy in Addison's disease (Johns Hopkins Hospital—64 patients).

(table 10). Nineteen of these 31 patients were males. All 19 of these male patients are employed *full time* at present (table 11). Sixteen patients (25 per cent) have been greatly improved by therapy but cannot be considered to have been restored completely to normal strength and activity; in five of these 16 patients there is a complicating disease which will prevent these patients from returning completely to normal health (table 10, footnote 2). Seven patients in the group of 64 have shown little or no improvement. In four of these patients there is a definite complication (table 10, footnote 3); in the remaining three there is no apparent reason for the failure of desoxycorticosterone acetate therapy. The therapeutic results which were achieved in the outside group of patients (94) approximated closely the results which were obtained in the Johns Hopkins Hospital group.

* The difference between means is significant when the value of this factor is greater than 2.
See footnote to table 22.

TABLE X

Summary of Present Status of 64* Patients with Addison's Disease (Johns Hopkins Hospital) Treated with Desoxycorticosterone Acetate

	Number	Per Cent
Striking improvement (fully rehabilitated)	31	48 } 75
Improved—but not fully rehabilitated†	17	27 }
No improvement‡	6	9
Deaths	10	16

* 62 of these patients have been treated with subcutaneously implanted pellets.

† This group includes 3 patients with tuberculosis and 2 patients with rheumatic heart disease.

‡ This group includes 1 patient with tuberculosis; 1 patient with coronary infarction; 1 patient with marked hypertension which antedated onset of Addison's disease.

The immediate causes of death in the 10 patients in the Hopkins group and in the 14 patients in the outside group have been listed in table 12. Acute intercurrent infections and cardiovascular accidents account for more than 50 per cent of the deaths. These complications will be considered in some detail later. The two patients who died from hypoglycemia represent, in our estimate, preventable deaths, if preparations with "carbohydrate-regulating" potency had been used. In neither instance was the patient able to afford supplementary extract therapy.

TABLE XI

Effect of Desoxycorticosterone Acetate Therapy on Rehabilitation of Male Patients with Addison's Disease (Johns Hopkins Hospital)

Total Number of Male Patients	Number now Employed Full time	Per Cent
34	19	56%

In addition to the disturbance in carbohydrate metabolism which persisted in patients adequately treated with desoxycorticosterone acetate certain other signs and symptoms of adrenal insufficiency also failed to respond to continued hormone therapy in a small proportion of the patients. Thus, four patients (approximately 6 per cent of the Johns Hopkins Hospital

TABLE XII

Immediate Causes of Death in 24 Patients with Addison's Disease (Entire Group of 158 Patients)

	Number	Per Cent
Acute intercurrent infections	7	29
Cardiovascular disease	7	29
Tuberculosis	4	17
Hypoglycemia	2	8
Discontinued therapy	1	4
Unexplained	3	13
TOTAL	24	

group) lost weight during a prolonged period of desoxycorticosterone acetate treatment (2.5 years, average duration of treatment). In six of the patients (approximately 10 per cent) an appreciable degree of muscular weakness and asthenia persisted. In three patients (approximately 5 per cent) anorexia, nausea, and occasionally vomiting were observed.

Disturbances in Carbohydrate Metabolism: Recent studies[11] have increased our understanding of the nature of the disorder in carbohydrate metabolism which occurs in patients with Addison's disease. It now appears that any or all of the following defects may be observed in these patients:

1. Decreased rate of absorption of glucose from the gastrointestinal tract (flat glucose curve).
2. Increased utilization of carbohydrate.
3. Impaired ability to form new carbohydrate from non-glucose sources, i.e., "impaired gluconeogenesis."
4. "2" and "3" facilitate depletion of liver glycogen reserves and consequently predispose to hypoglycemia.
5. Lowered threshold at which signs and symptoms of hypoglycemia become evident.

Patients with Addison's disease vary widely in the extent to which disturbances in carbohydrate metabolism complicate their illness. Some patients develop hypoglycemia only during the course of intercurrent infections, prolonged fasting, or other stresses, whereas other patients have been known to display signs and symptoms of hypoglycemia after a brief postponement of a meal. To detect underlying disturbances in carbohydrate metabolism we have tested 52 of our patients with an intravenous glucose tolerance test * in which the development of moderate or severe signs and symptoms of *hypoglycemia* two to three hours after the intravenous administration of glucose signifies the presence of a rather profound disturbance in carbohydrate metabolism.[11] Of the group of 52 patients tested, 39 developed marked signs and symptoms of hypoglycemia two to three hours after the glucose solution had been injected intravenously (table 13). Twenty-six of these 39 patients had experienced similar episodes of hypoglycemia spontaneously. In 13 of the patients the positive reaction to this test constituted the first clinical evidence of a disturbance in carbohydrate metabolism. Thirteen patients in the group of 52 gave no evidence of the existence of any disturbance in carbohydrate metabolism by this test, and no history of spontaneous hypoglycemic episodes.

* *Standard Intravenous Glucose Tolerance Test.* Glucose, 0.5 gm. per kg. body weight, is injected intravenously as a 20 per cent solution in *distilled water.* The rate of flow is so adjusted that the infusion is completed in 30 minutes. Capillary blood for sugar determinations is taken in the fasting state and at 30 minute intervals for three to four hours following the completion of the infusion. Urine specimens are collected at appropriate intervals and analyzed for sugar.

It is of interest to note that restoration of plasma volume, plasma electrolyte concentration and blood pressure to normal levels by means of desoxycorticosterone acetate therapy does not correct the underlying disturbance in carbohydrate metabolism.[11] Only the gastrointestinal absorption of glucose is facilitated by synthetic hormone therapy, whereas treatment with adrenal cortex extract (large doses [50 c.c.] by injection) or certain, naturally occurring, crystalline adrenal steroid compounds (corticosterone, dehydrocorticosterone, 17-hydroxy-dehydrocorticosterone) promotes gluconeogenesis, depresses glucose utilization, increases liver glycogen stores

TABLE XIII

Incidence of Abnormal Carbohydrate Metabolism in 52 Patients with Addison's Disease (Johns Hopkins Hospital)

	Number of Patients	Per Cent
Spontaneous hypoglycemia	26	50
Hypoglycemia induced by intravenous glucose tolerance test	39	75
No evidence of disturbance in carbohydrate metabolism	13	25

and raises blood sugar levels.[11, 12] Unfortunately adrenal steroids with "carbohydrate-regulating" potency are not as yet available for clinical use, and adrenal cortical extract in quantity sufficient to affect carbohydrate metabolism significantly cannot be afforded by most patients. Thus, with the exception of the use of adrenal cortex extract therapy in patients in crisis, the treatment of hypoglycemia consists primarily in attempting to prevent its occurrence by the use of frequent feedings of a diet high in readily available carbohydrate content.

Treatment of Adrenal Crisis: In most instances intercurrent infections were responsible for the precipitation of adrenal crises in patients treated with desoxycorticosterone acetate. In a few patients the development of hypoglycemia, spontaneously, acted as the exciting factor. Of all infections, those due to streptococcus appeared to be the most frequent and most severe. Because of the rapidity with which crisis is precipitated during the onset of acute respiratory infections, treatment must be instituted immediately, if possible. The use of sulfadiazine is of great aid in the treatment of streptococcus infections in patients with Addison's disease.[13]

The aims of therapy in patients in crisis or in impending crisis may be summarized as follows:

1. Support of plasma volume and blood pressure by

(*a*) Intravenous infusion of sodium chloride (0.9 per cent solution) and dextrose (5 to 10 per cent solution).

(*b*) Aqueous adrenal cortex extract (intravenously and subcutaneously) in large quantities.

(*c*) Synthetic desoxycorticosterone acetate in oil (intramuscularly) to supplement maintenance dose.
(*d*) Epinephrine in oil (0.5 c.c.) intramuscularly if systolic blood pressure falls below 90 mm. Hg.

2. Prevention of hypoglycemia.

(*a*) Infusions of dextrose (see 1 *a*).
(*b*) Frequent feedings of readily available carbohydrate as soon as tolerated
(*c*) Large quantities of adrenal cortex extract (1 *b*).

3. Antibacterial chemotherapy whenever indicated.
4. Plasma and whole blood transfusions are not recommended as routine procedures.

Suggested Outline of Therapy: 1. The patient is placed in a warm bed with adequate blankets and *is immediately given an intravenous infusion of 1,000 to 1,500 c.c. of sodium chloride 0.9 per cent and glucose 5 to 10 per cent.* This is repeated in 12 hours and is given subsequently at least once daily until the temperature has reached normal or until the patient is taking fluids and eating well.

2. Twenty-five c.c. of aqueous adrenal cortex extract are added to the infusion and in addition 10 c.c. of extract are injected subcutaneously. The subcutaneous injection of 5–10 c.c. of aqueous extract (Wilson, Upjohn or Parke, Davis) is repeated every two to four hours until fever subsides, then every four to eight hours until the patient is eating well.

3. Twenty milligrams of desoxycorticosterone acetate in oil are injected intramuscularly in divided doses immediately; and thereafter 5 to 10 mg. are given once daily depending upon blood pressure, quantity of saline solution which has been administered, appearance of excessive fluid retention, etc.

4. One c.c. of epinephrine in oil injected intramuscularly is indicated if the level of systolic blood pressure falls below 90 mm. Hg.

5. Blood pressure determinations are made at intervals of one to two hours, day and night. Small quantities of fruit juice with added lactose, or ginger ale, are given at frequent intervals if tolerated. Since 1,500 c.c. of saline and dextrose solution are given intravenously at 8 to 12 hour intervals, additional fluid or sodium chloride by mouth is not essential during the first 24 hours of treatment. A fall in blood pressure without signs of excessive sodium chloride and water retention is a definite indication for increasing the infusions of sodium chloride and for giving additional desoxycorticosterone acetate intramuscularly (5 to 10 mg.). A fall in blood pressure in the presence of excessive sodium chloride and water retention is a definite indication for reducing the number of infusions, for discontinuing the desoxycorticosterone acetate therapy and for *increasing* the quantity of adrenal cortex extract, i.e., 10 c.c. every hour. *At this time a plasma transfusion*

should be seriously considered. Our experience with the unfavorable reaction of patients with Addison's disease to whole blood transfusions suggests that this therapeutic procedure should be withheld unless other measures fail.

As a precautionary measure we urge that all patients with Addison's disease keep on hand *at all times or have immediate access to the following:*

Emergency Kit:

1. 1000 c.c. of 0.9 per cent NaCl and 5 to 10 per cent glucose solution for intravenous administration.
2. Sulfadiazine tablets.
3. Adrenal cortex extract, *50 c.c.* (Wilson, Upjohn, Parke-Davis).
4. Synthetic desoxycorticosterone acetate in oil, 10 c.c. (Percorten, Ciba; Cortate, Schering; Doca, Hoffmann-LaRoche).

Complications Which May Arise During Desoxycorticosterone Acetate Therapy.

1. *Non-specific:* Hypoglycemia occurs not infrequently in patients treated with desoxycorticosterone acetate alone. This complication has already been referred to (see "Disturbances in carbohydrate metabolism"). Treatment consists in frequent feedings of a diet high in readily available carbohydrate and supplementary injections of aqueous adrenal cortex extract, 5 to 10 c.c. every four to six hours.

In two patients intramuscular injections of desoxycorticosterone acetate in sesame oil (Percorten) were accompanied by localized redness, pain and tenderness at the site of the injection, as well as fever and malaise. It was demonstrated subsequently that these reactions were due to the injection of sesame oil and not to synthetic hormone.[5] Both patients did well when pellets of crystalline hormone were implanted.

On four occasions in over 200 pellet implantations pellets were extruded from the site of the incision. Such complications may be avoided by placing the pellets a distance of at least 2.5 cm. from the margin of the incision. In no instance thus far has a local infection occurred at the site of the implantations.

2. *Specific:* Most of the complications which occur in patients with Addison's disease treated with desoxycorticosterone acetate (intramuscular injections of hormone in oil, pellets of crystalline hormone implanted subcutaneously or hormone administered sublingually) may be accounted for by one factor, i.e., *excessive retention of sodium chloride and water.* The extent to which untoward signs and symptoms develop is dependent upon

(*a*) the dose of hormone;
(*b*) the amount of sodium chloride in the diet and the supplementary sodium chloride therapy;
(*c*) predisposing factors in certain patients, such as heart disease, hypertension, hypoproteinemia, etc.

The nature of the complications which have arisen in 64 patients (Johns Hopkins Hospital) treated with synthetic hormone is summarized in table 14. *Hypertension* was noted at some time during therapy in 22 or 35 per cent of the patients. In most instances the hypertension was of a transient nature and occurred only during a period of excessive hormone and supplementary

TABLE XIV

Incidence of Complications Associated with Desoxycorticosterone Acetate Therapy (Johns Hopkins Hospital—64 Patients)

	Number of Patients	Per Cent
Hypertension*	22	34
Edema	17	27
Cardiac decompensation	5	8
Tendon "contractures"	2	3
Transient paralysis	1	2

* Systolic blood pressure exceeding 150 mm. Hg or diastolic blood pressure exceeding 100 mm. Hg or both, at some time during course of therapy.

sodium chloride therapy. In patients with Addison's disease in whom some degree of hypertension existed prior to the onset of adrenal cortical insufficiency there was a great predilection for the blood pressure to return to high levels and to remain there with only moderate doses of hormone.

Transient edema was noted in 14 (23 per cent) of the patients during desoxycorticosterone acetate therapy. In three of these patients the edema was rather extensive (anasarca). Edema was most frequently observed during the early weeks of therapy when an attempt was being made to determine the patient's optimum maintenance dose of hormone. The edema subsided rapidly following a reduction in the dose of hormone or upon withdrawing supplementary sodium chloride medication. In patients with long standing thrombophlebitis or lymphatic obstruction it was difficult to administer the optimum maintenance dose of hormone without at the same time inducing a moderate degree of localized edema in the affected part.

In five patients (8 per cent) continued synthetic hormone therapy accompanied by a marked increase in plasma volume, body weight, blood pressure and physical activity, ultimately induced signs and symptoms of circulatory failure. This complication occurred only in elderly patients or in patients in whom there had been some evidence of preëxisting myocardial damage or vascular disease. Circulatory failure may usually be avoided if care is exercised in restricting sodium chloride intake and in restricting activity during the early period of therapy during which blood volume, blood pressure and body weight are increasing rapidly. Treatment for this complication consists in absolute bed rest, digitalization, reduction in hormone and elimination of sodium chloride from diet. Subsequent rehabilitation should proceed slowly.

The long continued administration of even moderately excessive quantities of desoxycorticosterone acetate, or the synthetic hormone in conjunction with supplementary sodium chloride therapy may result in the excessive retention of sodium and chloride in the blood serum and tissues [14] associated with an abnormally low concentration of potassium. The resulting disturbance in sodium-potassium ratio, which is just the antithesis of the ratio which obtains in adrenal insufficiency (table 15) may give rise to unusual complications characterized by disturbances in neuromuscular function. In one patient (J. Z.) transient peripheral extensor motor paralysis was observed in conjunction with a low serum potassium concentration.[5] The

TABLE XV

Changes in Sodium to Potassium Ratio Which May Occur During Excessive Desoxycorticosterone Acetate Therapy

	Serum Sodium m.eq./l.	Serum Potassium m.eq./l.	Sodium / Potassium
Adrenal crisis	120	8.0	15
Adequate treatment	140	4.6	30
Excessive treatment	145	3.2	45

rapidity of onset, the absence of sensory disturbances and the rapid recovery without sequelae suggested an episode similar to that which is observed in familial periodic paralysis. Experimentally, similar disturbances have been noted in dogs treated with excessive doses of synthetic hormone in conjunction with supplementary sodium chloride.[15] As might be anticipated, a diet low in potassium content (of the type formerly recommended in the treatment of Addison's disease before the advent of desoxycorticosterone acetate) would facilitate these changes. For this reason it is urged that patients with Addison's disease treated with desoxycorticosterone acetate *not be given a diet of low potassium content!*

A second type of complication which has been observed in two of the 64 patients in our group, and in one patient in the outside group of 94 patients, consists of a painful and disabling contracture of the thigh muscles and tendons. The onset of this complication has occurred after several weeks or months of continued hormone therapy. Thus far it has been observed only in patients who have been incapacitated because of marked weakness or because of arthritic involvement of the knee joints. At the onset, because of the periarticular reference of the pain, it was thought that the patients were suffering from a relapse of the underlying arthritis. During the progress of the illness, the thighs slowly became flexed on the abdomen and the patients were unable to walk because of inability to straighten their legs. Roentgenograms of the joints revealed no evidence of progressive articular change. Although contractures conforming to this type have been seen in a patient with Addison's disease prior to therapy, it seemed probable that synthetic hormone therapy might have been a precipitating factor, since in all three of these patients the onset of symptoms occurred after a continued period of hormone therapy. It is possible that this complication may be caused by excessive sodium and chloride retention in tissues, particularly tendons. No doubt inactivity and preëxisting joint disease predispose a patient to these changes.

Treatment of this complication, thus far, has been unsatisfactory. Obviously, sudden withdrawal of hormone would precipitate a crisis. Elimination of added sodium chloride therapy, reduction of synthetic hormone to a minimum maintenance dose, and supplementary potassium medication (potassium citrate solution 10 per cent; 30 to 45 c.c. in fruit juice daily) would be indicated if it could be proved that excessive sodium retention actually induced the change. In one patient we have resorted to orthopedic measures (traction followed by manipulation under anesthesia), since a trial on the above regimen, and a continued period of adrenal cortex extract therapy did not result in any appreciable improvement in this patient. Attention is called to this condition particularly because of the ease with which it may be confused with the muscular pains (low-sodium cramps) which are commonly observed in patients in adrenal insufficiency. For the latter, sodium chloride and hormone are specific.

Although desoxycorticosterone is closely related chemically to progesterone we have not, to date, observed any evidence of progestational changes in female patients with Addison's disease who have been treated for long periods of time with the synthetic adrenal cortical hormone. Several patients have noted increased turgor of the breasts. It seems reasonable to assume that this change may be accounted for by an increased accumulation of extracellular fluid which occurs during adrenal cortex hormone therapy.

Cardiac Changes in Addison's Disease: It has long been known that the heart in patients with Addison's disease is smaller than normal [7] and that the electrocardiogram in many of these patients shows abnormalities suggesting disease of the myocardium.[16, 17] Recent studies [4, 18, 19, 20] have demonstrated that progressive cardiac enlargement may occur in patients with Addison's disease following overdosage with desoxycorticosterone acetate. It seems probable that preëxisting cardiac disease may play an important rôle in predisposing certain patients to myocardial failure following excessive desoxycorticosterone acetate therapy. The poor physical condition of untreated patients with Addison's disease makes a study of cardiac reserve difficult, if not impossible, prior to therapy. Investigation of the effect of synthetic hormone therapy on cardiac function, therefore, is dependent chiefly on a study of the progressive changes in electrocardiograms and teleroentgenograms.

The effect of synthetic hormone therapy on changes in cardiac diameter was followed closely in 46 of our 64 patients studied (table 16). In no patient did the heart-to-chest ratio exceed 50 per cent prior to therapy. In two patients during therapy the ratio exceeded 50 per cent and both of these

TABLE XVI

Effect of Desoxycorticosterone Acetate Therapy on Cardiac Diameter (46 patients)

	Heart to Chest Ratio	Range
Prior to treatment	38.6%	(28–46)
Maximum measurement during treatment	42.2%	(32–55)
Present status (approx. 2 yrs. therapy)	41.3%	(32–50)

patients were among the five who developed signs of circulatory insufficiency. With care in the regulation of the dose of hormone and supplementary sodium chloride medication, only a moderate increase in heart size occurred during a period of approximately two years of treatment, viz., 38.6 per cent heart-to-chest ratio prior to therapy; present status 41.3 per cent heart-to-chest ratio.

Electrocardiograms were analyzed in 58 of our 64 patients to determine the incidence of abnormal changes without regard to therapy (tables 17 and 18). There were significant electrocardiographic changes in 35 of the patients (60 per cent). In 17 patients (29 per cent) the changes suggested definite myocardial damage. A high incidence of abnormal electrocardiograms appeared in all age groups (table 17). It is interesting to note that 19 of the patients (54 per cent) with abnormal electrocardiograms were under 40 years of age.

The group of 35 patients with abnormal electrocardiograms included one patient with clinical evidence of arteriosclerotic heart disease and two patients with clinical evidence of rheumatic heart disease. There was clinical evidence of arteriosclerosis in seven patients and of rheumatic heart disease in three patients in the entire group of 64 patients.

TABLE XVII

Electrocardiographic Findings in Addison's Disease (58 patients)

Age Group (years)	Number of Patients	Electrocardiographic Interpretation			
		Normal	"Borderline" *	Myocardial Damage †	Per Cent Abnormal
20–29	16	7	5	4	56
30–39	18	8	4	6	56
40–49	13	6	4	3	54
50–59	8	1	3	4	88
60–69	3	1	2	0	67
TOTAL	58	23	18	17	60

* The term "borderline" has been used to indicate the presence of abnormal electrocardiographic changes which are believed to be significant, although not indisputable evidence of myocardial damage. These changes were as follows: PR interval over .21 second; prolonged QT interval (by formula of Ashman and Hull [21]); QRS voltage less than 5 mm. in Leads I, II, III and/or Lead IV F; isoelectric T_1 or T_2; negative T_4; initial upward QRS deflection in Lead IV F absent or less than 1 mm.; ST segment deviation of less than 1 mm.

† As indicated by inverted T_1 and/or T_2, isoelectric T-waves in all leads, or the presence of combinations of three or more of the "borderline" changes.

TABLE XVIII
Incidence of Electrocardiographic Changes in Addison's Disease (58 patients)

Change	Number of Patients	Per Cent
Prolonged PR interval*	12	21
Prolonged QT interval*	15	26
Low voltage (QRS)*		
Leads I, II, III	11	19
Lead IV F	9	16
Low or isoelectric		
T_1	19	33
T_2	19	33
T_4	4	7
Diphasic or Negative		
Ti	5	9
T_2	11	19
T_3	39	67
T_4	19	33

* See footnote to table 17.

The preponderance of females among the patients with abnormal electrocardiograms is of interest. Twenty (57 per cent) of the 35 patients with significant electrocardiographic changes were females (chart 5). Of the 26 females studied 77 per cent had abnormal electrocardiograms, whereas only 47 per cent of the males were in this group. The explanation for this

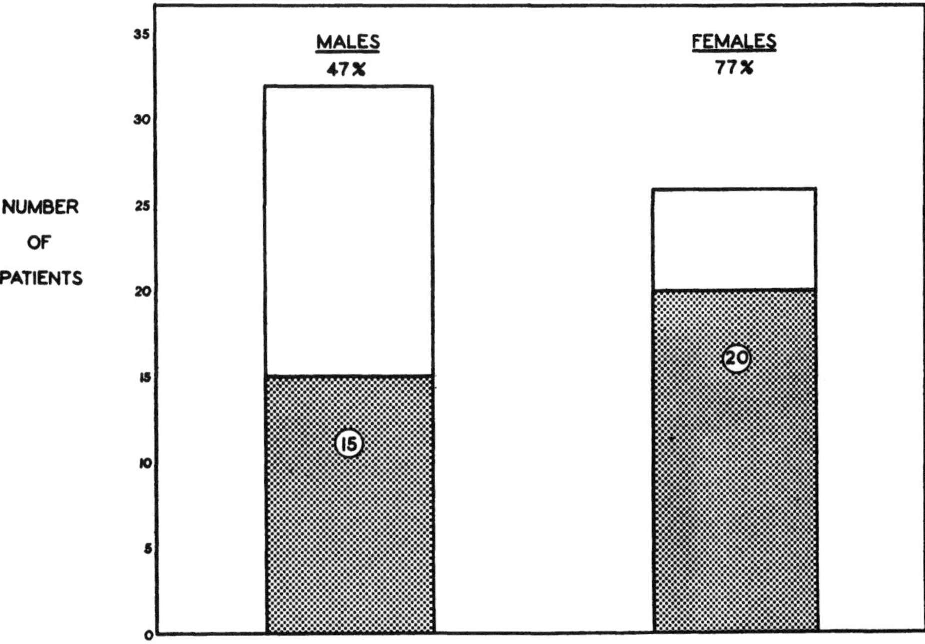

CHART 5. Electrocardiographic abnormalities in Addison's disease (sex incidence) ▩ patients with abnormal electrocardiograms.

Males: "borderline" changes—9; myocardial damage—6. Females: "borderline" changes —9; myocardial damage—11.

greater frequency of abnormal electrocardiographic changes in the females is not apparent. However, in support of this apparently higher incidence of cardiac abnormalities in female patients is the fact that five of the seven deaths which could be attributed to cardiovascular disease (entire group of 158 patients, table 12) occurred in female patients.

There appeared to be no pattern of electrocardiographic changes specific for Addison's disease. A wide variation characterized the changes, viz., prolonged PR and QT intervals, low QRS voltage, and low or inverted T-waves. The incidence of these findings in this group of patients was considerably higher than that reported recently for a normal population.[22, 23] Other significant electrocardiographic changes observed less frequently were: an absence of the initial upward QRS deflection in the chest lead (two patients), small initial upward QRS deflection in the chest lead (seven patients), sinus bradycardia with cardiac rate of less than 50 per minute (five patients), premature ventricular contractions (four patients) and ST segment depression of less than 1 mm. (four patients).

In no instance was an electrocardiogram included in this series which had been taken during digitalis therapy or within three weeks after digitalis therapy had been discontinued. Since no attempt was made to standardize the position of patients during the recording of electrocardiograms, it is possible that in some instances inversion of T_2 actually represented a change related to the sitting position.[24] In no patient in this series, however, did the interpretation of myocardial damage depend solely upon the presence of inversion of T_2.

Effect of Desoxycorticosterone Therapy upon the Electrocardiogram in Addison's Disease: The relation of potassium retention to changes in the electrocardiogram has been reported in experimental adrenal insufficiency.[25] The abnormal electrolyte pattern is restored to normal in adrenalectomized animals and in patients with Addison's disease by desoxycorticosterone acetate therapy. Excessive desoxycorticosterone acetate therapy can produce an abnormal electrolyte pattern in both the blood serum and tissues, i.e., high sodium, low potassium.[14] Presumably changes in the electrocardiogram could accompany these disturbances in electrolyte concentration. Changes in the electrocardiogram associated with low serum potassium have been observed in a patient with familial periodic paralysis.[26] The relation of the disturbances in electrolyte metabolism to changes in carbohydrate metabolism and cardiac function is not fully understood.

Electrocardiograms were recorded in 28 patients before desoxycorticosterone therapy was begun and repeated during therapy (1.4 years, average duration of therapy—tables 19 and 20). In 13 additional patients electrocardiograms were taken after desoxycorticosterone therapy had been begun. Of this total group of 41 patients, seven showed significant improvement in the electrocardiogram during therapy, whereas 14 showed an increase in the number and extent of the abnormalities. Five of the seven instances of improvement were related to recovery from periods of inadequate therapy or of overdosage with hormone. In contrast, only two of the 14 instances of impairment of the electrocardiogram coincided with a period of unfavorable clinical response. The remaining 12 patients showed a moderate to marked improvement in well-being, at the time that the electrocardiogram

TABLE XIX

Changes in Electrocardiograms Which Occurred During Desoxycorticosterone Acetate Therapy (Addison's Disease)

	Number of Patients	Electrocardiographic Interpretation			
		Normal	"Borderline" *	Myocardial Damage	Per Cent Abnormal
Prior to hormone therapy	28	19	6	3	32
Following 1.4 years of continuous hormone therapy	28	12	8	8	57

* See footnote to table 17.

TABLE XX

Incidence of Electrocardiographic Changes in 28 Patients with Addison's Disease Prior to and During Desoxycorticosterone Acetate Therapy

	* Prolonged PR Interval	* Prolonged QT Interval	* Low QRS Voltage		Low or Isoelectric			Diphasic or Negative			
			I II III	IV	T_1	T_2	T_4	T_1	T_2	T_3	T_4
Prior to desoxycorticosterone acetate therapy	0	2	4	2	4	2	3	0	4	11	4
During desoxycorticosterone acetate therapy (1.4 yrs.)	9	10	5	2	6	5	2	5	11	19	8

* See footnote to table 17.

was giving evidence of progressive myocardial involvement. The most striking abnormalities developing under desoxycorticosterone therapy were prolongation of the PR interval (10 patients) and prolongation of the QT interval (10 patients). No patients showed a prolonged PR interval before receiving synthetic hormone (table 20). T-wave inversion suggesting diffuse myocardial damage or coronary insufficiency appeared in six patients, three of whom had had normal and three of whom had had "borderline" electrocardiograms before treatment.

The number of patients showing myocardial damage increased from three to eight during desoxycorticosterone therapy in the group of 28 patients in whom records were available prior to treatment with synthetic hormone (table 19). No increase in the number of patients with electrocardiographic abnormalities occurred in the smaller group of 13 patients in whom records were made only during the period of desoxycorticosterone

TABLE XXI

Summary of Electrocardiographic Findings in Patients with Addison's Disease prior to and during Desoxycorticosterone Acetate Therapy

	Number of Patients	Duration of Hormone Therapy (years)	Electrocardiographic Interpretation							
			Normal		* Borderline		Myocardial Damage		Abnormalities	
			1st ECG	Present	1st ECG	Present	1st ECG	Present	1st ECG	Present
Serial electrocardiograms prior to and during hormone therapy	28	1.4	19	12	6	8	3	8	32%	57%
Serial electrocardiograms during hormone therapy (no record prior to therapy)	13	2.1	4	4	7	8	2	1	69%	69%
Single electrocardiograms prior to hormone therapy (none since)	9	0	6	—	3	—	0	—	38%	—
Single electrocardiograms during hormone therapy	8	0.8	—	5	—	1	—	2	—	38%
Total: electrocardiograms prior to hormone therapy	37	—	25	—	9	—	3	—	32%	—
Total: electrocardiograms during hormone therapy	49	1.5	—	21	—	17	—	11	—	57%

*See footnote to table 17.

therapy (table 21). This difference in the two groups did not appear to be related to the duration of Addison's disease or to the clinical response to therapy, but may indicate that electrocardiographic abnormalities make their appearance early during the period of rapid clinical improvement which follows the *initiation* of desoxycorticosterone therapy. It is possible that in untreated patients myocardial disease may be masked by the decreased demands made on the heart by the lowered arterial pressure and reduced blood volume of patients in adrenal insufficiency. By elevating blood pressure and restoring blood volume, desoxycorticosterone therapy disturbs this balance, increases the cardiac load, and may thereby lead to electrocardiographic abnormalities in patients with latent myocardial damage.

Electroencephalographic Changes in Addison's Disease: Electroencephalograms * were recorded in 36 of the 64 patients under our observation. Definite abnormalities were noted in 25 or 69 per cent of these 36 patients. The abnormal features in most instances consisted of one or more of the following changes:

(1) regular occurrence of oscillations slower than the normal alpha rhythm with a predilection for the frontal areas, not influenced by opening the eyes.

(2) absence of, or greatly decreased number of low voltage, fast frequency waves (beta waves).

(3) increased sensitivity to hyperventilation.

Unfortunately in the majority of patients it was not possible to obtain electroencephalographic records prior to synthetic hormone therapy. However, in two of the three patients who were studied before therapy had been instituted, changes similar to those noted above were observed. The effect of desoxycorticosterone therapy on the electroencephalographic records was unpredictable. Four patients with normal electroencephalograms, early in the course of therapy, also had normal tracings after 4 to 27 months of continued hormone therapy. Four patients with abnormalities in the electroencephalograms early in the course of synthetic hormone therapy showed no progression of the abnormal changes during the subsequent 12 months of treatment. Three patients, however, showed a pronounced increase in the abnormal electroencephalographic features during a 12 month period of desoxycorticosterone acetate treatment. In contrast to these evidences of progressive change in the resting pattern of the electroencephalogram during hormone therapy, four patients were observed to have a pronounced decrease in the abnormal sensitivity to hyperventilation during a 12 month period of synthetic hormone therapy.

The situation in relation to the changes in the electroencephalogram of patients with Addison's disease treated with desoxycorticosterone acetate is

* We are greatly indebted to Dr. W. Christie Hoffmann of the Henry Phipps Psychiatric Clinic for the encephalographic records. A complete study of the electroencephalographic changes in these patients has been prepared for publication.[27]

somewhat analogous to that which was observed in relation to the abnormal electrocardiographic changes in the same group of patients. In both instances typical abnormalities were present before synthetic hormone therapy was instituted, and in most instances continued synthetic hormone therapy failed to correct the abnormalities despite striking evidence of clinical improvement. Although in both instances it was thought likely that the extensive and progressive changes in electrocardiogram and electroencephalogram might be correlated with the degree to which carbohydrate metabolism was impaired in these patients, such a correlation was not present in all cases. A higher incidence of abnormal electroencephalograms was noted in male patients in contrast to the predominance of abnormal electrocardiograms which was observed in female patients.

Metabolic Studies

A. Plasma Electrolytes and Plasma Volume: A striking increase in plasma volume is one of the first changes which is noted in patients with Addison's disease under desoxycorticosterone acetate treatment.[2] If not measured directly, some idea of the magnitude of the increase in plasma volume can be obtained from the changes in hematocrit, red blood cell count and serum protein concentration which occur during the first few days of therapy. In addition to the prompt increase in plasma volume there is also a restoration of the plasma concentration of sodium, chloride, potassium and non-protein nitrogen to normal levels. During treatment with synthetic hormone the renal excretion of sodium and chloride is decreased (positive balance), whereas the excretion of potassium and inorganic phosphorus is increased (negative balance). Withdrawal of hormone therapy is followed rapidly by increased excretion of sodium, chloride and water, weight loss, decrease in plasma volume, decrease in *total plasma content* of sodium and chloride, retention of potassium and inorganic phosphorus associated with an increase in the concentration of potassium in plasma.[2] Patients may improve remarkably during the early period of therapy without necessarily showing any increase in plasma concentration of sodium and chloride; ultimately, however, these values attain normal levels. Conversely, sudden withdrawal of hormone therapy may temporarily precipitate a crisis without necessarily effecting a significant reduction in the concentration of sodium and chloride in the plasma. This apparent lack of correlation between changes in clinical state and changes in plasma concentration of electrolytes can be understood if plasma volume measurements are made during these periods, since it can be readily demonstrated that during the early period of treatment there is an appreciable *increase in the total plasma content of sodium and chloride* and that immediately following withdrawal of therapy there is a *reduction in the total plasma content of these ions.* Whether or not corresponding changes take place in the plasma concentration of these ions depends upon the relative gain or loss of water.

The changes which occurred in blood sugar and non-protein nitrogen levels, as well as plasma sodium, potassium, chloride and carbon dioxide combining power, hematocrit and serum protein concentration during desoxycorticosterone acetate in 44 of our 64 patients are summarized in table 22. It is of particular interest to note that the fasting blood sugar level

TABLE XXII

Blood Chemical Changes in Patients with Addison's Disease During Desoxycorticosterone Acetate Therapy

Number of Patients	Blood Chemical Constituent	Mean Value Prior to Therapy	Mean Value during Therapy	Difference Between Means * / Standard Deviation of the Distribution of the Means
40	Serum sodium m.eq./l.	132.3	141.3	4.5
41	Serum chloride m.eq./l.	97.5	104.3	4.2
38	Carbon-dioxide combining capacity	24.2	26.0	2.9
44	Serum potassium m.eq./l.	5.7	4.4	5.0
42	Non-protein nitrogen mg./100 c.c.	34	28	3.6
42	Blood sugar mg./100 c.c.	87	81	2.7
42	Hematocrit (per cent cell volume)	41.4	36.5	4.5
37	Serum protein gm./100 c.c.	6.3	5.7	3.7

* The difference between means is significant when the value of this factor is greater than 2.

$$\sqrt{\frac{\sigma_0^2}{N}}$$

Standard deviation of the distribution of means of individual changes.

N = Number in series

$\sigma_0 = \sqrt{\frac{(X_1 - X_2)^2}{N}}$ = Standard deviation of the distribution of individual changes

$(X_1 - X_2)^2$ = Sum of squares of difference in means in series 1 and 2 (the two series being compared)

N = number in series

$\bar{X}_1$ = Mean of series 1

$\bar{X}_2$ = Means of series 2

If $\dfrac{\bar{X}_1 - \bar{X}_2}{\sqrt{\frac{\sigma_0^2}{N}}} > 2$, difference of $\bar{X}_1 - \bar{X}_2$ is significant.

(Note that N occurs in this formula twice—once as a part of γ_0^2.)

prior to desoxycorticosterone acetate therapy was significantly higher than during therapy. This suggests that not only does desoxycorticosterone acetate lack the carbohydrate-stimulating quality of certain adrenal cortical steroids, but that it may actually exert a slight insulin-like action. The changes in serum electrolyte concentration which occurred during synthetic hormone therapy were significant and were consistent with the changes reported previously.[2]

B. Basal Metabolic Rate: In an earlier report [11] it was shown that a basal metabolic rate of less than — 20 per cent of standard was unusual in patients with Addison's disease uncomplicated by thyroid or pituitary deficiency. Furthermore, it was shown that in a group of seven patients no significant change in basal metabolic rate was noted following continued treatment with desoxycorticosterone acetate, the average value before treatment being — 10 per cent (18 determinations) and during treatment — 12 per cent (10 determinations). The basal metabolic rates of 55 of the 64 patients in the Johns Hopkins Hospital group have been measured on several

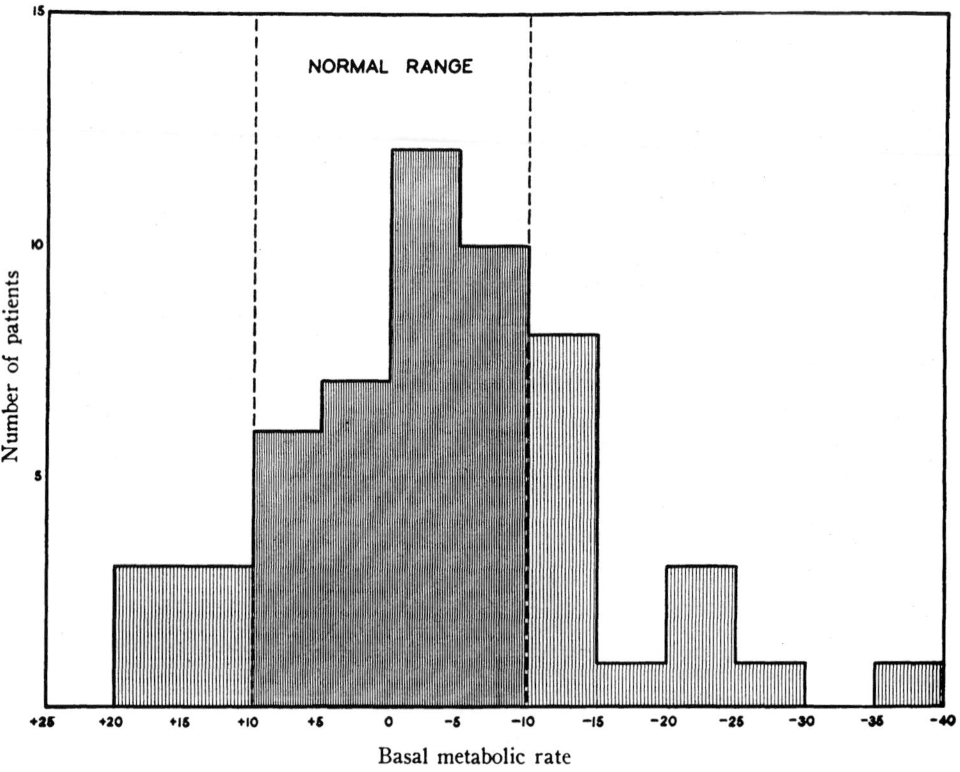

CHART 6. Basal metabolic rate in fifty-five patients with Addison's disease (Johns Hopkins Hospital) during treatment with desoxycorticosterone acetate.

occasions during desoxycorticosterone acetate therapy. The average value of these determinations for each patient is presented in chart 6. It is to be noted that the values for 35 patients or 64 per cent of the group lie between + 10 per cent and — 10 per cent of standard. In six patients the values exceeded + 10 per cent and in 14 patients the values were below — 10 per cent, five of the latter being below — 20 per cent. All five of this latter group presented definite clinical evidence of thyroid deficiency.

C. Pigmentation: Abnormal pigmentation was present in 60 (94 per cent) of the 64 patients in our group. Vitiligo was present in eight, or 13 per cent, of these 60 patients. The occurrence of vitiligo in the presence of adrenal cortical deficiency was pointed out by Addison in his original monograph.[7]

In considering the type of abnormal pigmentation which may occur in patients with Addison's disease it may be helpful to list the variety of changes which have been observed in the present group of patients, viz.:

1. Bluish-black discolorations which appear on the lips, gums and on the mucous membranes of the mouth, rectum and vagina. It should be pointed out that this type of pigmentation occurs normally in negroes and in certain southern European races.
2. A diffuse tan over the non-exposed as well as the exposed portions of the body.
3. Hyperpigmentation of the extensor surfaces of the body, pressure points, scars and lines on the palms of the hands.
4. Multiple black freckles, distributed most commonly over the forehead, face, neck, shoulders and arms.
5. Areas of vitiligo or leukoderma. The appearance of these areas is usually striking because of the hyperpigmentation of the surrounding skin.

It is not possible to predict what change, if any, may occur in the pigmentation of patients with Addison's disease during treatment with desoxycorticosterone acetate. In all patients there is a noticeable lightening of the complexion within a few days after hormone therapy is instituted. This immediate change reflects the hemodilution and increase in peripheral circulation which has occurred as a result of sodium, chloride and water retention, increase in plasma volume and increase in blood pressure. During periods of insufficient therapy patients rapidly assume a much darker complexion.

In the majority of patients during long continued hormone therapy there has been some decrease in the intensity of the abnormal pigmentation (table 23) and in a few patients there has been complete disappearance of small localized areas of increased pigmentation. In two patients, despite continued hormone therapy, there has been a slow but progressive increase in pigmentation.

It is well known that the margins of scars which occur in patients with Addison's disease are a frequent site for increased pigment deposition. For this reason the small scars which are made in the infrascapular region during the implantation of pellets may provide an excellent indicator of the change in pigment metabolism which occurs during therapy. A striking pigmentation of the margins of these scars following the implantation of pellets of desoxycorticosterone acetate strongly suggests that the abnormality in pigment metabolism has not been corrected by synthetic hormone therapy, whereas failure of the margins of these scars to become pigmented suggests that the progress of the abnormal process has been arrested.

D. Creatine Metabolism: The presence of spontaneous creatinuria associated with a decrease in creatine tolerance has been observed in untreated patients with Addison's disease.[7, 28] Treatment with whole adrenal cortex extract was followed by improved appetite, increased ingestion of food, gain in weight and improved clinical condition. Under these circumstances spontaneous creatinuria disappeared and creatine tolerance improved.[29] It was not known whether the beneficial effect of adrenal cortex extract represented a specific effect of certain adrenal steroids on phosphocreatine metabolism or whether the improvement was merely a reflection of the improved nutritional state induced by hormone therapy.

TABLE XXIII

Changes in Pigmentation Which Occurred in 64 Patients (Johns Hopkins Hospital) with Addison's Disease during Desoxycorticosterone Acetate Therapy

	Number of Patients	Per Cent of Total of 64 Patients
Abnormal pigmentation	60	94
Vitiligo	8	13
No significant change in pigmentation during therapy	33	52
Definite decrease in pigmentation	25*	40
Complete restoration to normal	0	0
Increase in pigmentation	1	2
First appearance of pigmentation *during* therapy	1	2

* Six patients in this group exhibited a striking decrease in pigmentation as a result of a marked increase in the extension of the areas of vitiligo.

With the exception of one patient (A. H., chart 7), it was not possible to study the disturbance in creatine metabolism prior to the institution of desoxycorticosterone acetate therapy. The status of creatine metabolism in 15 patients, however, was investigated at a later date (following one year of continuous synthetic hormone therapy). In seven of the 16 patients (44 per cent) spontaneous creatinuria of more than 100 mg. per day was observed at this time. (The patients were maintained on a creatine-low diet during these tests.) The nutritional state and appetite of the patients at the time of these observations were good. Retention of administered creatine (chart 7) was definitely impaired in 10 of the 16 patients or 63 per cent during synthetic hormone therapy, as well as in patient A. H., prior to the institution of therapy (chart 7).

It is evident from these data that creatine metabolism was abnormal during synthetic hormone therapy in a high proportion of the patients who were tested. There was no indication that prolonged treatment resulted in progressive improvement in creatine metabolism. In two patients who received long continued therapy with adrenal cortex extract (5 to 10 c.c. daily) a high normal retention of administered creatine (97.0 and 94.9 per cent respectively) was noted.

It appears probable that the abnormality in creatine metabolism which occurs in patients with Addison's disease is aggravated by anorexia and

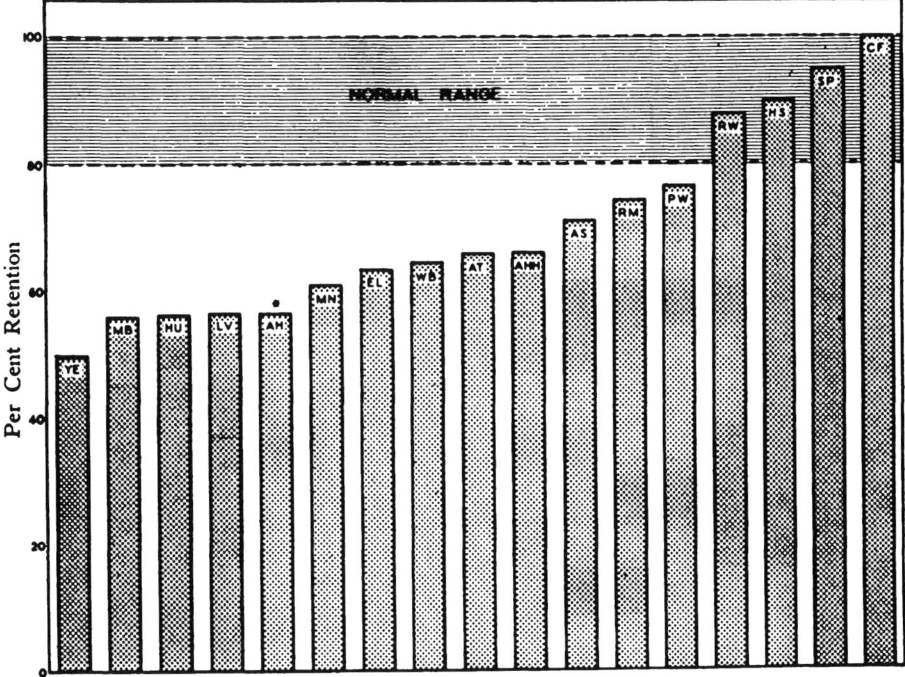

CHART 7. Creatine tolerance test * in patients with Addison's disease treated with desoxycorticosterone acetate. Creatine retention following test dose 2.64 gm.

inanition but is certainly not dependent upon these factors. Desoxycorticosterone acetate therapy does not correct the abnormality in creatine metabolism, whereas earlier studies [28, 29] and the studies on two patients in the present series suggest that treatment with adequate quantities of whole adrenal cortex extract may correct the underlying disturbance in creatine metabolism.

E. Renal Function: Renal function may be temporarily reduced during adrenal crisis as a consequence of reduced blood volume and reduced blood pressure. At this time there may occur a rise in blood non-protein nitrogen. Treatment with adrenal cortex extract or synthetic desoxycorticosterone acetate is followed by a rapid improvement in renal function.

One practical difficulty which arises in carrying out renal function tests in patients with Addison's disease is the inability in many instances to obtain a satisfactory rate of urine formation. This may result from the fact that these patients frequently experience considerable difficulty in ingesting large quantities of water, and furthermore, the absorption of water from the intestinal tract may occur at a rate slower than normal.

* Patients were maintained on a diet of low creatine content for a period of at least 72 hours prior to these determinations. On the day of the creatine tolerance test 2.64 gm. of creatine were administered by mouth. Details of the test and the technical methods employed have been described elsewhere.[30]

Patient A. H. was tested prior to the institution of therapy.

A summary of the results of the phenolsulphonphthalein and urea clearance tests in 55 of the 64 patients in our group is presented in table 24. Inulin and diodrast clearances were not measured in these patients. Talbott, recently, has made a number of very careful observations on the status of renal function in patients with Addison's disease.[31] He has demonstrated that although the phenolsulphonphthalein excretion and urea clearance may appear to be normal, more exact methods frequently demonstrate an appreciable degree of renal insufficiency.

TABLE XXIV

Summary of Renal Function Tests in 55 Patients with Addison's Disease Treated with Desoxycorticosterone Acetate (Johns Hopkins Hospital)

Phenolsulphonphthalein Test

	Number of Patients	Per Cent of Total of 55 Patients
Less than 40% excretion in 1 hour	5	9
Less than 60% excretion in 2 hours	9	16
Urea Clearance		
Less than 60% standard clearance	3	5

F. Hepatic Function: It is well known that the tolerance of adrenalectomized animals and patients with Addison's disease to various toxic agents is greatly reduced. One theory regarding the action of adrenal cortical hormone postulates that an important function of this hormone is its ability to assist the body in processes involving the detoxification of noxious substances.[32]

Rowntree and Snell [7] investigated hepatic function in patients with Addison's disease by studying the bilirubin content of the serum and retention of bromsulphthalein. The serum bilirubin level was uniformly normal, but the results of the bromsulphthalein test suggested slight impairment of liver function. We have studied the excretion of hippuric acid after intravenous injection of a standard dose of sodium benzoate in nine patients with Addison's disease during treatment with desoxycorticosterone acetate. In all instances the values obtained were distinctly below those observed in normale subjects (chart 8). It is of interest that four of the nine patients showed moderate splenomegaly. In no instance was there evidence of impaired renal function. It is possible that the impaired conversion of sodium benzoate to hippuric acid may reflect a defect in hepatic function occasioned by prolonged glycogen depletion or may be the result of impaired amino acid metabolism (glycine).

Intercurrent Infections: In the group of 64 patients treated in the Johns Hopkins Hospital, intercurrent infections played a significant rôle (a) as a precipitating factor in the original episode of adrenal insufficiency, (b) as a complication in the course of subsequent hormone therapy, and (c) as one of the chief causes of death. Ten patients definitely dated the onset of Addi-

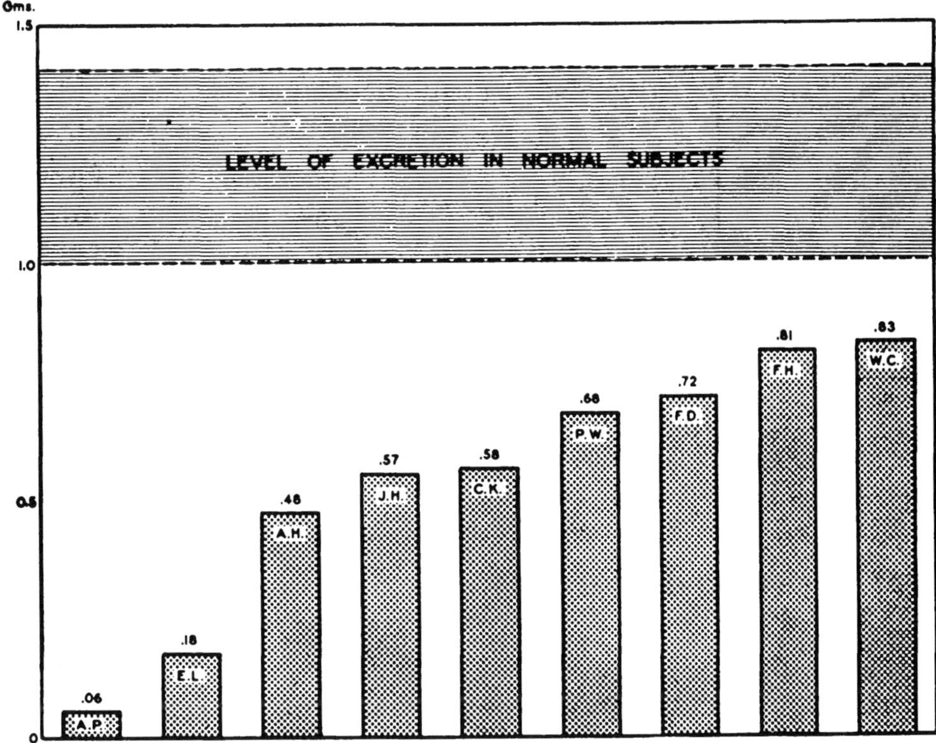

CHART 8. Hippuric acid excretion in patients with Addison's disease treated with desoxycorticosterone acetate. Excretion of hippuric acid patients.

son's disease to an acute febrile episode which was diagnosed in eight cases as "influenza," in one case as scarlet fever, and in one case as infectious mononucleosis. Exacerbation of adrenal insufficiency following acute infections occurred in 16 of the patients during treatment with synthetic hormone. In several of these patients repeated exacerbations of the disease occurred with successive bouts of infection. In five of the patients (8 per cent) crises induced by acute infections led to death. Infections due to hemolytic streptococci were one of the most common types encountered.

A striking characteristic of the response of patients with Addison's disease to acute infections was the extreme rapidity with which they became prostrate. On several occasions severe adrenal crisis with shock occurred within 48 hours of the onset of the acute infection. The increase in hormone requirement was very great during this period. Thus the problem of immediate and intensive early treatment had to be met. It is to be noted that although patients treated with synthetic hormone may experience a crisis induced by an acute intercurrent infection, the convalescence of these patients is very rapid in comparison with the prolonged period of invalidism previously observed in patients with Addison's disease.

Extremely encouraging results have been obtained recently in two patients with acute hemolytic streptococcus infection in which *sulfadiazine* was used in conjunction with adrenal cortex extract, desoxycorticosterone acetate and intravenous infusion of sodium chloride and glucose solution.[13] Sulfadiazine appears to be the most desirable of the sulfonamide drugs in treating patients with Addison's disease because of the low incidence of nausea and vomiting associated with its administration. The basic routine treatment which was employed in these two patients is similar in every respect to that outlined in "the treatment of adrenal crisis," the only difference being the addition of sulfadiazine therapy. An initial dose of 4 to 5 gm. of the sodium salt was given intravenously in conjunction with the infusion of saline and glucose solutions as soon as the patient was seen. Subsequently 1 gm. of sulfadiazine was given by mouth every four to six hours and an attempt was made to maintain a blood level of 10 to 20 mg. per 100 c.c. as long as fever persisted. In the event that sulfadiazine could not be taken by mouth, the intravenous injection of sodium salt of sulfadiazine (2 gm.) was repeated at 8 to 12 hour intervals. The importance of administering large quantities of adrenal cortex extract at frequent intervals, in conjunction with saline and glucose infusions and a supplementary dose of desoxycorticosterone acetate has been pointed out. The prompt recognition of infections and the appreciation of the necessity for immediate hospitalization with intensive therapy should do much toward reducing the relatively high mortality rate from hemolytic streptococcus infections in patients with Addison's disease. It is apparent that the hormone requirement of patients who have recently experienced an acute infection may be temporarily and even permanently increased.

Effect of Pregnancy: In one patient (H. B.) signs of adrenal insufficiency became manifest during pregnancy. In two other patients (K.D., and M.P.) an increase in pigmentation which was not considered to be beyond normal was noted during pregnancy. However, following the termination of pregnancy, the pigmentation in these two patients became progressively more intense instead of diminishing. In two patients (R. G., and M. P.) the first episode of adrenal crisis was precipitated by delivery. In one patient (A. K.) interruption of pregnancy was followed by septicemia and death. At present one patient (K. D.) is again pregnant.

The early weeks of pregnancy are especially difficult for patients with Addison's disease because of the associated nausea and vomiting. During this period it may be necessary to supplement desoxycorticosterone acetate treatment with daily injections of adrenal cortex extract and infusions of saline and glucose. The latter months of pregnancy should be rather well tolerated because of the sodium-retaining effect of the sex hormones,[33] and the secretion of the fetal adrenal. It has been demonstrated repeatedly that the hormone requirement of adrenalectomized animals is greatly reduced during pregnancy,[34, 35] and the beneficial effect of progesterone on the life maintenance of adrenalectomized animals is well known.[36] Desoxycorticosterone acetate treatment during the latter months of pregnancy should be regulated carefully to prevent excessive sodium and chloride retention.

The period immediately following delivery may prove to be a very critical one for patients with Addison's disease. Blood loss, the removal of supplementary adrenal cortical hormone provided by the fetus and the rapid decrease in titer of sex hormones may readily induce a crisis. Collapse at the time of delivery may result in hemorrhage into the anterior pituitary with resulting pituitary deficiency.[37] Therefore, patients with Addison's disease should be treated for impending crisis immediately prior to delivery (see section on preoperative therapy).

Although pregnancy is distinctly contraindicated in patients with Addison's disease, once established, it is probably much safer to attempt to carry the pregnancy to termination unless very unusual complications supervene. The need for hospitalization and careful supervision at the time of delivery should be emphasized.

Surgery in Addison's Disease: Patients with Addison's disease have long been known to represent extremely poor surgical risks.[7] Minor operative procedures such as dental extractions have been known to precipitate a crisis, and major operative procedures frequently resulted in death. Several factors contribute to the poor response of patients with Addison's disease to surgical procedures:

1. Lowered tolerance to narcotics and anesthetics.
2. Hypotension.
3. Dehydration and reduced plasma volume.
4. Depleted carbohydrate reserves.
5. Myocardial damage.

The first four of these disturbing factors may be corrected by adequate treatment with adrenal cortex extract, desoxycorticosterone acetate and intravenous infusions of saline and glucose solutions. At present with the improved management of patients it is possible to carry patients successfully through major operative procedures. A comparison has been made between the effect of surgery on patients prior to therapy (and in some instances prior to the diagnosis of Addison's disease) and subsequently (table 25). All seven patients did very poorly following operative procedures which were carried on prior to specific therapy. In five of these seven patients it appeared that the operative procedure hastened the development of the classical clinical picture of the disease (table 25, Section *A*). Of the seven treated patients (table 25, Section *B*), six had an uneventful postoperative course with the exception, in one patient, of a rather mild hypoglycemic episode during the second postoperative day. The seventh patient died on the forty-first postoperative day following a therapeutic abortion complicated by perforation of the uterus, pelvic vein thrombophlebitis, mul-

TABLE XXV

Complications of Surgical Operations in Patients with Addison's Disease

A.

Patient	Sex	Present Age	Operation	Hormone Therapy	Remarks
F. H.	M	24	Appendectomy	0	Precipitated adrenal crisis.
R. G.	F	28	Hysterectomy	0	Crisis, onset of Addison's disease.
R. M.	F	36	Tonsillectomy	0	Crisis, onset of Addison's disease.
E. V.	M	43	Cholecystectomy	0	Stormy postoperative period, onset of Addison's disease.
A. H.	F	40	Dental extraction	0	Crisis.
H. S.	M	49	Tonsillectomy	0	Stormy postoperative period, onset of Addison's disease.
A. S.	F	46	Hysterectomy	0	Prolonged convalescence, onset of Addison's disease.

B.

Patient	Sex	Present Age	Operation	Hormone Therapy	Remarks
D. B.	M	36	Herniorrhaphy	Desoxycorticosterone acetate	Uneventful convalescence.
E. F.	F	50	Dental extraction	Desoxycorticosterone acetate	No complications.
F. H.	M	24	Tonsillectomy	Desoxycorticosterone acetate+adrenal cortex extract.	Uneventful convalescence.
A. H.	F	41	Hemorrhoidectomy	Desoxycorticosterone acetate+adrenal cortex extract.	Uneventful convalescence.
A. K.	F	32	Therapeutic abortion	Desoxycorticosterone acetate	Septicemia, death.
F. G.	F	32	Appendectomy	Desoxycorticosterone acetate.	Uneventful convalescence.
J. P.	M	22	Nephrectomy	Desoxycorticosterone acetate+adrenal cortical extract.	Immediate postoperative course excellent, late convalescence complicated by excessive sodium retention, present health excellent.
A. S.	M	35	Epididymectomy	Desoxycorticosterone acetate+adrenal cortex extract.	Uneventful convalescence.

tiple pulmonary infarcts, severe pyelitis and *B. coli* bacteremia. It is of interest to note that this patient's blood pressure was maintained at a level of 125 mm. Hg systolic and 80 mm. diastolic until shortly before death.

Technic for Preparing Patients with Addison's Disease for Surgery: Local anesthesia is used whenever possible. When necessary a general anesthetic may be used, but care should be taken not to use anesthetic agents which *induce an appreciable degree of anoxia.* The ideal general anesthetic for patients with Addison's disease is yet to be discovered. It is possible that cyprethylene may prove to be the best for these patients. Cyclopropane has been used successfully, although the undesirable features of using this anesthetic in general operating rooms is well known. Pre-anesthetic morphine is given in reduced dosage, i.e., 5 to 10 mg. instead of 10 to 15 mg. It is our custom to give adrenal cortex extract and desoxycorticosterone acetate in increased doses for 24 to 48 hours prior to operation in an effort to increase liver glycogen, plasma volume and blood pressure. Adrenal cortex extract, 5 c.c. every four hours day and night for 48 hours preceding operation and 10 mg. of desoxycorticosterone acetate, once daily, is a safe routine. Early on the morning of operation, an intravenous infusion of 1000 c.c. of sodium chloride, 0.9 per cent, and glucose, 5 to 10 per cent, is given as well as a supplementary dose of 10 to 15 c.c. of adrenal cortex extract and 10 mg. of desoxycorticosterone acetate. A second infusion of saline and glucose is instituted at the time that the anesthetic is started, and 25 c.c. of adrenal cortex extract are added directly to the infusion. Additional extract is given during the operation if the systolic blood pressure falls below 120 mm. Hg. Epinephrine is given immediately (0.5 c.c.) subcutaneously if the systolic blood pressure falls below 100 mm. Hg. Following operation the patient is treated in a manner similar to that described under "treatment of adrenal crisis." Care should be taken not to give large doses of desoxycorticosterone acetate when the fluid requirement during the postoperative period is being provided by saline and glucose infusions.

Discussion

An analysis of the etiological factors responsible for adrenal cortical insufficiency in this group of 158 patients suggests that the incidence of tuberculosis is appreciably lower than that previously reported. This fact is of significance in relation to the therapeutic response which may be expected, since patients with active tuberculosis or extensive, healed tuberculosis present complications which are not encountered in the non-tuberculous group.

There is no evidence to show that a daily intramuscular injection of synthetic hormone in oil regularly taken is inferior to pellet therapy except in relation to the quantity of hormone which is required. However, the implantation of pellets of crystalline hormone has definite advantages in the treatment of patients who are unable or unwilling to coöperate by continuing daily injections of hormone indefinitely. Sublingual administration of hormone is not practical in most instances because hormone must be taken frequently throughout the day (four to six times daily) and relatively large quantities of hormone are required, hence the cost of therapy is excessively high.

The results of therapy in the present group of patients are striking as judged by survival at 1.5 years and by the extent to which these patients have been rehabilitated. However, it must be pointed out that the present good state of the majority of these patients is the result of intensive therapy with synthetic hormone, supplemented in crisis or during the course of intercurrent infections with adrenal cortex extract therapy and parenteral

Table XXVI

Summary of Observations on 64 Patients Treated with Desoxycorticosterone Acetate

Patient	Sex	Age	Occupation	Etiology of Addison's Disease	Duration of Disease (years)	Complications	Blood Pressure * Admission	Blood Pressure Present	Body Weight * Admission	Body Weight Present	Duration of Hormone Therapy (years)	Carbohydrate Defect	Electroencephalogram	Electrocardiogram	Present Therapy: Desoxycorticosterone Acetate	Present Therapy: Added Sodium Chloride gm.	Present Therapy: Adrenal Cortex Extract	Present Condition ‡
M. A.	F	48	Housewife	Tuberculous	14.0	Preëxisting hypertension	136/84	133/86	55.0	58.9	0.4	−−	—	"Borderline"	Pellets	3	0	A
I. B.	F	48	Housewife	Non-tuberculous	7.0	Cirrhosis, arthritis	110/74	180/110	48.0	50.0	2.8	0	—	Normal	Pellets	9	0	C
†J. B.	F	38	Housewife	Non-tuberculous	7.0	Rheumatic heart disease	100/70	130/80	53.0	60.0	0.3	++	—	—	Pellets	0	0	D
S. B.	M	22	Clerk	Non-tuberculous	3.0	None	100/75	140/80	45.5	56.0	0.7	−−	Abnormal	Normal	Pellets	0	0	A
B. B.	F	53	Housewife	Non-tuberculous	3.0	Arthritis, anemia	90/60	150/100	47.3	42.2	1.3	0	—	"Borderline"	Pellets	0	0	B
W. B.	M	21	Clerk	Non-tuberculous	4.0	Hypothyroidism	92/74	150/112	41.5	50.9	2.6	++	Abnormal	Myocardial damage	Pellets	3	0	A
D. W. B.	F	28	Housewife	Non-tuberculous	9.0	None	105/70	118/80	60.0	60.5	2.3	−−	Normal	—	Pellets	0	0	A
†M. B.	F	31	Teacher	Non-tuberculous	5.0	Hypothyroidism, anemia	90/66	102/60	49.4	52.9	1.0	+++	—	"Borderline"	Pellets	0	0	D
B. B.	M	22	Salesman	Non-tuberculous	4.0	None	120/76	120/70	56.3	60.5	1.7	+	—	Normal	Pellets	2	0	A
D. B.	M	35	Printer	Non-tuberculous	4.0	Inguinal hernia	108/70	168/98	64.7	68.6	2.9	++	—	Normal	Pellets	6	0	A
J. B.	M	56	Engineer	Non-tuberculous	2.0	None	96/82	150/92	60.0	88.6	0.8	−−	—	—	Pellets	2	0	A
W. C.	M	24	Truckdriver	Non-tuberculous	4.0	None	80/50	112/82	50.0	56.0	1.1	++	Abnormal	Normal	Pellets	5	0	B
C. C.	F	43	Housewife	Non-tuberculous	4.0	Anxiety neurosis	124/76	118/74	43.1	44.5	2.4	0	—	"Borderline"	Pellets	0	5 c.c.	C
W. J. C.	M	27	Unemployed	Non-tuberculous	8.0	Hypothyroidism	98/60	130/82	64.1	72.8	1.3	++	Abnormal	"Borderline"	Pellets	0	0	A
K. D.	F	19	Housewife	Non-tuberculous	2.0	Pregnancy	105/60	115/65	38.8	40.9	1.3	+	Normal	Normal	Pellets	5	0	A
F. D.	M	43	Writer	Non-tuberculous	5.0	None	96/58	108/70	66.8	66.4	3.0	++	Abnormal	Normal	Pellets	5	0	B
M. D.	M	29	Clerk	Non-tuberculous	3.0	None	80/60	116/78	50.1	66.6	2.8	++	Abnormal	"Borderline"	Pellets	0	0	B
†J. D.	M	68	Unemployed	Non-tuberculous	2.0	Arthritis	108/70	120/80	62.5	69.0	0.2	−−	—	"Borderline"	Percorten	10	0	D
†C. E.	M	67	Mail Carrier	Non-tuberculous	6.0	Arteriosclerosis, senility	104/78	132/78	51.2	48.0	1.7	0	—	"Borderline"	Pellets	8	0	D
Y. E.	F	39	Housewife	Non-tuberculous	4.0	Rheumatic heart disease	102/74	105/65	51.9	56.4	2.6	++	—	"Borderline"	Pellets	0	3 c.c.	B
C. F.	M	33	Mechanic	Tuberculous	3.0	Active tuberculosis	90/60	120/80	55.9	68.2	1.2	++	Abnormal	Normal	Pellets	0	0	A
J. F.	M	21	Student	Tuberculous	1.0	Active tuberculosis	80/60	140/100	68.2	72.3	0.3	−−	Normal	Normal	Pellets	3	0	B
E. F.	F	49	Housewife	Non-tuberculous	2.0	Arthritis	90/50	142/98	78.2	59.6	1.3	++	Normal	"Borderline"	Pellets	3	0	B
R. G.	F	27	Teacher	Non-tuberculous	2.0	Hypothyroidism	107/60	120/80	38.3	46.0	1.5	++	Abnormal	Myocardial damage	Pellets	1	0	A
A. H. G.	M	52	Mechanic	Tuberculous	1.0	Healed pulmonary tbc.	105/70	122/76	88.1	87.3	0.3	++	Abnormal	Normal	Pellets	0	0	A
F. G.	F	30	Clerk	Non-tuberculous	3.0	None	104/65	110/70	46.8	47.7	2.6	++	Normal	"Borderline"	Pellets	5	0	A
A. G.	F	51	Housewife	Tuberculous	6.0	Anemia	116/70	135/78	44.9	54.7	1.2	+	Abnormal	Myocardial damage	Pellets	5	0	A
J. H.	M	22	Clerk	Non-tuberculous	4.0	None	100/60	110/65	63.2	68.2	2.9	0	Abnormal	Normal	Pellets	3	0	A
F. H.	M	24	Clerk	Non-tuberculous	3.0	Splenomegaly	95/54	150/100	59.5	66.4	2.3	++	Abnormal	"Borderline"	Pellets	0	5 c.c.	A
A. W. H.	F	20	Housewife	Tuberculous	3.0	Active tuberculosis	108/76	120/88	58.1	59.1	1.8	0	Abnormal	Myocardial damage	Pellets	0	0	A
A. H.	F	40	Housewife	Non-tuberculous	4.0	None	90/60	120/80	45.0	47.3	1.1	0	Normal	"Borderline"	Pellets	3	0	B
I. H.	F	36	Teacher	Tuberculous	5.0	None	108/70	107/70	53.0	53.0	2.3	++	Abnormal	Normal	Pellets	0	0	A
A. H. H.	F	38	Housewife	Non-tuberculous	5.0	Splenomegaly	90/58	118/76	40.0	44.9	2.5	++	Abnormal	Myocardial damage	Pellets	3	0	B
†H. H.	M	38	Salesman	Non-tuberculous	1.0	None	120/74	120/78	80.5	85.0	0.6	−−	—	Normal	Pellets	0	0	D
C. K.	M	45	Service Mgr.	Tuberculous	7.0	Active tuberculosis	80/60	130/90	65.6	76.0	1.5	+	Abnormal	Myocardial damage	Pellets	0	0	B

TABLE XXVI—*Continued*

Patient	Sex	Age	Occupation	Etiology of Addison's Disease	Duration of Disease (years)	Complications	Blood Pressure		Body Weight		Duration of Hormone Therapy (years)	Carbohydrate Defect	Electroencephalogram	Electrocardiogram	Present Therapy			Present Condition ‡
							* Admission	Present	* Admission	Present					Desoxycorticosterone Acetate	Added Sodium Chloride gm.	Adrenal Cortex Extract	
E. K.	F	47	Stenographer	Tuberculous	8.0	Preëxisting hypertension	190/130	170/110	42.9	44.5	1.2	0	Abnormal	Normal	Pellets	0	0	C
†A. K.	F	32	Housewife	Non-tuberculous	1.0	Puerperal sepsis	90/60	125/80	54.8	59.4	0.2	− −	—	—	Percorten	8	0	D
E. L.	F	51	Bookkeeper	Tuberculous	7.0	None	88/50	136/92	43.5	46.1	1.8	++	Normal	Myocardial damage	Percorten	0	0	C
†M. M.	F	27	Housewife	Non-tuberculous	3.0	None	85/72	120/80	51.3	54.5	2.8	++	—	Myocardial damage	Pellets	10	0	D
F. M.	M	32	Laborer	Non-tuberculous	4.0	Hypothyroidism	92/60	130/80	61.2	62.7	3.2	+++	Normal	Myocardial damage	Pellets	5	0	A
H. M.	M	44	Mechanic	Non-tuberculous	5.0	None	96/54	100/60	66.0	68.2	2.1	− −	Normal	Normal	Pellets	0	0	A
R. M.	F	35	Housewife	Non-tuberculous	4.0	Urticaria	60/40	120/90	49.6	62.7	2.6	+	—	"Borderline"	Pellets	3	0	A
C. N.	F	34	Housewife	Non-tuberculous	5.0	Hypoproteinemia	94/60	110/70	55.9	54.7	3.3	+++	—	Myocardial damage	Pellets	0	0	A
M. N.	F	37	Housewife	Non-tuberculous	2.0	Anemia	90/58	100/84	47.1	42.7	1.0	+	Abnormal	Normal	Pellets	3	0	B
O. O.	M	43	Manager	Tuberculous	11.0	None	88/70	100/80	58.3	63.6	1.8	+	—	Normal	Pellets	4	0	A
M. P.	F	35	Housewife	Non-tuberculous	4.0	Pregnancy	102/80	110/78	71.8	69.3	2.3	0	Normal	Normal	Pellets	3	0	A
A. P.	M	45	Professor	Non-tuberculous	7.0	None	106/76	120/80	72.0	70.0	1.1	+++	Abnormal	"Borderline"	Pellets	0	6 c.c.	A
J. P.	M	19	—	Tuberculous	5.0	Active tuberculosis	85/60	138/92	39.3	47.7	3.3	++	—	Normal	Pellets	0	0	A
S. P.	M	28	Foreman	Non-tuberculous	3.0	None	120/75	130/90	70.9	71.1	2.3	0	—	"Borderline"	Pellets	0	0	A
†O. Q.	M	62	Farmer	Non-tuberculous	2.0	Arthritis, arteriosclerosis	80/62	132/80	50.8	54.7	0.5	−	—	Normal	Pellets	10	0	D
J. S.	M	29	Clerk	Non-tuberculous	5.0	Peptic ulcer	92/70	160/100	55.2	70.7	2.3	−	—	Normal	Pellets	0	0	A
M. S.	F	38	Housewife	Non-tuberculous	3.0	None	80/60	150/106	50.2	58.2	1.3	+	Abnormal	Myocardial damage	Pellets	3	3 c.c.	B
†A. B. S.	M	32	Bookkeeper	Tuberculous	5.0	Active tuberculosis	104/68	146/104	57.4	59.2	1.8	+	—	Normal	Pellets	10	0	D
A. S.	M	40	—	Tuberculous	1.0	Active tuberculosis	80/50	130/80	52.7	52.3	0.3	—	—	Myocardial damage	Pellets	0	0	C
A. C. S.	F	44	Housewife	Non-tuberculous	2.0	Diverticulosis of sigmoid	90/65	115/65	52.7	59.6	2.1	0	—	—	Pellets	0	0	A
H. S.	M	48	Unemployed	Tuberculous	6.0	Active tuberculosis	124/76	138/82	81.0	83.6	1.0	0	Abnormal	Normal	Pellets	6	0	B
A. T.	M	49	Innkeeper	Tuberculous	5.0	Healed pulmonary tbc.	118/80	140/88	60.0	68.2	2.3	++	Abnormal	"Borderline"	Pellets	0	0	B
H. U.	F	34	Housewife	Non-tuberculous	2.0	Rheumatic heart disease	100/50	108/60	40.7	41.0	0.9	+	Abnormal	Myocardial damage	Pellets	4	0	B
†L. V.	F	43	Housewife	Non-tuberculous	2.0	None	100/60	112/75	41.5	43.1	0.2	+	Normal	Myocardial damage	Pellets	0	0	D
E. V.	M	39	Tailor	Non-tuberculous	6.0	None	94/60	118/82	54.4	63.6	3.3	++	Abnormal	"Borderline"	Pellets	0	0	A
P. W.	M	34	Clergyman	Non-tuberculous	9.0	None	95/60	140/90	51.0	58.1	3.3	++	Abnormal	Myocardial damage	Pellets	5	0	B
S. W.	F	55	Housewife	Non-tuberculous	3.0	Arthritis	120/78	158/90	58.5	66.1	2.8	+	Normal	Myocardial damage	Pellets	0	3 c.c.	B
R. W.	M	58	Unemployed	Non-tuberculous	4.0	Coronary occlusion	108/70	122/78	71.2	75.5	2.8	+	—	Myocardial damage	Pellets	7	0	C
B. W.	M	26	Accountant	Non-tuberculous	3.0	Healed pulmonary tbc.	80/60	140/80	57.3	61.4	1.8	0	—	—	Pellets	5	0	A

* Values at the time desoxycorticosterone acetate treatment was instituted or substituted for some other form of therapy.

† Indicates patients who have succumbed. Data for "present weight" and "blood pressure" are the values reported shortly before death. Under "present therapy" are listed the hormone and sodium chloride requirements during the period of survival on desoxycorticosterone acetate therapy.

‡ A = greatly improved. B = improved. C = unimproved. D = dead.

administration of saline and glucose solutions. That the results of therapy are not due primarily to the extract and supplementary sodium chloride therapy is indicated by the mortality rate of 42 per cent which was reported in a group of 34 patients treated with extract and sodium chloride alone (chart 3) and by the fact that at least 60 patients in the present group are receiving only desoxycorticosterone acetate without supplementary sodium chloride or extract therapy.

It is unfortunate that at present commercial adrenal cortex extracts are not assayed for their "carbohydrate-regulating" potency since the benefits to be derived from this factor constitute one of the principal reasons for administering extract to patients in crisis and during the course of intercurrent infections. Furthermore, it has recently been demonstrated [38] that certain adrenal steroids which possess "carbohydrate-regulating" potency actually facilitate sodium and chloride excretion in contrast to the well known sodium and chloride-retaining effect of desoxycorticosterone acetate. It appears probable that a combination of these steroid compounds in correct proportions may not only supplement the deficiency of desoxycorticosterone acetate in respect to "carbohydrate-regulating" potency but may also decrease the tendency for excessive sodium and chloride retention which frequently occurs with rather moderate maintenance doses of desoxycorticosterone acetate.

Studies of electrolyte metabolism, plasma volume, carbohydrate metabolism, electrocardiogram, electroencephalogram, renal, hepatic, muscle and gastrointestinal function emphasize the widespread damage which may occur in patients with adrenal insufficiency. Since many of these changes appear to be irreversible, every effort should be made to establish the diagnosis as early as possible in the course of the disease. Diagnosis of Addison's disease at the time of its onset, however, presents an extremely difficult problem. The use of "deprivation" tests, such as the Cutler-Power-Wilder test,[39] is justified if the patient can be kept in a hospital under very careful supervision. A test described more recently by Robinson, Power and Kepler [40] presents several advantages over the Cutler-Power-Wilder test, and it is certainly advisable to consider applying this test before carrying out procedures which entail much greater risk. Glucose tolerance tests, particularly the response to intravenously administered glucose,[11] and a study of the 17-ketosteroid excretion are of considerable aid.[41] When carefully controlled with adequate periods of placebo medication, we have found the response to sodium chloride and hormone therapy (desoxycorticosterone acetate 2 to 5 mg. daily or adrenal cortex extract, 5 to 10 c.c. daily) to be helpful. More specific, however, is the speed and extent of *relapse which follows the sudden withdrawal of therapy after it has been* maintained for a period of one to two weeks.[42]

Summary

1. One hundred and fifty-eight patients with Addison's disease have been treated with synthetic desoxycorticosterone acetate of whom 148 have re-

ceived subcutaneous implantations of crystalline pellets of synthetic hormone. An analysis of the entire group revealed the following:

(*a*) Tuberculosis appeared to be the etiological factor responsible for the adrenal cortical insufficiency in less than 50 per cent of the patients.
(*b*) Approximately 80 per cent of the total number of cases occurred in patients 20 to 50 years of age.
(*c*) The difference in incidence between sexes was not great, i.e., males 56 per cent.
(*d*) Presenting symptoms were as follows: weakness and fatigability in 100 per cent; increasing pigmentation in 94 per cent; anorexia in 91 per cent.

2. Approximately 90 per cent of the patients required 1 to 5 mg. daily of hormone in oil, injected intramuscularly, or 2 to 10 pellets (125 mg. each) implanted subcutaneously. The average duration of therapy was 1.7 years.

3. The mortality rate for the entire group of 156 patients was 15.4 per cent during the present period of therapy (1.7 years); 46 per cent of the deaths were due to infections and 29 per cent to cardiovascular disease. Sixty of these patients are now receiving desoxycorticosterone acetate treatment alone, 66 patients are receiving synthetic hormone and supplementary sodium chloride medication, and six patients are receiving supplementary daily injections of adrenal cortical extract.

4. A detailed analysis of the results of therapy in 64 patients studied in the Johns Hopkins Hospital revealed that 48, or 75 per cent, of the group were definitely improved, and that 56 per cent of the male patients have now been restored to full time employment. In this group of 64 patients an average gain in weight of 4 kg., and a rise in blood pressure from 100 mm. Hg systolic and 66 mm. diastolic to 126 mm. Hg systolic and 70 mm. diastolic were noted. The effect of synthetic hormone on the abnormal pigmentation was neither striking nor consistent.

5. A high proportion of patients with Addison's disease was observed to show:

(*a*) abnormalities in carbohydrate metabolism (75 per cent).
(*b*) abnormal electrocardiograms (60 per cent).
(*c*) abnormal electroencephalograms (69 per cent).
(*d*) abnormalities in creatine metabolism (69 per cent).
(*e*) reduced hippuric acid excretion (100 per cent).

These abnormalities persisted despite continued desoxycorticosterone acetate, and in certain instances the extent or incidence of the abnormalities increased during the period of therapy.

6. Desoxycorticosterone acetate treatment was followed by transient hypertension (34 per cent), transient edema (27 per cent), circulatory insufficiency (8 per cent), tendon and muscular contractions (4 per cent) and transient peripheral motor paralysis (2 per cent). Practically all

of the over dosage phenomena may be explained on the basis of excessive retention of sodium and chloride. For this reason the dose of supplementary sodium chloride medication, if used at all in conjunction with desoxycorticosterone acetate, must be regulated carefully. A diet of low potassium content is definitely contraindicated in patients under treatment with desoxycorticosterone acetate. The incidence of undesirable complications may be reduced greatly by care in the regulation of the dose of synthetic hormone and by an appreciation of the mechanism by which complications are initiated.

Conclusion

The use of desoxycorticosterone acetate in the treatment of a large group of patients with Addison's disease has been associated with the rehabilitation of approximately 50 per cent of the patients. A striking reduction in mortality rate was observed at the end of 1.5 years of therapy. The disturbances in function which may persist despite desoxycorticosterone acetate therapy have been indicated and the undesirable effects of excessive doses of synthetic hormone have been described. If reasonable care is employed in regulating the dose of hormone, complications resulting from overdosage may be greatly reduced. The functional changes which develop in the heart, brain, liver, kidney, muscle, gastrointestinal tract and skin of patients with longstanding adrenal cortical deficiency demonstrate the protean nature of the disease and indicate the great need for early diagnosis.

Acknowledgments

This report would not have been possible without the continued coöperation of a large group of physicians who were kind enough to provide us with information relating to the hormone assay, implantation of pellets and subsequent clinical course of patients under their care. We also wish to acknowledge the assistance of Miss Rachel Fee, nurse in charge of the metabolism unit, Miss Janet Ruth Engebretson, dietitian-in-charge, and Drs. Marshall Clinton, Jr., and John Arthur Luetscher, Jr. We are indebted to Dr. Warfield M. Firor, Associate Professor of Surgery, for implanting pellets in the patients who were studied in the Johns Hopkins Hospital.

BIBLIOGRAPHY

1. Thorn, G. W., Howard R. P., Emerson, Kendall, Jr., and Firor, W. M.: Treatment of Addison's disease with pellets of crystalline adrenal cortical hormone (synthetic desoxycorticosterone acetate) implanted subcutaneously, Bull. Johns Hopkins Hosp., 1939, lxiv, 339.
2. Thorn, G. W., Howard, R. P., and Emerson, Kendall, Jr.: Treatment of Addison's disease with desoxycorticosterone acetate, a synthetic adrenal cortical hormone (preliminary report), Jr. Clin. Invest., 1939, xviii, 449.
3. Cleghorn, R. A., Fowler, J. L. A., and Wenzel, J. S.: The treatment of Addison's disease by synthetic adrenal cortical hormone (desoxycorticosterone acetate), Canad. Med. Assoc. Jr., 1939, xli, 226.
4. Ferrebee, J. W., Ragan, Charles, Atchley, D. W., and Loeb, R. F.: Desoxycorticosterone esters: certain effects in the treatment of Addison's disease, Jr. Am. Med. Assoc., 1939, cxiii, 1725.
5. Thorn, G. W., and Firor, W. M.: Desoxycorticosterone acetate therapy in Addison's disease. Clinical consideration, Jr. Am. Med. Assoc., 1940, cxiv, 2517.

6. CONYBEARE, J. J., and MILLIS, G. C.: Observations on 29 cases of Addison's disease treated in Guy's Hospital between 1904 and 1923, Guy's Hosp. Rep., 1924, lxxiv, 369.
7. ROWNTREE, L. G., and SNELL, A. M.: A clinical study of Addison's disease, Mayo Clin. Monographs, 1931, W. B. Saunders Co., Philadelphia.
8. RICHTER, C. P.: Sodium chloride and dextrose appetite of untreated and treated adrenalectomized rats, Endocrinology, 1941, xxix, 115.
9. ANDERSON, E., HAYMAKER, W., and HENDERSON, E.: Successful sublingual therapy in Addison's disease, Jr. Am. Med. Assoc., 1940, cxv, 2167.
10. THORN, G. W., GREIF, R. L., COUTINHO, S. O., and EISENBERG, H.: Relative effectiveness of several methods of administering desoxycorticosterone acetate, Jr. Clin. Endocrinol., 1941, i, 967.
11. THORN, G. W., KOEPF, G. F., LEWIS, R. A., and OLSEN, E. F.: Carbohydrate metabolism in Addison's disease, Jr. Clin. Invest., 1940, xix, 813.
12. LEWIS, R. A., KUHLMANN, D., DELBUE, C., KOEPF, G. F., and THORN, G. W.: The effect of the adrenal cortex on carbohydrate metabolism, Endocrinology, 1940, xxvii, 971.
13. THORN, G. W., and LEWIS, R. A.: Acute hemolytic streptococcus infections complicating Addison's disease. Treatment with sulfadiazine and adrenal cortex extract: report of 2 cases, Jr. Am. Med. Assoc., 1942, cxviii, 214.
14. BUELL, M. V., and TURNER, E.: Cation distribution in the muscles of adrenalectomized rats, Am. Jr. Physiol., 1941, cxxxiv, 2.
15. KUHLMANN, D., RAGAN, C., FERREBEE, J. W., ATCHLEY, D. W., and LOEB, R. F.: Toxic effects of desoxycorticosterone esters in dogs, Science, 1939, xc, 496.
16. DUQUE SAMPAYO, A., LOPEZ MORALES, J. M., and LAFUENTE, A.: Studien über Physiopathologie der Nebennieren. Der Zustand des Herzens bei der chronischen Nebenniereninsuffizienz (Addison'sche Krankheit), Endocrinologie, 1934, xiv, 22.
17. MATTIOLI, M.: L'electrocardiogramma nella sindrome di Addison, Cuore e Circol., 1937, xxi, 406.
18. MCCULLAGH, E. P., and RYAN, E. J.: Use of desoxycorticosterone acetate in Addison's disease, Jr. Am. Med. Assoc., 1940, cxiv, 2530.
19. MCGAVACK, T. H.: Changes in heart volume in Addison's disease and their significance, Am. Heart Jr., 1941, xxi, 1.
20. WILLSON, D. M., RYNEARSON, E. H., and DRY, T. J.: Cardiac failure following treatment of Addison's disease with desoxycorticosterone acetate, Proc. Staff Meet. Mayo Clin., 1941, xvi, 168.
21. ASHMAN, R. and HULL, E.: Essentials of electrocardiography, 2nd Edition, 1941, MacMillan Co., New York.
22. CHAMBERLAIN, E. N., and HAY, J. D.: Normal electrocardiogram, Brit. Heart Jr., 1939, i, 105.
23. LARSEN, K., and SKULASON, T.: Study of 2400 electrocardiograms of apparently healthy males, Am. Heart Jr., 1941, xxii, 625.
24. WHITE, P. D., CHAMBERLAIN, F. L., and GRAYBIEL, A.: Inversion of the T-waves in Lead II caused by a variation in position of the heart, Brit. Heart Jr., 1941, iii, 233.
25. NICHOLSON, W. M., and SOFFER, L. J.: Cardiac arrhythmia in experimental suprarenal insufficiency in dogs, Bull. Johns Hopkins Hosp., 1935, lvi, 236.
26. STEWART, H. J., SMITH, J. J., and MILHORAT, A. T.: Electrocardiographic and serum potassium changes in familial periodic paralysis, Am. Jr. Med. Sci., 1940, cxcix, 789.
27. HOFFMANN, W. C., LEWIS, R. A., and THORN, G. W.: The electroencephalogram in Addison's disease, Bull. Johns Hopkins Hosp., 1942, lxx, 335.
28. THORN, G. W.: Creatine studies in thyroid disorders, Endocrinology, 1936, xx, 628.
29. THORN, G. W.: Unpublished data.
30. THORN, G. W., and TIERNEY, N. J.: Myasthenia gravis complicated by thyrotoxicosis: creatine studies, Bull. Johns Hopkins Hosp., 1941, lxix, 469.

31. Talbott, J. H., Pecora, L. J., Melville, R. S., and Consolazio, W. V.: Renal function in patients with Addison's disease and in patients with adrenal insufficiency secondary to pituitary pan-hypopituitarism, Jr. Clin. Invest., 1942, xxi, 107.
32. Perla, D., and Marmorston, J.: Natural resistance and clinical medicine, 1940, Little, Brown & Co., Boston.
33. Thorn, G. W., and Harrop, G. A.: The "sodium-retaining effect" of the sex hormones, Science, 1937, lxxxvi, 40.
34. Roggoff, J. M., and Stewart, G. N.: Studies on adrenal insufficiency; influence of "heat" on survival period of dogs after adrenalectomy, Am. Jr. Physiol., 1928, lxxxvi, 20.
35. Swingle, W. W., Parkins, W. M., Taylor, A. R., Hays, H. W., and Morrell, J. A.: Effect of estrus (pseudo pregnancy) and certain pituitary hormones on life span of adrenalectomized animals, Am. Jr. Physiol., 1937, cxix, 675.
36. Gaunt, R., and Hays, H. W.: Life-maintaining effect of crystalline progesterone in adrenalectomized ferrets, Science, 1938, lxxxviii, 576.
37. Sheehan, H. L.: Simmond's disease due to post partum necrosis of anterior pituitary, Quart. Jr. Med., 1939, viii, 277.
38. Thorn, G. W., Engel, L. L., and Lewis, R. A.: The effect of 17-hydroxycorticosterone and related adrenal cortical steroids on sodium and chloride excretion, Science, 1941, xciv, 348.
39. Cutler, H. H., Power, M. H., and Wilder, R. M.: Concentration of chloride, sodium and potassium in urine and blood, Jr. Am. Med. Assoc., 1938, cxi, 117.
40. Robinson, F. J., Power, M. H., and Kepler, E. J.: Two new procedures to assist in the recognition and exclusion of Addison's disease: a preliminary report, Proc. Staff Meet. Mayo Clin., 1941, xvi, 577.
41. Fraser, R. W., Forbes, A. P., Albright, F., Sulkowitch, H., and Reifenstein, E. C., Jr.: Colorimetric assay of 17-ketosteroids in urine, Jr. Clin. Endocrinol., 1941, i, 234.
42. Thorn, G. W.: Adrenal insufficiency and the use of synthetic adrenal cortical hormone, Proc. Inter-State Postgraduate Medical Assembly of North America, Oct. 14–18, 1940.

ANNALS OF
INTERNAL MEDICINE

VOLUME 44 JANUARY, 1956 NUMBER 1

PRIMARY ALDOSTERONISM, A NEW CLINICAL ENTITY * †

By JEROME W. CONN, M.D., F.A.C.P., and LAWRENCE H. LOUIS, ScD., *Ann Arbor, Michigan*

ALDOSTERONE, the newly discovered normal adrenal secretory product,[1-6] has attracted the attention of a great many clinical investigators because of its apparent rôle in the pathogenesis of a number of clinical disorders. This extremely potent sodium-retaining corticoid has been found to be present in excessive amounts in the urine of edematous nephrotics,[7, 8] cardiacs with congestive failure,[9, 10] patients with decompensated hepatic cirrhosis [11-13] and women with eclampsia.[14-16] All of these conditions manifest marked edema, but it is obvious that the *primary* difficulty in each condition is *not* due to increased activity of a sodium-retaining steroid. It seems reasonable to assume that in the course of the development of each of these conditions a metabolic event occurs which is common to them and which triggers the production of excessive quantities of aldosterone. We would therefore classify such conditions as being associated with *secondary aldosteronism.*

Primary aldosteronism, by which we mean that the disease originates in the adrenal gland, is *not* associated with edema, and in its pure state manifests itself in the form of an interesting complex of symptoms and a fascinating disturbance of electrolyte metabolism.

The data to be presented have been obtained in the course of an extensive metabolic balance study upon a *single patient.* The investigation extends from April, 1954, to April, 1955, and includes 227 days of rigid metabolic control. It appears to establish the existence of a new clinical syndrome, which we have named "primary aldosteronism." [17, 18] The data afford a reasonable explanation for the abnormality of electrolyte metabolism which

* Presented at the Thirty-sixth Annual Session of the American College of Physicians, Philadelphia, Pennsylvania, April 27, 1955.

From the Division of Endocrinology and Metabolism, Department of Internal Medicine, University of Michigan Medical School, Ann Arbor, Michigan.

† This study has been supported in part by a grant from the Research and Development Board, Office of the Surgeon General, U. S. Army.

is involved. Perhaps of greater significance is the fact that these patients can be relieved of a disease formerly called "potassium-losing nephritis" [19, 20] by surgical removal of an adrenal cortical adenoma. We say *these patients* because we are now aware of 12 additional cases, recognized by others [21–30] since our preliminary report (October, 1954 [17]). Of the 13 cases, nine have been cured by removal of an adrenal cortical adenoma and one by bilateral adrenalectomy. The remaining three cases were recognized in retrospect, having had the clinical picture and having disclosed an adrenal cortical adenoma at autopsy.

Case Report

Clinical Findings and Initial Laboratory Data: A 34 year old white housewife was admitted to the Metabolic Research Unit of the University Hospital on April 27, 1954. She stated that for seven years she had been having attacks of intense generalized muscular weakness. Occasionally these attacks would be so severe as to result in complete "paralysis" of both lower extremities. The first episode of this nature had occurred in October, 1947, when she suddenly became paralyzed from the hips down. The "paralysis" persisted for two days and then disappeared within a few hours. Four other attacks of this degree of severity had occurred over the seven year period. No clear-cut precipitating factors could be elicited, although the patient felt certain that on one occasion exposure to cold (two hours as a spectator at a hockey game) had brought on a severe attack. Except for vague, intermittent general muscular weakness, she had been quite well between attacks.

A secondary complaint, also involving the muscular system but not necessarily related temporally to episodes of weakness, was "spasms of the muscles." These attacks occurred frequently and, in character, were typical of tetany involving mainly the upper extremities but occasionally the lower extremities as well. Intravenous calcium gluconate administered at a local hospital was said to have relieved several of the more severe attacks of tetany.

The patient was told in 1950 that her blood pressure was "180." Since then it had varied between "180 and 190." Over this same period of time proteinuria had been found repeatedly. Polydipsia, polyuria and nocturia (two to three times) had existed for years.

There was no history of vomiting or diarrhea, or of the habitual use of cathartics or other drugs.

The essential findings on physical examination were as follows: Well developed musculature (figure 1), general distribution of body fat and no cutaneous striae. Blood pressure, 176/104 mm. of Hg. Normal heart size. No edema. Positive Chvostek's and Trousseau's signs. Hyperactivity of all tendon reflexes. The remainder of the examination disclosed no abnormalities.

The initial laboratory values are summarized in table 1. In addition, glucose tolerance was found to be perfectly normal, and a battery of liver function tests revealed normal hepatic function. Urine volume averaged 4 liters per day. Electrocardiograms showed changes compatible with hypokalemia.

It was clear that we were dealing with a hypernatremic, hypokalemic alkalosis associated with alkaline urine. The muscular weakness was explainable on a hypokalemic basis, and the tetany on the basis of severe alkalosis. But we were anxious to determine, if possible, the mechanism of production of this abnormality of electrolyte metabolism. The situation was obviously not Cushing's syndrome, since eosinophils and 17-hydroxycorticoids were normal. (Subsequently, over 200 such determinations gave normal values.)

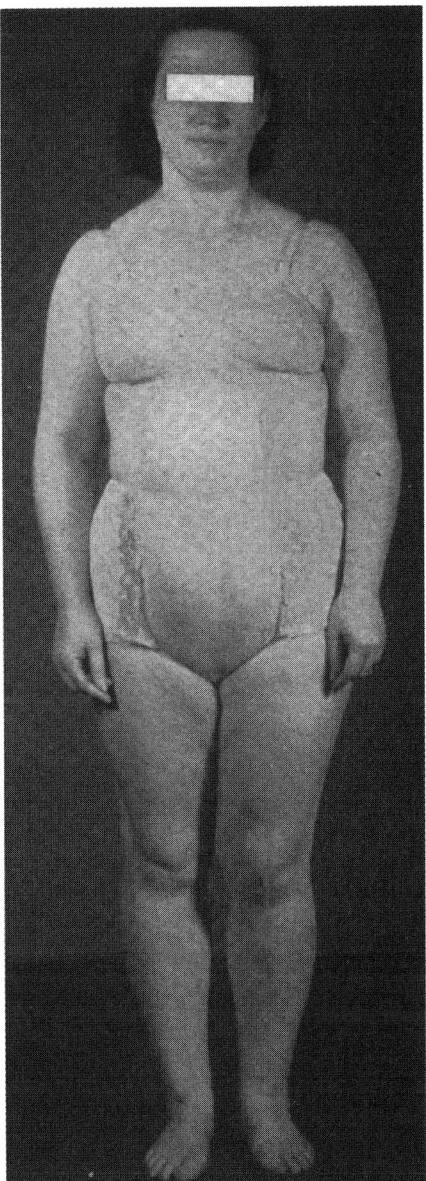

FIG. 1.

The renal status, too, was of great interest, since the major functional defect consisted of hyposthenuria unaffected by administration of Pitressin. We attributed this (deficient tubular reabsorption of water) to the presence of chronic hypokalemia, an association described by Schwartz and Relman in 1953.[31] It was also apparent that if the hypokalemia was due to excessive urinary loss of potassium (the most likely possibility), the tubules had retained their capacity to reabsorb sodium and calcium normally. This suggested a functional lesion, probably hormonal, since it would be expected that in degenerative renal tubular disease ions other than, and in addition to, potassium would be involved.

We suggested, therefore, that excessive amounts of aldosterone could be the cause of the entire disturbance, and proceeded to study the patient from this point of view.

Metabolic Studies: The data can be divided conveniently into three parts, namely, preoperative data, data obtained at the time of operation, and postoperative data.

1. *Preoperative studies:* Metabolic balance data and their interpretation covering the first 70 days of the preoperative period have already been reported in detail.[17] Those results can be summarized as follows:

(A) Assays of urine for sodium-retaining corticoid, presumably aldosterone, gave values four to 30 times greater than those found in the urine of normal adults.

(B) The concentrations of sodium and chloride of 60 samples of thermal sweat were found to be extremely low. Earlier we [32, 33] had described this test as an index of the activity of sodium-retaining corticoids, whether of exogenous or endogenous origin.

TABLE 1

Initial Laboratory Values, M. W., F, 34

Blood Values		Urinary and Renal Values
1. Counts normal, Hb.	14.4 gm.	1. Urine protein 0 to tr., sed. neg.
2. Eosin.	198/cu. mm.	2. pH 7.17–7.54
3. Serum creatinine	0.54–1.02	3. End. creat. clearance 125–170 L./day
4. NPN	33–38 mg. %	4. PSP 50% in 15 min., 80% in 2 hr.
5. Sugar	84 mg. %	5. 18 hour concentration test sp. gr. 1.011 18th h 10 mg. Pitressin. 20th h sp. gr. 1.011
6. Serum Protein	6.9%, alb. 4.9%	
7. Serum Ca	10.2 mg. %	6. Ca 122 mg./day with intake 137 mg./day
8. Serum Inorg. P	2.4 mg. %	7. 17-ketosteroids 5.7 mg./day
9. Serum Cl	101–103 mEq./L.	8. 17-hydroxysteroids 5.0 mg./day
10. Serum Na	146–151 mEq./L.	9. K-U/P 13 at serum K-2.5 mEq.
11. Serum K	1.6–2.5 mEq./L.	
12. Serum pH	7.62	Metabolic alkalosis with hypokalemia and tetany
13. CO_2 comb. power	82 vols. %	
		Possibilities
		1. Excessive activity of aldosterone
		2. Specific renal tubular lesion with K loss

Program: To have complete balance study with assays for aldosterone

(C) A similar number of samples of saliva gave sodium-potassium ratios indicative of great activity of a sodium-retaining corticoid.[34]

(D) Hypernatremia, hypokalemia and marked elevation of blood pH and of CO_2 combining power were persistent and were not influenced by administration at 230 mEq. of potassium daily for 28 days. Serum chloride was normal.

(E) Mean blood pressure for 60 days was 170/100 mm. of Hg. A small amount of protein (usually less than 1 gm. daily) was found in the urine constantly. Chvostek's and Trousseau's signs were positive daily.

(F) Balance data showed an average daily loss of 12 mEq. of potassium while the patient's intake of potassium was 100 mEq./day. Stool potassium was normal. There existed sodium and nitrogen equilibrium. Urinary 17-hydroxycorticoids and 17-ketosteroids were normal constantly.

(G) Repeatedly, administration of ACTH or hydrocortisone produced perfectly normal responses with respect to changes in 17-ketosteroids, 17-hydroxycorticoids, eosinophils, nitrogen and carbohydrate metabolism. Thus, on the basis of the usual indices one would have no reason to suspect abnormal adrenal cortical function.

(H) There was, however, a paradoxic response to ACTH and hydrocortisone with respect to electrolyte metabolism. Upon administration of either Compound F or ACTH there ensued two to three days of sodium and chloride retention, followed by a sharp diuresis of sodium and chloride while the hormones were still being given. This is reminiscent of what often happens in nephrosis under hormonal treatment, and suggests some kind of peripheral antagonism between Compound F and aldosterone when activity of the latter is abnormally high.

Another paradox was observed in the immediate post-hormone periods, where sharp sodium and chloride retention occurred at a time when adrenal function was at its lowest, i.e., when urinary 17-hydroxycorticoid excretion reached its lowest levels.

(I) Several attempts at repletion of potassium were made, using as much as 300 mEq./day of potassium. Under such circumstances one could demonstrate sig-

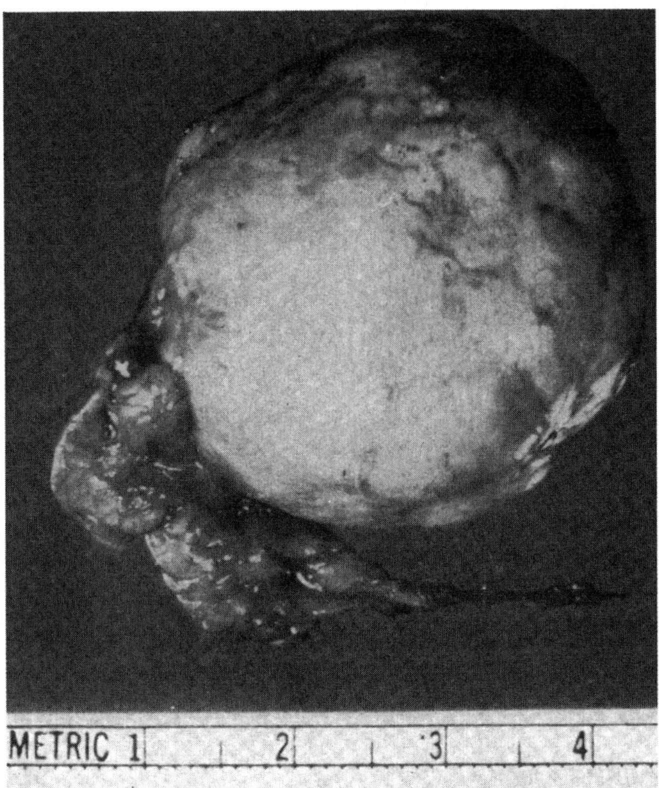

FIG. 2.

nificant but short-lived retention of potassium, accompanied by loss of sodium. Upon cessation of supplementary potassium there ensued abrupt retention of sodium and loss of potassium. It appeared that an abnormal type of electrolyte equilibrium was dominant, and that great resistance to repletion of potassium existed.

We interpreted the entire syndrome as being due to production of excessive amounts of aldosterone; theorized that resistance to repletion of potassium was the result of an intracellular overabundance of sodium, held there by excessive activity of aldosterone; and concluded as follows: "From a therapeutic point of view and in the light of present knowledge these data indicate that total adrenalectomy followed

TABLE 2

Approximation of Aldosterone Content of Tumor by Bioassay

	Sodium-Output Bioassay μg. DOC/kilo	Aldosterone μg./kilo
Tumor tissue (M. W.)	261,800	8,727*
† Beef adrenal		40–95
† Hog adrenal		765
† Tumor tissue (Cushing's Syndrome)		285

* Assuming aldosterone to be 30 × more potent than DOC on Na retention.
† Wettstein—Experientia, **10**: 397, 1954.

by substitution therapy should abolish the entire metabolic abnormality. We hope to report other studies as well as the results of adrenalectomy at a later date."[17]

Further preoperative studies were carried out following a 60 day period during which the patient had been at home. She had ingested 200 mEq./day of potassium in addition to that contained in an average diet. Upon her return to the Metabolic Unit she was somewhat improved symptomatically. This time she was found to be in negative potassium balance to the extent of 45 mEq./day while taking essentially

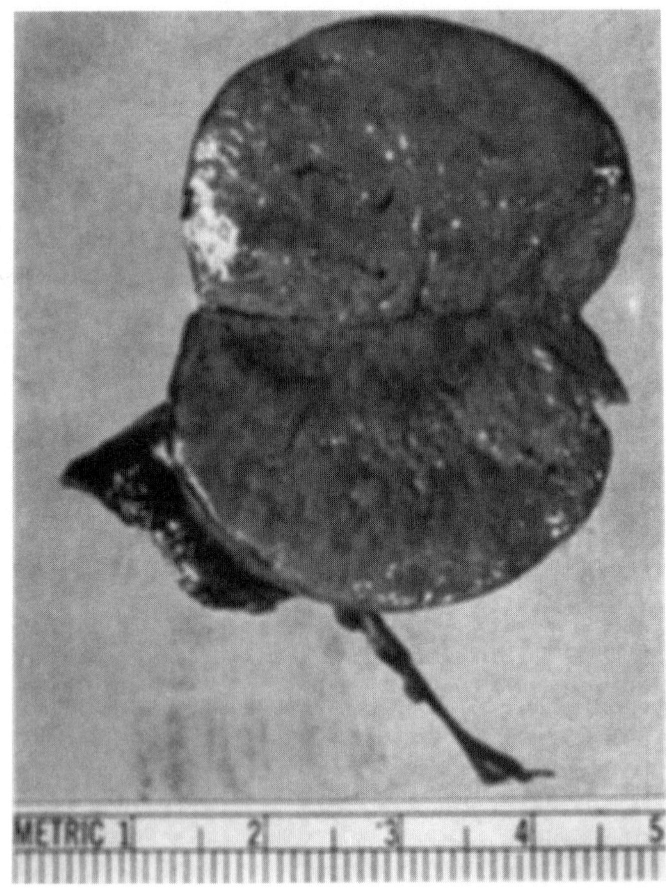

FIG. 3.

the same diet as that given during the previous balance studies (K content, 100 mEq./day). She was in sodium equilibrium. The remainder of the data were found to be similar to those obtained in the earlier study outlined above.

2. *Data obtained at the time of operation, December 10, 1954:* As already stated, the plan was to remove both adrenal glands. In addition, the surgeon (Dr. William C. Baum, Department of Surgery, University Hospital) had agreed to obtain a surgical biopsy from each kidney and to take large samples of lumbar muscle bilaterally, the latter for the purpose of determining directly the content of sodium and potassium in muscle. Since preoperative preparation of the patient with adrenal steroids could alter the concentrations of electrolytes in muscle, hydrocortisone intravenously was begun in the operating room immediately after the muscle biopsies had been obtained. Both adrenals were then exposed simultaneously.

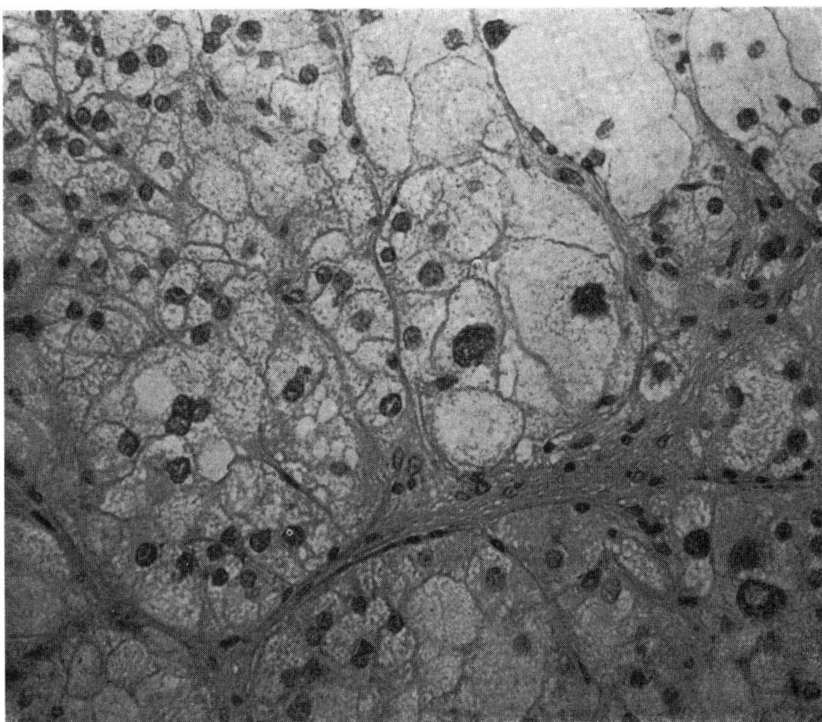

Fig. 4.

To our surprise and delight a cortical adenoma, 4 cm. in diameter, was observed to be arising from the right adrenal gland (figure 2). A right adrenalectomy which included the tumor was performed. The contralateral adrenal, which appeared normal grossly, was left in situ after a wedge biopsy had been obtained.

Figure 3 shows the tumor on cut section, and figure 4 demonstrates its microscopic appearance. The cells are laden with lipid material.

Bio-assays for sodium-retaining corticoid were carried out on extracts of the tumor tissue. Table 2 demonstrates the results. If one can judge from the results of the bio-assays, the tumor tissue, on a per gram basis, contains 100 to 200 times as much aldosterone as does beef adrenal, 10 times as much as hog adrenal, and 30 times as much as Wettstein [6] found in an adrenal tumor that had produced Cushing's syndrome. Paper chromatographic study of extracts of the tumor of our patient indicates a large quantity of material which is not Compounds F, E, B or DOC, and which migrates at the same speed as pure aldosterone. Short of chemical isolation, the combination of intense sodium-retaining activity and an aldosterone migration rate on paper makes it almost certain that the material is aldosterone.

The biopsy obtained from the contralateral adrenal showed a cortex which was somewhat thinner than normal. Microscopically, the atrophy was limited to the zona fasciculata. This finding is highly suggestive that aldosterone is made in the cells of the fascicular zone.

Biopsies of both kidneys disclose a major tubular lesion (figure 5). This is characterized by a diffuse vacuolar change in tubular epithelium which in some

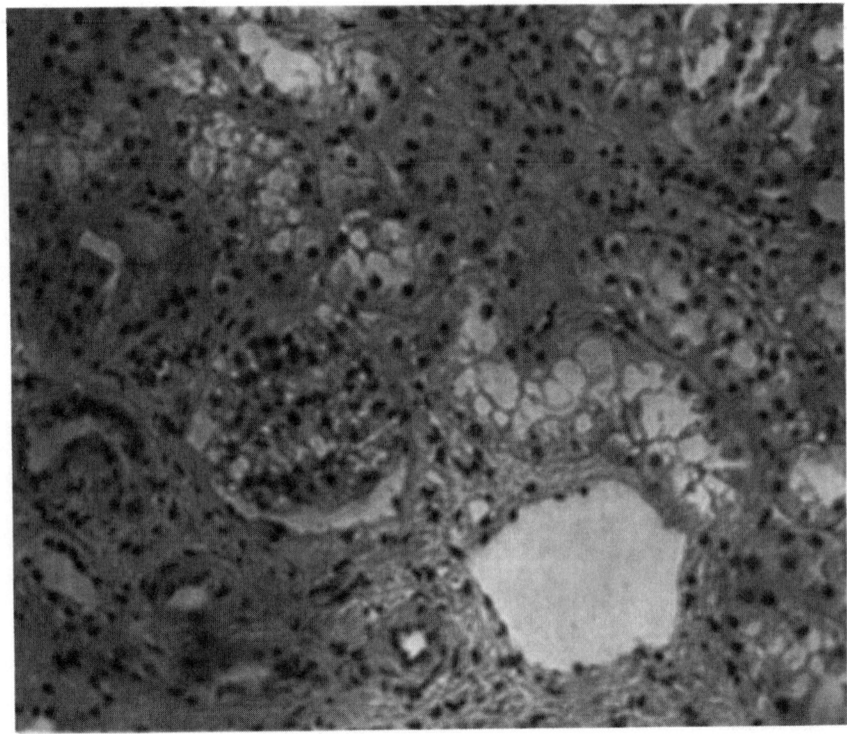

FIG. 5.

areas has progressed to necrosis. In other areas calcium salts have been deposited. The vacuoles in tubular epithelium do not take up fat or glycogen stains and are therefore regarded as representing hydropic change. This is the so-called "vacuolar nephropathy," or "clear cell nephrosis," already recognized [35] as being associated with severe depletion of potassium. In addition to the tubular lesion, a severe degree of renal arteriolosclerosis is evident (figure 6). In this connection, it is of considerable interest that the muscle biopsies showed no evidence of any form of vascular lesion.

It will be observed in table 3 that the muscle tissue contains far above normal amounts of sodium and much below normal amounts of potassium.

3. *Postoperative studies:* Figure 7 gives a running account of some of the changes which took place following removal of the tumor. The observations shown on this

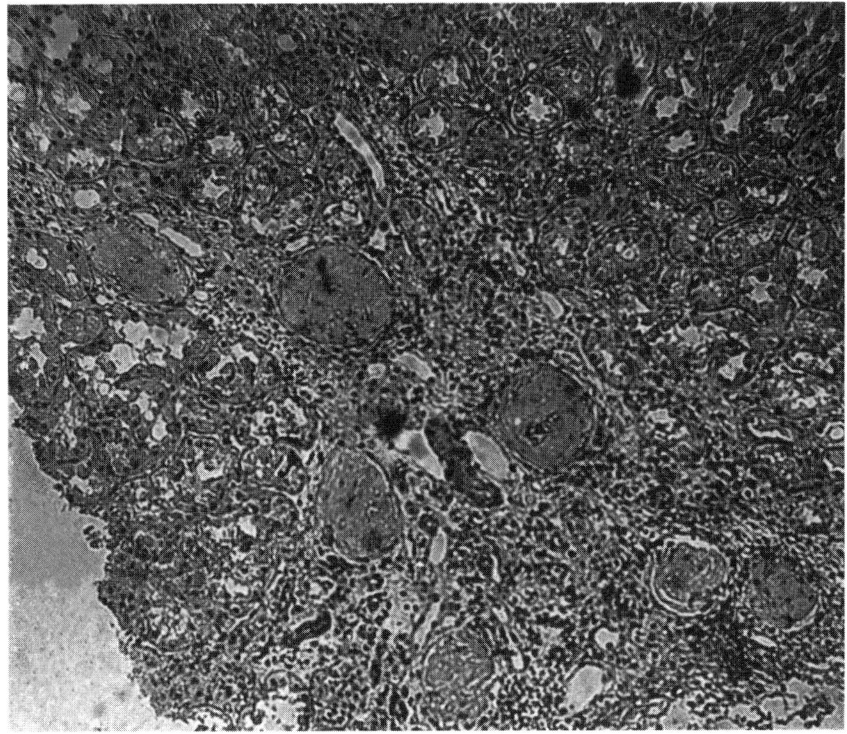

Fig. 6.

Table 3

Chemical Composition* of Muscle Obtained at Operation (M. W.)

	Water %	Nitrogen %	Potassium mEq./kilo	Sodium mEq./kilo	Phosphorus mEq./kilo
Dry ashing					
Left lumbar	72.3	3.0	58	43	
Right lumbar	72.1	3.0	66	47	
Wet ashing					
Left lumbar		2.8	61	54	70
Right lumbar		3.1	54	53	62
Farago et al. 1951 Human lumbar			106	21	
Baldwin et al. 1952 Human muscle			95		60
Shohl 1949 Human muscle			93	31	71
Hastings 1952 Rat muscle	76.0	3.5	107	28	80

* Expressed in terms of wet weight.

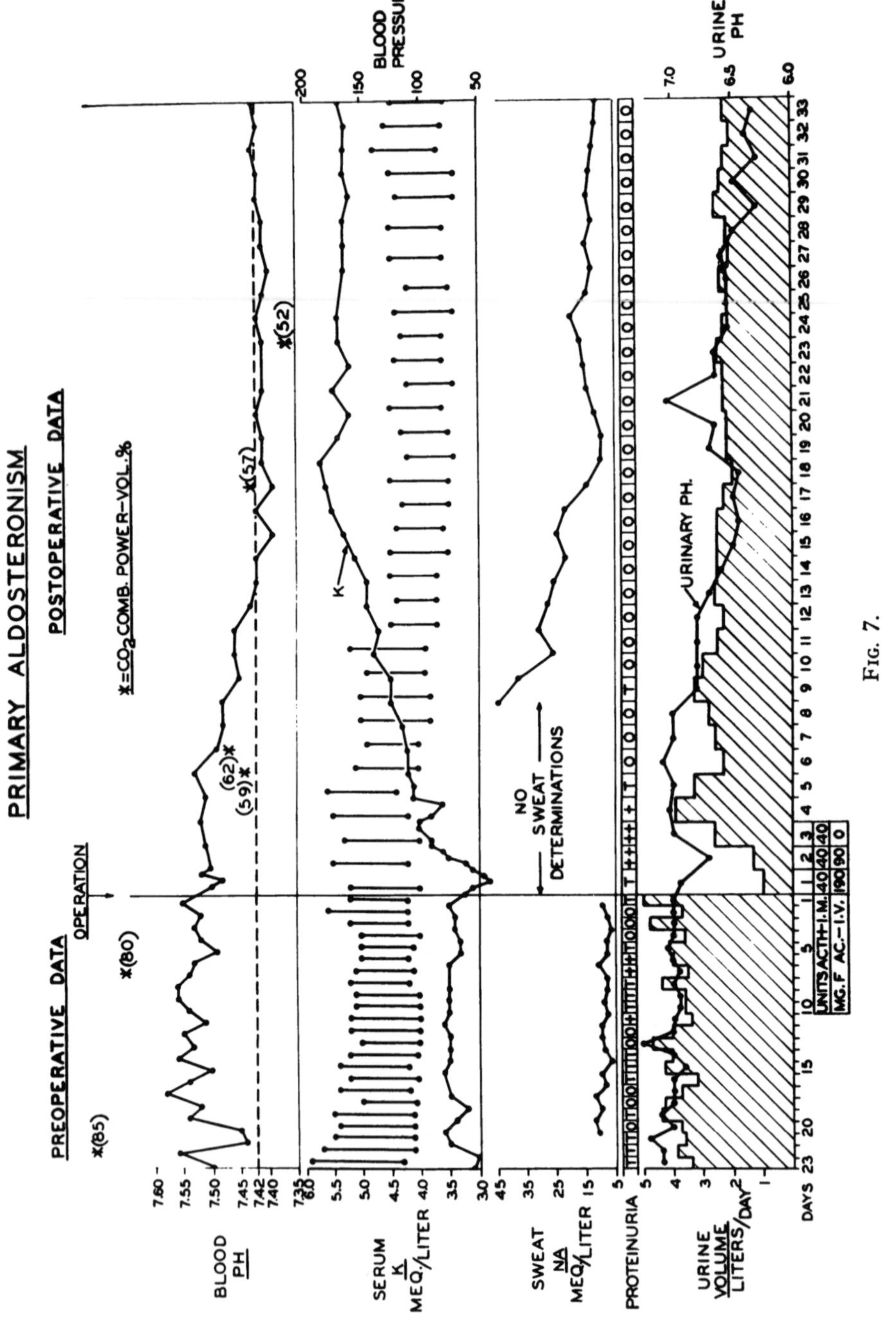

PRIMARY ALDOSTERONISM
PREOPERATIVE DATA
POSTOPERATIVE DATA
OPERATION
✱=CO2 COMB. POWER-VOL.%
BLOOD PH
SERUM K MEQ./LITER
SWEAT NA MEQ./LITER
NO SWEAT DETERMINATIONS
PROTEINURIA
URINE VOLUME LITERS/DAY
DAYS
BLOOD PRESSURE
URINE PH
URINARY PH.
UNITS ACTH-I.M.
MG. F AC.-I.V.

Fig. 7.

figure begin 23 days before operation and continue for 33 days postoperatively. It will be observed that blood pH, CO_2 combining power, serum potassium, blood pressure, sweat sodium, urinary volume and urinary pH had all returned to normal values by the fourteenth postoperative day (December 24, 1954). The last trace (T) of proteinuria was observed on the ninth postoperative day. Polydipsia, polyuria and nocturia disappeared abruptly on the sixth postoperative day. This constituted a great surprise and relief to the patient, since these symptoms had been present for years. During the first 16 postoperative days there existed negative balance for sodium and positive balance for potassium, after which time external equilibrium for both of these ions was established. Electrocardiograms have been normal since the fifth postoperative day.

A total of 112 days of continuous metabolic balance studies have been carried out since operation. The data can be summarized as follows:

1. Sodium and potassium equilibrium continues.
2. Blood pressure remains normal, and proteinuria has not recurred.
3. Blood pH, CO_2 combining power, serum sodium and potassium, sweat sodium, urinary volume and pH continue to be normal.
4. Daily determinations of 17-hydroxycorticoids, 17-ketosteroids and circulating eosinophils remain normal, as they were preoperatively.
5. Renal concentrating ability has improved but is still below normal. Nevertheless, polydipsia, polyuria and nocturia are absent.

TABLE 4

Postoperative Bioassays of Urinary Sodium Retaining Corticoid

Days Postop.	Procedure	Sodium Output Bioassay µg. DOC/day
35	0	47
36	0	neg.*
38	0	neg.
65	0	neg.
88	0	neg.
	Aldosterone/day	
89	1 mg.	
90	1 mg.	
91	1 mg. } Average/day	103
92	0.9 mg.	

* Means effect opposite from DOC, i.e., increased Na output.

Finally, table 4 shows that in the postoperative period little sodium-retaining corticoid could be detected in the urine by bio-assay. However, when aldosterone * was administered in a continuous, intravenous drip for four days (delivering 1 mg. of aldosterone per 24 hour period), the average daily excretion of sodium-retaining corticoid was found to be at the upper limit of normal. Preoperatively, there had been three to 23 times this amount in the urine. Thus, it seems clear that the tumor was producing considerably more aldosterone than 1 mg. per day.

During the four day period of administration of aldosterone some of the biochemical indices moved in the direction of the preoperative abnormality, but the changes were very slight compared with those presented by the patient originally.

* We are greatly indebted to Dr. Harold Mason, Mayo Foundation, Rochester, Minnesota, Dr. Harold Hailman, The Upjohn Company, Kalamazoo, Michigan, and Dr. Robert Gaunt, Ciba, Inc., Summit, New Jersey, for contributing the aldosterone used in this study.

Comment

It would appear to us that the syndrome of primary aldosteronism is now firmly established. It is likely that the condition, which descriptively has been called "potassium-losing nephritis," is a manifestation of primary aldosteronism. A case recently described in England as potassium-losing nephritis [36] is now recognized as one of primary aldosteronism,[19, 20] a large amount of sodium-retaining corticoid having been found in the urine.[37] †

The major clinical manifestations of this syndrome consist of periodic severe muscular weakness, intermittent tetany and paresthesia, polyuria and polydipsia, and hypertension. There is no edema. The characteristic biochemical alteration in the blood is comprised of hypokalemia, hypernatremia and alkalosis (elevation of pH and CO_2 combining power). Total serum calcium is normal.

Hyposthenuria unresponsive to Pitressin, persistently alkaline urine, and mild proteinuria are observed. 17-hydroxycorticoids and 17-ketosteroids are consistently normal.

Despite the periodic occurrence of severe muscular weakness, one is impressed with the relative lack of important symptoms at extremely low levels of serum potassium. Another striking manifestation of this syndrome is the great resistance which it offers against attempts at potassium repletion. With very large amounts of supplementary potassium, serum potassium rises, but only mildly.

It is recommended that patients exhibiting such clinical and laboratory manifestations be subjected to adrenal surgery. To date, all 12 cases of which we are personally aware have disclosed an adrenal cortical adenoma at operation or at autopsy. Nine have been cured of primary aldosteronism by surgical removal of the adenoma. The other three were recognized in retrospect at autopsy. We believe, however, that in some patients with this syndrome an adenoma will not be found at operation. Under these circumstances a total or extensive subtotal adrenalectomy (pending future experience) should be performed. The case reported by Wyngaarden et al.,[38] typical of primary aldosteronism, disclosed no adenoma at autopsy. One case is said to have been cured by bilateral adrenalectomy.[27]

Finally, this study raises a number of questions that demand intensive investigation. Without attempting to speculate upon them, we list them as follows:

1. What is the stimulus for secretion of aldosterone? It is clear from our data that large amounts of aldosterone produced by a tumor for a long period of time failed to depress endogenous production of conventional ACTH. Yet it did suppress something which affects adrenal size, since a significant degree of atrophy was found in the zona fasciculata of the contralateral gland.

† An adrenal cortical adenoma recently has been removed from this patient.[30]

2. What are the physiologic functions of aldosterone in addition to its capacity to produce a positive external balance for sodium and a negative one for potassium?

3. By what mechanisms do large doses of ACTH or hydrocortisone produce diuresis of sodium in either primary or secondary aldosteronism?

4. What is the relationship of hyperaldosteronism to hypertension?

5. What is the relationship of hyperaldosteronism to the production of renal arteriolosclerosis?

6. Is aldosterone involved in the production of the so-called "diseases of adaptation" (Selye)? Nature has now provided for study a condition in man which manifests not only chronic and excessive production of the naturally occurring mineralocorticoid but also biochemical evidence of an intense mineralocorticoid effect in the body. It would be difficult to conceive of a more profound, hormonally produced disturbance of sodium and potassium metabolism. There is obvious "imbalance" between mineralocorticoid and glucocorticoid activity, since the latter has been shown to be quite normal. The condition is associated with hypertension and renal arteriolosclerosis, the former disappearing as the electrolyte disturbance is corrected by removal of excessive amounts of aldosterone.

If the effects in man of chronic, excessive and "unbalanced" mineralocorticoid activity are sought (and this is postulated as the predominant factor in the evolution of "diseases of adaptation"), primary aldosteronism is a good place to look.

Summario in Interlingua

Es demonstrate que le fascinante disturbation del metabolismo electrolytic que esseva previemente describite como "nephritis a perdita de kalium" es causate per un excesso in le production del novemente discoperite sodium-retenente steroide adreno-cortical, aldosterona. Le syndrome es producite per un adenoma adreno-cortical que secerne aldosterona; illo pote esser curate per le ablation del tumor. Nos ha designate iste syndrome como "aldosteronismo primari" pro distinguer lo nettemente ab altere conditiones que es associate con un augmento del production de aldosterona—per exemplo nephrosis, congestive disfallimento cardiac, cirrhosis hepatic con ascites, e eclampsia. In casos de iste secunde gruppo nos usa le termino "aldosteronismo secundari."

Depost nostre reporto initial (octobre 1954), multe casos de aldosteronismo primari ha essite identificate, e al minus octo casos ha essite curate per le ablation de un adenoma adreno-cortical. In su forma pur le morbo ha nulle del characteristicas del syndrome de Cushing.

Le major manifestationes clinic de aldosteronismo primari consiste de periodic, sever debilitate muscular, intermittente tetania e paresthesia, polyuria e polydipsia, e hypertension. Il non ha edema. Le characteristic lesion biochimic in le sanguine consiste de hypokalemia, hypernatremia, e alcalosis (elevation de pH e del potentia combinatori pro CO_2). Le calcium total del sero es normal.

Il ha hyposthenuria (que non responde a pitressina), persistente alcalinitate del urina, e leve proteinuria. Le nivellos del 17-hydroxycorticoides e 17-cetosteroides es persistentemente normal. Le corpore resiste fortemente a effortios a replenar su kalium. Le urina contine grande quantitates de aldosterona.

Post ablation del tumor, omne anormalitates biochimic dispare intra duo septimanas, e le pression sanguinee deveni normal. Le urina non plus contine excessos de aldosterona.

Le tumor mesme contine un tremende quantitate de aldosterona. Sub le examine microscopic le renes exhibi un forma classic de "nephropathia vacuolar" que es debite a chronic depletion de kalium. Le substantia muscular contine grande excessos de natrium e inadequatissime quantitates de kalium.

Il es a recommendar que patientes qui exhibi iste manifestationes clinic e laboratorial es subjicite a chirurgia adrenal.

BIBLIOGRAPHY

1. Simpson, S. A., Tait, J. F., Wettstein, A., Neher, R., Von Euw, J., and Reichstein, T.: Isolierung eines neuen kristallisierten Hormons aus Nebennieren mit besonders hoher Wirksamkeit auf den Mineralstoffwechsel, Experientia **9**: 333, 1953.
2. Simpson, S. A., Tait, J. F., Wettstein, A., Neher, R., Von Euw, J., Schindler, O., and Reichstein, T.: Konstitution des Aldosterons, des neuen Mineralocorticoid, Experientia **10**: 132, 1954.
3. Simpson, S. A., Tait, J. F., Wettstein, A., Neher, R., Von Euw, J., Schindler, O., and Reichstein, T.: Aldosteron, Isolierung und Eigenschaften. Über Bestandteile der Nebennierenrinde und verwandte Stoffe, Helv. chim. acta **37**: 1163, 1954.
4. Simpson, S. A., Tait, J. F., Wettstein, A., Neher, R., Von Euw, J., Schindler, O., and Reichstein, T.: Die Konstitution des Aldosterons. Über Bestandteile der Nebennierenrinde und verwandte Stoffe, Helv. chim. acta **37**: 1200, 1954.
5. Harman, R. E., Ham, E. A., DeYoung, J. J., Brink, N. G., and Sarett, L. H.: Isolation of aldosterone (electrocortin), J. Am. Chem. Soc. **76**: 5035, 1954.
6. Wettstein, A.: Advances in the field of adrenal cortical hormones, Experientia **10**: 397, 1954.
7. Deming, Q. B., and Luetscher, J. A., Jr.: Bioassay of desoxycorticosterone-like material in urine, Proc. Soc. Exper. Biol. and Med. **73**: 171, 1950.
8. Luetscher, J. A., Jr., Neher, R., and Wettstein, A.: Isolation of crystalline aldosterone from the urine of a nephrotic patient, Experientia **10**: 456, 1954.
9. Singer, B., and Wener, J.: Excretion of sodium-retaining substances in patients with congestive heart failure, Am. Heart J. **45**: 795, 1953.
10. Luetscher, J. A., Jr., and Johnson, B. B.: Observations on the sodium-retaining corticoid (aldosterone) in the urine of children and adults in relation to sodium balance and edema, J. Clin. Investigation **23**: 1441, 1954.
11. Luetscher, J. A., Jr.: Symposium on adrenal function of infants and children, State University of New York, Syracuse, November, 1954, p. 57.
12. Chart, J. J., and Shipley, E. S.: The mechanism of sodium retention in cirrhosis of the liver, J. Clin. Investigation **32**: 560, 1953.
13. Pechet, M. M., Duncan, L. E., Jr., Liddle, G. W., and Bartter, F. C.: Studies on a salt-retaining factor prepared from human urine, J. Clin. Investigation **33**: 957, 1954.
14. Chart, J. J., Shipley, E. G., and Gordon, E. S.: Evidence for a sodium retaining factor in toxemia of pregnancy, Proc. Soc. Exper. Biol. and Med. **78**: 244, 1951.
15. Gordon, E. S., Chart, J. J., Hagedorn, D., and Shipley, E. G.: Mechanism of sodium retention in preeclamptic toxemia, Obst. and Gynec. Surv. **4**: 39, 1954.
16. Venning, E. G., Singer, B., and Simpson, G. A.: Adrenocortical function in toxemia of pregnancy, Am. J. Obst. and Gynec. **67**: 542, 1954.
17. Conn, J. W.: Primary aldosteronism, a new clinical syndrome, J. Lab. and Clin. Med. **45**: 6, 1955.
18. Conn, J. W.: Primary aldosteronism, J. Lab. and Clin. Med. **45**: 661, 1955.
19. Conn, J. W.: Potassium-losing nephritis, Brit. M. J. **2**: 1415, 1954.

20. Cope, C. L., and Milne, M. D.: Primary aldosteronism, Brit. M. J. **1**: 969, 1955.
21. Mader, J. P., and Iseri, L.: Am. J. Med., in press.
22. Crane, M. G.: Personal communication (Los Angeles, California), in press, J. Lab. and Clin. Med.
23. Bartter, F. C.: Personal communication (Bethesda, Maryland).
24. Keutman, E. H.: Personal communication (Rochester, New York).
25. Eales, L.: Personal communication (Capetown, S. Africa).
26. Steinbeck, A. W.: Personal communication (Brisbane, Australia).
27. Iseri, L., quoted in editorial, Conn's syndrome, Lancet **1**: 1167, 1955.
28. Hewlett, J.: Personal communication concerning three proven cases (Cleveland, Ohio), in press, J. A. M. A.
29. Milne, M. D.: Personal communication (London, England).
30. Meiselas, L. E.: Personal communication (Brooklyn, N. Y.).
31. Schwartz, W. B., and Relman, A. S.: Metabolic and renal studies in chronic potassium depletion resulting from overuse of laxatives, J. Clin. Investigation **32**: 258, 1953.
32. Conn, J. W.: The mechanism of acclimatization to heat, *in* Advances in internal medicine, Vol. 3, 1949, Interscience Publishers, Inc., New York, pp. 372–393.
33. Conn, J. W., and Louis, L. H.: Production of endogenous salt-active corticoids as reflected in the concentrations of sodium and chloride of thermal sweat, J. Clin. Endocrinol. **10**: 12, 1950.
34. Simpson, S. A., and Tait, J. F.: Some recent advances in methods of isolation and the physiology and chemistry of electrocortin, Recent Progress in Hormone Research, in press.
35. Schwartz, W. B.: Potassium and the kidney, in press.
36. Evans, B. M., and Milne, M. D.: Potassium-losing nephritis presenting as a case of periodic paralysis, Brit. M. J. **2**: 1067, 1954.
37. Cope, C. L., and Gardcia-Llaurado, J.: The occurrence of electrocortin in human urine, Brit. M. J. **1**: 1290, 1954.
38. Wyngaarden, J. B., Keitel, H. G., and Isselbacker, J.: Potassium depletion and alkalosis. Their association with hypertension and renal insufficiency, New England J. Med. **250**: 597, 1954.

Nonenzymatic Glycosylation and the Pathogenesis of Diabetic Complications

MICHAEL BROWNLEE, M.D.; HELEN VLASSARA, M.D.; and ANTHONY CERAMI, Ph.D.; New York, New York

Glucose chemically attaches to proteins and nucleic acids without the aid of enzymes. Initially, chemically reversible Schiff base and Amadori product adducts form in proportion to glucose concentration. Equilibrium is reached after several weeks, however, and further accumulation of these early nonenzymatic glycosylation products does not continue beyond that time. Subsequent reactions of the Amadori product slowly give rise to non-equilibrium advanced glycosylation end-products which continue to accumulate indefinitely on longer-lived molecules. Excessive formation of both types of nonenzymatic glycosylation product appears to be the common biochemical link between chronic hyperglycemia and a number of pathophysiologic processes potentially involved in the development of long-term diabetic complications. The major biological effects of excessive nonenzymatic glycosylation include: inactivation of enzymes; inhibition of regulatory molecule binding; crosslinking of glycosylated proteins and trapping of soluble proteins by glycosylated extracellular matrix (both may progress in the absence of glucose); decreased susceptibility to proteolysis; abnormalities of nucleic acid function; altered macromolecular recognition and endocytosis; and increased immunogenicity.

OVER THE LAST 15 years, data from many clinical, morphologic, and biochemical investigations have established that hyperglycemia is the single metabolic consequence of insufficient insulin action most responsible for the development of chronic diabetic complications (1-3). Clinicians have responded to this emerging consensus by advocating intensive diabetic treatment regimens as a preventive therapeutic measure (4). Unfortunately, recent clinical trials suggest that when complications are already present, improvement of glycemic control alone may not be sufficient to prevent the continued progression of these pathologic processes (5, 6). For this common clinical problem, optimal future therapy may require pharmacologic agents that directly interfere with the self-perpetuating component of hyperglycemia-initiated tissue damage. Before such new drugs can be developed, the biochemical basis of progressive diabetic complications must be better understood.

There appear to be two general pathophysiologic mechanisms by which hyperglycemia leads to irreversible tissue damage. Intracellular hyperglycemia can result, by increased flux through different metabolic pathways, in altered steady-state levels of metabolites and synthetic products that may ultimately affect function adversely. This mechanism gives rise to quantitative and qualitative changes in glomerular basement membrane glycoprotein and proteoglycan components, biochemical alterations in peripheral nerve myelin composition, disturbances in platelet prostanoid production, and abnormalities in somatomedin and growth hormone secretion. A particularly well-studied example of this mechanism is the polyol pathway. In lens and nerve, two tissues that do not require insulin for glucose transport, increased activity of this glucose-consuming pathway has been implicated in the pathogenesis of acute diabetic cataracts and early peripheral neuropathy (7, 8). Increased polyol pathway activity results in several metabolic changes, including decreased levels of NADPH, glutathione, and myoinositol. Each of these components may have a role in the development of some diabetic complications. These processes and others that may contribute to the development of diabetic complications are reviewed elsewhere (3).

▶ From the Laboratory of Medical Biochemistry, The Rockefeller University; New York, New York.

The other major consequence of hyperglycemia is excessive nonenzymatic glycosylation of proteins. In this process glucose chemically attaches to proteins without involvement of enzymes. The stable products thus formed accumulate inside insulin-independent cells, and outside on cell membrane proteins, circulating proteins, and structural proteins. Formation of glycosylated hemoglobin inside erythrocytes is the best known example of nonenzymatic protein glycosylation in vivo (9). Elucidation of the biochemical and physiologic factors involved in glycosylated hemoglobin formation led to the rapid development of clinical assays that provide previously unobtainable information about mean blood glucose levels in diabetic patients. Glycosylated adducts (the Amadori product) similar to that formed on hemoglobin have been subsequently reported in a large number of mammalian proteins (10).

Recent chemical studies of nonenzymatic glycosylation have focused on important new glycosylation adducts, advanced glycosylation end-products, which form very slowly from the Amadori product through a series of further reactions and rearrangements. In contrast to the Amadori product, these adducts, once formed, are irreversible, and continue to accumulate indefinitely on longer-lived proteins. New biological investigations over the past few years have explored major functional consequences of excessive nonenzymatic glycosylation. In this review, similarities and differences between the familiar Amadori products and the less well-known advanced glycosylation end-products will be presented first, along with a description of the factors that determine the extent of nonenzymatic glycosylation. With this information as background, major physiologic processes altered by non-

Annals of Internal Medicine. 1984;**101**:527-537.

I. PROTEINS WITH T½ OF DAYS TO WEEKS

$$\text{Glucose} + NH_2\text{-Protein} \underset{K_{-1}}{\overset{K_1}{\rightleftharpoons}} \text{Schiff Base} \underset{K_{-2}}{\overset{K_2}{\rightleftharpoons}} \text{Amadori Product}$$

II. LONG-LIVED STRUCTURAL PROTEINS

$$\text{Glucose} + NH_2\text{-Protein} \underset{K_{-1}}{\overset{K_1}{\rightleftharpoons}} \text{Schiff Base} \underset{K_{-2}}{\overset{K_2}{\rightleftharpoons}} \text{Amadori Product} \xrightarrow{K_n} \text{Advanced Glycosylation Endproducts}$$

ADVANCED GLYCOSYLATION ENDPRODUCTS (BROWN FLUORESCENT PIGMENTS WHICH CROSSLINK PROTEINS)

Figure 1. Formation of early reversible and advanced irreversible nonenzymatic glycosylation products. Steady-state levels of the reversible Schiff base and Amadori product are reached within hours and weeks, respectively. In contrast, irreversible advanced glycosylation end-products continue to accumulate over long periods of time.

enzymatic glycosylation will be discussed, and the possible relationship of these to diabetic complications will be considered. The central concept that emerges is that excessive nonenzymatic glycosylation appears to be the common biochemical link between chronic hyperglycemia and a number of pathophysiologic processes potentially involved in the development of long-term diabetic complications.

Types of Nonenzymatic Glycosylation

PROTEINS WITH HALF-LIVES OF DAYS TO WEEKS

Nonenzymatic glycosylation begins in all cases with glucose attachment to protein amino groups via nucleophilic addition with formation of a Schiff base (Figure 1). The labile Schiff base rapidly reaches an equilibrium level in vivo reflecting ambient glucose concentration. The rate of Schiff base formation (k_1) is approximately equal to the rate of dissociation (k_{-1}). Over a period of weeks, a slow chemical rearrangement of the Schiff base occurs (k_2 is approximately equal to 1.6% of k_1), which results in the accumulation of a stable but chemically reversible sugar-protein adduct, the Amadori product (11). Accumulation of Amadori products does not continue indefinitely, however, even on long-lived proteins, because equilibrium is reached over a period of several weeks. After equilibrium is attained, measured levels of Amadori products reach a constant steady-state value that does not increase as a function of time beyond that point. The chemistry of Amadori nonenzymatic glycosylation products formed in vivo has been extensively studied using human hemoglobin as a model protein (10, 11).

LONG-LIVED STRUCTURAL PROTEINS

In contrast to proteins whose turnover time is equal to or less than the time required to reach equilibrium amounts of the Amadori product, proteins that turn over at a much slower rate such as crystallins, collagen, elastin, and myelin accumulate post-Amadori nonenzymatic glycosylation products (10). These advanced glycosylation end-products form very slowly from Amadori products, through a series of further reactions, rearrangements, and dehydrations. Advanced glycosylation end-products are qualitatively identified by their characteristic brown pigment, fluorescence, and participation in protein-protein crosslinking (12, 13). Structure has been determined for only one advanced glycosylation end-product compound formed under physiologic conditions [2-furoyl-4(5)-(2-furanyl)-1*H*-imidazole]. Although the rate of formation of these products under physiologic conditions is extremely slow, advanced glycosylation end-product derivatives, unlike the Amadori products, are chemically irreversible once formed. As a result, the quantity of the advanced glycosylation end-product continues to accumulate for the life of the protein at a rate proportional to the equilibrium concentration of the reversible Amadori product.

In vitro and in vivo, nonenzymatic glycosylation has been shown in a large number of biologically relevant proteins (Table 1) (9, 14-35). Methodologic difficulties limited earlier studies to isolated proteins such as hemoglobin, the lens protein crystallins, and albumin. Subsequently developed techniques made it possible to accurately quantitate nonenzymatic glycosylation in complex biological samples such as tissue homogenates, using either affinity chromatography or high pressure liquid chromatography (36-38). Only Amadori products are detected by current methods used to quantitate the extent of nonenzymatic glycosylation, however. The effect of diabetes-induced hyperglycemia on levels of Amadori products in various tissue proteins is remarkably similar to its effect on levels of Amadori products formed on hemoglobin. A twofold to threefold increase is consistently seen when diabetic tissue proteins are compared with

Table 1. Nonenzymatic Glycosylation of Proteins

Protein	Physiologic Function
Hemoglobin	Oxygen exchange
Red cell membrane	Deformability in microvasculature
Antithrombin III*	Inhibition of excessive coagulation
Fibrinogen	Plasma viscosity and clot formation
Fibrin*	Clot maintenance
Endothelial cell membrane*	Maintenance of vascular integrity
Lens crystallins†	Transmission of light to retina
Lens capsule	Focusing of light on retina
Myelin†	Nerve impulse conduction
Tubulin	Axonal transport
Glomerular basement membrane	Renal filtration barrier
Collagen†	Tissue structural properties; scar and plaque formation
Coronary artery proteins	Vessel integrity for myocardial perfusion
Low density lipoprotein	Lipid transport and metabolism
High density lipoprotein*	Lipid transport and metabolism
Albumin	Osmotic regulation; transport of metabolites
Cathepsin B*	Intracellular protein degradation
Beta-NAc-D-glucosaminidase*	Glycoprotein sugar removal
Pancreatic RNase*	Hydrolysis of RNA
Ferritin*	Iron storage

* Not yet evaluated in vivo.
† Presence of advanced glycosylation end-products documented.

normal proteins despite different lengths of exposure to hyperglycemia ranging from 18 weeks in experimental animals to years in human autopsy specimens (28, 37). These values represent equilibrium levels of Amadori products reached relatively quickly on all proteins whose survival time is not shorter than the time required for equilibrium to be achieved.

Detection of accumulated advanced glycosylation end-products in biological macromolecules can be accomplished using spectroscopic and fluorescence techniques, but direct quantitation of specific, chemically defined products has not been possible. This inability to obtain information about the level of nonenzymatic glycosylation products beyond the Amadori product has deprived both clinical investigation and clinical practice of a means for assessing time-averaged exposure of patients' long-lived proteins to glucose over extended periods (months to years). As a result, clinical studies correlating the extent of total nonenzymatic protein glycosylation with degree of complications have not yet been feasible. Recently, determination of exact chemical structure has been accomplished for the first successfully isolated advanced glycosylation end-product protein hydrolysis product. Development of an advanced glycosylation end-product analytic method based on this work should greatly expand the scope of future research.

Factors Determining the Extent of Nonenzymatic Glycosylation

For a given protein, the extent of nonenzymatic glycosylation is determined by the sum of effects of a number of independently acting variables (10) (Table 2). The first four of these variables are fixed and constant in living systems. In vitro, pH has a profound influence. Experimentally, significant formation of the Amadori product is not seen below pH 7.0. Increasing pH over the range of 7.0 to 9.0 results in a concomitant increase in the concentration of the Amadori product reached at equilibrium. This observation is consistent with the chemical prediction that only uncharged amino groups on the protein can participate in this type of addition reaction with glucose. Increasing temperature produces a proportional acceleration of Amadori product formation rate, similar to that seen in other nonenzymatic chemical reactions. Two other factors constant in vivo are protein concentration and amino group microenvironment. With higher protein concentration, the absolute number of amino groups potentially available to react with glucose increases, whereas the protein's local environment in the areas immediately surrounding each amino group has a direct effect on that amino group's reactivity with glucose. These last factors may explain the non-random pattern of amino group glycosylation seen within a given protein, as well as differences in susceptibility to nonenzymatic glycosylation seen between different proteins (39, 40).

Glucose concentration and incubation time are the most clinically relevant variables affecting the extent of nonenzymatic glycosylation, because only these two variables have counterparts that also differ in vivo. Increasing glucose concentrations (via mass action) cause the level of accumulated Amadori products on proteins to rise in a parallel fashion. Length of incubation time is also critical, for two reasons. The first reason is that Amadori products continue to accumulate as a function of time until equilibrium is reached. The degree of pre-equilibrium or equilibrium excessive glycosylation of amino groups caused by exposure to hyperglycemia (either Schiff base or Amadori product) may be sufficient to significantly impair important functional properties of several critical proteins. The second reason is that even though steady-state levels of Amadori products do not increase beyond the time required for equilibrium to occur at a particular mean blood glucose level, advanced glycosylation end-products continue to accumulate over the entire lifetime of proteins that turn over slowly or not at all. Significant clinical consequences of continuous net advanced glycosylation end-product accumulation would be expected to arise from altered physiologic processes related to increased crosslinking within and between protein molecules, as well as from other glycosylation-associated structural changes. Accumulation of advanced glycosylation end-products on proteins such as collagen appears to occur at a rather slow rate in patients with normal glucose tolerance, and at a significantly faster rate in patients with juvenile onset diabetes (27). This information is consistent with the clinically recognized time scales over which both age-associated degenerative vascular disease in nondiabetics and hyperglycemia-accelerated atherosclerosis in diabetics develop.

Table 2. In-vitro Variables That Determine the Extent of Nonenzymatic Glycoslation and Their In-vivo Counterparts

In Vitro	In Vivo
pH	Constant
Temperature	Constant
Protein concentration	Constant
NH_2 microenvironment	Constant
Glucose concentration	Mean blood glucose level
Incubation time	Duration of hyperglycemia and protein half-life

Physiologic Processes Altered by Nonenzymatic Glycosylation

The studies shown in Table 1 demonstrate that nonenzymatic glycosylation occurs on many proteins throughout the body. These studies also confirm that the hyperglycemia of diabetes produces elevated levels of the Amadori glycosylation product on these proteins, as it does with hemoglobin. Relative increases in advanced glycosylation end-products have been seen on several diabetic long-lived structural proteins as well. The functional consequences of such excessive nonenzymatic glycosylation were essentially unknown until quite recently, however. Only now has information about the biological effects of excessive protein glycosylation accumulated to a point where a conceptual schema organizing this material can be constructed, as shown in Table 3.

ENZYME ACTIVITY

From the discussion in previous sections, it may seem

Table 3. Physiologic Processes Altered by Nonenzymatic Glycosylation

Enzyme activity
Binding of regulatory molecules
Crosslinking of proteins
Susceptibility to proteolysis
Function of nucleic acids
Macromolecular recognition and endocytosis
Immunogenicity

that nonenzymatic glycosylation would not occur to an appreciable extent on enzymes, because most of these proteins have relatively short half-lives. However, reversible glucose-protein Schiff base compounds form quite rapidly under physiologic conditions (Figure 1), and an increased concentration of these compounds in vivo could significantly alter the catalytic properties of certain types of enzymes. The most likely inactivation mechanism would involve glucose attachment to a lysine epsilon-amino group essential for normal function at the active site. In ribonuclease A, for example, loss of a single lysine at position 41 is known to cause total loss of enzyme activity. Incubation of this enzyme with glucose for 24 hours results in a 50% loss of initial enzymatic activity, associated with nonenzymatic glycosylation of two lysine residues per molecule (34). Similar results would be predicted for a number of decarboxylases and aldolases, because their mechanism of action requires formation of reversible covalent intermediates involving unsubstituted active-site lysine amino groups (41).

A second type of enzyme whose activity appears to be influenced by nonenzymatic glycosylation is the so-called sulfhydryl protease. Enzymes of this type, such as cathepsin B from animal cells and papain from plants, are proteases that resemble in their reaction mechanism the serine proteases trypsin, thrombin, and plasmin. These enzymes differ, however, in having a cysteine rather than a serine at the active site to form covalent intermediates with substrates (41). The activity of cathepsin B isolated from human liver cells is completely abolished after incubation for 2 weeks with a glucose concentration of 300 mg/dL (32). Similarly, papain activity is reduced 70% to 90% after nonenzymatic glycosylation. In contrast, the serine proteases trypsin and chymotrypsin retain full activity after identical glucose incubations (42). The presence of critical lysine residues only in the extended active site areas of sulfhydryl proteases may explain this differential effect of glycosylation on enzyme activity.

Studies of the glycoconjugate-degrading enzyme beta-*N*-acetyl-D-glucosaminidase from kidney provide evidence that loss of activity associated with nonenzymatic glycosylation may also result from conformational changes in the molecule (33). Loss of enzyme activity was shown to progress as a function of both incubation time and glucose concentration. After 15 days incubation in 44.4 mmol glucose, activity of isoenzyme A decreased to 20% of its initial activity. This glucose-induced decrease in enzyme activity was accompanied by an increase in apparent molecular weight of the enzyme from 130 000 to 250 000, suggesting that glucose-induced changes in protein aggregation and crosslinking may contribute to loss of enzyme activity in some cases.

BINDING OF REGULATORY MOLECULES

Steady-state levels of metabolites are maintained in vivo by constant modulation of protein functional activity. One general mechanism by which maintenance is accomplished involves reversible interaction with metabolites or cofactors that are not involved in the primary reaction. Binding of these regulatory molecules alters the equilibrium between different conformational states of the protein, each of which is associated with a defined level of function. In cases where the binding of regulatory molecules requires unsubstituted N-terminal or lysine epsilon-amino groups, nonenzymatic glycosylation would be expected to inhibit effector-molecule binding.

The reversible binding of 2,3-diphosphoglycerate to hemoglobin is a well-studied model of regulatory molecule binding. In the erythrocyte, where 2,3-diphosphoglycerate and hemoglobin are found in equimolar concentrations, this negatively charged organic phosphate binds to properly oriented positively charged amino groups on tetrameric hemoglobin contributed by the N-terminal valine, lysine 82, and histidine 143 of the beta chains. Binding of 2,3-diphosphoglycerate to hemoglobin stabilizes the deoxy form and decreases the affinity of hemoglobin for oxygen. Conversely, hemoglobin structural changes induced by oxygen binding reduce the affinity of hemoglobin for 2,3-diphosphoglycerate. An equilibrium exists, therefore, between hemoglobin, 2,3-diphosphoglycerate, and oxygen, which serves as a sensitive control of oxygen exchange (43).

The functional properties of nonenzymatically glycosylated hemoglobins differ significantly from those described above for normal studied hemoglobin A_0. The first glycosylated hemoglobins to be recognized and studied were minor hemolysate components that appeared to be more negatively charged than the single major hemoglobin, Hb A_0. The functional properties of four of these components, designated Hb A_{1a1}, Hb A_{1a2}, Hb A_{1b}, and Hb A_{1c}, have been evaluated (44). Compared to Hb A_0, Hb A_{1a1} and Hb A_{1a2} have low oxygen affinities, Hb A_{1b} has high affinity, and Hb A_{1c} has moderately high affinity. Removal of organic phosphate increases the oxygen affinities of Hb A_{1b} and Hb A_{1c}, whereas the affinities of Hb A_{1a1} and Hb A_{1a2} remain low. Addition of organic phosphates substantially decreases the oxygen affinity of Hb A_{1b} and Hb A_{1c}, although to a much smaller degree than that of Hb A_0. Hemoglobin A_{1a1} and Hb A_{1a2} are essentially unaffected by addition of organic phosphate. In the presence of high concentrations of organic phosphate, all of the glycohemoglobins are still 50% saturated with oxygen at partial pressures where Hb A_0 has given up most of its oxygen. Although compensatory mechanisms in vivo essentially restore oxygen affinity of diabetic whole blood to normal (45), these studies are important because they show that nonenzymatic glycosylation of proteins can significantly interfere with the binding of critical regulatory molecules.

Another protein whose regulatory activity is modified

by nonenzymatic glycosylation is antithrombin III. This factor, after binding catalytic amounts of heparin to critical lysine residues, functions as the major inhibitor of activated serine-protease coagulation factors in plasma (46). Binding of heparin to lysine amino groups in the antithrombin III molecule is the initial and rate-determining step of the antithrombin III and thrombin reaction. This heparin-binding step, which is independent of thrombin, enhances the rate of inhibition of thrombin by antithrombin III nearly 1000-fold (47).

Nonenzymatic glycosylation of antithrombin III produces a significant decrease in thrombin-inhibiting activity in vitro (15). The degree of antithrombin III activity loss correlates with both factors determining the extent of nonenzymatic glycosylation, glucose concentration, and incubation time. Nonenzymatic glycosylation-induced inhibition of heparin-catalyzed human antithrombin III activity can be completely overcome, however, by addition of a large molar excess of heparin to the glycosylated antithrombin III before assay. This observation suggests that the antithrombin III molecule contains a lower-affinity binding site for heparin after nonenzymatic glycosylation. Nonenzymatic attachment of glucose to antithrombin III thus reduces the affinity of antithrombin III for heparin, but does not eliminate its heparin-binding capacity. Inhibition of heparin binding to human antithrombin III in hyperglycemic patients would result in a transient functional deficiency of this protein. This finding could explain the significant in-vivo inhibition of biological function of human antithrombin III that occurs in both type II and type I diabetic patients (48, 49). In type I patients the degree of reduction in antithrombin III activity was directly related to the level of both Hb A_{1c} and fasting blood glucose. Glycosylation-induced interference with antithrombin III activity could explain the accelerated disappearance rate of fibrinogen that is normalized by improving glucose control in hyperglycemic diabetic patients (50). A specific effect of nonenzymatic glycosylation on antithrombin III heparin binding affinity would also explain why infused heparin alone corrected the accelerated disappearance of fibrinogen in poorly controlled diabetics.

In vivo, the glucose-induced defect in heparin binding to antithrombin III may well be accentuated by a markedly reduced heparan sulfate content in several diabetic tissues (51). This inhibition of heparin-catalyzed antithrombin III activity by nonenzymatic glycosylation, in conjunction with glycosylation-induced changes in susceptibility of fibrin to degradation, could play a role in the abnormal accumulation of fibrin reported to occur in several diabetic tissues affected by long-term complications (52-55).

CROSSLINKING OF PROTEINS

Extensive early studies of nonenzymatic glycosylation showed that this process ultimately gave rise to pigmented, fluorescent, glucose-derived protein crosslinks (12, 13). The incubation conditions used in these studies were nonphysiologic, however, and a degree of uncertainty existed concerning the formation of glucose-derived crosslinks under diabetic conditions. The ability of hyperglycemia to aggregate and crosslink proteins under physiologic conditions in vitro and in vivo was first shown using the lens protein crystallins (56). Incubation of lens proteins with glucose or glucose-6-phosphate resulted in opacification of clear protein solutions as nonenzymatic glycosylation of lysine epsilon-amino groups increased. This opacification was shown to be a consequence of high molecular weight, light-scattering protein aggregate formation. Addition of disulfide-bond reducing agents such as dithiothreitol substantially reduced the degree of glucose-induced protein aggregation. Similar data were obtained from in-vivo studies with diabetic animals (19). These observations suggest that protein conformational changes induced by nonenzymatic glycosylation render some previously unexposed sulfhydryl groups susceptible to oxidation. In vivo, lens proteins are normally protected against oxidation-induced crosslink formation by intracellular reduced glutathione. In the diabetic lens, decreased levels of reduced glutathione resulting from increased polyol pathway activity may act synergistically with nonenzymatic glycosylation to cause accelerated formation of disulfide bonds (57).

Lens proteins examined after longer-term incubation under physiologic conditions showed the presence of covalent crosslinks that were not disulfide in nature (20). Concomitantly, these glycosylated protein solutions developed pigment and showed spectroscopic properties similar to those of lens proteins from brunescent human cataracts. More rapid accumulation of these glucose-derived crosslinks could contribute to accelerated senile cataract formation in diabetic patients.

Extensive glucose-derived crosslink formation may also contribute to the reversible defects in axoplasmic transport seen in experimental diabetic neuropathy (58). In vitro, rapid formation of non-reducible, high molecular weight protein aggregates occurs during nonenzymatic glycosylation of the neuronal microtubular protein, tubulin (23). In vivo, tubulin prepared from diabetic rats shows an increased quantity of nonreducible, high molecular weight material, corresponding to a dramatic increase in the amount of nonenzymatic glycosylation. Despite this nonenzymatic glycosylation-induced increase in tubulin aggregate formation, however, guanosine triophosphate-dependent tubulin polymerization is profoundly inhibited, because normal polymerization of monomers into functional microtubules requires unsubstituted lysine residues.

Glucose-derived crosslinks also form when reactive groups generated by nonenzymatic glycosylation of long-lived structural proteins trap potentially damaging nonglycosylated soluble proteins. Experimentally, addition of serum albumin or IgG to nonenzymatically glycosylated collagen washed free of glucose resulted in binding of both these proteins to the collagen (59). Furthermore, the albumin and anti-bovine serum albumin IgG that bound to nonenzymatically glycosylated collagen retained their ability to form immune complexes in situ with the corresponding free antibody and antigen (Figure 2). These observations provide a biochemical expla-

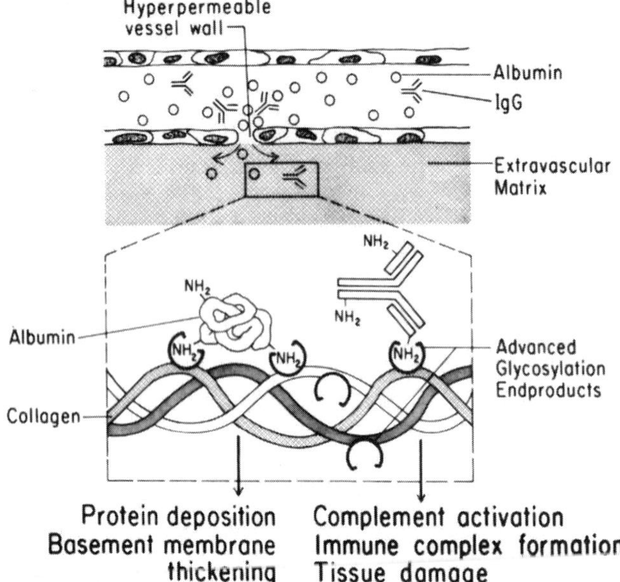

Figure 2. Covalent trapping of potentially damaging nonglycosylated plasma proteins by advanced glycosylation end-products on collagen. Increased diabetic vascular permeability would accelerate this process.

nation for the intense linear immunofluorescent staining for albumin and IgG characteristically seen in diabetic extravascular membranes (60). Binding of these serum proteins to diabetic kidney has been shown to be essentially undissociable. Persistent accumulation of circulating proteins such as albumin, may contribute to the characteristic thickening of diabetic basement membranes, and trapping of IgG may be responsible for the activated-complement (poly C9) membrane-attack complex deposition that occurs in diabetic kidneys (61). In addition, covalent attachment of soluble proteins by nonenzymatically glycosylated collagen may be the first step in a process of in situ formation of immune complexes in some diabetic tissues, where discontinuous granular ("lumpy-bumpy") deposits of immunoglobulins have been identified as immune complexes by electron microscopy (62). The reported production of pseudodiabetic glomerular basement membrane thickening in normal mice after repeated injections of glucosylated proteins may involve glucose-derived crosslinks with free amino groups in the glomerular extracellular matrix (63), but direct evidence for this has not been obtained. Binding of plasma protein constituents to nonenzymatically glycosylated perivascular structural proteins may be enhanced in vivo by the well-described increase in vascular permeability associated with diabetes in both animals and humans.

The ability of nonenzymatically glycosylated collagen to trap soluble proteins after being washed free of glucose suggests that glucose itself may not be a required participant in protein crosslinking. The clinical implications of this possiblity are sobering. If glucose-derived protein crosslink formation can progress in the absence of glucose, then perfect correction of hyperglycemia in diabetic patients in the future may not prevent the continued progression of diabetic complications. In-vitro evidence has recently come from a model system using the protein RNase A (34). After extensive nonenzymatic glycosylation of this protein, the rate of continuing crosslink formation was determined in both the absence and presence of glucose. The observed rates of continued protein crosslinking were essentially identical. If continuing crosslink formation occurs in vivo, then additional pharmacologic approaches may ultimately be required to directly interfere with these processes.

To develop such pharmacologic approaches, more complete chemical information will be needed about glucose-derived protein crosslinks formed under physiologic conditions. A recent advance towards this end has been the isolation of an advanced glycosylation end-product-protein hydrolysis product involved in crosslinking, followed by determination and confirmation of its exact chemical structure (64). The isolated product has spectral properties identical to those that characterize intact advanced glycosylation end-product proteins. From nuclear magnetic resonance, mass spectroscopy, and chemical derivatization studies, this compound has been assigned the novel structure 2-furoyl-4(5)-(2-furanyl)-1*H*-imidazole (FFI). This compound is a condensation product of two glucose molecules and two lysine-derived amino groups into a conjugated system of three aromatic heterocycles (Figure 3). Formation of FFI could occur through interaction of two Amadori products, but this would not explain the previously discussed ability of advanced glycosylation end-product proteins to trap other unglycosylated proteins. The FFI crosslinks between glycosylated and nonglycosylated protein amino groups could form, however, if nonglycosylated protein amino groups reacted with either a monoglycosylated Amadori product, followed by addition of a second glucose molecule, or with a diglycosylated Amadori product alone.

SUSCEPTIBILITY TO PROTEOLYSIS

Accumulation of collagen-related proteins in the glomerular extravascular matrix is the central pathologic alteration that characterizes diabetic nephropathy. Continual accumulation over many years ultimately results in progressive renal failure due to progressive glomerular capillary occlusion. In experimental animals, some of the morphologic features of diabetic renal disease are reversible by islet transplantation. Diabetes-induced glomerular basement membrane thickening does not regress, however, suggesting that its susceptibility to physiologic degradative mechanisms may be abnormally low (65, 66). In vitro, susceptibility of nonenzymatically glycosylated glomerular basement membrane preparations to digestion by nonspecific general proteases such as pepsin, papain, and trypsin, is considerably reduced (67). Similarly, susceptibility of tendon collagen from diabetic patients to digestion by nonspecific protease activities such as bacterial collagenase and pepsin is also significantly reduced (68). The collagen cleavage products released by pepsin have more high molecular weight components, and the pepsin-resistant portion more associated Amadori glycosylation products, than the corresponding fractions from normal subjects.

In collagen from normal subjects, an age-related increase in diabetic-like changes is seen. Both basement membrane and the structurally related collagens undergo nonenzymatic glycosylation in vitro and in vivo (21, 24-26). Collagen from nondiabetics shows an age-related linear increase in advanced glycosylation end-product pigment accumulation, and associated age-related changes in collagen mechanical properties consistent with increased crosslink formation (27, 69, 70). The acceleration of both of these processes by diabetes could result in reduced susceptibility of diabetic glycosylated basement membrane and collagen to in-vivo proteolysis. Further studies using the appropriate mammalian enzymes will be necessary to demonstrate this finding, however. Abnormal accumulation of several other proteins in particular diabetic tissues may reflect the same general pathophysiologic mechanism.

One such protein appears to be fibrin. Excessive nonenzymatic glycosylation of circulating fibrinogen has been shown in diabetic patients, and after fibrin deposition, the degree of glycosylation could increase even further (16). This nonenzymatic glycosylation of fibrin would be expected to reduce susceptibility to degradation by the specific fibrinolytic enzyme plasmin, because this protease cleaves only at substrate arginine and lysine peptide bonds. Using both a fibrin plate assay and a fluorogenic synthetic plasmin substrate assay, it was found that glucose blocking of the epsilon-amino group of lysines in the fibrinogen and fibrin molecule interferes with the specific fibrinolytic enzyme-substrate interaction (17). Acetylation and carbamylation had qualitatively similar effects, showing that chemical modification of lysine amino groups, rather than crosslink formation, is the underlying phenomenon responsible for the degradative defect produced by glucose. Experimental conditions that increased the rate of nonenzymatic protein glycosylation were associated with correspondingly greater degrees of resistance to degradation by plasmin. Analogous reductions in susceptibility to degradation would be expected consequences of excessive nonenzymatic glycosylation in other proteins cleaved preferentially at substrate lysine residues. Extensive glucose-derived crosslinking of long-lived structural proteins discussed above may also reduce susceptibility to degradation by proteases cleaving at non-lysine residues.

Defective fibrin degradation induced by excessive nonenzymatic glycosylation in vivo could lead to the fibrin accumulation seen in various diabetic tissues. In the diabetic kidney, immunohistochemical studies have shown the presence of fibrin in glomerular capillary basement membrane (52). Local responses to mesangial and endothelial fibrin trapping may represent the initial phase of Kimmelsteil-Wilson nodule development (71), and persistence of this fibrin may contribute to the capillary occlusion and progressive glomerular drop-out of long-term diabetes. Fibrin deposition has also been reported in diabetic retinal capillaries (53), and in small epineurial arterioles from patients with long-standing diabetic neuropathy (54). In the arterial wall, fibrin appears to enhance the proliferation of arterial smooth muscle cells, whereas

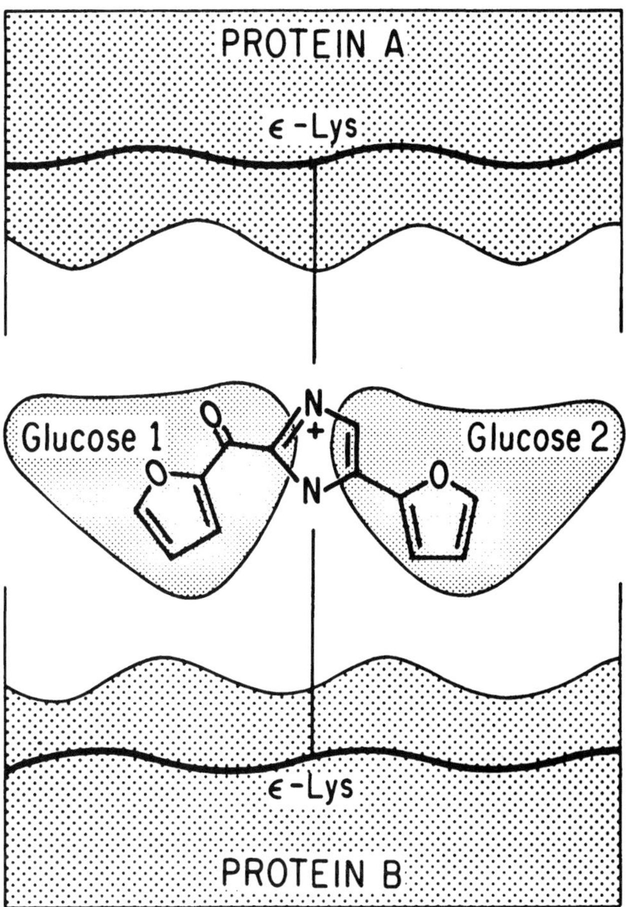

Figure 3. Glucose-derived protein crosslink formed under physiologic conditions. This compound, 2-furoyl-4(5)-(2-furanyl)-1*H*-imidazole, is a condensation product of two glucose molecules and two lysine-derived amino groups.

fibrin degradation products (fragments D and E) inhibit the proliferation of smooth muscle cells (72). Defective degradation of nonenzymatically glycosylated fibrin could thus play an important role in the development of several major diabetic complications.

FUNCTION OF NUCLEIC ACIDS

Although the primary amino groups of nucleotides are chemically less reactive toward reducing sugars than epsilon-amino groups of lysine, nonenzymatic glycosylation of nucleic acid bases can occur, with resultant abnormalities of DNA template function (73). The spectral and fluorescent properties of DNA advanced glycosylation end-products were similar to those of advanced glycosylation end-product proteins. Such nonenzymatic glycosylation reduced the ability of viral DNA fl to transfect *Escherichia coli* at a rate proportional to both incubation time and sugar concentration. Loss of transfection potential was related primarily to DNA glycosylation itself, rather than to a subsequently occurring strand scission reaction. Reducing sugars also have been found to act as mutagens for DNA. Incubation of glucose-6-phosphate with the plasmid pBR322 containing ampicillin- and tetracycline-resistance genes resulted in the occurrence of mutants that were antibiotic sensitive (BUCALA R, MODEL P, CERAMI A. Unpublished observations.).

Although DNA, like protein, reacts with glucose-6-phosphate at a much faster rate than with glucose, it was found that the DNA-glucose reaction could be greatly accelerated by the presence of lysine (73). After an initial lag period, the rate of DNA inactivation increased to that seen with glucose-6-phosphate. This finding implies that a common intermediate is formed initially between the lysine and the glucose or glucose-6-phosphate that can react subsequently with DNA. Such glucose-derived crosslinking of amino acids to nucleic acids may be the mechanism by which increasing amounts of proteins become covalently attached to DNA as persons age (74).

Because nucleic acids are long-lived molecules in the resting cell, in-vivo advanced glycosylation end-products would progressively accumulate on DNA over time. Such accumulation may be responsible for age-dependent changes in the genetic material that include chromosomal aberrations, DNA strand breaks, and a decline in DNA repair, replication, and transcription (75-79). Acceleration of this process by diabetic hyperglycemia would result in an earlier onset of cellular senescence. The decrease in diabetic fibroblast replicative capacity resembling that associated with normal aging may be one example (80, 81). Nonenzymatic glycosylation of nucleic acids may also be responsible for the increased frequency of congenital abnormalities in children of diabetic mothers. The exposure of the early embryo to high glucose concentrations could lead to an increased reaction of glucose or a glucose metabolite with DNA at critical developmental stages, causing chromosomal breaks and mutagenesis. Fetal abnormalities similar to those produced by diabetic pregnancy have been reported after exposure to mutagens.

MACROMOLECULAR RECOGNITION AND ENDOCYTOSIS

Most mammalian cells have various unique surface structures that recognize particular chemical signals such as hormones and neurotransmitters. High-affinity binding of such chemical signals to their specific cell-surface receptors initiates a response within the cell that contributes to the maintenance of organismal homeostasis. In a few cell types, such as capillary endothelial cells and monocyte plus macrophages, binding of certain ligands to sites on the cell membrane stimulates rapid interiorization and intracellular processing. Consequences of ligand-induced endocytosis seen experimentally include unidirectional protein transport, alterations in intracellular enzyme activities, and extracellular secretion of neutral proteases (82). Although macromolecular recognition is not well understood at the biochemical level, carbohydrate structure and protein conformation have been identified as two potentially critical factors in this process. Modification of proteins by nonenzymatic glycosylation may therefore be expected to alter macromolecular recognition and endocytosis significantly.

The effects of nonenzymatic glycosylation on endocytic ingestion were first studied using serum albumin and isolated microvessels (18). Unmodified albumin was excluded from ingestion by microvessel endothelial cells, whereas glycosylated albumin was rapidly taken up by endocytosis. Concentrations of glycosylated albumin similar to those found in diabetic plasma appeared to stimulate the ingestion of unmodified albumin as well. Similar recognition and endocytosis of nonenzymatically glycosylated albumin by capillary endothelial cells may be involved in the blood-retinal barrier dysfunction which occurs soon after the onset of diabetes.

In nondiabetic patients, endocytosis of cholesterol-rich low-density lipoprotein (LDL) is thought to influence the development of atherosclerosis by affecting both the rate of accumulation and the rate of removal of tissue cholesterol deposits (83, 84). The existence of high-affinity LDL receptors on fibroblasts allows these and many other nonhepatic cells to be supplied with adequate amounts of cholesterol (required for membrane synthesis) while maintaining the lowest possible level of plasma LDL. Low plasma LDL is critical, because the rate of cholesterol deposition in tissues increases linearly with plasma LDL concentration. When normal LDL receptor function is impaired, compensatory increases in plasma LDL concentrations lead to accelerated atherogenesis. Removal of deposited lipoprotein cholesterol appears to involve tissue macrophages that recognize and ingest both beta-very-low-density lipoproteins, and LDL that has been modified by endothelial cells (85). In vitro, the modified LDL receptor also interacts with lipoproteins whose lysine residues have been modified using formaldehyde, gluteraldehyde, malondialdehyde, acetylation, acetoacetylation, carbamylation, and maleylation (84).

Nonenzymatic glycosylation of LDL from diabetic patients exceeds that of normal persons (29). The absolute amount of glycosylation is relatively small, however, because the apolipoproteins have short half-lives. More extensive nonenzymatic glycosylation of LDL can be readily accomplished in vitro. This hyperglycosylated LDL is internalized and degraded by cultured human fibroblasts significantly less than control LDL, and the fractional catabolic rate of this material is reduced in guinea pigs (86, 87). These studies confirm earlier work showing that extensive chemical modification of LDL lysine residues interferes with recognition and uptake by fibroblasts (88). The extent to which similar changes occur in vivo is unclear, however, because the abnormally high plasma LDL levels associated with genetic disorders of LDL-receptor function are not a characteristic feature of diabetes (89). Although degradation of glycosylated LDL by mouse peritoneal macrophages did not occur via the acetyl-LDL mechanism, this may indicate only that the required threshold level of recognizable modifications had not been reached (90). In vivo, advanced glycosylation end-products would continue to accumulate on LDL trapped in the extracellular matrix, and recognition of these by macrophages may contribute to the pathogenesis of atherosclerosis.

In contrast to the plasma proteins discussed above, structural proteins with long half-lives accumulate advanced glycosylation end-products. Recently, these advanced glycosylation end-products have been shown to mediate specific macrophage recognition and uptake of proteins glycosylated both in vitro and in vivo (91). Long-term exposure of peripheral nerve myelin proteins to glucose markedly altered the way in which myelin interacts with elicited macrophages. Myelin that had been incubated with glucose in vitro for 8 weeks reached a steady-state accumulation within thioglycolate-elicited macrophages that was five times greater than myelin incubated without glucose (Figure 4a). Similarly, myelin isolated from rats having diabetes for 1.5 to 2.0 years had a steady-state level that was nine times greater than that of myelin from young rats, and 3.5 times greater than myelin from age-matched controls (Figure 4c). In contrast, myelin isolated from rats having diabetes for 4 to 6 weeks had the same degree of accumulation as did myelin from age-matched normal rats (Figure 4b). These data suggest that the amount of increased nonenzymatic glycosylation seen in the myelin of short-term diabetic rats had not yet resulted in the significant accumulation of advanced glycosylation end-product myelin present both in vitro and in the long-term diabetic rats. The addition of increasing amounts of unlabeled normal unmodified myelin failed to compete with ^{125}I-advanced glycosylation end-product myelin accumulation, whereas the addition of unlabeled advanced glycosylation end-product myelin competed effectively.

Formation of irreversible advanced glycosylation end-product adducts on myelin appears to promote recognition and uptake by macrophages. This interaction between advanced glycosylation end-product myelin and macrophages could initiate or contribute to the segmental demyelination associated with diabetes and the normal aging of peripheral nerve by mechanisms that remain to be elucidated. Demyelination may result in part from augmented secretion of proteolytic enzymes triggered by interaction of advanced glycosylation end-product myelin with its receptor. Macrophage secretion of several neutral proteases has already been reported in response to maleylated albumin binding (92).

IMMUNOGENICITY

Covalent attachment of small molecules to autologous proteins can produce conjugates that are capable of inducing an immune response in the host. Formation of specific glucose-derived adducts on body proteins could function in a similar fashion, leading to potentially damaging autoantibody formation in diabetic patients. The Amadori product of nonenzymatic glycosylation has been shown experimentally to be a poor immunogen, however. The LDL-Amadori products, for example, induce low titers of low affinity antibodies in guinea pigs, even when given with complete Freund's adjuvant. In contrast, when similar immunization is done using lipoproteins whose Amadori products have been chemically converted in vitro to a hexitolamino derivative, high titers of region-specific antibodies are generated that do not cross-react with any of the Amadori product proteins (93). Qualitatively similar results have been obtained in preliminary studies using the chemically produced hexitolamino derivative of collagen Amadori products (94).

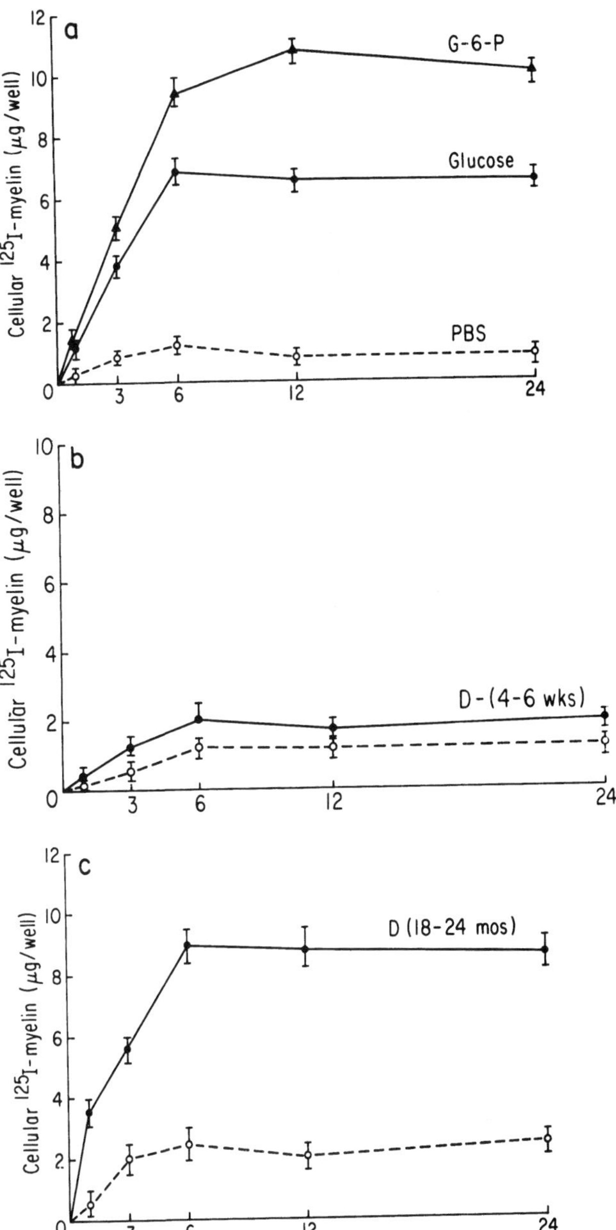

Figure 4. Macrophage recognition and uptake of peripheral nerve myelin proteins glycosylated both in vitro and in vivo. **Figure 4a.** Proteins from 8-week incubations in 50 mmol/L glucose (*closed circle*), 50 mmol/L glucose-6-phosphate (*triangle*), or phosphate-buffered saline (*open circle*). **Figure 4b.** Proteins from rats having diabetes for 4 to 6 weeks (*closed circle*) and from age-matched normal rats (*open circle*). **Figure 4c.** Proteins from rats having diabetes for 1.5 to 2.0 years (*closed circle*) and from age-matched normal rats (*open circle*).

These data suggest that in vivo, a structural analog of the open-chain hexitolamino Amadori product derivative would have greater immunogenic potenial than the Amadori product itself. Such glucose-derived open-chain structures probably occur in vivo during formation of the advanced glycosylation end-product FFI. Direct experimental evidence for the immunogenicity of advanced glycosylation end-products on long-lived structural proteins has not yet been provided, however.

Potential Clinical Applications of Research on Nonenzymatic Glycosylation

New knowledge about nonenzymatic glycosylation may lead to significant advances in both diagnosis and therapy. Diagnostically, the isolation and identification of FFI now make possible the development of an analytical method for measuring accumulated advanced glycosylation end-products in clinical samples. This information about patients' long-term, time-averaged exposure to glucose may help identify subsets of clinically indistinguishable diabetic patients who differ in inherent susceptibility to hyperglycemia-induced tissue damage. Epidemiologic evidence suggests that for any given level of sustained hyperglycemia, some patients appear to be at greater risk. Although the presence of HLA-DR4 may be associated with this additional risk (1, 95), there is at present no laboratory procedure that can be used to determine prognosis.

Therapeutically, new agents may be required to directly interfere with the self-perpetuating component of glycosylation-mediated tissue damage, if perfect correction of hyperglycemia in some diabetic patients will not prevent the continued progression of diabetic complications. These new pharmacologic developments must be based on increased understanding of the biochemistry of advanced glycosylation end-product formation on proteins of diabetic tissues, because attempts at preventing Amadori product formation by nonspecific chemical modification of protein amino groups would result in pathophysiologic changes similar to those produced by diabetes itself (96).

ACKNOWLEDGMENTS: Grant support: in part by a grant from the American Diabetes Association-New York Diabetes Affiliate, and grant R01-AM19655 from the National Institutes of Health. Dr. Vlassara is the recipient of a Research Scientist Development Award (1-K01-AG00148) from the National Institute of Arthritis, Diabetes, and Digestive and Kidney Diseases, and the National Institute of Aging.

▶ Requests for reprints should be addressed to Michael Brownlee, M.D.; Laboratory of Medical Biochemistry, The Rockefeller University, 1230 York Avenue; New York, NY 10021.

References

1. CUDWORTH AG, BODANSKY HJ, WEST KM. Genetic and metabolic factors in relationship to the prevalence and severity of diabetic complications. In: KEEN H, JARRETT J, eds. *Complications of Diabetes.* 2nd edition. London: Edward Arnold (Publishers) Ltd.;1982:1-18.
2. PIRART J. Diabetes mellitus and its degenerative complications: prospective study of 4,400 patients observed between 1947 and 1973. *Diabetes Care.* 1978;**1**:168-88;252-63.
3. BROWNLEE M, CERAMI A. The biochemistry of the complications of diabetes mellitus. *Annu Rev Biochem.* 1981;**50**:385-432.
4. SHADE DS, SANTIAGO JV, SKYLER JS, RIZZA RA. *Intensive Insulin Therapy.* Princeton, New Jersey: Medical Examination Publishing Co., Inc.;1983:1-341.
5. LAURITZEN T, FROST-LARSEN K, LARSEN HW, DECKERT T. Effect of 1 year of near-normal blood glucose levels on retinopathy in insulin-dependent diabetics. *Lancet.* 1983;**1**:200-4.
6. VIBERTI GC, BILOUS RW, MACKINTOSH D, BENDING JJ, KEEN H. Long term correction of hyperglycaemia and progression of renal failure in insulin-dependent diabetics. *Br Med J (Clin Res).* 1983;**286**:598-602.
7. CLEMENTS RS JR. The role of abnormal polyol metabolism in diabetic complications. In: BRODOFF BN, BLEICHER SJ. *Diabetes Mellitus and Obesity.* Baltimore: Williams and Wilkins; 1982:117-28.
8. GREENE DA. Metabolic abnormalities in diabetic peripheral nerve: relation to impaired function. *Metabolism.* 1983;**32**:118-23.
9. KOENIG RJ, CERAMI A. Hemoglobin A_{Ic} and diabetes mellitus. *Annu Rev Med.* 1980;**31**:29-34.
10. MONNIER VM, CERAMI A. Nonenzymatic glycosylation and browning of proteins in vivo. In: WALLER GR, FEATHER MS, eds. *The Maillard Reaction in Foods and Nutrition.* American Chemical Society Symposium Series No. 215. Washington, D.C.: The American Chemical Society; 1983:431-9.
11. HIGGINS PJ, BUNN HF. Kinetic analysis of the nonenzymatic glycosylation of hemoglobin. *J Biol Chem.* 1981;**256**:5204-8.
12. REYNOLDS TM. Chemistry of nonenzymatic browning: I. *Adv Food Res.* 1963;**12**:1-52.
13. REYNOLDS TM. Chemistry of nonenzymatic browning: II. *Adv Food Res.* 1965;**14**:167-283.
14. MILLER JA, GRAVALLESE E, BUNN HF. Nonenzymatic glycosylation of erythrocyte membrane proteins: relevance to diabetes. *J Clin Invest.* 1980;**65**:896-901.
15. BROWNLEE M, VLASSARA H, CERAMI A. Inhibition of heparin-catalyzed human antithrombin III activity by nonenzymatic glycosylation: possible role in fibrin deposition in diabetes. *Diabetes.* 1984;**33**:532-5.
16. MCVERRY BA, THORPE S, JOE F, GAFFNEY P, HUEHNS ER. Nonenzymatic glycosylation of fibrinogen. *Haemostasis.* 1981;**10**:261-70.
17. BROWNLEE M, VLASSARA H, CERAMI A. Nonenzymatic glycosylation reduces the susceptibility of fibrin to degradation by plasmin. *Diabetes.* 1983;**32**:680-4.
18. WILLIAMS SK, DEVENNY JJ, BITENSKY MW. Micropinocytic ingestion of glycosylated albumin by isolated microvessels: possible role in pathogenesis of diabetic microangiopathy. *Proc Natl Acad Sci USA.* 1981;**78**:2393-7.
19. MONNIER VM, STEVENS VJ, CERAMI A. Nonenzymatic glycosylation, sulfhydryl oxidation, and aggregation of lens proteins in experimental sugar cataracts. *J Exp Med.* 1979;**150**:1098-107.
20. MONNIER VM, CERAMI A. Nonenzymatic browning in vivo: possible process for aging of long-lived proteins. *Science.* 1981;**211**:491-3.
21. COHEN MP, URDANIVIA E, SURMA M, CIBOROWSKI CJ. Nonenzymatic glycosylation of basement membranes: in vitro studies. *Diabetes.* 1981;**30**:367-71.
22. VLASSARA H, BROWNLEE M, CERAMI A. Excessive nonenzymatic glycosylation of peripheral and central nervous system myelin components in diabetic rats. *Diabetes.* 1983;**32**:670-4.
23. WILLIAMS SK, HOWARTH NL, DEVENNY JJ, BITENSKY MW. Structural and functional consequences of increased tubulin glycosylation in diabetes mellitus. *Proc Natl Acad Sci USA.* 1982;**79**:6546-50.
24. COHEN MP, URDANIVIA E, SURMA M, WU VY. Increased glycosylation of glomerular basement membrane collagen in diabetes. *Biochem Biophys Res Commun.* 1980;**95**:765-9.
25. ROSENBERG H, MODRAK JB, HASSING JM, AL-TURK WA, STOHS SJ. Glycosylated collagen. *Biochem Biophys Res Commun.* 1979;**91**:498-501.
26. SCHNIDER SL, KOHN RR. Glucosylation of human collagen in aging and diabetes mellitus. *J Clin Invest.* 1980;**66**:1179-81.
27. MONNIER VM, KOHN RR, CERAMI A. Accelerated age-related browning of human collagen in diabetes mellitus. *Proc Natl Acad Sci USA.* 1984;**81**:583-7.
28. VOGT BW, SCHLEICHER ED, WIELAND OH. Epsilon-amino-lysine-bound glucose in human tissues obtained at autopsy: increase in diabetes mellitus. *Diabetes.* 1982;**31**:1123-7.
29. SCHLEICHER E, DEUFEL T, WIELAND OH. Non-enzymatic glycosylation of human serum lipoproteins: elevated epsilon-lysine glycosylated low density lipoprotein in diabetic patients. *FEBS Lett.* 1981;**129**:1-4.
30. WITZTUM JL, FISHER M, PIETRO T, STEINBRECHER UP, ELAM RL. Nonenzymatic glucosylation of high-density lipoprotein accelerates its catabolism in guinea pigs. *Diabetes.* 1982;**31**:1029-32.
31. DAY JR, THORPE SR, BAYNES JW. Nonenzymatically glucosylated albumin: in vitro preparation and isolation from normal human serum. *J Biol Chem.* 1979;**254**:595-7.
32. CORADELLO H, POLLACK A, PUGNANO M, LEBAN J, LUBEN G. Nonenzymatic glycosylation of cathepsin B: possible influence on conversion of proinsulin to insulin. *IRCS Med Sci.* 1981;**9**:766-7.
33. DOLHOFER R, SIESS EA, WIELAND OH. Inactivation of bovine kidney beta-N-acetyl-D-glucosaminidase by nonenzymatic glucosylation. *Hoppe Seylers Z Physiol Chem.* 1982;**363**:1427-36.
34. EBLE AS, THORPE SR, BAYNES JW. Nonenzymatic glucosylation and glucose-dependent cross-linking of protein. *J Biol Chem.* 1983;**258**:9506-12.
35. ZAMAN Z, VERWILGHEN RL. Non-enzymatic glycosylation of horse spleen and rat liver ferritins. *Biochem Biophys Acta.* 1981;**669**:120-4.
36. VLASSARA H, BROWNLEE M, CERAMI A. Nonenzymatic glycosylation of peripheral nerve protein in diabetes mellitus. *Proc Natl Acad Sci USA.* 1981;**78**:5190-2.
37. YUE DK, MCLENNAN S, TURTLE JR. Non-enzymatic glycosylation of tissue protein in diabetes in the rat. *Diabetologia.* 1983;**24**:377-81.
38. SCHLEICHER E, SCHELLER L, WIELAND OH. Quantitation of lysine-bound glucose of normal and diabetic erythrocyte membranes by HPLC analysis of furosine [epsilon-N(L-furoylmethyl)-L-lysine]. *Biochem Biophys Res Commun.* 1981;**99**:1011-9.

39. Garlick RL, Mazer JS, Higgins PJ, Bunn HF. Characterization of glycosylated hemoglobins: relevance to monitoring of diabetic control and analysis of other proteins. *J Clin Invest.* 1983;**71**:1062-72.
40. Garlick RL, Mazer JS. The principal site of nonenzymatic glycosylation of human serum albumin in vivo. *J Biol Chem.* 1983;**258**:6142-6.
41. Walsh C. *Enzymatic Reaction Mechanisms.* San Francisco: W.H. Freeman and Company; 1979:1-928.
42. Coradello H, Lubec G, Pollak A, Sternberg M. [Enzyme activities of native non-enzymatically glucosylated trypsin, chymotrypsin and papain]. *Padiatr Padol.* 1982;**17**:457-64.
43. Perutz MF. Regulation of oxygen affinity of hemoglobin. *Annu Rev Biochem.* 1979;**48**:327-86.
44. McDonald MJ, Bleichman M, Bunn HF, Noble RW. Functional properties of the glycosylated minor components of human adult hemoglobin. *J Biol Chem.* 1979;**254**:702-7.
45. Samaja M, Melotti D, Carenini A, Pozza G. Glycosylated haemoglobins and the oxygen affinity of whole blood. *Diabetologia.* 1982;**23**:399-402.
46. Bick RL. Clinical relevance of antithrombin III. *Semin Throm Hemost.* 1982;**8**:276-87.
47. Pletcher CH, Nelsestuen GL. The rate-determining step of the heparin-catalyzed antithrombin/thrombin reaction is independent of thrombin. *J Biol Chem.* 1982;**257**:5342-5.
48. Banerjee RN, Sahni AL, Kumar V, Arya M. Antithrombin 3 deficiency in maturity onset diabetes mellitus and atherosclerosis. *Thromb Diath Haemorrh.* 1974;**31**:399-45.
49. Sowers JR, Tuck ML, Sowers DK. Plasma antithrombin III and thrombin generation time: correlation with hemoglobin A1 and fasting serum glucose in young diabetic women. *Diabetes Care.* 1980;**3**:655-8.
50. Jones RL, Peterson CM. Reduced fibrinogen survival in diabetes mellitus: a reversible phenomenon. *J Clin Invest.* 1979;**63**:485-93.
51. Brown DM, Klein DJ, Michael AF, Oegema TR. ^{35}S-glycoaminoglycan and ^{35}S-glycopeptide metabolism by diabetic glomeruli and aorta. *Diabetes.* 1982;**31**:418-25.
52. Ireland JT, Viberti GC, Watkins PJ. The kidney and renal tract. In: Keen H, Jarrett J, eds. *Complications of Diabetes.* London: Edward Arnold Publishing Co.; 1982:137-98.
53. Cunha-Vaz JG. Pathophysiology of diabetic retinopathy. *Br J Ophthalmol.* 1978;**62**:351-5.
54. Timperly WR, Ward JD, Preson FE, et al. Clinical and histological studies in diabetic neuropathy. *Diabetologia.* 1976;**12**:237-43.
55. Haust MD, Wyllis JC, More RH. Electron microscopy of fibrin in human atherosclerotic lesions. *Exp Mol Pathol.* 1965;**4**:205-16.
56. Stevens VJ, Rouzer CA, Monnier VM, Cerami A. Diabetic cataract formation: potential role of glycosylation of lens crystallins. *Proc Natl Acad Sci USA.* 1978;**75**:2918-22.
57. Cerami A, Stevens VJ, Monnier VM. Role of nonenzymatic glycosylation in the development of the sequelae of diabetes mellitus. *Metabolism.* 1979;**28**:431-9.
58. Sidenius P. The axonopathy of diabetic neuropathy. *Diabetes.* 1982;**31**:356-63.
59. Brownlee M, Pongor S, Cerami A. Covalent attachment of soluble proteins by nonenzymatically glycosylated collagen: role in the *in situ* formation of immune complexes. *J Exp Med.* 1983;**158**:1739-44.
60. Miller K, Michael AF. Immunopathology of renal extracellular membranes in diabetes: specificity of tubular basement-membrane immunofluorescence. *Diabetes.* 1976;**25**:701-8.
61. Falk RJ, Kin Y, Tsai CH, et al. Renal deposition of poly C9 neoantigen of the membrane attack complex (MAC). *Kidney Int.* 1983;**23**:194.
62. Cavallo T, Pinto JA, Abbott LC, Rajaraman S. Immune complex disease complicating diabetic glomerulosclerosis. *Lab Invest.* 1983;**48**:13A.
63. McVerry BA, Fisher C, Hopp A, Huehns ER. Production of pseudodiabetic renal glomerular changes in mice after repeated injections of glucosylated proteins. *Lancet.* 1980;**1**:738-40.
64. Pongor S, Ulrich PC, Bencsath FA, Cerami A. Aging of proteins: isolation and identification of a fluorescent chromophore from the reaction of polypeptides with glucose. *Proc Nat Acad Sci USA.* 1984;**81**:2684-8.
65. Lee CS, Mauer SM, Brown DM, Sutherland DE, Michael AF, Najarian JS. Renal transplantation in diabetes mellitus in rats. *J Exp Med.* 1974;**139**:793-800.
66. Steffes MW, Brown DM, Basgen JM, Matas AJ, Mauer SM. Glomerular basement membrane thickness following islet transplantation in the diabetic rat. *Lab Invest.* 1979;**41**:116-8.
67. Lubec G, Pollak A. Reduced susceptibility of nonenzymatically glucosylated glomerular basement membrane to proteases: is thickening of diabetic glomerular basement membranes due to reduced proteolytic degradation? *Renal Physiol.* 1980;**3**:4-8.
68. Schnider SL, Kohn RR. Effects of age and diabetes mellitus on the solubility and nonenzymatic glucosylation of human skin collagen. *J Clin Invest.* 1981;**67**:1630-5.
69. Andreassen T, Seyer-Hansen K, Bailey AJ. Thermal stability, mechanical properties and reducible cross-links of rattail tendon in experimental diabetes. *Biochem Biophys Acta.* 1981;**677**:313-7.
70. Yue DK, McLennan S, Delbridge L, Handelsman DJ, Reeve T, Turtle JR. The thermal stability of collagen in diabetic rats: correlation with severity of diabetes and non-enzymatic glycosylation. *Diabetologia.* 1983;**24**:282-5.
71. Farquhar A, MacDonald MR, Ireland JT. The role of fibrin deposition in diabetic glomerulosclerosis: a light, electron and immunofluorescence microscopy study. *J Clin Pathol.* 1972;**25**:657-67.
72. Ishida T, Tanaka K. Effects of fibrin and fibrinogen-degradation products on the growth of rabbit aortic smooth muscle cells in culture. *Atherosclerosis.* 1982;**44**:161-74.
73. Bucala R, Model P, Cerami A. Modification of DNA by reducing sugars: a possible mechanism for nucleic acid aging and age-related dysfunction in gene expression. *Proc Natl Acad Sci USA.* 1984;**81**:105-9.
74. Bojanovic JJ, Jevtovic AD, Pantic VS, Dugandzic SM, Javonovic DS. Thymus nucleoproteins: thymus histones in young and adult rats. *Gerontologia.* 1970;**16**:304-12.
75. Saksela E, Moorhead PS. Aneuploidy in the degenerative phase of serial cultivation of human cell strains. *Proc Natl Acad Sci USA.* 1963;**50**:390-5.
76. Price GB, Modak SP, Makinodan T. Age-associated changes in the DNA of mouse tissue. *Science.* 1971;**171**:917-20.
77. Karran P, Ormerod MG. Is the ability to repair damage to DNA related to the proliferative capacity of a cell? The rejoining of x-ray produced strand breaks. *Biochem Biophys Acta.* 1973;**299**:54-64.
78. Petes TD, Farber RA, Tarrant GM, Holliday R. Altered rate of DNA replication in aging human fibroblast cultures. *Nature.* 1974;**251**:434-6.
79. Berdyshev GD, Zhelabovskaya SM. Composition, template properties and thermostability of liver chromatin from rats of various age at deproteinization by NaCl solutions. *Exp Gerontol.* 1972;**7**:321-30.
80. Goldstein S, Littlefield JW, Soeldner JS. Diabetes mellitus and aging: diminished plating efficiency of cultured human fibroblasts. *Proc Natl Acad Sci USA.* 1969;**64**:155-60.
81. Vracko R, Benditt EP. Restricted replicative life-span of diabetic fibroblasts in vitro: its relation to microangiopathy. *Fed Proc.* 1975;**34**:68-70.
82. Silverstein SC, Steinman RM, Cohn ZA. Endocytosis. *Annu Rev Biochem.* 1977;**46**:669-722.
83. Goldstein JL, Brown MS. The low-density lipoprotein pathway and its relation to atherosclerosis. *Annu Rev Biochem.* 1977;**46**:897-930.
84. Brown MS, Goldstein JL. Lipoprotein metabolism in the macrophage: implications for cholesterol deposition in atherosclerosis. *Annu Rev Biochem.* 1983;**52**:223-61.
85. Steinberg D. Lipoproteins and atherosclerosis: a look back and a look ahead. *Arteriosclerosis.* 1983;**3**:283-301.
86. Gonen B, Baenziger J, Schonfeld G, Jacobson D, Farrar P. Nonenzymatic glycosylation of low density lipoproteins in vitro: effects on cell-interactive properties. *Diabetes.* 1981;**30**:875-8.
87. Witztum JL, Mahoney EM, Branks MJ, Fisher M, Elam R, Steinberg D. Nonenzymatic glucosylaton of low-density lipoprotein alters its biologic activity. *Diabetes.* 1982;**31**:283-91.
88. Weisgraber KH, Innerarity TL, Mahley RW. Role of the lysine residues of plasma lipoproteins in high affinity binding to cell surface receptors on human fibroblasts. *J Biol Chem.* 1978;**253**:9053-62.
89. Briones ER, Mao SJT, Palumbo WM, O'Fallon WM, Chenoweth W, Kottke BA. Analysis of plasma lipids and apolipoproteins in insulin-dependent and noninsulin-dependent diabetics. *Metabolism.* 1984;**33**:42-9.
90. Haberland ME, Fogelman AM, Edwards PA. Specificity of receptor-mediated recognition of malondialdehyde-modified low density lipoproteins. *Proc Natl Acad Sci USA.* 1982;**79**:1712-6.
91. Vlassara H, Brownlee M, Cerami A. Accumulation of diabetic rate peripheral nerve myelin by macrophages increases with extent and duration of nonenzymatic glycosylation. *J Exp Med.* 1984;**160**:197-207.
92. Johnson WJ, Pizzo SV, Imber MJ, Adams DO. Receptors for maleylated proteins regulate secretion of neutral proteases by murine macrophages. *Science.* 1982;**218**:574-6.
93. Witztum JL, Steinbrecher UP, Fisher M, Kesaniemi A. Nonenzymatic glucosylation of homologous low density lipoprotein and albumin renders them immunogenic in the guinea pig. *Proc Natl Acad Sci USA.* 1983;**80**:2757-61.
94. Bassiouny AR, Rosenberg H, McDonald TL. Glucosylated collagen is antigenic. *Diabetes.* 1983;**32**:1182-4.
95. Dornan TL, Ting A, McPherson CK, et al. Genetic susceptibility to the development of retinopathy in insulin-dependent diabetics. *Diabetes.* 1982;**31**:226-31.
96. Peterson CM, Tsairis P, Ohnishi A, et al. Sodium cyanate-induced polyneuropathy in patients with sickle-cell disease. *Ann Intern Med.* 1974;**81**:152-8.

Section V

Gastroenterology

Serum glutamic oxalacetic transaminase activity as an index of liver cell injury: a preliminary report.

Wróblewski F, LaDue JS. Ann Intern Med. 1955;43:345-60.

Until Wróblewski and LaDue's article was published, liver cell injury or inflammation was often difficult to diagnose. Of the established tests of the day, only the relatively insensitive cephalin flocculation and thymol turbidity tests indicated liver injury or inflammation. An elevated serum bilirubin level often reflected such damage, but it also reflected states of intrahepatic or extrahepatic bile stasis without acute or chronic injury to hepatocytes. Other commonly used tests at the time—serum albumin and globulins, or bromsulfophthalein excretion—were measures of liver function, not of the degree of injury or inflammation. The advent of aminotransferase (or "transaminase") measurement by Karmen and colleagues in 1954 and their demonstration of significantly elevated serum levels following damage to heart and liver (1) set the stage for more accurate diagnosis and management of patients with a wide variety of liver injuries.

Wróbelwski and LaDue's 1955 report clearly documented the value of increased activity of serum aspartate aminotransferase (AST) in detecting liver injury. An earlier study (2) had shown the same for acute injury to the myocardium, the organ with the highest concentration of this cytosolic enzyme. Both AST and alanine aminotransferase (ALT) catalyze the transformation of the α-amino groups of aspartate and alanine to pyruvate and oxaloacetate, respectively. At the time, determining whether an increase in AST level was due to heart or liver damage depended on ancillary clinical information that could be determined (sometimes imprecisely) only by concomitant symptoms, signs, or laboratory data pointing to the heart or liver. The most complicated situation occurred when both organs were injured, as in hepatic anoxia associated with shock liver due to severe hypotension from massive bleeding or acute myocardial infarction.

Distinguishing between injuries to the liver or heart become possible with measurement of ALT (1). A 1956 article clearly showed the specificity of serum ALT for liver injury and inflammation (3). The concentration of this enzyme is highest in mitochondria of hepatocytes and is low in myocardial cells. Thus, its activity reflects the state of the liver and is considered its most specific indicator of injury.

Alanine aminotransferase is the best indicator of hepatic injury due to many toxic agents, particularly acetaminophen; pathophysiologic events, such as shock liver of acute heart failure or hypotension; trauma; the spectrum of fatty liver and toxemia of pregnancy (HELLP syndrome); alcoholic or immune hepatitis; Wilson disease; septic cholangitis; nonalcoholic steatohepatitis; and, most prominently, viral hepatitis (although levels may be normal in some patients with hepatitis C) (4–7). However, ALT often does not correlate with other common tests of liver disease, particularly those of liver function. Striking ALT elevations characterize the most acute injuries due to drug, toxin, virus, and shock, although the magnitude of elevation often correlates neither with degree of necrosis nor prognosis. Measuring ALT at appropriate intervals is very useful, particularly in determining the efficacy of such therapies as interferon and ribavirin for hepatitis C, nucleosides for hepatitis B, corticosteroids for autoimmune hepatitis and acute alcoholic hepatitis, and *N*-acetylcysteine for acetaminophen toxicity.

References

1. **Karmen A, Wróblewski F, LaDue JS.** Transaminase activity in human blood. J Clin Invest. 1955;34:126-131.
2. **LaDue JS, Wróblewski F, Karmen A.** Serum glutamic oxaloacetic transaminase activity in human acute transmural myocardial infarction. Science. 1954;120:497-499.
3. **Wróblewski F, LeDue JS.** Serum glutamic pyruvic transaminase SGP-T in hepatic disease: a preliminary report. Ann Intern Med. 1956;45: 801-811.
4. **Wróblewski F.** The clinical significance of transaminase activities of serum. Am J Med. 1959;27:911-923.
5. **Zimmerman HJ, West M.** Serum enzyme levels in the diagnosis of hepatic disease. Am J Gastroenterol. 1963;40:387-404.
6. **Van Waes L, Lieber S.** Glutamate dehydrogenase: a reliable marker of liver cell necrosis in the alcoholic. Br Med J. 1977;2:1508-1510.
7. **Ellis G, Goldberg DM, Spooner RJ, Ward AM.** Serum enzyme tests in diseases of the liver and biliary tree. Am J Clin Pathol. 1978;70:248-258.
8. **Diehl AM, Potter J, Boitnott J, Van Duyn MA, Herlong HF, Mezey E.** Relationship between pyridoxal 5'-phosphate deficiency and aminotransferase levels in alcoholic hepatitis. Gastroenterology. 1984;86:632-636.

Risk for serious gastrointestinal complications related to use of nonsteroidal anti-inflammatory drugs. A meta-analysis.

Gabriel SE, Jaakkimainen L, Bombardier C. Ann Intern Med. 1991; 115:787-796.

Nonsteroidal anti-inflammatory agents (NSAIDs) are arguably more prescribed worldwide than any other medication. Up to 17 million Americans use them to treat a variety of inflammations, most commonly arthritis. The safe and intelligent use of NSAIDs requires that physicians and patients understand the harmful effects of these agents, as established through accurate clinical observation and meticulous assessment (1).

This report by Gabriel and associates was the first to use meta-analysis, as defined by Chalmers (2), to document clearly the risk of serious complications of the gastrointestinal tract due to NSAID use. Although the meta-analysis did not cover every NSAID, its conclusions encompass all of them, because they all have the same pharmacological effects: inhibition of prostaglandin H synthetases 1 and 2 or cyclooxygenases (COX) 1 and 2 (3,4).

NSAIDs cause peptic ulcers of the gut, particularly of the stomach and duodenum. In 1984, Levy (5) reported a clear relationship between hospitalization for upper gastrointestinal bleeding and peptic ulcer disease due to aspirin ingestion, and Langman (6) confirmed shortly thereafter the association of anti-inflammatory drugs with peptic ulcer. These adverse effects were predictable from the known biological functions of these enzymes, which are an integral component of the breakdown of membrane arachidonic acid into prostaglandins and thromboxanes. The former, particularly prostaglandins G_2 and H_2, protect mucosal integrity, mainly of the stomach, and the diminution of these prostaglandins by inhibition of COX1 would jeopardize it (7).

Gabriel and associates statistically combined data from 16 studies over 15 years after doing a qualitative summary of study characteristics and a critical appraisal of study quality, as required for inclusion in a meta-analysis. The overall odds ratio for complications due to NSAID use was about 3. People older than 60 years; those with a history of gastrointestinal problems, particularly peptic ulcer; and those who concomitantly used corticosteroids had greater risk. Of interest, the risk is greatest during the first month of treatment with NSAIDs.

The search for protection against the adverse effects of NSAIDs, first with COX-2 inhibitors and now with proton-pump inhibitors, is in part the result of this classic clinical outcome study of these compounds. A change in the design of NSAIDs so that they inhibit only COX-2 may reduce the incidence of ulcers in the stomach, duodenum, and small intestines, provided that they are not administered with aspirin or corticosteroids. Unfortunately, the specter of cardiovascular complications, particularly myocardial infarction, severely limits their usefulness (8). However, proton-pump inhibitors offer protection to patients taking NSAIDs with or without concomitant aspirin (9).

Continuing study has confirmed that the risk of ulceration and bleeding with NSAID use is increased in patients older than 60 years, those taking high doses, those with a history of NSAID toxicity or peptic ulcer disease, and those concomitantly taking corticosteroids. *Helicobacter pylori* is an additional hazard and should be treated at the start of NSAID therapy. Risk also is increased in people who are concomitantly taking anticoagulants and, possibly, those taking selective serotonin reuptake inhibitors (10).

References

1. **Pirmohamed M, James S, Meakin S, et al.** Adverse drug reactions as cause of admission to hospital: prospective analysis of 18 820 patients. BMJ. 2004;329:15-19.
2. **Chalmers TC, Berrier J, Hewitt P, Berlin J, Reitman D, Nagalingam R, et al.** Meta-analysis of randomized controlled trials as a method of estimating rare complications of non-steroidal anti-inflammatory drug therapy. Aliment Pharmacol Ther. 1988;2 Suppl 1:9-26.
3. **Vane JR.** Inhibition of prostaglandin synthesis as a mechanism of action for aspirin-like drugs. Nat New Biol. 1971;231:232-235.
4. **Meade EA, Smith WL, DeWitt DL.** Differential inhibition of prostaglandin endoperoxide synthase (cyclooxygenase) isozymes by aspirin and other non-steroidal anti-inflammatory drugs. J Biol Chem. 1993;268:6610-6614.
5. **Levy M.** Aspirin use in patients with major upper gastrointestinal bleeding and peptic-ulcer disease. A report from the Boston Collaborative Drug Surveillance Program, Boston University Medical Center. N Engl J Med. 1974;290:1158-1162.
6. **Langman MJ.** Epidemiologic evidence on the association between peptic ulceration and antiinflammatory drug use. Gastroenterology. 1989;96: 640-646.
7. **Cryer B, Feldman M.** Cyclooxygenase-1 and cyclooxygenase-2 selectivity of widely used nonsteroidal anti-inflammatory drugs. Am J Med. 1998; 104:413-421.
8. **Silverstein FE, Faich G, Goldstein JL, et al.** Gastrointestinal toxicity with celecoxib vs nonsteroidal anti-inflammatory drugs for osteoarthritis and rheumatoid arthritis: the CLASS study: A randomized controlled trial. Celecoxib Long-term Arthritis Safety Study. JAMA. 2000;284:1247-1255.
9. **Wallace JL, Reuter B, Cicala C, McKnight W, Grisham MB, Cirino G.** Novel nonsteroidal anti-inflammatory drug derivatives with markedly reduced ulcerogenic properties in the rat. Gastroenterology. 1994;107: 173-179.
10. **Lanza FL.** A guideline for the treatment and prevention of NSAID-induced ulcers. Members of the Ad Hoc Committee on Practice Parameters of the American College of Gastroenterology. Am J Gastroenterol. 1998;93:2037-2046.
11. **Yuan Y, Tsoi K, Hunt RH.** Selective serotonin reuptake inhibitors and risk of upper GI bleeding: confusion or confounding? Am J Med. 2006; 119:719-727

Effect of treatment of *Helicobacter pylori* infection on the long-term recurrence of gastric or duodenal ulcer. A randomized, controlled study.

Graham DY, Lew GM, Klein PD, et al. Ann Intern Med. 1992;116: 705-708.

Graham and associates provided further conclusive evidence that *Helicobacter pylori* caused peptic ulcer disease by demonstrating endoscopically that eradication of the organism by antibiotics is curative. They showed that 50% of patients with active gastric or duodenal ulcers treated only with histamine-2 blocker had relapses of ulcers within 12 weeks of healing, compared with only 12% of those treated with triple therapy antibiotics. This finding further substantiated Marshall and Warren's postulate (1) that an organism was the cause of peptic ulcer and that its eradication would heal gastritis and peptic ulcer. In addition, ulcer recurrence in the group treated with antibiotics was associated either with failure to eradicate *H. pylori* or concurrent use of a nonsteroidal anti-inflammatory drug.

The long search for an infectious cause of peptic ulcer, which began more than 100 years ago, ended with Marshall and Warren's discovery of *Campylobacter* in the stomachs of patients with gastritis and peptic ulcer (1). Marshall and colleagues satisfied the Koch postulates for establishing a bacterium as the cause of a disease by inducing gastritis, clinically and histologically, in Marshall by injecting the organism into his stomach (2).

The discovery of *Campylobacter pylori,* later reclassified as *H. pylori*, also answered the vexing riddle of the 75% relapse rate of peptic ulcer disease. For more than a century, one agent or another had been implicated (1). In the early 1940s, A. Stone Freedberg described a curved bacterium in slides of gastric tissue stained with silver in surgically resected stomachs, including a specimen from a patient with a gastric ulcer; however, investigators could not grow the organism in culture (3). At about the same time, W.B. Castle, finding urease in gastric juice, seemed certain that a bacterium somehow infects the stomach (Schmid R, personal communication).

Within a few years after Marshall and Warren discovered *H. pylori* (which won them the Nobel Prize), the pathogenesis of the disease was reasonably well worked out. *Helicobacter pylori* infection leads to hypersecretion of hydrochloric acid by increasing the release of gastrin and sensitivity of parietal cells to it, and by decreasing the release of somatostatin, which normally acts to reduce gastrin release (4, 5). Most important, duodenal mucosa develops gastric metaplasia, making it much more susceptible to the damage of hyperacidity (6–8). In most cases, the CaGA^{+} strain of *H. pylori* is the cause (9).

By confirming *H. pylori* as the cause of peptic ulcer disease and linking its eradication with permanent healing of the ulcers, Graham and associates' well-controlled study stimulated a sort of "working backwards" to explain the pathophysiology of peptic ulcer disease and severe gastritis. This reasoning led to valuable information about the development of mucosa-associated lymphoid tumor lymphoma (MALT) and gastric adenocarcinoma, which are also caused by *H. pylori* (10–12). Fortunately, *H. pylori* gastritis and MALT are treatable with the accepted antibiotic regimens that promise, by eradicating the organism, to prevent the later appearance of gastric adenocarcinoma.

References

1. **Marshall BJ, Warren JR.** Unidentified curved bacilli in the stomach of patients with gastritis and peptic ulceration. Lancet. 1984;1:1311-1315.
2. **Marshall BJ, Armstrong JA, McGechie DB, Glancy RJ.** Attempt to fulfil Koch's postulates for pyloric Campylobacter. Med J Aust. 1985;142:436-439.
3. **Freedberg AS, Barron LE.** The presence of spirochetes in human gastric mucosa. Ann J Dig Dis. 1940;7:443.
4. **Mégraud F.** Transmission of Helicobacter pylori: faecal-oral versus oral-oral route. Aliment Pharmacol Ther. 1995;94. Mégraud F. Transmission of Helicobacter pylori: faecal-oral versus oral-oral route. Aliment Pharmacol Ther. 1995;9 Suppl 2:85-91.
5. **el-Omar EM, Penman ID, Ardill JE, Chittajallu RS, Howie C, McColl KE.** Helicobacter pylori infection and abnormalities of acid secretion in patients with duodenal ulcer disease. Gastroenterology. 1995; 109:681-91.
6. **Logan RP.** Adherence of Helicobacter pylori. Aliment Pharmacol Ther. 1996;10 Suppl 1:3-15.
7. **Yamaoka Y, Kita M, Kodama T, Sawai N, Kashima K, Imanishi J.** Induction of various cytokines and development of severe mucosal inflammation by cagA gene positive Helicobacter pylori strains. Gut. 1997;41: 442-451.
8. **Wyatt JI, Rathbone BJ, Dixon MF, Heatley RV.** Campylobacter pyloridis and acid induced gastric metaplasia in the pathogenesis of duodenitis. J Clin Pathol. 1987;40:841-848.
9. **Mobley HL.** Defining Helicobacter pylori as a pathogen: strain heterogeneity and virulence. Am J Med. 1996;100:2S-9S.
10. **Lynch DA, Mapstone NP, Clarke AM, et al.** Cell proliferation in Helicobacter pylori associated gastritis and the effect of eradication therapy. Gut. 1995;36:346-350.
11. **Wotherspoon AC, Ortiz-Hidalgo C, Falzon MR, Isaacson PG.** Helicobacter pylori-associated gastritis and primary B-cell gastric lymphoma. Lancet. 1991;338:1175-1176.
12. **Huang JQ, Zheng GF, Sumanac K, Irvine EJ, Hunt RH.** Meta-analysis of the relationship between cagA seropositivity and gastric cancer. Gastroenterology. 2003;125:1636-1644.

SERUM GLUTAMIC OXALACETIC TRANSAMINASE ACTIVITY AS AN INDEX OF LIVER CELL INJURY: A PRELIMINARY REPORT * †

By Felix Wróblewski, M.D., and John S. LaDue, M.D., Ph.D., F.A.C.P., *New York, N. Y.*

Introduction

Glutamic oxalacetic transaminase is widely distributed in animal tissues. Its greatest concentration, however, is in heart muscle, skeletal muscle, brain, liver and kidney, in decreasing order.[1] We have already shown that, when measured in serum, this enzyme is elevated after acute myocardial infarction.[2] This finding led us to study its concentration in liver diseases, since the enzyme is present in relatively high concentration in liver.

Glutamic oxalacetic transaminase is present in all human sera and will henceforth be referred to as SGO-T. Comparable concentrations are found whether chromatographic or spectrophotometric methods are employed.[3] When serum is added to excesses of aspartic acid and alpha ketoglutaric acid buffered at optimal pH in the presence of coenzyme 1 ($DPNH_2$) and malic dehydrogenase, SGO-T can be measured in a spectrophotometer by the decrease in optical density resulting from the oxidation of $DPNH_2$ to DPN (figure 1). One unit of SGO-T activity represents a change in optical density of 0.001/ml./min. at wave lengths of 340 mu. All tests done in this series of patients were performed with 0.5 ml. or 0.2 ml. of serum.

The range of SGO-T in normal adult individuals was ascertained by random and serial determinations on the sera of 500 persons without regard to the fasting state. The mean value of the normal range (5 to 40 units) was found to be 22.1 units, with a standard deviation of $\pm$ 6.8 units.

The studies following myocardial infarctions indicate that the enzyme is liberated into the blood stream following injury to the cell.[4] If the enzyme is also released from damaged liver cells, the SGO-T level should provide an index of liver cell destruction. The level and persistence of increased activity might then provide an index of active liver cell disease.[5]

SGO-T has not been found to be increased in patients with infectious, neoplastic, degenerative, metastatic, reactive, allergic or congenital disease states unless evidence of acute damage to liver tissue, heart muscle or skeletal muscle has been evident. Patients with pneumonia, active pulmonary

* Received for publication April 13, 1955.

From the Sloan-Kettering Institute, Division of Clinical Investigation, and the Medical Service of the Memorial Center for Cancer and Allied Diseases, New York, N. Y.

† Supported in part by a grant from the National Institutes of Health.

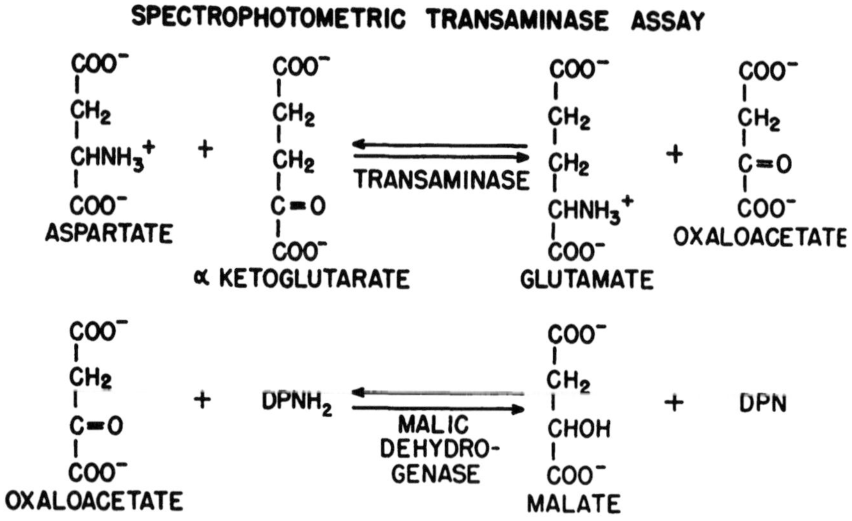

SPECTROPHOTOMETRIC TRANSAMINASE ASSAY

$COO^- - CH_2 - CHNH_3^+ - COO^-$ (ASPARTATE) + $COO^- - CH_2 - CH_2 - C{=}O - COO^-$ (α KETOGLUTARATE) $\rightleftharpoons$ (TRANSAMINASE) $COO^- - CH_2 - CH_2 - CHNH_3^+ - COO^-$ (GLUTAMATE) + $COO^- - CH_2 - C{=}O - COO^-$ (OXALOACETATE)

$COO^- - CH_2 - C{=}O - COO^-$ (OXALOACETATE) + $DPNH_2$ $\rightleftharpoons$ (MALIC DEHYDROGENASE) $COO^- - CH_2 - CHOH - COO^-$ (MALATE) + DPN

Fig. 1. Summary of the chemical reactions involved in the spectrophotometric assay of SGO-T.

tuberculosis, infections of the genitourinary tract, empyema and other infections have had SGO-T levels within normal limits. Many patients with neoplastic disease of many varieties have had normal levels of SGO-T in the presence of widespread metastases when the liver is not involved. The disease states in which the SGO-T has been followed over a period of time and found to be within normal limits are listed in table 1.

The purpose of this paper is to report the variation in SGO-T activity following acute liver cell destruction, such as that seen after carbon tetrachloride (CCl_4) poisoning in man and animals, and its activity during the course of acute infectious and homologous serum jaundice; and to compare

Table 1

Diseases in Which the SGO-T Has Been Found to Be Within Normal Limits in the Absence of Damage to the Liver, Heart or Skeletal Muscle

Infectious

Pneumonia
Tuberculosis
Cystitis
Pyelonephritis
Wound infection
Empyema
Acute cholecystitis
Pancreatitis
Pericarditis
Thrombophlebitis

Neoplastic

Carcinoma
Melanomas
Osteogenic sarcomas
Lymphomas
Teratomas

Allergic

Hay fever
Asthma
Urticaria
Allergic dermatitis

Degenerative

Cerebral arteriosclerosis
Cerebral thrombosis
Cerebral hemorrhage
Multiple sclerosis
Muscular dystrophies
Nephrosclerosis
Osteoporosis
Osteoarthritis

Reactive

Rheumatoid arthritis
Rheumatic fever without carditis
Chorea
Lupus erythematosus
Polyarteritis nodosum

Congenital

Congenital heart disease

Metabolic

Hypothyroidism or hyperthyroidism
Addison's disease
Panhypopituitarism
Uremia
Uremic pericarditis

the levels noted in these disorders with SGO-T activity in patients with cirrhosis of varying degree, with obstructive jaundice and with metastatic carcinoma of the liver. We were interested in finding out whether the degree of SGO-T elevation is related to the amount of liver cell destruction; whether the enzyme concentration will help differentiate medical from surgical jaundice; whether SGO-T activity in chronic liver disorders indicates active liver cell destruction; whether the height and length of elevation bear any relation to prognosis; what correlation there may be between the SGO-T activity and the various tests of liver dysfunction; and whether changes in SGO-T reflect the presence of liver metastases.

Method and Material

SGO-T activity was determined spectrophotometrically on serum stored for from a few minutes to seven days at 0° C.[3] Patients with CCl_4 poisoning, acute infectious and homologous serum hepatitis, cirrhosis, obstructive jaundice, and metastatic and primary carcinoma of the liver had blood withdrawn at varying intervals during their illness. SGO-T levels as well as determinations of serum bilirubin, cephalin flocculation, thymol turbidity, A/G ratio, alkaline phosphatase, cholesterol and esters, Bromsulphalein retention and prothrombin time were done.

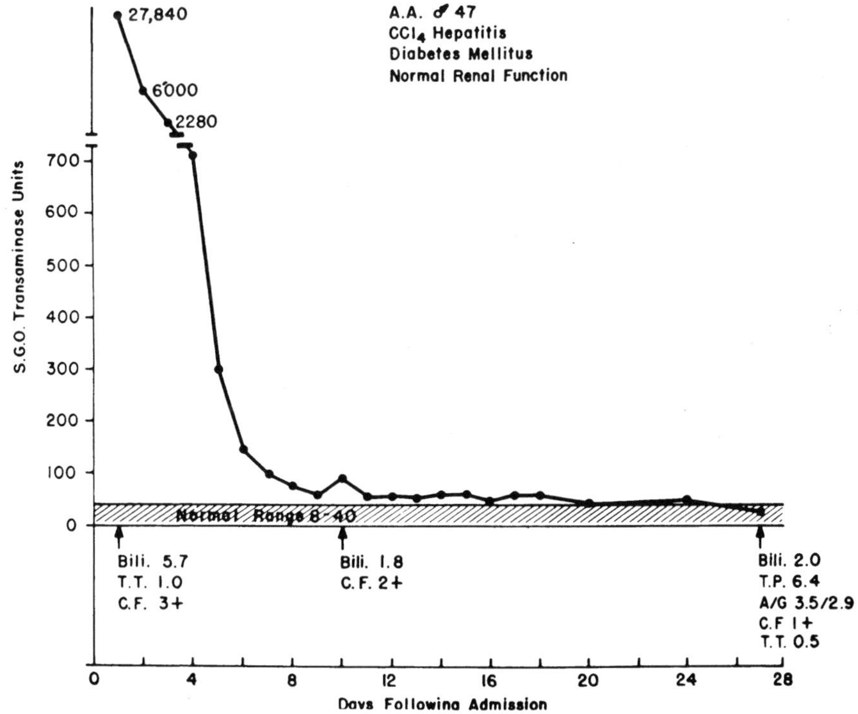

Fig. 2. SGO-T activity following CCl_4 poisoning, together with the results of some of the usual liver function tests.

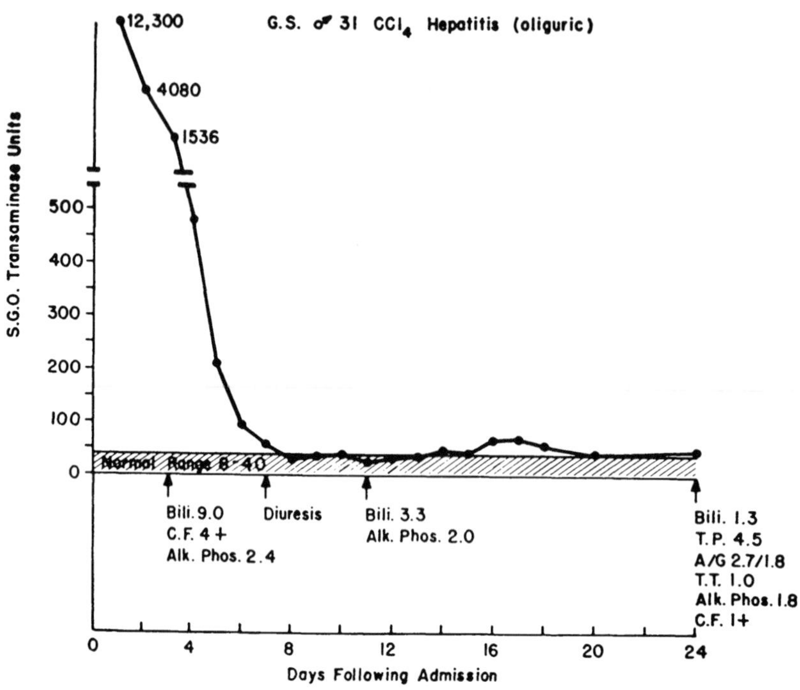

Fig. 3. SGO-T activity after CCl_4 poisoning in G. S. who, contrary to A. A. in figure 2, was oliguric. Both curves are similar.

Acute Liver Cell Destruction (Toxic)

Two patients had been exposed to CCl_4 fumes two days prior to admission to the hospital. They complained of nausea, vomiting, headache and generalized malaise. Both were moderately icteric and presented with minimal enlargement of the liver. Their course is summarized in figures 2 and 3. The tremendous elevation of the SGO-T transaminase to 27,840 and 12,340 units respectively 48 hours after exposure was striking; the enzyme activity then rapidly fell to normal within one week. The bilirubin rose to 5.7 and 9.0 mg., respectively, and the cephalin flocculation, originally abnormal, fell to 1 plus at the time of discharge. Both patients recovered.

Homologous Serum Hepatitis and Infectious Hepatitis

Ten patients had homologous serum hepatitis, in six apparently transmitted during various injections and in four following transfusions. Anorexia, nausea, emesis, pruritus, dark urine and, in some instances, light-colored stools were the symptoms proffered by these patients. All had hepatomegaly and jaundice of varying degree; in two the spleen was palpable. Hospital admission was within 10 days of the onset of illness in three patients, and after 20 to 30 symptom days in the remainder. Figure 4 represents the course of illness in N. P., a 32 year old physician admitted to the hospital after one week complaining of generalized malaise of one week's duration. On the second hospital day his SGO-T was 2,140, falling gradually within 20 days to normal. All liver function tests were abnormal on the day of admission, three remaining abnormal for 40 or more days, with persistent elevation of the bilirubin to 3.0 mg. more than two months

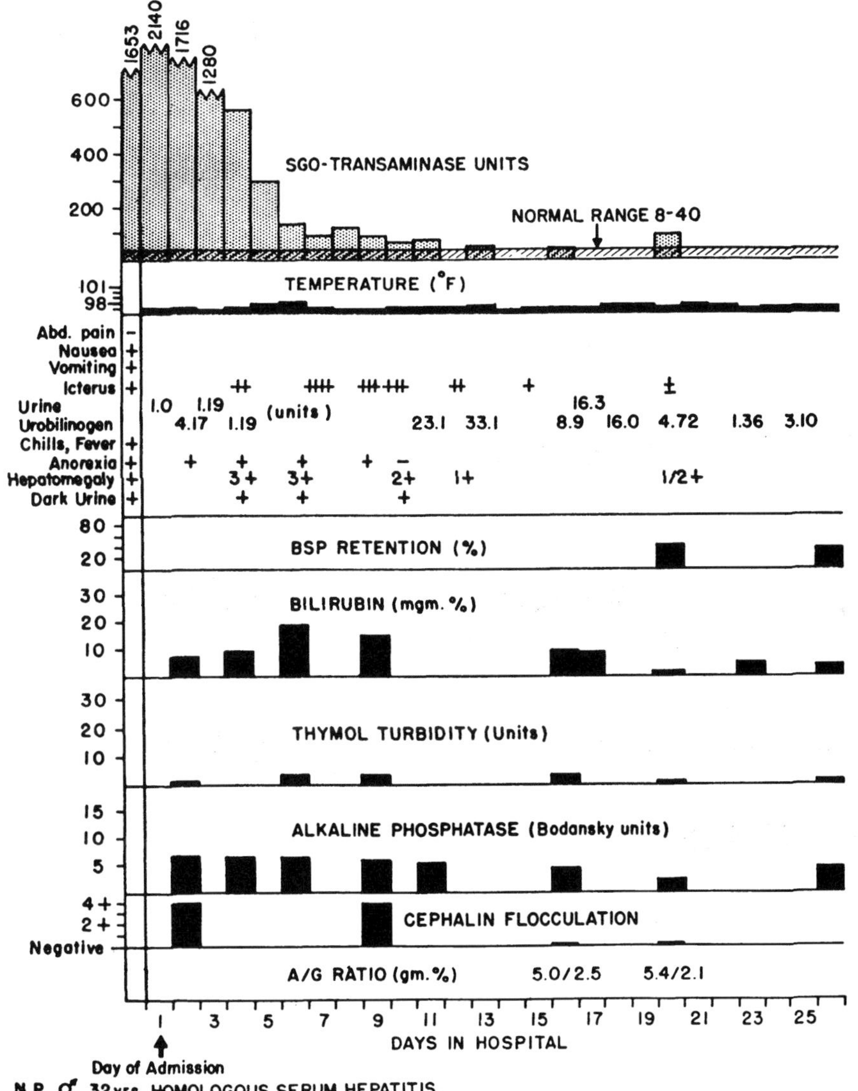

FIG. 4. Summary of the SGO-T activity, together with the values for urinary urobilinogen (Ehrlich units), blood bilirubin, thymol turbidity, alkaline phosphatase, cephalin flocculation, A/G ratio and Bromsulphalein excretion over a 26 day period in a patient with acute homologous serum hepatitis.

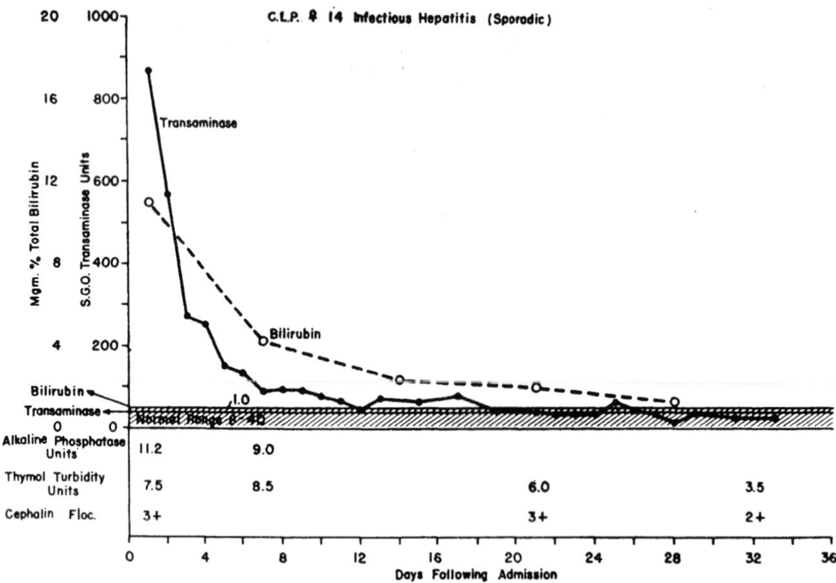

FIG. 5. SGO-T activity and bilirubin, thymol turbidity and cephalin flocculation over a 36 day period in a patient with infectious hepatitis.

later. When he left the hospital he did not rest, as suggested, and his SGO-T promptly rose to 98 units, returning to normal after two additional weeks of bed-rest.

In five of these patients the usual liver function tests remained abnormal for from 10 days to three months longer than it took for the SGO-T to return to normal limits. Three patients had levels of 2,000 or more units, four of 750 to 1,500 units, and in the remaining the level taken after 10 or more days of illness was 220 units, 176 units and 76 units. Two patients died. In one the SGO-T activity remained at 250 units during the five months of her illness. The second died on the one hundred fiftieth day of her illness of hepatic failure complicated by cardiac decompensation. The SGO-T fell from 1,245 to 50 units on the thirty-eighth hospital day, only to rise to 921 eight days before death.

Five patients had infectious hepatitis, and in four symptoms were present for one week prior to hospitalization, the fifth having been ill for five weeks.* The symptoms consisted of anorexia, nausea, vomiting and generalized malaise. All of the patients were jaundiced; three had moderate enlargement of the liver; none had splenomegaly. In three patients the SGO-T was 800 or more units on admission; in the fourth the level was 564 during the sixth week of the illness, and in the last the level was 60 on the twenty-third day of his sickness. Figures 5 and 6 represent the course of the disease which was typical for this group. In four patients the SGO-T had

* None of these patients had received injections or been given transfusions or had any contact with fresh human blood for at least one year prior to their present illness.

fallen to normal by the fourth week, and in the patient admitted during the fifth week of his illness the SGO-T had dropped to normal on the nineteenth hospital day. The tests of liver function, grossly abnormal on admission, were still far from normal at the time the SGO-T had fallen to 40 units in four of the five patients. All patients recovered and will be restudied at a later date.

Cirrhosis

Twenty-eight patients with cirrhosis of the liver (19 proved by biopsy) were studied. In eight the level of SGO-T was within normal limits; in 14 the activity was 41 to 100 units, and in six the level was more than 100 units. Table 2 indicates the percentile incidence of hepatomegaly, splenomegaly, ascites and abnormal liver function tests in the three groups. This can be stated another way by noting that in two of the eight patients with normal SGO-T activity two of the conventional liver function tests were abnormal; two had more than two abnormal tests, and four had only an abnormal cephalin flocculation test. In patients with SGO-T between 41 and 100 units three had only one abnormal test of liver function, four had two, and seven had more than two tests indicating liver dysfunction. All the six patients with SGO-T levels of 101 to 1,600 units had two or more abnormal tests of liver function. Of the last group, three patients had biliary cirrhosis.

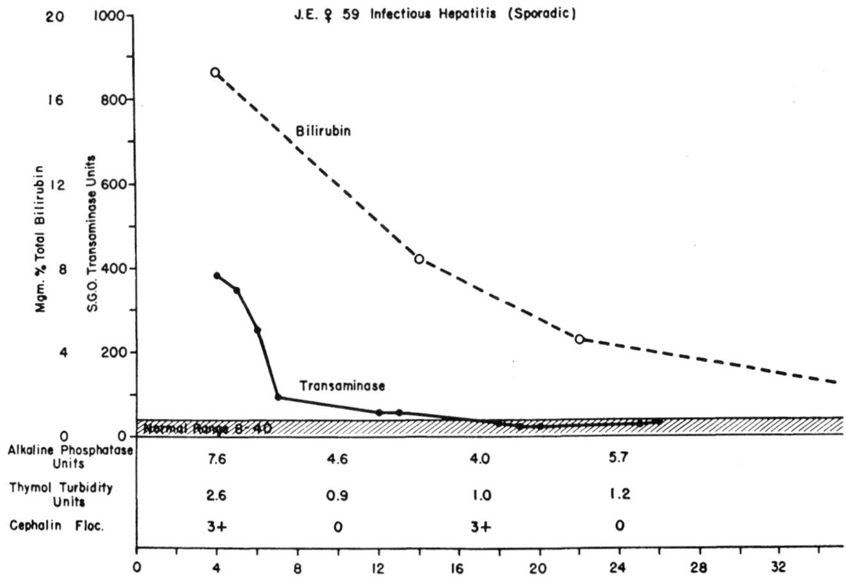

Fig. 6. Comparison of the SGO-T activity with the bilirubin, alkaline phosphatase, thymol turbidity and cephalin flocculation. Note the persistent elevation of the serum bilirubin and cephalin flocculation when the SGO-T was within normal limits.

TABLE 2

Comparison of the Incidence in Per cent of Hepatosplenomegaly, Ascites and Abnormal Liver Function Tests in 28 Patients with Cirrhoses According to the SGO-T Activity

SGO-T Units	Enlarged Liver	Palpable Spleen	Ascites Present	Abnormal						
				Bili-rubin	Cephalin Flocc.	Thymol Turbidity	BSP	Total Protein	Albu-min	Alkaline Phospha-tase
40 or less (8 patients)	50	25	63	17	100	76	67	0	13	67
41 to 100 (14 patients)	50	14	43	77	90	93	80	0	23	33
Greater than 100 (6 patients)	67	17	67	83	100	100	100	0	33	100

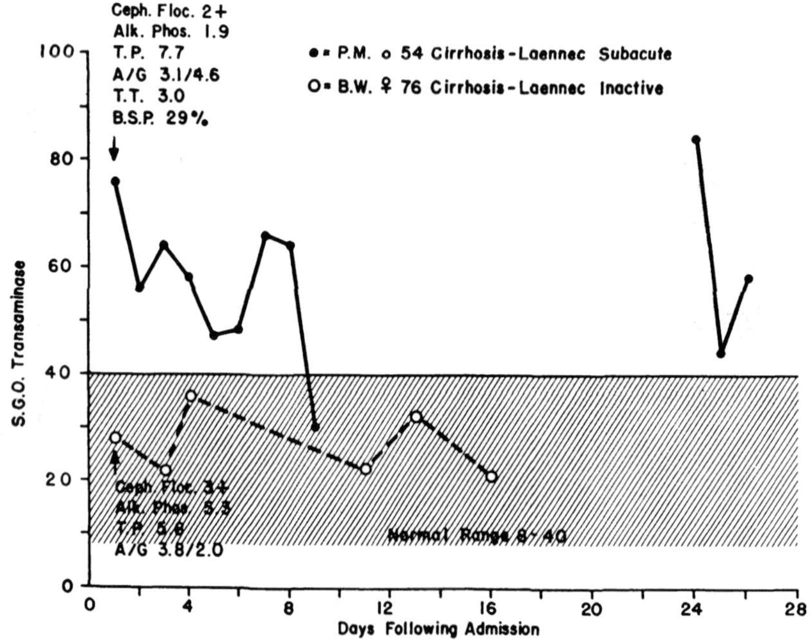

FIG. 7. Comparison of the SGO-T activity and the liver functions of two patients with Laennec's cirrhosis. See text for discussion.

Figure 7 shows the level of SGO-T in two patients with Laennec's cirrhosis—one who was asymptomatic (B. W.), and another (P. M.) who was admitted to the hospital with increasing jaundice, anorexia, nausea and generalized malaise which cleared after adequate bed-rest. Of interest in these patients was the fact that one was obviously sick with active liver disease and the other was asymptomatic. It appeared that the SGO-T level in Case P. M. may have represented active liver cell injury.

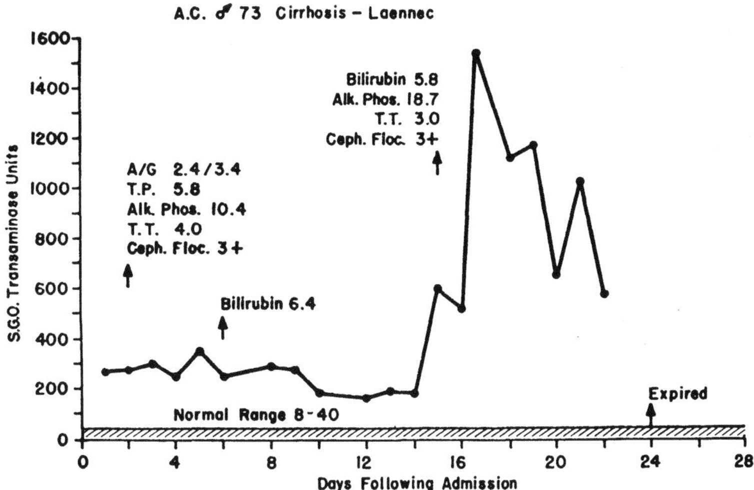

FIG. 8. This figure demonstrates the persistently abnormal levels of SGO-T in a patient with cirrhosis of the liver who died on the 24th hospital day.

Figure 8 also demonstrates this dissociation between values of the conventional liver function tests and the SGO-T in a patient with Laennec's cirrhosis who, while chronically ill the first two weeks of his hospitalization, became acutely and critically ill from the fourteenth to the twenty-fourth day, when he died. During this period the SGO-T rose precipitously. Autopsy revealed Laennec's cirrhosis with superimposed acute hepatitis.

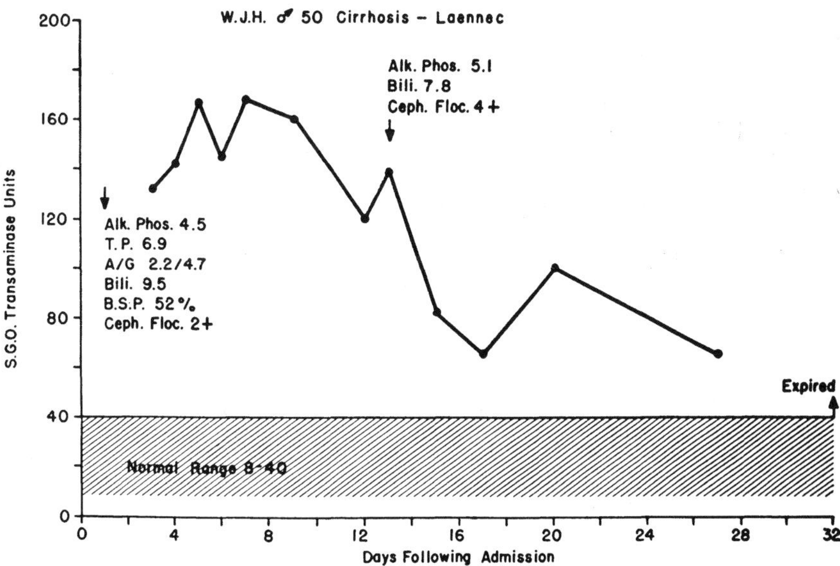

FIG. 9. Decreasing but persistently abnormal SGO-T activity in a patient with Laennec's cirrhosis who died on the 32nd hospital day.

Figure 9 shows the course of another patient with Laennec's cirrhosis who died in liver coma after a slowly downhill illness of three months' duration. Autopsy showed Laennec's cirrhosis.

Metastatic Carcinoma of the Liver

Twenty of 22 patients with proved metastatic involvement of the liver from various types of carcinoma showed increased SGO-T activity on one or more determinations. The usual liver function tests were run concomitantly, and it is interesting that in seven patients increased SGO-T activity, with levels varying from 46 to 140 units, was the only sign of liver involvement. In 13 patients the SGO-T varied from 60 to 230 units, but the alkaline phosphatase and, at times, other liver function tests were also abnormal. In two instances with small areas of metastasis both the SGO-T and all other liver function tests were normal. The level of the SGO-T elevation did not correlate with the levels of the bilirubin, alkaline phosphatase, A/G ratio, Bromsulphalein, cholesterol and esters, or any other laboratory study. It is also of interest that 20 patients who had moderate

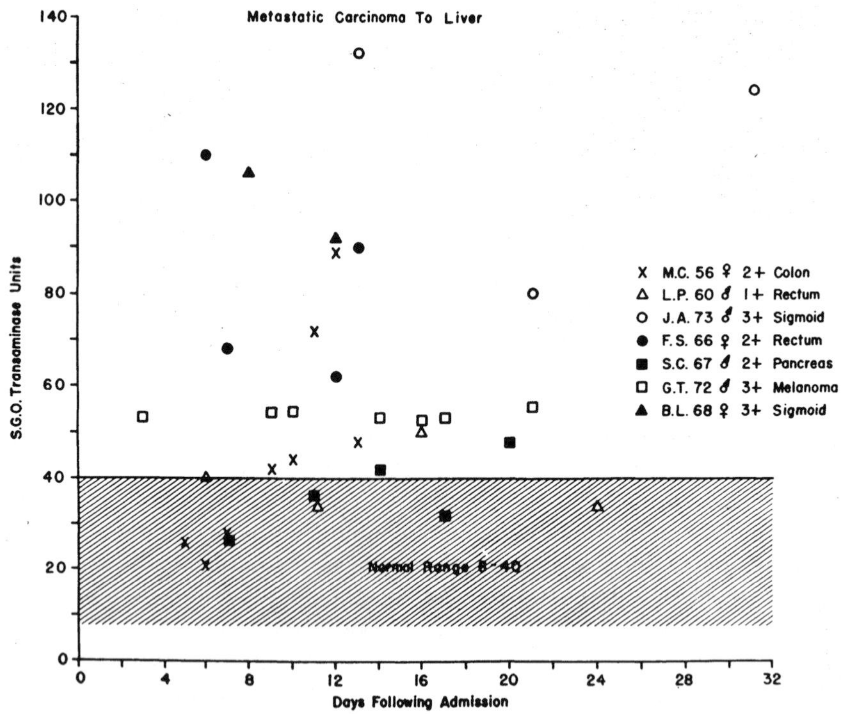

Fig. 10. SGO-T activity in seven patients with proved metastatic carcinoma of the liver followed over a four week period. Note that at some time during the study the SGO-T activity was elevated in all the patients.

to marked elevation of the alkaline phosphatase secondary to bone metastases in the absence of hepatic dysfunction all had normal SGO-T activity.

The variable level of SGO-T activity in seven patients with metastatic carcinoma of the liver is shown in figure 10. If similar symbols are connected it will be seen that at some time during the hospital study the SGO-T was elevated.

Figure 11 shows the SGO-T levels in a patient with proved primary hepatoma whose bilirubin was 5.2 mg. %, alkaline phosphatase 8.3 Bodansky units, and cephalin flocculation 2 plus. Persistent evidence of liver cell destruction was again noted and confirmed at autopsy.

It was interesting to study the enzyme alterations in a female with metastatic disease involving most of the right lobe of the liver which was resected. Preoperative levels were 60 to 80 units, but rose to 200 after resection of the right lobe of the liver and fell to normal with recovery of the patient four weeks later.

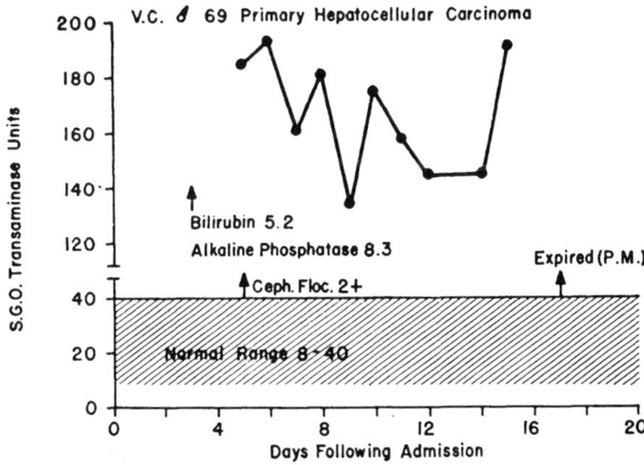

FIG. 11. SGO-T activity in a patient with primary liver carcinoma who died on the 17th day. See text for discussion.

Obstructive Jaundice

Five patients with obstructive jaundice were studied. Four had proved cancer of the pancreas, with jaundice of from two weeks' to three months' duration. In two the SGO-T activity was 120 units preoperatively, falling to normal in 14 days in one and in less than 10 days in the other. Figure 12 shows the SGO-T levels together with values for the bilirubin, thymol turbidity, cephalin flocculation, alkaline phosphatase and A/G ratio preoperatively and postoperatively in one patient with cancer of the pancreas. The second patient had a similar course. Note the lack of correlation between the SGO-T and other laboratory studies. The third had inoperable disease with liver metastases, and his SGO-T has varied between 60 and 80 units for six weeks, his bilirubin from 20 to 30 mg., and his alkaline phosphatase 20 to 45 units during the period of observation. The cephalin flocculation and thymol turbidity stayed within normal limits. The fourth had a normal SGO-T despite obstructive jaundice of four weeks' duration.

The single patient with jaundice due to common duct stones had a preoperative SGO-T of 70 units, which fell to normal two days postoperatively after the insertion of a T tube into the common duct (figure 13). This is as rapid a return to normal as one could expect, since following any operative procedure in which muscle is cut or damaged the SGO-T usually remains elevated for one to four days.*

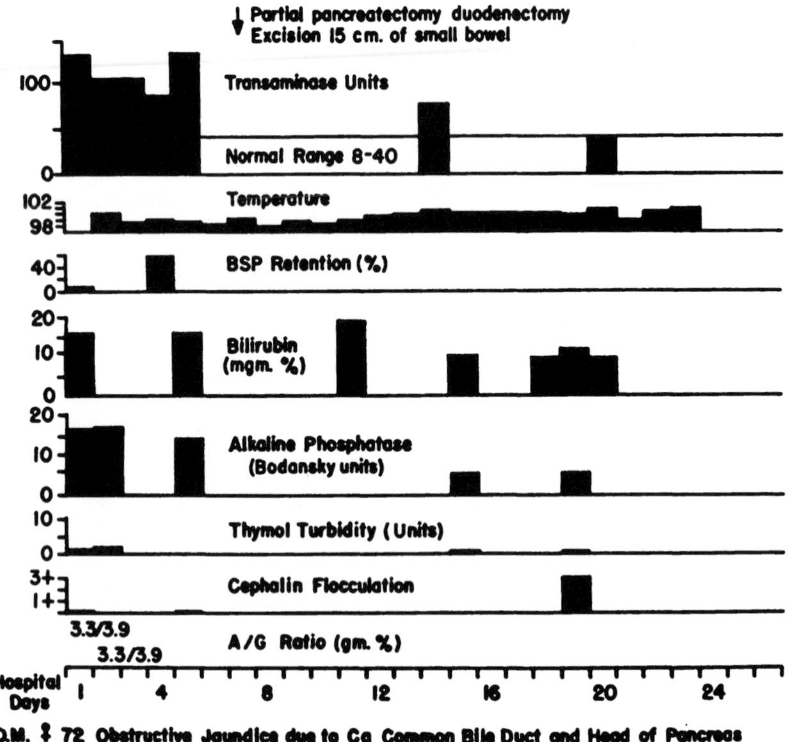

FIG. 12. Variations in SGO-T activity in a patient with obstructive jaundice due to carcinoma of the common bile duct and head of the pancreas, relieved by partial pancreatectomy and duodenectomy.

DISCUSSION

The clinical data reported here are too meager to permit any conclusions relative to the correlation, if any, between the height of the SGO-T elevation and the amount of liver cell damage. However, in collaboration with Dr. David Molander, graded damage of liver tissue was produced in rats by giving them carbon tetrachloride, 0.3 c.c./dose.[6] Figure 14 shows that

* Unpublished data.

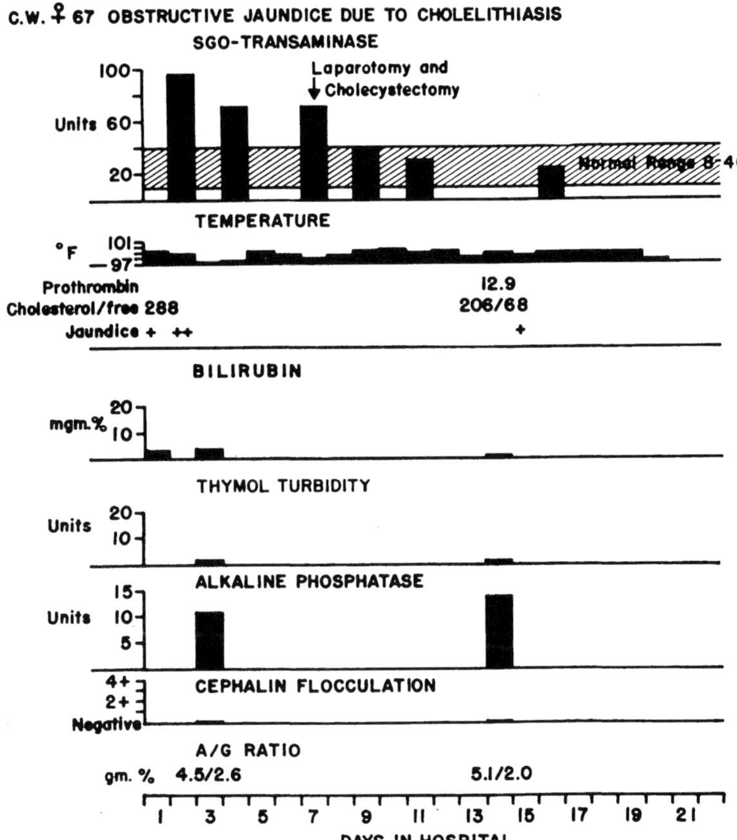

FIG. 13. SGO-T levels in a patient with obstructive jaundice due to cholelithiasis preoperatively and postoperatively.

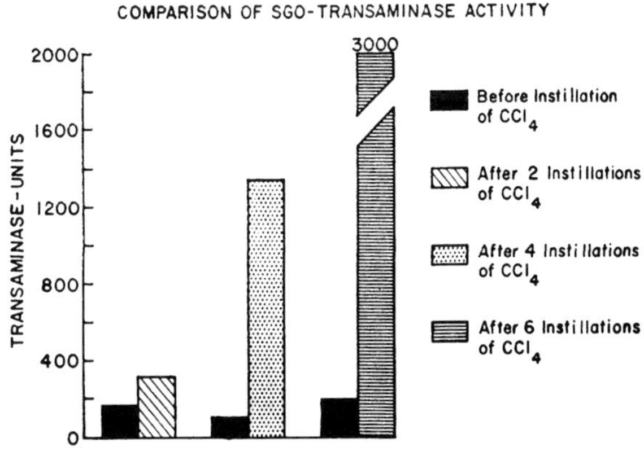

FIG. 14. Comparison of the SGO-T activity in three groups of rats intubated with 0.3 c.c. of carbon tetrachloride. One group received two instillations, the second four and the third six.

there is a close parallel between the amount of CCl_4 given to the rats and the level of the SGO-T elevation. It was our impression from the clinical course that there was a rough relationship between the severity of infectious and homologous serum hepatitis and the SGO-T activity.

Serum glutamic oxalacetic transaminase levels of from 600 to 22,500 units, with a falling titer over a period of from five to 10 days, were seen in hepatitis and acute liver cell damage due to CCl_4. In the few instances of obstructive jaundice that we have studied the SGO-T activity was not above 300 units and remained relatively constant, or increased slowly until the mechanical obstruction was relieved (figures 12 and 13). It thus appears that infectious or homologous serum jaundice can be differentiated from obstructive jaundice if SGO-T activity is measured early and serially in the course of the disease. Patients with cirrhosis or with metastases to the liver, however, cannot be separated from obstructive jaundice due to stone, cancer or other cause by study of the SGO-T activity alone.

Too few patients with cirrhosis have been followed over any period of time to state whether changes in SGO-T activity with time are common, or what might be their significance. Secondary rises in two patients with superimposed hepatitis, however, preceded rapid liver decompensation and death. Persistent elevation of SGO-T activity has been associated with a poor prognosis in the patients we have had an opportunity to observe (figure 9).

The SGO-T activity does not alter in the same direction, magnitude or time as any of the currently employed liver function tests. This has been emphasized in the presentation of the data on patients with acute toxic cell damage, in those with hepatitis and in those with cirrhosis or metastatic carcinoma of the liver. There was no correlation between the SGO-T activity and the erythrocyte sedimentation rate, white blood count, temperature, C-reactive protein or antistreptolysin titers in patients with various infectious diseases whose SGO-T activity has been studied, or in our patients with liver disease. Changes in the level of SGO-T, therefore, cannot be considered as those of a nonspecific reactant. Hence the SGO-T activity is not related to the physiologic causes for changes in the erythrocyte sedimentation rate, white blood count or C-reactive protein.

In our hands the SGO-T activity has been a sensitive index of metastatic carcinoma. In seven of 22 patients with proved metastatic carcinoma of the liver all the tests for liver function which were done were within normal limits but the SGO-T was significantly elevated. This experience has been extended to more than 30 such instances. In addition, the test has been of use in evaluating the significance of alkaline phosphatase elevation, since the SGO-T is normal when the phosphatase is elevated as a result of bone disease or bone metastasis but rises when concomitant alkaline phosphatase elevation is due to liver disease including liver metastases.

Conclusions

1. Serum glutamic oxalacetic activity is impressively elevated following acute liver cell injury due to CCl_4 poisoning, infectious hepatitis or homologous serum hepatitis.

2. The SGO-T activity in patients with acute liver cell damage is usually many times that seen in obstructive jaundice.

3. Cirrhosis of the liver may be associated with normal SGO-T activity with mildly elevated levels and with high activity. Further study is needed to explain the significance of variation in SGO-T activity associated with cirrhosis of the liver.

4. Serum glutamic oxalacetic transaminase activity appears to be an index of liver cell injury and does not necessarily correlate with the usual tests of liver dysfunction.

5. An increase in SGO-T activity appears to be a relatively sensitive index of liver metastases.

6. The level of the SGO-T activity in liver disease has not been found to parallel or correlate with the tests of liver function commonly in use. When elevated, the SGO-T activity appears to indicate liver cell destruction and not liver cell function.

Acknowledgments

The authors are indebted to Dr. David P. Barr, Dr. Rulon Rawson and Dr. Edwin P. Maynard for permission to study clinical material at New York Hospital, Memorial Center for Cancer and Allied Diseases, and Brooklyn Hospital, respectively.

We are indebted to Dr. I. J. Van Elk, Dr. Robert J. Zullo and Dr. Gordon McGill for their close clinical coöperation and for collection of some of the data, and to Dr. David E. Molander, who collaborated with us on the experiments upon rats given carbon tetrachloride.

We also wish to express our appreciation for the technical help of Mr. Martin Podgainy and Mr. Albert Friedman.

Summario in Interlingua

Transaminase oxalacetic glutamic es extensemente distribuite in texitos animal. Illo occurre in concentrationes major in le musculo cardiac e—in ordine retrogradente—in le musculos skeletal, le cerebro, le hepate, e le renes. Omne le seros human que esseva essayate per nos monstrava un activitate de transaminase oxalacetic glutamic. In le caso de seros ab individuos normal le activitate variava ab 5 a 40 unitates.

Le activitate enzymic esseva determinate spectrophotographicamente per un simple e rapide methodo. Le nivello de transaminase oxalacetic glutamic del sero es marcatemente elevate post acute lesiones del cellulas hepatic causate per toxicosis a tetrachlorido de carbon, per hepatitis infectiose, e per hepatitis a sero homologe. Alterationes significative del transaminase oxalacetic glutamic del sero esseva observate in patientes con obstruction biliari extrahepatic, con cirrhosis, e con primari o metastatic morbo neoplastic del hepate. Le nivello del transaminase oxalacetic glutamic del sero pare esser un indice del lesion del cellulas hepatic, sed illo reflecte un parametro de morbo hepatic non identic con le parametro reflectite per le currente essayos laboratorial del functionamento hepatic. Excepte in casos de evidente lesiones del texito hepatic o del musculo cardiac o skeletal, le nivello del transaminase oxalacetic glutamic del sero non se monstrava elevate in patientes con morbose conditiones infectiose, neoplastic, degenerative, metastatic, reactive, o congenite. Usate como adjuncto laboratorial, le determination de transaminase oxalacetic glutamic del sero pare esser un promittente technica in le studio de morbo hepatic experimental e clinic.

BIBLIOGRAPHY

1. Awapara, J., and Seale, H.: Distribution of transaminase in rat organs, J. Biol. Chem. **194**: 497, 1952.
2. LaDue, J. S., Wróblewski, F., and Karmen, A.: Serum glutamic oxalacetic transaminase activity in human acute transmural myocardial infarction, Science **120**: 497, 1954.
3. Karmen, A., Wróblewski, F., and LaDue, J. S.: Transaminase activity in human blood, J. Clin. Investigation **34**: 126, 1955.
4. Nydick, I., Wróblewski, F., and LaDue, J. S.: Evidence for increased serum glutamic oxalacetic transaminase activity following graded myocardial infarction in dogs, in press (Circulation).
5. Wróblewski, F., and LaDue, J. S.: Serum glutamic oxalacetic transaminase activity as an index of liver destruction and disease, Clin. Res. Proc. **3**.
6. Molander, D., Wróblewski, F., and LaDue, J. S.: Transaminase compared with cholinesterase and alkaline phosphatase as an index of hepatocellular integrity in the white rat, Clin. Res. Proc. **3**.

Risk for Serious Gastrointestinal Complications Related to Use of Nonsteroidal Anti-inflammatory Drugs

A Meta-analysis

Sherine E. Gabriel, MD, MSc; Liisa Jaakkimainen, MSc; and Claire Bombardier, MD

■ *Objective:* To describe the relative risk for serious gastrointestinal complications due to nonaspirin nonsteroidal anti-inflammatory drug (NSAID) exposure among NSAID users as well as in selected subgroups.
■ *Design:* Overview and meta-analysis.
■ *Data Identification:* A literature search of English-language studies examining the association between NSAIDs and adverse gastrointestinal events for the period 1975 to 1990 identified using MEDLINE and communicating with three internationally recognized experts.
■ *Data Analysis:* A qualitative summary of study characteristics and a critical appraisal of study quality were done. The results of 16 primary studies were selected and combined statistically. Summary estimates were weighted by sample size and quality score.
■ *Main Results:* The overall odds ratio of the risk for adverse gastrointestinal events related to NSAID use, summarized from 16 studies (9 case-control and 7 cohort) was 2.74 (95% CI, 2.54 to 2.97). The summary odds ratios were as follows: elderly patients, (aged ≥ 60 years), 5.52 (CI, 4.63 to 6.60); patients under 65 years of age, 1.65 (CI, 1.08 to 2.53); women, 2.32 (CI, 1.91 to 2.82); and men, 2.40 (CI, 1.85 to 3.11). The summary odds ratio for NSAID users receiving concomitant corticosteroids compared with NSAID users not receiving corticosteroids was 1.83 (CI, 1.20 to 2.78). The summary odds ratio for the first gastrointestinal event was 2.39 (CI, 2.16 to 2.65). The relative risk for a subsequent or unspecified gastrointestinal event was 4.76 (CI, 4.05 to 5.59). The summary odds ratio for less than 1 month of NSAID exposure was 8.00 (CI, 6.37 to 10.06); for more than 1 month but less than 3 months of exposure, the summary odds ratio was 3.31 (CI, 2.27 to 4.82); and for more than 3 months of exposure, the summary odds ratio was 1.92 (CI, 1.19 to 3.13).
■ *Conclusions:* Users of NSAIDs are at approximately three times greater relative risk for developing serious adverse gastrointestinal events than are nonusers. Additional risk factors include age greater than 60 years, previous history of gastrointestinal events, and concomitant corticosteroid use. Another possible risk factor is the first 3 months of NSAID therapy. The risk for serious gastrointestinal events appears to be equal among men and women. These data represent summary statistics from 16 studies and cannot be considered generalizable to all NSAID users.

Annals of Internal Medicine. 1991;**115**:787-796.

From the Mayo Clinic and Mayo Foundation, Rochester, Minnesota; and Wellesley Hospital, Toronto, Ontario. For current author addresses, see end of text.

Nonsteroidal anti-inflammatory drugs (NSAIDs) are the most widely used agents for the treatment of musculoskeletal and arthritic syndromes (1). Use of these agents has been increasingly associated with gastrointestinal toxicity, including mild dyspepsia, as well as more serious gastrointestinal reactions such as bleeding, perforation, and other events leading to hospitalization or death. Although researchers agree that an increased risk for gastrointestinal toxicity exists with NSAID use, the size of the reported risk has varied markedly, and there is little agreement on the definition of "high risk" groups (2-19).

We reviewed the literature on NSAID-related adverse gastrointestinal events. First, we summarized study characteristics and appraised study quality. We then did a meta-analysis of all controlled trials that examined the risks for serious gastrointestinal events among NSAID users. Our primary objective was to estimate a summary odds ratio or relative risk for serious gastrointestinal complications due to nonaspirin NSAID exposure.

Methods

A comprehensive search of the English-language literature from 1975 to 1990 was conducted using MEDLINE and searching the following terms: anti-inflammatory agents, non-steroidal; gastropathy, toxicity, adverse effects, or side effects; peptic ulcer or dyspepsia; gastric erosion, gastritis, gastric ulcer, gastric mucosa, endoscopy; and human. We also searched for specific NSAIDs by name.

Five hundred twenty-six references were obtained. These were reviewed by one of the authors, and any citation that mentioned NSAID-related gastrointestinal events was selected (Figure 1). One hundred forty-two articles met this criterion and were entered into "Reference Manager" (20). Five additional articles were identified by communication with three investigators (Marie Griffin, MD; Michael Langman, MD; and Richard Hunt, MD) from the United States, United Kingdom, and Canada, respectively. These 5 articles were added to the data set, for a total of 147 articles.

From the 147 articles in the data set, 40 studies were selected that examined the association between NSAIDs and adverse gastrointestinal events. Specific inclusion and exclusion criteria were applied to these studies independently by two of the authors. All studies that contained a comparison group and provided an estimate of risk for serious gastrointestinal complications (defined as bleeding, perforation, or other adverse gastrointestinal events resulting in hospitalization or death) in NSAID users compared with nonusers, regardless of underlying disease, were included in the meta-analysis. A study was excluded if its primary objective was to assess effectiveness, if it involved the treatment of children (under 18 years of age), if it described fewer than ten patients, if the only NSAID studied was salicylate, or if the outcome examined was

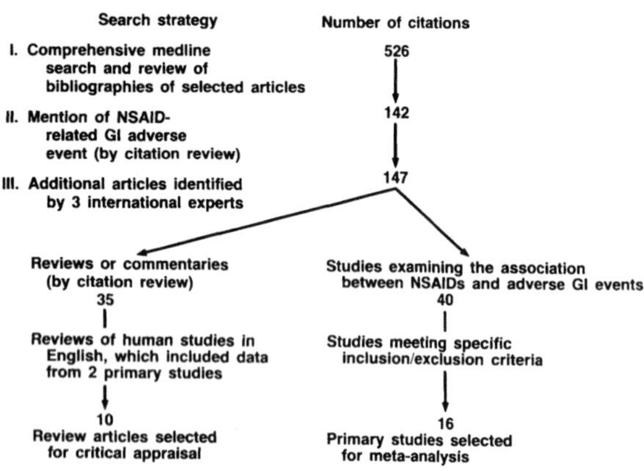

Figure 1. Selection of studies and reviews.

the identification of ulcer rather than the presence of serious gastrointestinal complications. Disagreements between the two reviewers were resolved by consensus. Sixteen studies were selected (21-36) for meta-analysis (*see* Figure 1).

Meta-analysis

The following criteria were used to evaluate the quality of the studies included in the meta-analysis: blinding, definition of outcome, case selection, control selection, matching technique, definition of exposure, and control for confounders (Appendix A). The Methods section of each study was photocopied, with care taken to exclude any mention of the authors' names, study results, or journal title. Study quality was evaluated in a blinded fashion by two of the investigators. Quality scores were assigned to each criterion according to its relative importance. A quality score of 0 indicated poor definitions and no attempt to avoid bias, and a score of 46 indicated the converse. The average score (between the two readers) among the first six categories constituted the baseline score for the study. For every 5 confounders identified in a primary study, 1 bonus point was awarded, to a maximum of 5 points for studies that identified more than 25 confounders. Thus, the maximum quality score attainable was 51. Agreement between the two readers regarding the quality score was evaluated using the kappa statistic (37).

Data from all articles were abstracted in duplicate to avoid errors. The two observers met, discussed each item, and resolved all disagreements and errors. A final copy of the completed data collection forms was then created and entered into a database (ORACLE, Oracle Corporation, Belmont, California) (38).

The results of the 16 primary studies were combined statistically using two different techniques. First, overall point estimates of the odds ratios and 95% confidence intervals (CIs) were calculated from the raw data of the 16 selected studies using the Mantel-Haenszel statistic (39). The second technique involved combining the published odds ratios and CIs directly across studies to produce an overall estimate of the odds ratio and 95% CI (40). The latter will hereafter be referred to as the "direct" method. The direct method was the primary statistical analysis technique used, and all results were calculated using this method unless otherwise stated.

The purpose of this analysis was not to estimate a common parameter, but rather to compute an average or summary statistic across the 16 selected studies. The CI for this statistic cannot, therefore, be generalized beyond the study samples. All summary estimates were weighted by sample size. The influence of the quality scores on the summary estimates was evaluated using logistic-regression analysis with quality score as a covariate.

Overall odds ratios for all studies included in the meta-analysis as well as odds ratios for various subgroups were calculated. The overall odds ratios referred to the odds ratios combined from the main research questions of each of the studies. Summary odds ratios for various subgroups were calculated from those studies which provided data on these subgroups. The method of Breslow and Day was used to test for homogeneity of the Mantel-Haenszel estimates (41). Tests of homogeneity were also performed for the direct method according to the method of Greenland (40).

Results

We selected 16 studies (9 case-control and 7 cohort) that specifically examined the risks for clinically defined, NSAID-related, adverse gastrointestinal events (21-36). The reported relative risks varied from 1.0 (34) (indicating no increased risk for gastrointestinal events) to 13.7 (29) (indicating a risk for NSAID users 13.7 times greater than that for nonusers). Two potential sources of variability were identified: differences in study characteristics and differences in study quality.

Study Characteristics

Study characteristics are shown in Appendix B. For both the case-control and cohort studies, serious gastrointestinal events were defined among hospital-based cases. Among the case-control studies, the ascertainment of gastrointestinal outcome was not done in a uniform manner. Gastrointestinal events were assessed based on the results of endoscopy, roentgenography, or surgery (27-29, 33, 35) or on a clinical diagnosis of hematemesis or melena (26, 30-32). Some case-control studies used community controls (31, 33, 35); others compared cases with hospital controls (28-30, 32) or used both types of controls (26, 27). Most studies matched controls directly with cases (26-28, 30, 31, 33). Two case-control studies used a nested case-control

Table 1. Study Quality Scores

Study (reference)	Baseline (range, 0-46)*	Bonus (range, 0-5)†	Total (range, 0-51)
Griffin et al. (33)	25.5	4.00	29.5
Levy et al. (32)	24.5	5.00	29.5
McIntosh et al. (35)	22.5	5.00	27.5
Somerville et al. (26)	22.5	4.00	26.5
Bartle et al. (27)	23.0	3.00	26.0
Henry et al. (30)	20.5	2.00	22.5
Jick et al. (31)‡	20.0	1.00	21.0
Carson et al. (24)‡	15.5	5.00	20.5
Guess et al. (25)‡	16.0	3.00	19.0
Bloom (22)‡	14.5	4.00	18.5
Beard et al. (23)‡	14.5	4.00	18.5
Beardon et al. (21)‡	13.5	2.00	15.5
Armstrong and Blower (29)	14.5	0.00	14.5
Collier and Pain (28)	13.5	1.00	14.5
Jick et al. (34)‡	10.0	2.00	12.0
Alexander et al. (36)	9.50	1.00	10.5

* Baseline scores were assigned based on an evaluation of the following design items: explicit definitions of exposure, outcome, case and control status as well as the use of blinding and matching.

† Bonus points were assigned based on the number of confounders, which were accounted for in the analysis. *See* text for method of bonus-point assignment.

‡ Cohort studies.

Figure 2. Individual study and summary odds ratios. Individual study odds ratios are arranged in order of increasing sample size (top to bottom). Individual study odds ratios were provided in the original studies (21-28, 30-32, 34, 36) or calculated from data provided in original studies (29, 33, 35). (●, Individual study odds ratio; ◆, summary odds ratio; the 95% confidence intervals are indicated by the extended lines; * cohort study; † case-control study; ‡ odds ratios summarized by "direct" technique [40]; numbers in parentheses are the number of studies combined.)

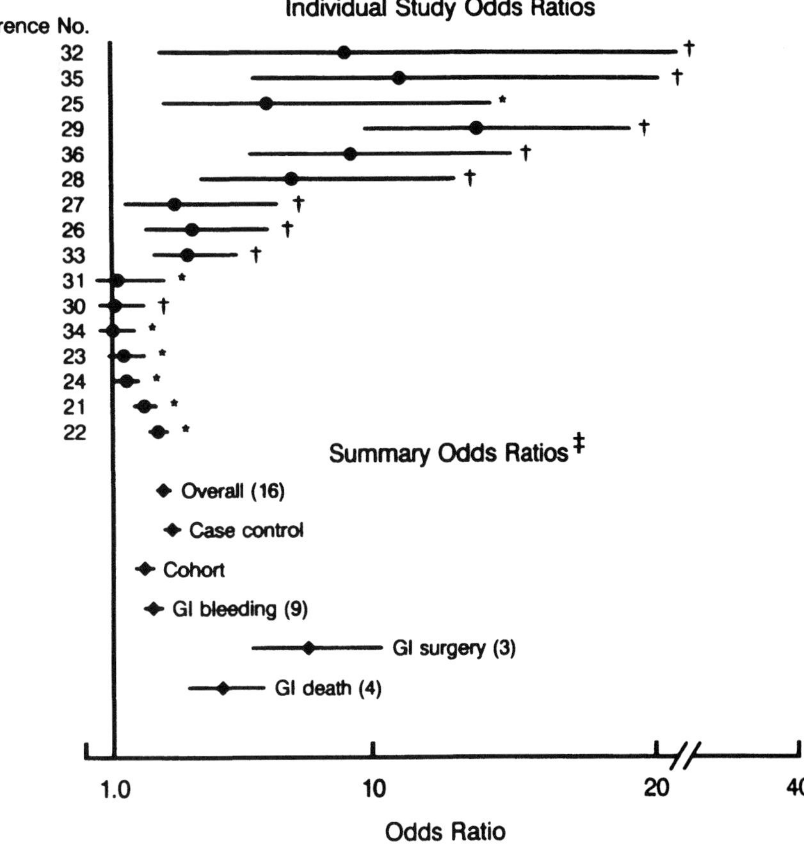

design (31, 33). Determinations of NSAID exposure were made by an unblinded review of clinical notes (28-30), a structured questionnaire with interviewers who were blinded (26, 27, 32, 35), or an extraction of prescription data from pharmacy computer files (31, 33). In all cohort studies, the assessment of NSAID exposure was based on prescription files. Estimates of the duration of NSAID exposure varied from 30 days (24, 25) to 90 days (22, 23, 31, 34). One cohort study (25) examined deaths from gastrointestinal causes, whereas the remainder looked at hospitalizations caused by gastrointestinal complications. Samples examined in the cohort studies included the Group Health Cooperative in Puget Sound; the Pennsylvania Medicaid group; the residents of Saskatchewan, Canada; and the residents of the Tayside Region, Scotland. The Puget Sound Group Health Cooperative represents a younger, employed population, the Medicaid group is elderly, and the Tayside and Saskatchewan groups represent residents of geographically diverse districts.

Study Quality

Table 1 shows the study quality scores. Methodologic assessment of the 16 studies showed acceptable agreement between two observers for the six study quality categories evaluated (mean kappa, 0.70; minimum, 0.56; maximum, 0.83). The mean kappa for the quality category of blinding was 0.67 (minimum, 0.0; maximum, 1.0); for case selection, 0.75 (minimum, 0.66; maximum, 0.90); for control selection, 0.68 (minimum, 0.4; maximum, 1.0); for definition of exposure, 0.74 (minimum, 0.59; maximum, 0.96); for matching technique, 0.83 (minimum, 0.66; maximum, 1.0); and for definition of outcome, 0.56 (minimum, 0.0; maximum, 1.0). Disagreements regarding control of confounders were reexamined and resolved by consensus. The six studies with the highest quality scores were case-control studies (Table 1). These studies gave more explicit definitions of cases, controls, and exposure and used blinding more frequently. The study quality score was not found to be a significant covariate in the regression model ($P > 0.2$).

Summary Odds Ratios

Published odds ratios and summary odds ratios from the primary studies are shown in Figure 2. The overall odds ratio of the risk for adverse gastrointestinal events related to NSAID use (summarized from 16 case-control and cohort studies) is 2.74 (CI, 2.54 to 2.97). The summary odds ratio (combined from 8 studies) for elderly persons is 5.52 (CI, 4.63 to 6.60). In the cohort studies, the term "elderly" refers to persons 65 years of age or older. In the case-control studies, "elderly" refers to persons 60 years of age or older. The summary odds ratio for nonelderly persons, combined from 3 studies, is 1.65 (CI, 1.08, 2.53). These data show a greater than threefold increase in relative risk for serious gastrointestinal events among elderly NSAID users when compared with nonelderly users.

Odds ratios were subdivided by gastrointestinal out-

Table 2. Comparison of Summary Odds Ratios and Confidence Intervals Obtained by Two Methods

Category	Number of Studies Combined	Summary Odds Ratio	95% CI
Overall	12*/16†	2.86*/2.74†	2.62 to 3.12*; 2.54 to 2.97†
Patient ≥ 60 years of age	6/8	6.24/5.52	5.21 to 7.48; 4.63 to 6.60
Patient < 60 years of age	2/3	3.07/1.65	1.62 to 5.82; 1.08 to 2.53
Gastrointestinal bleeding	7/9	2.71/2.39	2.26 to 3.24; 2.11 to 2.70
Gastrointestinal surgery	3/3	7.04/7.75	5.34 to 9.29; 5.83 to 10.31
Gastrointestinal cause of death	3/4	4.22/4.79	3.24 to 5.50; 3.64 to 6.22
Unspecified adverse gastrointestinal event	2/3	2.68/1.79	2.42 to 2.98; 1.70 to 1.90

* Mantel-Haenszel technique for case-control studies only.
† Direct technique method of Greenland (reference 40).

come. The odds ratio for gastrointestinal bleeding, combined from nine studies, was 2.39 (CI, 2.11 to 2.70). The odds ratio for gastrointestinal surgery, combined from three studies, was 7.75 (CI, 5.83 to 10.31). The summary odds ratio for gastrointestinal death, combined from four studies, was 4.79 (CI, 3.64 to 6.22). Thus, the relative risk for surgical or fatal outcomes among NSAID users is 2- or 3-fold higher than the relative risk for gastrointestinal bleeding.

The summary odds ratio for women was 2.32 (CI, 1.91 to 2.82), whereas the summary odds ratio for men was 2.40 (CI, 1.85 to 3.11). The summary odds ratio for women compared with men was 1.15 (CI, 0.89 to 1.50). These data do not support gender as an independent risk factor. The risk for first compared with subsequent gastrointestinal event was also examined. The summary odds ratio for the first gastrointestinal event, combined from six studies, was 2.39 (CI, 2.16 to 2.65). The relative risk for subsequent or unspecified gastrointestinal event, combined from the remaining 10 studies, was 4.76 (CI, 4.05 to 5.59). These data suggest that patients with a history of gastrointestinal events may have an increased relative risk for further events. The use of concomitant corticosteroids was also examined. The summary odds ratio for NSAID users receiving concomitant corticosteroids compared with NSAID users not receiving corticosteroids was 1.83 (CI, 1.20 to 2.78). This finding suggests an approximately twofold increase in the relative risk among NSAID users who are receiving corticosteroids compared with NSAID users not receiving corticosteroids.

Summary odds ratios were also obtained using the Mantel-Haenszel statistic. A comparison of the results obtained by the two statistical techniques showed that the direct method enabled the use of data from more studies, resulting in narrower CIs. Summary odds ratios by both methods were similar in most categories (Table 2).

Summary odds ratios calculated according to individual NSAID used and duration of NSAID exposure were as follows: piroxicam, 11.12 (CI, 6.19 to 20.23); indomethacin, 4.69 (CI, 2.97 to 7.41); aspirin, 3.38 (CI, 2.26 to 5.01); naproxen, 2.84 (CI, 1.68 to 4.82); and ibuprofen, 2.27 (CI, 1.85 to 2.80). There is substantial overlap in the CIs among NSAIDs. The duration of NSAID consumption may be related to the size of the odds ratio (Figure 3). The summary odds ratio for less than 1 month of NSAID exposure was 8.00 (CI, 6.37 to 10.06); for longer than 1 month but less than 3 months, 3.31 (CI, 2.27 to 4.82); and for longer than 3 months, 1.92 (CI, 1.19 to 3.13). The highest odds ratios were obtained from studies in which the duration of NSAID consumption was less than 1 month.

Data were also subdivided by gastrointestinal event and age (Table 3). The relative risk for gastrointestinal surgery for nonelderly individuals, combined from three studies, was 0.44 (CI, 0.29 to 0.66), whereas the risk for gastrointestinal surgery among elderly persons, combined from three studies, was 10.42 (CI, 7.40 to 14.66). These data suggest a tenfold increase in relative risk for gastrointestinal surgery among elderly users when compared with younger users.

Estimates of the prevalence of serious gastrointestinal events among NSAID users were summarized from four cohort studies (7, 23, 25, 34). The summary, 1-year prevalence among NSAID users was 1 per 1000; the prevalence among elderly users (≥ 65 years of age) was 3.2 per 1000; and the prevalence among younger users (< 65 years of age) was 0.39 per 1000.

Sources of Heterogeneity

Tests for homogeneity were statistically significant ($P < 0.05$) for all analyses, indicating that the differ-

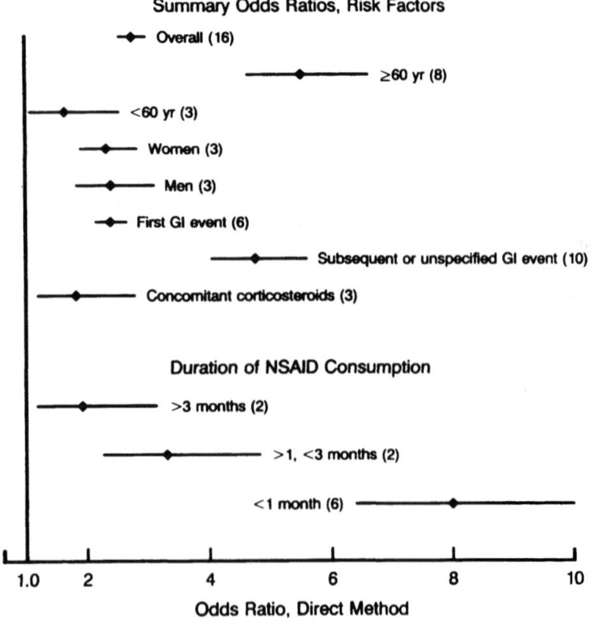

Figure 3. Summary odds ratios and risk factors. (◆, Summary odds ratio; the 95% confidence intervals are indicated by the extended line; numbers in parentheses are the number of studies combined.)

ences among the results of individual studies are greater than can be expected on the basis of chance alone.

We did two different types of analyses to identify sources of heterogeneity. Heterogeneity across studies is composed of intrastudy heterogeneity and inter-study heterogeneity. In an effort to describe intra-study heterogeneity, tests of homogeneity were conducted for several subgroups across studies. These subgroups were subdivided according to gastrointestinal outcome, age, age and gastrointestinal outcome, and use of individual NSAIDs. Each of these subgroups accounted for a portion of the variability, thus reducing the test statistic for homogeneity. There was, however, no subgroup identified that accounted for most of the observed heterogeneity. In an effort to describe interstudy heterogeneity, we did a multivariate regression analysis using the log of the study odds ratio as the dependent variable and study design, duration of NSAID use, gastrointestinal outcome, and average age as the independent variables. The regression was weighted using the individual study variances. The four independent variables accounted for approximately half of the interstudy variability.

Discussion

Two research designs have been used to study the risk for gastrointestinal events related to NSAID therapy: retrospective cohort and case-control studies. Most of the cohort studies used secondary analysis of health insurance registries in which data were collected primarily for billing purposes. The computerized case definition for gastrointestinal events is subject to substantial misclassification (42-44). Misclassification rates of up to 29% were noted in studies using retrospective chart review to confirm computerized diagnoses (23, 31, 34), resulting in contamination of the case group by controls and of the control group by cases and thus reducing the relative-risk estimate. Similarly, the information on NSAID exposure obtained from these registries may not have been of optimal quality. The duration of NSAID exposure is often unknown and assumptions are made from prescription registries regarding the average duration of NSAID use. Some studies estimated an average prescription duration of 90 days with full patient compliance (23, 31, 34). Such an assumption may overestimate the duration of NSAID exposure, biasing the results toward a falsely low relative risk. The frequency of NSAID use in a study sample determines the power of that study to detect a statistically significant relative risk (45). Nonsteroidal anti-inflammatory drug use among patients with prepaid health plans may be lower than that of the general population, further underestimating the relative risk. These factors contribute to the lower relative risks reported by the cohort studies when compared with the case-control studies.

In two case-control studies, different techniques were used to determine NSAID exposure among case patients and controls (28, 29). Physicians hospitalizing patients with gastrointestinal bleeding are more likely to inquire about NSAID use than are physicians questioning controls or their relatives. Such differences in the determination of NSAID exposure bias the results toward a falsely large relative risk. The use of a structured interview administered by an investigator who is blinded to the status (case patient or control) of the patient results in more valid estimates of relative risk (17, 26). Well-designed, nested, case-control studies minimize the selection bias, inherent in hospital-based case-control studies (33).

Although there have been many studies examining the gastrointestinal risks of NSAID use, important methodologic limitations and differences in study characteristics contribute to the conflicting results. Retrospective cohort studies probably underestimate the relative risk, whereas some case-control studies probably overestimate it. The aggregation of the results from observational studies is controversial (46). The strongest studies are those that defined cases, controls, outcome, and exposure accurately and reproducibly (26, 27, 32, 33, 35), as reflected by the quality-assessment scores in this meta-analysis (Table 1).

We conducted a structured overview of all previous reviews of NSAID-related adverse gastrointestinal events. The quality of the 10 reviews selected (3, 6-12, 18, 19) was assessed according to several criteria: the comprehensiveness of the literature search, the minimization of bias in the selection of primary studies, the assessment of the quality of the primary studies, the appropriateness of the techniques used in data synthesis, and the validity of the conclusions made by the authors as supported by the data. Most of the published reviews on this topic cite only a portion of the available literature, do not provide a critical assessment of the quality of the studies cited, and fail to combine the results of these studies statistically. Only 1 of the 10 reviews used a clearly defined, comprehensive search strategy (6). Inclusion criteria were stated for 2 of the 10 reviews (6, 8). A quality assessment of the studies was done in only 1 review (6). Appropriate, explicitly stated methods of data synthesis were given in only 2 reviews (6, 19).

Table 3. Subgroup Odds Ratios Combined from Case Control and Cohort Studies Using the "Direct" Method*

Variable	Number of Studies Combined	Summary Odds Ratio	95% CI
Gastrointestinal event by age*			
< 60 years			
Gastrointestinal bleeding	1	1.03	0.60 to 1.76
Gastrointestinal surgery	3	0.44	0.29 to 0.66
≥ 60 years			
Unspecified gastrointestinal adverse event	3	1.78	1.69 to 1.87
Gastrointestinal bleeding	9	2.38	2.10 to 2.69
Gastrointestinal surgery	3	10.42	7.40 to 14.66
Gastrointestinal cause of death	4	4.40	3.35 to 5.79

* Gastrointestinal events occurring in hospitalized patients.

Meta-analysis is a systematic, quantitative, strategy of reviewing and summarizing data from the literature to address a specific research question. It differs from the traditional review article in that it uses explicit inclusion and exclusion criteria, incorporates a standardized quality assessment, and provides a quantitative estimate of effect size. In this way, meta-analysis reduces the potential for error and bias implicit in the traditional review article (47).

Meta-analyses have been criticized for their emphasis on statistical techniques and their lack of attention to critical descriptions of methodologic and substantive issues discussed in the individual studies. The "best-evidence synthesis" method combines the strengths of quantitative meta-analytic techniques with detailed, qualitative analysis of study characteristics typical of traditional review articles (48). We have examined critically the study characteristics and quality and have provided a quantitative summary of the relative risks.

Because meta-analysis is a retrospective form of research, it is limited by any biases inherent in the primary studies. As with any review article, meta-analysis is subject to the preferential selection of studies demonstrating significant results (49). This publication bias is most problematic in studies of effectiveness in which it is assumed that studies showing no effect are less attractive to publishers and, therefore, remain unpublished. Such bias is less likely in studies of risk, in which the protective effect of an exposure on health status is of equal interest as the negative effect. Studies showing a protective effect of NSAIDs on the gastrointestinal mucosa would be of great interest. Studies showing no risk for gastrointestinal complications associated with NSAIDs would also be of interest. Using the data from the 16 studies in this overview, we determined that it would require having missed approximately 300 studies showing no gastrointestinal effect of NSAIDs to bring the summary odds ratio to unity. We believe such a scenario to be unlikely.

An assumption underlying most meta-analyses is that of homogeneity, the belief that differences among studies are due to sampling variation alone (50). Statistical tests for homogeneity examine systematic differences among study results depending on study characteristics. The statistical power of these tests depends on the sum of study sample sizes. In this meta-analysis, studies of large samples were combined, resulting in a sample size of approximately 1.7 million persons. Under these circumstances, statistical tests for homogeneity have a large amount of power to detect relatively modest heterogeneity. In this meta-analysis, tests for homogeneity were significant, suggesting important heterogeneity among these studies. Our results, therefore, cannot be considered generalizable to the overall sample of NSAID users. Rather, they represent summary statistics for the distribution of odds ratios in the selected studies.

Data from the primary studies were combined using two different methods: the Mantel-Haenszel statistic and the "direct" method (39, 40). The Mantel-Haenszel statistic is the most widely used meta-analysis technique (47). When compared with the Mantel-Haenszel statistic, the direct method has the advantage of retaining the standardization, stratification, and regression modeling used in the calculation of the odds-ratio estimates in the individual studies. This technique also allows the inclusion of studies in which the raw data were not published. Finally, this technique has the advantage of allowing the combination of odds ratios from case-control and cohort studies. For these reasons, the direct method may provide a more accurate estimate of the true overall odds ratio.

Summary data from 10 studies showed an inverse relation between the duration of NSAID consumption (estimated from prescription registries) and the relative risk for serious gastrointestinal events, suggesting that the period of greatest risk occurs during the first 3 months of NSAID therapy. This finding, which has recently been confirmed by others (51), may result from gastric mucosal adaptation: Endoscopic studies have shown that gastric mucosal damage lessens with continued aspirin therapy (52, 53). This relation, however, could be confounded by rates of compliance, because compliance with NSAID therapy, and thus exposure, is likely to be greatest early in the course of therapy.

One-year prevalence estimates were summarized from four cohort studies with varying durations of exposure (30 days to 1 year) by assuming that the risk for serious gastrointestinal events remained constant for 1 year. If, as the above data suggest, the risk is greatest during the first 3 months of therapy, this assumption would result in an overestimate of the true 1-year prevalence of NSAID-related gastrointestinal events. Alternatively, the methodologic limitations of the cohort studies suggest that an underestimate of the true risks for gastrointestinal events related to NSAID use may exist.

In summary, we conclude that NSAID users are at approximately three times greater relative risk than nonusers for developing serious adverse gastrointestinal events. Additional risk factors suggested by this analysis were age greater than 60 years, previous history of gastrointestinal events, concomitant corticosteroid use, inclusion in the first 3 months of NSAID therapy, and possibly use of piroxicam. Gender was not found to be an independent risk factor. Further studies are needed that provide an accurate estimate of the absolute risk for NSAID-related adverse gastrointestinal events and that examine the risk factors for such events.

Acknowledgments: The authors thank Kent R. Bailey, PhD, and Vern Farewell, PhD, for statistical consultation; Andrew Oxman, MD, MSc for advice on clinical epidemiology; and Elizabeth Ryan for preparation of the manuscript.

Requests for Reprints: Sherine E. Gabriel, MD, MSc, Department of Health Sciences Research, Mayo Clinic, 200 First Street SW, Rochester, MN 55905.

Current Author Addresses: Dr. Gabriel: Department of Health Sciences Research, Mayo Clinic, 200 First Street SW, Rochester, MN 55905.
Ms. Jaakkimainen: Clinical Epidemiology Unit, Room 650 Turner Wing, 160 Wellesley Street East, Toronto, Ontario, Canada M4Y 1J3.
Dr. Bombardier: Clinical Epidemiology Unit, Room 650 Turner Wing, 160 Wellesley Street East, Toronto, Ontario, Canada M4Y 1J3.

Appendix A. Study Quality Assessment Data Collection Form

Blinding				
Blinded assessment of eligibility of cases and controls	Yes	No	Unknown	
Blinded assessment of outcome	Yes	No	Unknown	
Blinded assessment of exposure	Yes	No	Unknown	
Definition of outcome				
Death due to gastric or duodenal ulcer defined surgically, endoscopically, by x-ray, or at autopsy				
Hospitalization due to gastric or duodenal ulcer defined by endoscopy or surgery				
Death or hospitalization due to gastric or duodenal ulcer defined or confirmed by chart review				
Hematemesis or melena defined by chart review				
Other				
Outcome defined as:				
First gastrointestinal event				
Any gastrointestinal event				
Unspecified				
Case selection				
Source of cases:				
All persons with disease in a defined segment of the population				
Medical care facility				
Health insurance registry				
Was computerized case definition verified by chart review?	Yes	No	Unknown	NA
Was there adjustment for case misclassification?	Yes	No	Unknown	NA
Control selection				
Source of controls				
Community				
Hospital				
Registry				
Unknown				
Sampling of controls				
Random				
Nonrandom				
Unknown				
Matching technique				
Were controls matched to cases?	Yes	No	Unknown	
What was the case-control ratio?				
1:1				
1:2-6				
1:> 6				
Unspecified				
NA				
Exposure				
Was duration of NSAID exposure defined?	Yes	No	Unknown	
NSAID use determined by:				
Direct patient inquiry or questionnaire				
Chart review				
Pharmaceutical registry				
Unknown				
Was NSAID use determined in the same manner for cases as for controls?	Yes	No	Unknown	NA
Was computerized ascertainment of exposure verified by chart review?	Yes	No	Unknown	NA
Was there adjustment for misclassification of exposure?	Yes	No	Unknown	NA
Control for confounders				
Aspirin use	Yes	No	M*	Unknown
Prednisone use	Yes	No	M	Unknown
Age	Yes	No	M	Unknown
Multiple NSAID use	Yes	No	M	Unknown
Past history of ulcer	Yes	No	M	Unknown
Past history of gastrointestinal bleeding	Yes	No	M	Unknown
Alcohol use	Yes	No	M	Unknown
Smoking	Yes	No	M	Unknown
Duodenal ulcer	Yes	No	M	Unknown
Health status	Yes	No	M	Unknown
Medical surveillance	Yes	No	M	Unknown
Anticoagulant use	Yes	No	M	Unknown
Sex	Yes	No	M	Unknown
Socioeconomic class	Yes	No	M	Unknown
Antacid or H_2-blocker use	Yes	No	M	Unknown
Indication for NSAID	Yes	No	M	Unknown

* M = measured but not used in the analysis; NA = not available.

Appendix B. Characteristics of Studies Used in the Meta-analysis*

Reference	Case Selection	Control Selection	Ascertainment of Exposure	Definition of Outcome
(35)†	Patients with bleeding gastric ulcer seen at outpatient endoscopic centers, Sydney, Australia; 1982 to 1985 (*n* = 63)	Randomly selected from Sydney electoral rolls (*n* = 411)	Telephone interview Structured questionnaire	Endoscopically proven gastric ulcer; hemorrhage-active bleeding or black clot at endoscopy, or hematemesis or melena
(28)†	Patients hospitalized for perforated peptic ulcer, Cambridge, England; 1973 to 1982 (*n* = 269)	Patients admitted for surgical emergencies, age and sex matched, etc. (*n* = 269)	Retrospective note review in cases. Not measured in controls, estimated by Intercontinental Medical Statistics for United Kingdom (1977 to 1982)	Perforation diagnosed by surgery, radiography, or necroscopy
(27)†	Consecutive patients hospitalized with non-variceal upper gastrointestinal bleeding, Toronto, Canada; 1982 to 1983 (*n* = 57)	Hospitalized patients and visitors, age and sex matched, visited physician within 2 months (*n* = 123)	Prospective interview	Hematemesis or melena on admission; all examined by endoscopy
(26)†	All patients (≥ 60y) hospitalized for bleeding peptic ulcer, Nottingham, England; 1983 to 1985 (*n* = 230)	Hospitalized controls without peptic ulcer; (*n* = 230); community controls (*n* = 230); age, sex, and general practice matched	Structured questionnaire, single interviewer	Clinical diagnosis of hematemesis or melena
(29)†	Consecutive patients who died or required emergency surgery for bleeding or perforated peptic ulcer, Cheshire, England; 1983 to 1985 (*n* = 235)	Hospitalized patients without peptic ulcer, unmatched (*n* = 1246)	Review of admitting physician note and direct patient questioning in cases. Direct questioning of controls or their relatives	Diagnosis by autopsy, endoscopy, or surgery
(30)†	Hunter Health Statistics Unit patients who died after peptic ulcer complication, New South Wales, Australia; 1980 to 1986 (*n* = 80)	Hunter Health Statistics Unit patients who survived bleeding or perforated peptic ulcer; matched for age, sex, ulcer site, and nature of complication (*n* = 160)	Review of clinical notes during week of admission	Diagnosis from database verified by chart review
(31)†	Group Health Cooperative (GHC) patients hospitalized for peptic ulcer perforation, Puget Sound, Washington (*n* = 54)	GHC controls matched for age, sex, and date of entry into plan (*n* = 324)	GHC pharmacy computer files	Diagnosis of perforation confirmed by review of discharge summaries
(32)†	Patients hospitalized for hematemesis or melena, U.S., Canada, and Israel; 1977-1984 (*n* = 57)	Patients hospitalized for conditions judged to be independent of antecedent analgesic use (*n* = 2417)	Trained nurse interviewer (cases and controls)	Diagnosis of hematemesis or melena by discharge summary
(33)†	Tennessee Medicaid patients (≥ 65y), death due to gastric or duodenal ulcer; 1976-84 (*n* = 122)	Tennessee Medicaid patients (≥ 65 years of age); stratified random sample, matched for age, sex, race, and nursing home status (*n* = 3897)	Medicaid formulary	Gastric or duodenal ulcer confirmed by surgery, endoscopy, or autopsy
(34)‡	GHC members ≥ 65 years who received an NSAID prescription for ≤ 90 d, 1977 to 1982	GHC members ≥ 65 years who did not receive an NSAID prescription	GHC prescription files	Hospitalizations for gastritis, bleeding peptic ulcer or hematemesis identified by computerized ICD codes
(23)‡	GHC members < 65 years who received an NSAID prescription for ≤ 90 d	GHC members < 65 years who did not receive an NSAID prescription	GHC prescription files	Hospitalization for gastritis, bleeding peptic ulcer or hematemesis identified by computerized ICD codes

Appendix B. Characteristics of Studies Used in the Meta-analysis*

Reference	Case Selection	Control Selection	Ascertainment of Exposure	Definition of Outcome
(31)‡	GHC members who received an NSAID prescription for ≤ 90 d, 1977 to 1983	GHC members who did not receive an NSAID prescription	GHC prescription files	Hospitalization for upper gastrointestinal perforation identified by computerized ICD codes confirmed by discharge summaries
(24)‡	Medicaid group, Michigan and Minnesota patients who received an NSAID prescription ≤ 30 d, 1980	Medicaid patients, Michigan and Minnesota patients who did not receive an NSAID prescription	Computerized pharmaceutical files	Upper gastrointestinal bleeding identified by Medicaid billing diagnoses, not verified by chart review
(25)‡	Saskatchewan Health Plan patients who received an NSAID prescription ≤ 90 d, 1983	Saskatchewan Health Plan patients matched for exposure time who did not receive an NSAID prescription	Saskatchewan drug formulary	Fatal upper gastrointestinal bleeding or perforation identified by computerized ICD codes, discharge summaries, and autopsy reports reviewed; misclassifications eliminated
(22)‡	Pennsylvania Medicaid population, patients who received an NSAID prescription ≤ 90 d, 1984-85	Pennsylvania Medicaid population matched for time of exposure who did not receive an NSAID prescription	Computerized Medicaid prescription files	Diagnoses of gastric, peptic, or duodenal ulcer and related conditions identified by computerized ICD codes, not verified by chart review
(21)‡	Users of one of five NSAIDs obtained from Prescription Pricing Division, Edinburgh, Tayside Region, Scotland, March-October 1983	NSAID nonusers in the Prescription Pricing Division, matched for age, sex, and general practitioner	Prescription files	Hospitalizations for gastrointestinal events identified by computerized ICD codes, not verified by chart review

* ICD = International Classification of Diseases; GHC = Group Health Cooperative of Puget Sound; NSAIDS = nonsteroidal anti-inflammatory drugs.
† Case-control studies.
‡ Cohort studies.

References

1. **Baum C, Kennedy DL, Forbes MB.** Utilization of nonsteroidal antiinflammatory drugs. Arthritis Rheum. 1985;28:686-92.
2. **Langman MJ.** Ulcer complications and nonsteroidal anti-inflammatory drugs. Am J Med. 1988;84(Suppl 2A):15-9.
3. **Barrier CH, Hirschowitz BI.** Controversies in the detection and management of nonsteroidal anti-inflammatory drug-induced side effects of the upper gastrointestinal tract. Arthritis Rheum. 1989;32: 926-32.
4. **Roth SH, Bennett RE.** Nonsteroidal anti-inflammatory drug gastropathy. Recognition and response. Arch Intern Med. 1987;147:2093-100.
5. **Gabriel SE, Bombardier C.** NSAID induced ulcers. An emerging epidemic? J Rheumatol. 1990;17:1-4.
6. **Chalmers TC, Berrier J, Hewitt P, Berlin J, Reitman D, Nagalingam R.** Meta-analysis of randomized controlled trials as a method of estimating rare complications of non-steroidal anti-inflammatory drug therapy. Alimentary Pharmacologic Therapy. 1988;2S:9-26.
7. **Fries JF, Miller SR, Spitz PW, Williams CA, Hubert HB, Bloch DA.** Toward an epidemiology of gastropathy associated with nonsteroidal antiinflammatory drug use. Gastroenterology. 1989;96:647-55.
8. **Langman MJ.** Epidemiologic evidence on the association between peptic ulceration and antiinflammatory drug use. Gastroenterology. 1989;96:640-6.
9. **Gibson T.** Nonsteroidal anti-inflammatory drugs—another look. Br J Rheumatol. 1988;27:87-90.
10. **Tenenbaum J.** Non-steroidal anti-inflammatory drugs (NSAIDs) cause gastrointestinal intolerance and major bleeding—or do they? Clin Invest Med. 1987;10:246-50.
11. **Carson JL, Strom BL.** The gastrointestinal side effects of the nonsteroidal anti-inflammatory drugs. J Clin Pharmacol. 1988;28:554-9.
12. **Butt JH, Barthel JS, Moore RA.** Clinical spectrum of the upper gastrointestinal effects of nonsteroidal anti-inflammatory drugs. Natural history, symptomatology, and significance. Am J Med. 1988; 84(Suppl 2A):5-14.
13. **Levy M.** Aspirin use in patients with major upper gastrointestinal bleeding and peptic-ulcer disease. A report from the Boston Collaborative Drug Surveillance Program. N Engl J Med. 1974;290: 1158-62.
14. **Clinch D, Banerjee AK, Levy DW, Ostick G, Faragher EB.** Nonsteroidal anti-inflammatory drugs and peptic ulceration. J R Coll Physicians Lond. 1987;21:183-7.
15. **McIntosh JH, Byth K, Piper DW.** Environmental factors in aetiology of chronic gastric ulcer: a case control study of exposure variables before the first symptoms. Gut. 1985;26:789-98.
16. **Martio J.** The influence of antirheumatic drugs on the occurrence of peptic ulcers. A controlled study of patients with chronic rheumatic diseases. Scand J Rheumatol 1980;9:55-9.
17. **Duggan JM, Dobson AJ, Johnson H, Fahey P.** Peptic ulcer and non-steroidal anti-inflammatory agents. Gut. 1986;27:929-33.
18. **Strom BL, Taragin MI, Carson JL.** Gastrointestinal bleeding from the nonsteroidal anti-inflammatory drugs. Agents Actions. 1990;29: 27-38.
19. **Hawkey CJ.** Non-steroidal anti-inflammatory drugs and peptic ulcers. BMJ. 1990;300:278-84.
20. Reference Manager, Version 4. Carlsbad, California: Research Information Systems, Inc; 1989.
21. **Beardon PH, Brown SV, McDevitt DG.** Gastrointestinal events in patients prescribed non-steroidal anti-inflammatory drugs: a controlled study using record linkage in Tayside. Q J Med. 1989;71: 497-505.
22. **Bloom BS.** Risk and cost of gastrointestinal side effects associated with nonsteroidal anti-inflammatory drugs. Arch Intern Med. 1989; 149:1019-22.
23. **Beard K, Walker AM, Perera DR, Jick H.** Nonsteroidal anti-inflammatory drugs and hospitalization for gastroesophageal bleeding in the elderly. Arch Intern Med. 1987;147:1621-3.
24. **Carson JL, Strom BL, Soper KA, West SL, Morse ML.** The association of nonsteroidal anti-inflammatory drugs with upper gastrointestinal tract bleeding. Arch Intern Med. 1987;147:85-8.
25. **Guess HA, West R, Strand LM, Helston D, Lydick EG, Bergman U, et al.** Fatal upper gastrointestinal hemorrhage or perforation among users and nonusers of nonsteroidal anti-inflammatory drugs in Saskatchewan, Canada 1983. J Clin Epidemiol. 1988;41:35-45.

26. **Somerville K, Faulkner G, Langman M.** Non-steroidal anti-inflammatory drugs and bleeding peptic ulcer. Lancet. 1986;1:462-4.
27. **Bartle WR, Gupta AK, Lazor J.** Nonsteroidal anti-inflammatory drugs and gastrointestinal bleeding. A case-control study. Arch Intern Med. 1986;146:2365-7.
28. **Collier DS, Pain JA.** Non-steroidal anti-inflammatory drugs and peptic ulcer perforation. Gut. 1985;26:359-63.
29. **Armstrong CP, Blower AL.** Non-steroidal anti-inflammatory drugs and life threatening complications of peptic ulceration. Gut. 1987; 28:527-32.
30. **Henry DA, Johnston A, Dobson AJ, Duggan JM.** Fatal peptic ulcer complications and the use of non-steroidal anti-inflammatory drugs, aspirin, and corticosteroids. BMJ [Clin Res]. 1987;295:1227-9.
31. **Jick SS, Perera DR, Walker AM, Jick H.** Non-steroidal anti-inflammatory drugs and hospital admission for perforated peptic ulcer. Lancet. 1987;2:380-2.
32. **Levy M, Miller DR, Kaufman DW, et al.** Major upper gastrointestinal tract bleeding. Relation to the use of aspirin and other nonnarcotic analgesics. Arch Intern Med. 1988;148:281-5.
33. **Griffin MR, Ray WA, Schaffner W.** Nonsteroidal anti-inflammatory drug use and death from peptic ulcer in elderly persons. Ann Intern Med. 1988;109:359-63.
34. **Jick H, Feld AD, Perera DR.** Certain nonsteroidal anti-inflammatory drugs and hospitalization for upper gastrointestinal bleeding. Pharmacotherapy. 1985;5:280-4.
35. **McIntosh JH, Fung CS, Berry G, Piper DW.** Smoking, nonsteroidal anti-inflammatory drugs, and acetaminophen in gastric ulcer. A study of associations and of the effects of previous diagnosis on exposure patterns. Am J Epidemiol. 1988;128:761-70.
36. **Alexander AM, Veitch GB, Wood JB.** Anti-rheumatic and analgesic drug usage and acute gastro-intestinal bleeding in elderly patients. J Clin Hosp Pharm. 1985;10:89-93.
37. **Fleiss JL.** Statistical Methods for Rates and Proportions. New York: Wiley; 1973:143-7.
38. Oracle Version 5.1.22. Belmont, California: ORACLE Corporation; 1987. ORACLE for PC/MS-DOS, Oracle Corporation, Version 5.1.
39. **Mantel N, Haenszel W.** Statistical aspects of the analysis of data from retrospective studies of disease. J Natl Cancer Inst. 1959;22: 719-48.
40. **Greenland S.** Quantitative methods in the review of epidemiologic literature. Epidemiologic Rev. 1987;9:1-30.
41. **Breslow NE, Day NE.** Statistical Methods in Cancer Research: Vol. 1. The Analysis of Case-Control Studies. Lyon, France: I.A.R.C.; 1980.
42. **Shapiro S.** The role of automated record linkage in postmarketing surveillance of drug safety. A critique. Clin Pharmacol Ther. 1989; 46:371-86.
43. **Faich GA, Stadel BV.** The future of automated record linkage for postmarketing surveillance: A response to Shapiro. Clin Pharmacol Ther. 1989;46:387-89.
44. **Strom BL, Carson JL.** Automated databases used for pharmacoepidemiology research. Clin Pharmacol Ther. 1989;46:390-4.
45. **Henry DA.** The relationship between non-steroidal anti-inflammatory drugs, the development of peptic ulcer and its complications—can we estimate risk? Agents Actions (Basel). 1985;17:105-17.
46. **Spitzer WO.** Meta-meta-analysis: unanswered questions about aggregating data. J Clin Epidemiol 1991;44:103-7.
47. **Mann C.** Meta-analysis in the breach. Science. 1990;249:476-80.
48. **Slavin HS.** Best-evidence synthesis: An alternative to meta-analysis of randomized controlled trials. N Engl J Med 1987;316:450-5.
49. **Dickerson K, Meinert CL.** Risk factors for publication bias: results of a follow-up study [Abstract]. Abstracts of the Society of Clinical Trials Eleventh Annual Meeting; Atlanta, Georgia. 1990:24.
50. **Hedges LV, Olkin I.** Statistical methods for meta-analysis. Orlando, Florida: Academic Press Inc.; 1985:122-7.
51. **Griffin MR, Piper JM, Daugherty JR, Snowden M, Ray WA.** Nonsteroidal anti-inflammatory drug use and increased risk for peptic ulcer disease in elderly persons. Ann Intern Med. 1991;114:257-63.
52. **Graham DY, Smith JL.** Aspirin and the stomach. Ann Intern Med. 1986;104:390-8.
53. **Graham DY, Smith JL, Spjut HJ, Torres E.** Gastric adaptation. Studies in humans during continuous aspirin administration. Gastroenterology. 1988;95:327-33.

1 May 1992 Volume 116 Number 9

Annals of Internal Medicine

Effect of Treatment of *Helicobacter pylori* Infection on the Long-term Recurrence of Gastric or Duodenal Ulcer

A Randomized, Controlled Study

David Y. Graham, MD; Ginger M. Lew, PA-C; Peter D. Klein, PhD; Dolores G. Evans, PhD; Doyle J. Evans, Jr., PhD; Zahid A. Saeed, MD; and Hoda M. Malaty, MD

■ *Objective:* To determine the effect of treating *Helicobacter pylori* infection on the recurrence of gastric and duodenal ulcer disease.

■ *Design:* Follow-up of up to 2 years in patients with healed ulcers who had participated in randomized, controlled trials.

■ *Setting:* A Veterans Affairs hospital.

■ *Participants:* A total of 109 patients infected with *H. pylori* who had a recently healed duodenal (83 patients) or gastric ulcer (26 patients) as confirmed by endoscopy.

■ *Intervention:* Patients received ranitidine, 300 mg, or ranitidine plus triple therapy. Triple therapy consisted of tetracycline, 2 g; metronidazole, 750 mg; and bismuth subsalicylate, 5 or 8 tablets (151 mg bismuth per tablet) and was administered for the first 2 weeks of treatment; ranitidine therapy was continued until the ulcer had healed or 16 weeks had elapsed. After ulcer healing, no maintenance antiulcer therapy was given.

■ *Measurements:* Endoscopy to assess ulcer recurrence was done at 3-month intervals or when a patient developed symptoms, for a maximum of 2 years.

■ *Results:* The probability of recurrence for patients who received triple therapy plus ranitidine was significantly lower than that for patients who received ranitidine alone: for patients with duodenal ulcer, 12% (95% CI, 1% to 24%) compared with 95% (CI, 84% to 100%); for patients with gastric ulcer, 13% (CI, 4% to 31%) compared with 74% (44% to 100%). Fifty percent of patients who received ranitidine alone for healing of duodenal or gastric ulcer had a relapse within 12 weeks of healing. Ulcer recurrence in the triple therapy group was related to the failure to eradicate *H. pylori* and to the use of nonsteroidal anti-inflammatory drugs.

■ *Conclusions:* Eradication of *H. pylori* infection markedly changes the natural history of peptic ulcer in patients with duodenal or gastric ulcer. Most peptic ulcers associated with *H. pylori* infection are curable.

Annals of Internal Medicine. 1992;**116:**705-708.

From Baylor College of Medicine, the Veterans Affairs Medical Center, and the U.S. Department of Agriculture/Agricultural Research Center Children's Nutrition Research Center. For current author addresses, see end of text.

Peptic ulcer disease is a chronic disease characterized by frequent recurrences. The continuation of antiulcer therapy after ulcer healing results in a reduced rate of ulcer recurrence but does not affect the natural history of the disease, because the expected pattern of rapid recurrence resumes when maintenance therapy is discontinued (1). Recent studies have suggested that the eradication of *Helicobacter pylori* infection affects the natural history of duodenal ulcer disease such that the rate of recurrence decreases markedly (2-6). However, the interpretation of these results has been complicated by the fact that several of the larger studies did not use control groups or any form of blinding (3, 5, 6). In addition, studies of the effect of *H. pylori* eradication in patients with gastric ulcer have not been done. We report the results of a randomized, controlled trial in which we evaluated the effect of therapy designed to eradicate *H. pylori* on the pattern of ulcer recurrence in patients with duodenal or gastric ulcer.

Methods

Our study took place between September 1988 and October 1990 at a single Veterans Affairs hospital. All patients whose *H. pylori*-associated active duodenal or gastric ulcer had healed during randomized trials comparing ranitidine and ranitidine plus "triple therapy" were invited to participate in this follow-up study. During the initial studies, patients were randomly assigned to either ranitidine alone (300 mg once daily in the evening) or to ranitidine plus triple therapy. Triple therapy consisted of bismuth subsalicylate and two antimicrobial agents: tetracycline hydrochloride, 500 mg four times a day and metronidazole, 250 mg thrice daily. Bismuth subsalicylate tablets containing 151 mg bismuth per tablet (Pepto-Bismol, Proctor & Gamble, Cincinnati, Ohio) were administered for the first 2 weeks of therapy, and patients received 5 or 8 tablets.

Two groups of patients were entered into our follow-up study. Patients with healed duodenal ulcers came from a randomized study of 146 patients, 105 of whom have been previously described (7); of these 146 patients, 112 experienced ulcer healing, 24 were lost to follow-up during the 16 weeks of therapy, and 10 had no ulcer healing after 16 weeks of treatment. Of the 112 patients in whom documented healing occurred, 83 (74%) agreed to enter the follow-up study. Patients with healed gastric ulcers came from a randomized trial of 41 patients; of these 41 patients, 31 had ulcer healing, 9 were lost to follow-up during the 16 weeks of therapy, and 1 patient had no ulcer healing after 16 weeks of treatment. Of the 31 patients in whom documented healing occurred, 26 (84%) agreed to enter the follow-up study. In sum, 109 patients with healed

Table 1. Demographic and Clinical Characteristics of Patients

Variable	Patients with Duodenal Ulcer		Patients with Gastric Ulcer	
	Ranitidine Alone	Triple Therapy plus Ranitidine	Ranitidine Alone	Triple Therapy plus Ranitidine
Patients, *n*	36	47	11	15
Median age (range), *y*	61 (31-85)	58 (29-79)	66 (43-76)	60 (27-67)
Male gender, %	97	100	100	100
Race, *n(%)*				
White	25 (69)	30 (64)	7 (64)	8 (53)
Black	11 (30)	17 (36)	3 (27)	7 (47)
Other	0	0	1 (9)	0
Recent NSAID* use, *n(%)*	6 (17)	11 (23)	2 (18)	5 (33)
Daily aspirin (1 tablet), *n(%)*	3 (8)	4 (8.5)	1 (9)	1 (6)
Smoker†, *n(%)*	17 (47)	34 (72)	6 (54)	11 (73)
Alcohol use				
1 or more drinks/wk, *n(%)*	7 (19)	15 (32)	2 (18)	4 (27)
H. pylori infection, %‡	100	100	100	100

* NSAID = nonsteroidal anti-inflammatory drugs.
† $P = 0.03$ for the difference between the ranitidine and triple therapy groups among patients with duodenal ulcer.
‡ Infection at entry into the ulcer healing study was confirmed by at least two of the following: urea breath test, histologic evaluation, culture, and serologic testing.

peptic ulcers (83 with duodenal ulcers and 26 with gastric ulcers) were included in our long-term follow-up study.

Patients were followed for up to 2 years. During this time, patients received no antiulcer medications (including antacids). Twenty-four patients regularly receiving nonsteroidal anti-inflammatory drugs were allowed to continue them if they wished. Patient follow-up visits were scheduled for 1 month after therapy, 3 months after therapy, and every 3 months for up to 2 years. Patients were also instructed to return for endoscopy if symptoms recurred. The endoscopist was blinded to the treatment status of the patients.

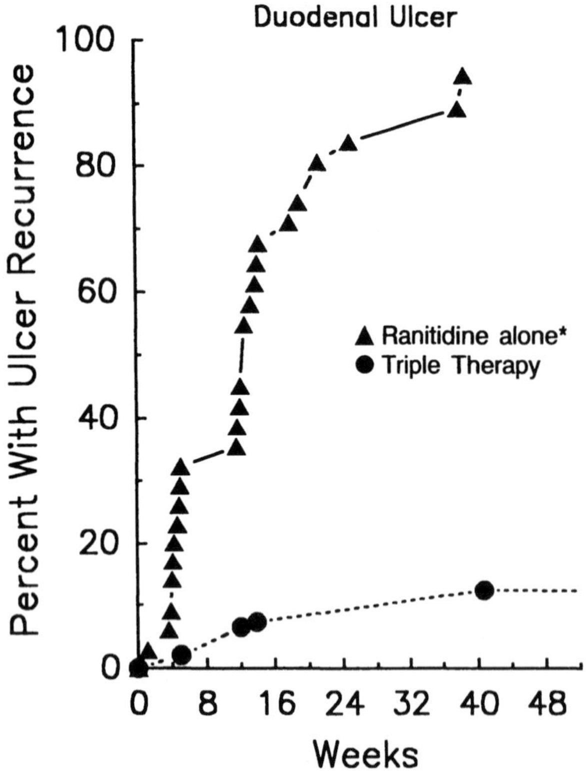

Figure 1. Lifetable recurrence of duodenal ulcers for the year after successful healing with ranitidine alone or triple therapy plus ranitidine. No maintenance therapy was given; the recurrence rate of ulcers in patients healed with ranitidine alone was significantly greater ($P < 0.01$) than in those who received triple therapy plus ranitidine. * The only patient in the ranitidine alone group who had not developed recurrent ulcer by October 1990 was then followed for a total of 16 months without ulcer recurrence (*see* text).

Patients originally assigned to receive ranitidine alone who experienced ulcer recurrence were crossed over to receive triple therapy plus ranitidine; after ulcer healing occurred with this latter therapy, patients were offered follow-up using the protocol described above. These patients were termed "cross-over follow-up" patients.

Ulcers were identified by endoscopy using Fujinon videoendoscopes (Fujinon, Inc., Wayne, New Jersey). A video still (ProMavica, Sony Corporation of America, Sony Park Ridge, New Jersey) of each ulcer was made so that the site and characteristics of the ulcer could be reviewed before subsequent endoscopic procedures. One video disk was assigned to each patient. An ulcer was defined as a circumscribed break in the duodenal mucosa that measured at least 5 mm in diameter, had apparent depth, and was covered by an exudate.

All patients were assessed for *H. pylori* infection by the ^{13}C-urea breath test (8, 9); by a sensitive and specific enzyme-linked immunosorbent assay (ELISA) for IgG antibody against the high-molecular-weight, cell-associated proteins of *H. pylori* (10); by culture; and by histologic evaluation of antral mucosal biopsy specimens. Eradication was defined by no evidence of *H. pylori* infection (by urea breath test, culture, or histologic evaluation) 1 or more months after discontinuing triple therapy. Patients were tested every 3 months and when symptomatic.

The protocol was approved by the Institutional Review Board at the Veteran Affairs Medical Center and Baylor College of Medicine. Written informed consent was obtained before patient entry.

Statistical Analysis

Ulcer recurrence was calculated by the lifetable method (Lifetest procedure, SAS/STAT software release 6.04, SAS Institute, Inc., Cary, North Carolina). Categorical data were evaluated by chi-square test with the Yates correction or by the Fisher exact test. All P values ≤ 0.05 (two-tailed) were considered to be significant. Ninety-five percent confidence intervals are given when appropriate.

Results

We followed 83 patients with duodenal ulcer and 26 patients with gastric ulcer (median age, 62 years). The sample was 98% men. The two groups of patients (assigned to ranitidine alone or ranitidine plus triple therapy) had similar demographic and clinical characteristics (Table 1). The percentage of smokers and alcohol users was higher in the group receiving triple therapy plus ranitidine than in the group receiving ranitidine alone. Only one significant difference was found between the treatment groups: Among patients with duodenal ulcer, the group receiving triple therapy had more smokers than the group receiving ranitidine alone (P = 0.03). All patients had active *H. pylori* infection before the start of ulcer therapy. All 47 patients treated with ranitidine alone were still infected at the end of therapy. In contrast, *H. pylori* was eradicated in 55 of 62 patients (89%) receiving triple therapy.

The lifetable probability of ulcer recurrence 1 year after ulcer healing (Figures 1 and 2) was significantly lower for patients who received triple therapy plus ranitidine (12% [CI, 1% to 24%] for patients with duodenal ulcer and 13% [CI, 4% to 31%] for patients with gastric ulcer) compared with those who received ranitidine alone (95% [CI, 84% to 100%] for patients with duodenal ulcer and 74% [CI, 44% to 100%] for patients with gastric ulcer) (P = 0.001). The median duration of follow-up for patients who had received triple therapy plus ranitidine was 38 weeks (range, 4 to 108 weeks) for patients with duodenal ulcer and 52 weeks (range, 12 to 95 weeks) for patients with gastric ulcer.

Fifty percent of patients with either duodenal or gastric ulcer who experienced healing with ranitidine alone had a recurrence within 12 weeks (*see* Figures 1 and 2). Seventy-five percent of recurrences were symptomatic. At the end of the study period, only three patients in the ranitidine alone group (one with duodenal ulcer and two with gastric ulcer) had not had ulcer recurrence. Follow-up on these three patients after the study was completed showed the following: One patient with duodenal ulcer was lost to follow-up after 16 months, and two patients with gastric ulcer were last seen at the 15-month follow-up visit (one was lost to follow-up and the other died of an unrelated illness).

Infection with *H. pylori* was a strong predictor of ulcer recurrence. All 47 patients whose ulcers healed while receiving ranitidine alone still had *H. pylori* infection at the end of therapy, and, by lifetable analysis, 95% of them developed recurrent ulcers by the end of 1 year. None of the patients in whom *H. pylori* was eradicated became reinfected during the study period. *Helicobacter pylori* infection was not eradicated in seven patients who received triple therapy. Of these seven patients, four experienced ulcer recurrence and three were lost to follow-up (two patients after 6 months and one patient after 1 year).

Three patients with duodenal ulcer in whom *H. pylori* infection was eradicated after triple therapy still developed recurrent duodenal ulcers (two patients after 3 months and one patient after 9 months). All three patients were using nonsteroidal anti-inflammatory drugs (ibuprofen, piroxicam, or salsalate). In addition, two patients with recurrent gastric ulcer who were also receiving such drugs had persistent *H. pylori* infection.

Ten patients with duodenal ulcer who experienced ulcer recurrence after healing with ranitidine alone were crossed over to receive ranitidine plus triple therapy after the completion of the randomized trial. Triple therapy resulted in the eradication of *H. pylori* infection in these patients. After ulcer healing, the patients were followed for a median of 44 weeks (range, 23 to 116 weeks), and none experienced ulcer recurrence. Four other patients with duodenal ulcer refractory to ranitidine alone were crossed over to receive ranitidine plus triple therapy. *Helicobacter pylori* infection was eradicated in all four patients. After ulcer healing, the patients were followed for a median of 40 weeks, and none experienced ulcer recurrence.

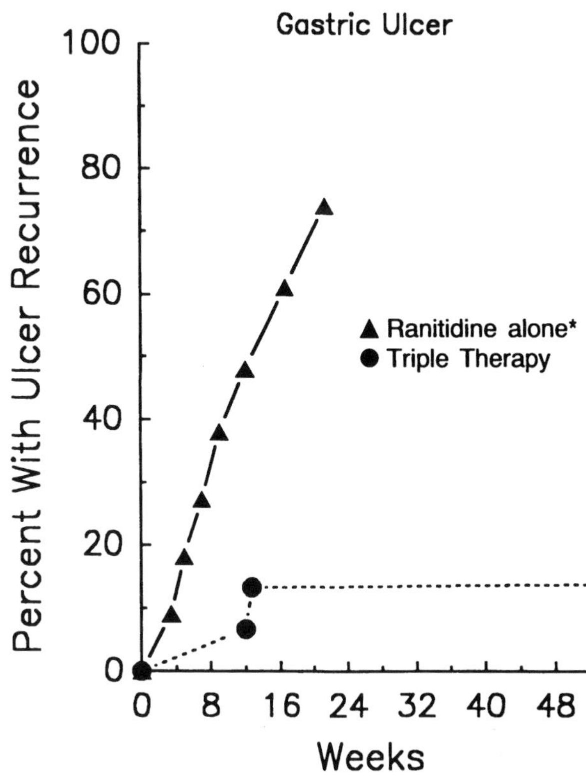

Figure 2. Lifetable recurrence of gastric ulcers for the year after successful healing with ranitidine alone or triple therapy plus ranitidine. No maintenance therapy was given; the recurrence rate of ulcers in patients healed with ranitidine alone was significantly greater ($P < 0.01$) than in those who received triple therapy plus ranitidine. * The two patients in the ranitidine alone group who had not developed recurrent ulcers by October 1990 were then followed for a total of 15 months without ulcer recurrence (*see* text).

Discussion

Recent studies have shown that the eradication of *H. pylori* infection is associated with healing of gastritis (11) and a marked reduction in the rate of recurrence of duodenal ulcers (2-6). The protocols of these studies have varied, but the results have been the same; the eradication of *H. pylori* infection changes the natural history of duodenal ulcer disease, and factors that contribute to rapid ulcer recurrence, such as smoking, seem to no longer to pose a risk (6). Our study confirms previous findings in patients with duodenal ulcers and extends the findings to patients with gastric ulcers. Patients in whom *H. pylori* infection was eradicated remained asymptomatic and ulcer free.

Smoking, alcohol use, and male gender have all been

described as risk factors for ulcer recurrence (1, 12). In our study, smoking and alcohol use were more frequent in the group that received triple therapy plus ranitidine, a factor that could have biased our results. However, our study confirms the observation that smoking is not a risk factor for ulcer recurrence after the eradication of *H. pylori* infection (6). In our patients, the only factors associated with ulcer recurrence were *H. pylori* infection and the continued use of nonsteroidal anti-inflammatory drugs.

Our study was single-blind, with the endoscopist blinded to initial therapy. Although some may argue that the lack of double-blinding introduced an important bias into our study, no objective data support such a contention, and we believe such a scenario extremely unlikely, especially considering the equipment now available for studying the gastroduodenal mucosa.

Three previous reports have used the word "cure" in the title or discussion (4-6). These studies, taken together, provide compelling evidence for the hypothesis that peptic ulcer, either duodenal or gastric, is the end result of a bacterial infection. We believe that, eventually, anti-*H. pylori* agents will be part of the therapy for *H. pylori*-associated ulcer disease. The universal introduction of such therapy may be delayed because several safe and effective therapies are currently available for healing peptic ulcers and because ulcer relapse can be greatly reduced by maintenance therapy with histamine-2-receptor antagonists (1, 12). In addition, there are still concerns that the benefits of therapy (that is, reduced recurrence) may not yet outweigh such side effects as antibiotic-associated diarrhea or the development of widespread antibiotic resistance in *H. pylori* and other bacteria (13). We have observed that triple therapy is often not effective in patients who have previously received metronidazole (unpublished data), and compliance with the complicated treatment protocols remains a major problem (14). Simpler protocols and improved therapies are needed. The eradication of the infection may also not yield a true cure because the patient vulnerable to additional *H. pylori* encounters may acquire a new infection and experience recurrence of the original disease. We recommend that patients with resistant ulcers (defined as failure to heal in 12 weeks), those with ulcer-associated complications, and those with symptoms severe enough to be candidates for surgery receive triple therapy for *H. pylori* infection.

Grant Support: In part by the Department of Veterans Affairs, by grant DK 39919 from the National Institute of Diabetes and Digestive and Kidney Diseases, by the U.S. Department of Agriculture/Agricultural Research Service Children's Nutrition Research Center, and by Hilda Schwartz.

Requests for Reprints: David Y. Graham, MD, Veterans Affairs Medical Center (111D), 2002 Holcombe Boulevard, Houston, TX 77030.

Current Author Addresses: Drs. Graham, Evans, Evans, Jr., Saeed, Malaty, and Ms. Lew: Veterans Affairs Medical Center (111D), 2002 Holcombe Boulevard, Houston, TX 77030.
Dr. Klein: Children's Nutrition Research Center, 1100 Bates Street, Houston, TX 77030.

References

1. **Sontag SJ.** Current status of maintenance therapy in peptic ulcer disease. Am J Gastroenterol. 1988;83:607-17.
2. **Coghlan JG, Gilligan D, Humphries H, McKenna D, Dooley C, Sweeney E, et al.** *Campylobacter pylori* and recurrence of duodenal ulcers—a 12-month follow-up study. Lancet. 1987;2:1109-11.
3. **Lambert JR, Borromeo M, Korman MG, Hansky J, Eaves ER.** Effect of colloidal bismuth (De-Nol) on healing and relapse of duodenal ulcers-role of *Campylobacter pyloridis* [Abstract]. Gastroenterology. 1987;92:1489.
4. **Marshall BJ, Goodwin CS, Warren JR, Murray R, Blincow ED, Blackbourn SJ, et al.** Prospective double-blind trial of duodenal ulcer relapse after eradication of *Campylobacter pylori*. Lancet. 1988;2:1437-42.
5. **Rauws EA, Tytgat GN.** Cure of duodenal ulcer associated with eradication of *Helicobacter pylori*. Lancet. 1990;335:1233-5.
6. **George LL, Borody TJ, Andrews P, Devine M, Moore-Jones D, Walton M, et al.** Cure of duodenal ulcer after eradication of *Helicobacter pylori*. Med J Aust. 1990;153:145-9.
7. **Graham DY, Lew GM, Evans DG, Evans DJ Jr, Klein PD.** Effect of triple therapy (antibiotics plus bismuth) on duodenal ulcer healing with ranitidine. A randomized controlled trial. Ann Intern Med. 1991;115:266-9.
8. **Graham DY, Klein PD, Evans DJ Jr., Evans DG, Alpert LC, Opekun AR, et al.** *Campylobacter pylori* detected noninvasively by the 13C-urea breath test. Lancet. 1987;1:1174-7.
9. **Klein PD, Graham DY.** *Campylobacter pylori* detection by the ^{13}C-urea breath test. In: *Campylobacter pylori* and Gastroduodenal Disease. Rathbone BJ, Heatley V, eds. Blackwell Scientific Publications, Oxford, 1989, pp. 94-106.
10. **Evans DJ Jr, Evans DG, Graham DY, Klein PD.** A sensitive and specific serologic test for detection of *Campylobacter pylori* infection. Gastroenterology. 1989;96:1004-8.
11. **Rauws EA, Langenberg W, Houthoff HJ, Zanen HC, Tytgat GN.** *Campylobacter pyloridis*-associated chronic active antral gastritis: a prospective study of its prevalence and the effects of antibacterial and antiulcer treatment. Gastroenterology. 1988;94:33-40.
12. **Van Deventer GM, Elashoff JD, Reedy TJ, Schneidman D, Walsh JH.** A randomized study of maintenance therapy with ranitidine to prevent the recurrence of duodenal ulcer. N Engl J Med. 1989;320:1113-9.
13. **Graham DY, Börsch GM.** The who's and when's of therapy for *Helicobacter pylori* [Editorial]. Am J Gastroenterol. 1990;85:1552-5.
14. **Graham DY, Lew GM, Malaty HM, Evans DG, Evans DJ Jr, Klein PD, et al.** Factors influencing the eradication of *Helicobacter pylori* with triple therapy. Gastroenterology. 1992;102:493-6.

Section VI

Hematology

The incidence and significance of the sickle cell trait.

Diggs LW, Ahmann CF, Bibb J. Ann Intern Med. 1933;7:769-778.

In a classic example of clinical research, Lemuel Diggs, an astute clinician and the director of the Clinical Laboratories at the University of Tennessee in Memphis, documented the important features of sickle cell trait before the molecular basis for the disease was known. Diggs, who joined the faculty at the University of Tennessee in 1929, recognized the problems of patients with sickle cell disease, and this became the focus of his career for the next 60 years.

Although sickle cell disease had been described in 1910, Diggs and colleagues state in their introduction that "The clinical importance of the sickle cell trait in the absence of anemia, and the relationship of the trait to sickle cell anemia, are subjects of controversy." Not so after publication of this article! Diggs and colleagues established the frequency of sickle cell trait, documented the absence of anemia and illness among subjects, identified the diminished sickling of red cells from erythrocytes in newborns, and defined the ratio of patients with sickle cell anemia to carriers of sickle cell trait. There could be no more controversy.

Diggs and colleagues studied 2539 black patients in Memphis and 674 black school children and teachers. For each subject, a drop of blood was placed on a slide under a sealed coverslip; microscopic observations were made each day for 3 days. Sickled cells were identified in 276 (8.6%) of the 3213 study participants; the frequency was equal in males and females. These data established the (still-current) prevalence of sickle cell trait among black Americans. Diggs and colleagues also documented that black newborns had a lower frequency of sickling and that the deformation of sickled red cells was less marked and developed more slowly. These observations predicted the transition from normal fetal hemoglobin to the abnormal adult hemoglobin with the sickle mutation in the β-globin chain after birth.

Furthermore, prior to Diggs' publication, it was generally assumed that persons with the sickle cell trait had a tendency to develop anemia. This Diggs disproved: Among 672 black school children, 65 had sickle cell trait; hemoglobin levels did not differ between the 65 children with sickle cell trait and the 607 children without it. Finally, over 30 months at the Memphis General Hospital, Diggs and colleagues identified 14 patients with sickle cell anemia. Comparing this number with the estimated number of patients with sickle cell trait among all hospital admissions, the ratio of sickle cell anemia to sickle cell trait was 1 to 40, exactly what would later be recognized as the homozygote/heterozygote ratio. Diggs concluded that ""The importance of sickle cell trait appears to be limited to the relatively small group who in addition to the trait has sickle cell anemia."

Diggs and colleagues' observations are an enduring lesson for clinical research: The investigators began with an important clinical question that could be answered using available laboratory methods. Their observations were not only remarkable for 1933 but also provided the clinical foundation for our current knowledge of the molecular genetics of sickle cell anemia. (JNG)

Immunologic mechanisms in idiopathic and neonatal thrombocytopenic purpura.

Harrington WJ, Sprague CC, Minnich V, Moore CV, Aulvin RC, Dubach R. Ann Intern Med. 1953;38:433-469.

William Harrington became one of hematology's most enduring legends in 1950 when, during his first year of hematology fellowship training at Washington University in St. Louis, he infused himself with whole blood from a patient with idiopathic thrombocytopenic purpura (ITP) and severe thrombocytopenia. The following day, Harrington was severely thrombocytopenic, with extensive purpura and gingival bleeding. The initial report of this experience (1) demonstrated acute thrombocytopenia following followed infusion of whole blood or plasma from eight patients with ITP Harrington and his colleagues. These observations, documenting the presence of a plasma factor that could cause platelet destruction, were the dramatic headline; Harrington's's *Annals* paper that followed two years later was a detailed investigation that described what happened and how it happened. The *Annals* article is a treasure trove of many clinical observations that led to our current understanding of the pathogenesis of ITP.

Harrington reported additional studies of infusion of blood and plasma from 27 ITP patients into healthy persons (including one "W.H."). An important point was the documentation that eight of the patients had no history of a previous pregnancy or transfusion, excluding the possibility of platelet isoagglutinins as the cause of thrombocytopenia in normal subjects. An in vitro method was established to demonstrate platelet agglutination caused by serum or plasma from patients with ITP. The severity of thrombocytopenia caused by infusion of ITP plasma into normal subjects seemed to correlate with the titer of the platelet agglutinin demonstrated in vitro. In four patients, the platelet agglutinins were demonstrated to be autoagglutinins: Plasma collected when the patients were thrombocytopenic agglutinated their own platelets after recovery occurred. Although tests for anti-platelet antibodies have never become an important clinical tool, these studies were an important correlation of in vitro and in vivo activity of the antibodies associated with ITP.

The role of the spleen was investigated by infusing plasma from a patient with ITP into two subjects, one normal and one who had been splenectomized. In two experiments, ITP plasma caused less severe thrombocytopenia in the splenectomized patient, demonstrating the role of the spleen in removing antibody-sensitized platelets. Demonstration that the platelet agglutinins became undetectable in some (but not all) patients who had a complete recovery after splenectomy suggested that the spleen was also was a source of antibody production. A final series of observations documented the clinical course of neonatal thrombocytopenia in infants born to women with ITP, even women who had a remission after splenectomy. In some infants, thrombocytopenia persisted for up to 12 weeks, much longer than the typical one 1-week duration of thrombocytopenia in normal subjects after infusion of ITP plasma. This may be related to the dose of plasma or to immaturity of splenic function.

Harrington and associates documented the immunologic etiology of ITP and demonstrated the role of the spleen, both as the site of platelet destruction and as a source of platelet autoantibodies. This type of study, of course, will never be repeated. It was undertaken near the end of a tradition of self-experimentation that had existed for centuries, an era foreign to our current concepts of ethics, informed consent, and human subject protection.

After his training at Washington University, William Harrington had a long and distinguished academic career, but he will be most remembered for his remarkable experiments that defined ITP. (JNG)

Reference

1. **Harrington WJ, Minnich V, Hollingsworth JW, Moore CV.** Demonstration of a thrombocytopenic factor in the blood of patients with thrombocytopenic purpura. J Lab Clin Med. 1951;38:1-10.

Combination chemotherapy in the treatment of advanced Hodgkin's disease.

DeVita VT Jr, Serpick AA, Carbone PP. Ann Intern Med. 1970;73: 881-895.

DeVita and colleagues' pioneering study was a landmark in the establishment of medical oncology as a medical specialty. It was the cornerstone on which members of this new specialty developed newer, more effective, and less toxic regimens. The authors described 43 patients with advanced stage Hodgkin's lymphoma, of whom 35 (81%) of the patients had stage IV disease with involvement of the liver and/or other organs in addition to lymph nodes. About ten years previously, dramatic reports had described the use of radiation therapy to cure Hodgkin's lymphoma with limited lymph node involvement. However, advanced-stage Hodgkin's lymphoma was still thought to be incurable. Therefore DeVita and colleagues' report was a revelation.

Patients were treated with chemotherapeutic combinations consisting of mustargen (nitrogen mustard), oncavine, procarbazine, and prednisone (MOPP regimen) or the same combination of drugs with cyclophosphamide substituted for mustargen (COPP regimen). The use of a combination of chemotherapy drugs to achieve a better cell kill rate was initially described in murine leukemia and was later successfully used in children with acute lymphoblastic leukemia. DeVita and colleagues were the first to use a combination of chemotherapeutic agents in adults with a nonleukemia form of cancer. Of the 43 patients enrolled in the study, 35 (81%) achieved a complete response and one half remained in remission for a median of about three years, an outcome totally unexpected by the hematology and oncology communities.

Another critically important aspect of this study was its meticulous study design. Although this study was performed more than 40 years ago, its quality matches or exceeds that of many current studies. Its strengths include 1) central review of all pathology specimens and the use of current classification criteria, 2) the use of informed consent, 3), extensive disease staging evaluation despite limited imaging capabilities, 4) detailed dose adjustment guidelines, 5) clear definition of end points, and 6) detailed qualitative and quantitative description of regimen toxicities.

This pioneering study was a landmark in the establishment of medical oncology as a medical specialty. It was the cornerstone upon which newer, more effective, and less toxic regimens were developed. The importance of this paper was far greater than its demonstration that advanced Hodgkin's lymphoma could be cured; it also helped change clinician attitudes about patients with advanced cancer, from one of pessimism and despair to one of optimism and hope with the aim of curing the patient. (JNG & AT)

THE INCIDENCE AND SIGNIFICANCE OF THE SICKLE CELL TRAIT *

By L. W. Diggs, M.D., C. F. Ahmann, Ph.D., and Juanita Bibb, A.B., *Memphis, Tennessee*

If one takes a drop of blood from each member of an unselected series of negroes, seals the drops under cover-slips, and examines them microscopically over a period of hours, he observes striking curved and pointed distortions of the erythrocytes in an appreciable number of the preparations. (Figure 1.) Erythrocytes assuming such bizarre stellate shapes are called " sickled cells " and individuals whose erythrocytes are capable of undergoing such a metamorphosis under suitable conditions are said to possess the " sickle cell trait." The anomaly is hereditary and is thought to be transmitted as a dominant Mendelian characteristic. Within the large group of those who inherit the sickle cell trait, an undetermined number, due to factors unknown, develop varying degrees of " sickle cell anemia," a hemolytic type of blood dyscrasia with characteristic clinical and pathological features.

Estimations of the frequency of occurrence of the sickle cell trait have been recorded by a number of observers, but the number of individuals examined has been relatively few; most of the studies have been made on hospital patients, and little attention has been given to the variable factors which play a part in the detection of the anomaly. The clinical importance of the sickle cell trait in absence of anemia, and the relationship of the trait to sickle cell anemia are subjects of controversy. For these reasons, it seems justifiable to present evidence revealed in our investigations which deals with the incidence and significance of the sickle cell trait.

Method

The individuals included in the surveys reported in this article were taken at random from groups of normal and hospital negroes and white people. One series examined by Ahmann consisted of negro school children and teachers in the grammar and high schools of Gainesville, Florida. Another series consisted of hospital negroes in the medical, surgical, obstetrical and pediatric wards, and in the out-patient clinic of the Memphis General Hospital, and in the medical wards of the Shelby County Hospital, Memphis, Tennessee. The white subjects examined for the presence of the sickle cell trait were medical students of the University of Tennessee and medical patients of the Memphis General Hospital.

Sealed moist preparations, used throughout the study as a means of detection of the sickle cell anomaly, were made in the following manner.

* Received for publication March 31, 1933.

From the Department of Clinical Pathology, University of Tennessee, Pathological Institute, Memphis, Tennessee, and from the Nutritional Division of the Experimental Station, University of Florida, Gainesville, Florida.

In the school series, new slides and new No. 0 and No. 1 cover-slips were boiled in cleaning solution, rinsed in distilled water and 95 per cent alcohol; then left in a mixture of alcohol and ether until dried for use. In the hospital series new slides and new No. 1 and No. 2 cover-slips were used. The method of cleaning varied; most of the glassware, however, was washed for 24 hours in running tap water and placed in 95 per cent alcohol, until dried for use. Capillary blood from alcohol cleaned fingers or heels was used for

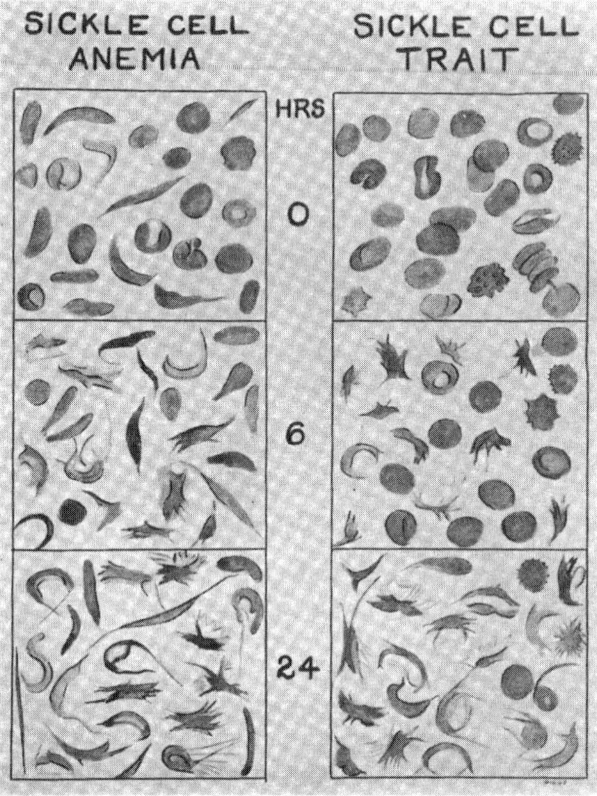

Fig. 1. Drawing showing the morphology of sickled erythrocytes in sickle cell anemia and in the sickle cell trait as revealed in sealed moist preparations at the time of making the preparations and after six hours and after 24 hours.

all preparations with the exception of those made in the out-patient department, where venous blood drawn for routine Wassermann tests was utilized. A small drop of blood was taken on a cover-slip, and the cover-glass placed drop-side down on a slide. The blood was allowed to spread without pressure, after which the edges of the cover-glass were rimmed with petrolatum. In the first 500 cases only one moist preparation was made per patient, but in the remaining hospital cases and in all of the school cases, two preparations per patient were made. The sealed drops were left at room temperature and examined under high dry magnification four times, once immediately after returning to the laboratory, and at 24 hour intervals thereafter for three days. The sickle cell trait for a given individual was recorded as positive when definite long tapering filaments and typical sickle cell distortions were observed. Crenated cells, elliptical cells, cells with blunt filaments and poikilocytosis of a questionable and non-specific nature were not considered as manifestations of the sickle cell phenomenon.

Results

The number of negroes examined in the hospital series was 2,539, of which number 211 or 8.3 per cent were demonstrated to have sickled cells in moist preparations. Of 674 negro school children and teachers examined, the sickle cell phenomenon was observed in 65 or in 9.6 per cent of the preparations. By combining our series with those previously recorded in the literature,[1-11] the average frequency of demonstration of the trait in negroes is found to be 7.3 per cent (619 in 8,453). (Table 1.) It is probable that the real incidence of the sickle cell trait is higher than this demonstrated average, because most of the sources of error in the method are on the side of not detecting the trait when it is present rather than in making false positive diagnoses.

Moist preparations were made with the blood of 309 white people and in no preparation was there any evidence of sickle cell distortion. Other sur-

Table I

Incidence of the Sickle Cell Trait

Negroes

Author	Place	Number Examined	Number with Trait	Per cent with Trait
Sydenstricker, Mulherin and Houseal	Ga.	300	13	4.3
Cooley and Lee	Mich.	400	30	7.5
Miyamoto and Korb	Mo.	300	19	6.3
Wollstein and Kreidel	N. Y.	150	13	8.6
Josephs	Md.	250	16	6.4
Smith	La.	100	5	5.0
Dolgopol and Stitt	N. Y.	77	4	5.2
Levy	N. Y.	213	12	5.6
Graham and McCarty	Ala.	1,500	122	8.1
Brandau	Tex.	150	10	6.7
Sydenstricker	Ga.	1,800	99	5.5
Diggs, Ahmann and Bibb	Tenn.	2,539	211	8.3
Ahmann	Fla.	674	65	9.6
Total		8,453	619	7.3
Whites				
Sydenstricker	Ga.	1,000	0	0.0
Miyamoto and Korb	Mo.	100	0	0.0
Diggs, Ahmann and Bibb	Tenn.	309	0	0.0
Total		1,409	0	0.0

veys of white people have likewise yielded negative results.[8,12] (Table 1.) The series reported by Lawrence,[13] which is falsely interpreted by some as being a proved demonstration of sickled erythrocytes in white people, is not included, for he describes and pictures elliptical cells and not true sickled cells. Wollstein and Kreidel[4] were unable to demonstrate the sickle cell phenomenon in white children, but fail to state the number examined.

Isolated instances of the sickle cell trait in white people have been placed on record by Castana,[14] Archibald,[15] Stewart,[16] Cooley and Lee,[17] Sights and Simon,[18] and by Rosenfeld and Pincus.[19] There is reason to suspect negro blood in the cases reported by Archibald and by Stewart. The claims of Castana and of Sights and Simon are contestable because of inadequate investigation of the families and because they did not prove conclusively by word description or illustration that they were dealing with the sickle cell trait. Cooley and Lee presented evidence of the sickle cell phenomenon in a Greek family, and Rosenfeld and Pincus demonstrated the presence of sickled cells in an Italian family. In both of these families there was no evidence of mixed blood. From these observations it is evident that the sickle cell trait is frequent in the negro race and quite rare in the white race, and that clearly established cases among white people have been limited to those of Mediterranean stock. If the sickle cell trait is a dominant characteristic, there will come from the interbreeding of the races an increasing number of cases with the sickle cell trait in those apparently white.[19] Whether or not the trait occurs in pure white strains will long remain a disputed point, and will be settled by preponderance of evidence rather than by single cases.

Examination of table 1 reveals slight differences in the incidence of the sickle cell trait as recorded by different observers, which is to be expected in any frequency estimation which deals with relatively small series and with many variable factors. Climate and geographical location do not seem to be important factors, as there are no significant or constant variations in the incidence in the widely separated localities where surveys have been conducted.

An analysis of the incidence according to sex discloses an even distribution of the sickle cell trait in males (8.4 per cent) and in females (8.1 per cent). (Table 2.)

An examination of the series to determine the incidence of the sickle cell trait according to age reveals the following findings. The lowest percentage occurred in new born babies, the sickle cell trait being demonstrated in only 3.1 per cent (6 in 159). It was also noted that the sickle cell distortion in this group was less marked and developed more slowly than in adults with the trait. In the negro school children the sickle cell phenomenon was demonstrated in 8.6 per cent (24 in 270) of those from 6 to 10 years of age, in 9.7 per cent (27 in 277) of those 11 to 15 years of age, and in 11.2 per cent (13 in 115) of the 16 to 20 year old group. This slight increase in incidence with advancing years is probably not significant. The

TABLE II

Incidence of the Sickle Cell Trait According to Sex

Females

Author	Number Examined	Number with Trait	Percentage
Miyamoto and Korb	196	14	7.1
Graham and McCarty	944	72	7.7
Diggs, Ahmann and Bibb	1,297	106	8.2
Ahmann	394	38	9.7
Total	2,831	230	8.1
Males			
Miyamoto and Korb	104	5	4.8
Graham and McCarty	556	50	8.7
Brandau	150	10	6.6
Diggs, Ahmann and Bibb	1,162	97	8.3
Ahmann	280	27	9.6
Total	2,252	189	8.4

frequency of demonstration of the sickle cell trait according to age for the entire group of negroes examined, including both the hospital and school series, is given in figure 2.

The youngest negro found to have sickled erythrocytes was a premature infant, and the oldest was 99 years of age. Twelve negroes who remembered incidents of slave days and the Civil War were still with us in spite of the sickle cell trait, which is rather definite evidence that the anomaly is compatible with life even beyond the period of life expectancy. These observations are not consistent enough to lead to very definite conclusions, but they suggest that the trait is least demonstrable in moist preparations in the newly born, most frequently observed in childhood and tends to decrease slightly with advancing years.

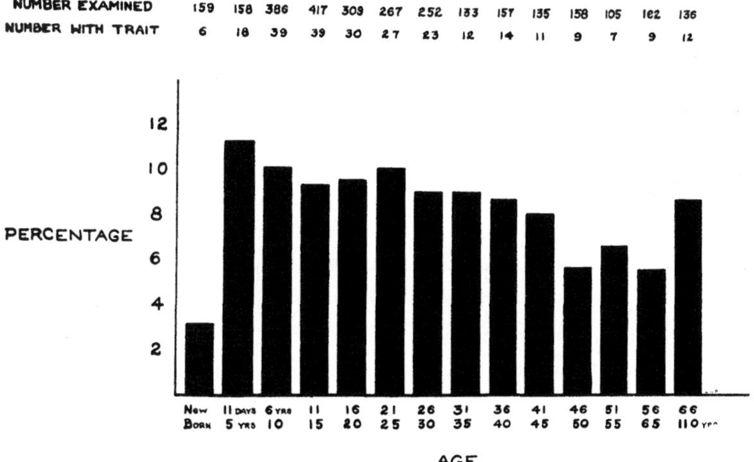

FIG. 2. The incidence of demonstration of the sickle cell trait in negroes according to age.

An evaluation of the effect of the mixture of white and negro blood on the incidence of the sickle cell trait was attempted by noting the frequency of occurrence of the trait in light and very light negroes as contrasted with dark and black types. It was found that 13.1 per cent (27 in 206) of the lightly pigmented negroes possessed the trait, whereas the percentage incidence in a comparable series of the deeply pigmented negroes was 7.1 per cent (51 in 701). The finding of an apparently significantly higher incidence in negroes with mixed blood than in pure negroid types must be confirmed before we speculate as to its cause, but it suggests avenues for further investigation.

In order to determine the effect of the state of health on the incidence of the sickle cell trait, comparisons were made of the frequency of occurrence of the trait in healthy negro school children and in hospital children of the same age. It was found that the incidence in the school series was 9.7 per cent (64 in 662) and in the hospital series the incidence was 9.8 per cent (44 in 450). These two series are not entirely comparable in that the examinations were made in different localities and the technic used was not exactly the same. Sydenstricker [11] demonstrated the sickling trait in 5.5 per cent of 1,800 presumably healthy negro children in the public schools, and Brandau [10] found that 6.7 per cent of 150 negro applicants for industrial work possessed the sickle cell trait. These figures are within the range of variation of similar series reported on hospital patients. From these findings we may conclude that a higher incidence of the sickle cell trait among sick negroes than among the healthy remains to be proved.

That the method of collection of blood may have an effect on the demonstrability of sickled cells is suggested by the fact that in a series of 823 preparations made with venous blood, sickled cells were observed in 10.2 per cent while in 1,716 preparations made with capillary blood the incidence was 7.4 per cent. It was found that the weight of the cover-slip was not a factor of importance in the determination of the sickle cell trait. Series of preparations made on the same patients, using No. 1 and No. 2 cover-slips, revealed a slower and a less complete development of the sickling phenomenon under the heavier cover-slip within the first few hours, but at 24 hours there was no consistent difference.

The Significance of the Sickle Cell Trait

A review of the literature dealing with the significance of the sickle cell trait shows that early workers [20, 21] considered the demonstration of sickled cells to be of definite clinical importance, but with increasing knowledge the general trend of opinion has been to assign to the sickle cell trait less and less significance. It is now generally conceded that the diagnosis of the sickle cell trait in absence of anemia can only be made by use of special methods such as the moist preparation or gas chamber, and that the history, physical signs and ordinary laboratory procedures do not give information which can be relied upon for recognition.[9, 10, 22, 23] Although many opinions have been expressed as to the significance of the sickle cell trait, there are few facts and figures. Observations made in our studies may elucidate certain disputed points.

Greenish-yellow discoloration of the sclerae is a common finding in patients with sickle cell anemia and is thought by some to be also characteristic of the sickle cell trait. The sclerae were examined in 438 negroes in our series on whom moist preparations were made. It was found to be extremely difficult accurately to describe the combinations of pigmentary change encountered. The sclerae of many individuals had background colors of gray, slate and brown, which were further complicated by black and brown macules, by dilatation of superficial vessels giving red appearances and by pingueculae. The sickle cell phenomenon was demonstrated in 28 and absent in 313 negroes who were considered to have scleral tints of green and of yellow. In 97 negroes with no definite discoloration, six were found to have sickled cells. From these investigations we come to the definite conclusion that the color of the sclerae in negroes cannot be used as a diagnostic aid in the detection of the sickle cell trait.

In order to determine whether patients with the sickle cell trait had leg ulcers more commonly than did those without the trait, the legs of 304 negroes were examined at the time moist preparations were made. It was noted that many negroes had scars and pigmentary changes of some kind on their legs, most of which could be accounted for by the trauma of barefoot years, industrial pursuits and superficial burns from huddling around fireplaces and red hot stoves. Only those cases with definite rounded scars who gave a history of delayed healing were recorded as positive. No open lesions were found. Of 258 negroes with no scars of the type found in sickle cell anemia, 21 (8.1 per cent) possessed the sickle cell trait, whereas within the group of 46 negroes with suspicious scars there were four negroes (8.7 per cent) in whom sickled cells were demonstrated. Although this series is too small and the criteria for judging the ulcerations too indefinite to draw conclusions, it does not support the idea that leg ulcers occur more commonly in those with the sickle cell trait than in normal individuals.

It has been generally assumed that negroes with the sickle cell trait have a tendency to develop anemia, but there is little evidence to support this idea, beyond the fact that a few have sickle cell anemia. Cooley and Lee [2] stated that " moderate anemia seems to be the rule among our colored children, and that there is practically no difference in this regard between those with and without sickled cells." Miyamoto and Korb [3] came to the same conclusion. Josephs [5] found no anemia in 16 children with characteristic sickle cell changes. In order to determine in a normal group whether or not those with the sickle cell trait were more anemic than those without the trait, hemoglobin determinations by the Dare method were made on 672 negro school children. Of 65 cases found to have the sickle cell trait, the highest hemoglobin reading was 103 per cent, the lowest 60 per cent and the average for the group 82.6 per cent. In the series of 607 without the trait, the highest hemoglobin was 108 per cent, the lowest 60 per cent and the average 81.4 per cent. Frequency distribution curves in percentage are given in graphic form. (Figure 3.) These findings indicate that the majority of individuals with the sickle cell trait are no more anemic than others in the same environment without the trait.

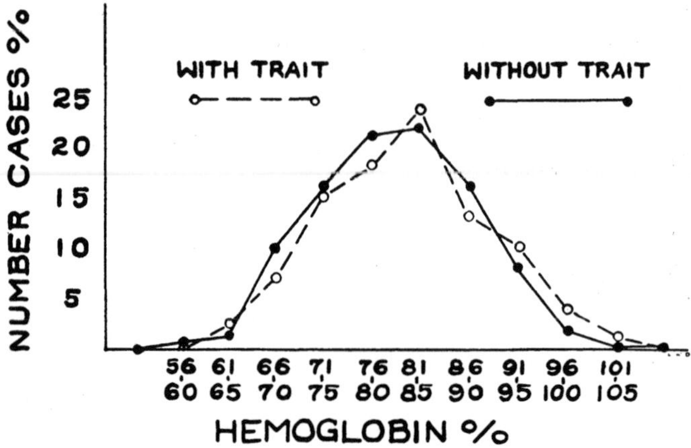

Fig. 3. Frequency distribution curve of hemoglobin determinations in 65 negro school children with the sickle cell trait and in 607 negro school children without the trait.

It is not as yet possible to estimate with any degree of accuracy how often sickle cell anemia develops within the group of those whose erythrocytes sickle. Severe cases of sickle cell anemia with characteristic symptoms and signs often are not recognized, and mild cases with less definite diagnostic signs are seldom detected. Sydenstricker [20] estimated that in hospital patients the ratio of anemia to the trait was one to nine. In a recent survey of school children, he found the ratio to be 1 to 50 and adds that " among children admitted to the hospitals and out-patient clinics the number is of course greater." On the medical and pediatric wards of the Memphis General Hospital during a 30 month period 14 cases of sickle cell anemia were recognized. Estimating the number of patients with the sickle cell trait as 7.4 per cent of the total number of admissions during the same period, the ratio of sickle cell anemia to the sickle cell trait is 1 to 40. These figures are merely rough estimates, but if approximately correct they indicate that sickle cell anemia is much more frequent than is commonly believed and that the number affected in the United States alone probably numbers in the tens of thousands.

Summary and Conclusions

1. The sickle cell trait was demonstrated by means of sealed moist preparations of whole blood in 8.3 per cent of 2,539 out-patient and hospital negroes examined at Memphis, Tennessee, and in 9.6 per cent of 674 negro school children and teachers at Gainesville, Florida.

2. The incidence of the sickle cell trait as demonstrated in moist preparations in the combined surveys reported in the literature and including the series reported in this paper is 7.3 per cent (619 in 8,453 examined).

3. The sickle cell trait has not been demonstrated in recorded surveys of white people, and the only reasonably proved instances of the sickle cell trait in families with unmixed blood have been limited to those of the Mediterranean stock.

4. Geographical location, sex and state of health do not appear to be factors affecting the incidence of the sickle cell trait.

5. In our series the frequency of demonstration of the sickle cell trait varied with age, degree of pigment and method of collection of blood, but the series are too small and the uncontrolled factors too numerous to draw definite conclusions.

6. That the sickle cell trait in absence of anemia is of little clinical significance is supported by the following observations:

(*a*) The trait is compatible with long life.

(*b*) The incidence in hospital cases has not been proved to be higher than in healthy individuals.

(*c*) Leg ulcers and greenish-yellow discoloration of the sclerae appear as frequently in those without the trait as in those with the trait.

(*d*) Hemoglobin determinations in a series of negro school children revealed parallel findings in those with and without the trait.

7. The ratio of sickle cell anemia to the sickle cell trait is estimated 1 to 40.

8. The importance of the sickle cell trait appears to be limited to the relatively small group who in addition to the trait have sickle cell anemia.

BIBLIOGRAPHY

1. Sydenstricker, V. P., Mulherin, W. A., and Houseal, R. W.: Sickle cell anemia, report of two cases in children, with necropsy in one case, Am. Jr. Dis. Child., 1923, xxvi, 132–156.
2. Cooley, T. B., and Lee, P.: Sickle cell phenomenon, Am. Jr. Dis. Child., 1926, xxxii, 334–340.
3. Miyamoto, K., and Korb, J. H.: Meniscocytosis (latent sickle cell anemia); its incidence in St. Louis, South. Med. Jr., 1927, xx, 912–916.
4. Wollstein, M., and Kreidel, K. V.: Sickle cell anemia, Am. Jr. Dis. Child., 1928, xxxvi, 998–1011.
5. Josephs, H.: Clinical aspects of sickle cell anemia, Bull. Johns Hopkins Hosp., 1928, xliii, 397–398.
6. Smith, J. H., Jr.: Sickle cell anemia, Med. Clin. N. Am., 1928, xi, 1171–1190.
7. Dolgopol, V. B., and Stitt, R. H.: Sickle cell phenomenon in tuberculosis patients, Am. Rev. Tuberc., 1929, xix, 454–460.
8. Levy, J.: Sicklemia, Ann. Int. Med., 1929, iii, 47–54.
9. Graham, G. S., and McCarty, S. H.: Sickle cell (meniscocytic) anemia, South. Med. Jr., 1930, xxiii, 598–607.
10. Brandau, G. M.: Incidence of sickle cell trait in industrial workers, Am. Jr. Med. Sci., 1930, clxxx, 813–817.
11. Sydenstricker, V. P.: Discussion of paper, South. Med. Jr., 1932, xxv, 620.

12. Sydenstricker, V. P.: Sickle cell anemia, South. Med. Jr., 1924, xvii, 177–183.
13. Lawrence, J. S.: Elliptical and sickle-shaped erythrocytes in the circulating blood of white persons, Jr. Clin. Invest., 1927, v, 31–49.
14. Castana, V.: I Gigantociti e le Anemie Semilunari, Pediatria, 1925, xxxiii, 431–440.
15. Archibald, R. G.: Sickle cell anemia in the Sudan, Tr. Roy. Soc. Trop. Med. and Hyg., 1926, xix, 389–393.
16. Stewart, W. B.: Sickle cell anemia; report of case with splenectomy, Am. Jr. Dis. Child., 1927, xxxiv, 72–80.
17. Cooley, T. B., and Lee, P.: Sickle cell anemia in a Greek family, Am. Jr. Dis. Child., 1929, xxxviii, 103–106.
18. Sights, W. P., and Simon, S. D.: Marked erythrocytic sickling in a white adult associated with anemia, syphilis and malaria; report of case, Jr. Med., 1931, xii, 177–178.
19. Rosenfeld, S., and Pincus, J. B.: Occurrence of sicklemia in white race, Am. Jr. Med. Sci., clxxxiv, 674 682.
20. Sydenstricker, V. P.: Further observations on sickle cell anemia, Jr. Am. Med. Assoc., 1924, lxxxiii, 12–17.
21. Graham, G. S., and McCarty, S. H.: Sickle cell anemia, Jr. Lab. and Clin. Med., 1927, xii, 536–547.
22. Steinberg, B.: Sickle cell anemia, Arch. Path., 1930, ix, 876–897.
23. Anderson, W. W., and Ware, R. L.: Sickle cell anemia, Jr. Am. Med. Assoc., 1932, xcix, 902–905.

ANNALS OF
INTERNAL MEDICINE

VOLUME 38 MARCH, 1953 NUMBER 3

IMMUNOLOGIC MECHANISMS IN IDIOPATHIC AND NEONATAL THROMBOCYTOPENIC PURPURA *

By WILLIAM J. HARRINGTON, M.D.,† *St. Louis, Missouri,* CHARLES C. SPRAGUE, M.D., *New Orleans, Louisiana,* VIRGINIA MINNICH, M.S., CARL V. MOORE, M.D., F.A.C.P., ROBERT C. AULVIN, B.S., and REUBENIA DUBACH, Ph.D., *St. Louis, Missouri*

THE mechanisms responsible for the low platelet count in idiopathic thrombocytopenic purpura are not well understood despite the careful studies by many competent investigators. The thrombocytopenia has been attributed to:

1. A decrease in the rate of platelet formation from megakaryocytes [1, 2] because of splenic inhibition of these cells; [3, 4, 5, 6]
2. An increase in the rate of platelet destruction by the spleen,[7, 8, 9, 10, 11, 12] and
3. A combination of damage to both megakaryocytes and circulating platelets.[13, 14]

Evidence to support the latter concept has been presented recently. A thrombocytopenic factor which damages circulating platelets and probably also suppresses the formation of platelets from megakaryocytes was demonstrated in the plasma of eight out of 10 patients with idiopathic purpura.[15, 16] In the present paper, observations are reported to indicate that the thrombocytopenic factor may be a platelet agglutinin, and that those patients with idiopathic thrombocytopenic purpura who do not have platelet antibodies develop their disease solely because of a deficiency in platelet production.

* Presented (in part) at the Thirty-third Annual Session of the American College of Physicians, Cleveland, Ohio, April 23, 1952.

From the Department of Internal Medicine, Washington University School of Medicine, St. Louis, Missouri.

This work was supported by Grant No. H-22 C (6) from the National Heart Council of the U. S. Public Health Service, Bethesda, Maryland.

† On assignment from the National Institute of Arthritis and Metabolic Diseases, U. S. Public Health Service.

The suggestion is made that idiopathic thrombocytopenic purpura is a syndrome which therefore may be caused by several different mechanisms. In addition, the rôle of the spleen in idiopathic thrombocytopenia is analyzed, the pathogenesis of neonatal thrombocytopenia is discussed, and evidence suggesting the existence of serologically distinguishable platelet types is described.

I. Case Material and Technics Employed

Thirty-five patients with idiopathic thrombocytopenic purpura have been studied. The diagnosis in each instance was made only after thorough examination of the peripheral blood and bone marrow, and exclusion of other etiologic factors. In 22 instances the syndrome was acute; in 13, it was chronic. There were 26 women, five men and four children. Pertinent data on each case are summarized in table 1.

In vivo and in vitro methods of investigation were employed. The former consisted of noting the effects produced by transfusing 500 c.c. of whole blood or its plasma equivalent obtained from 26 of these patients into volunteer recipients who were either normal subjects from the laboratory or patients with inoperable malignant neoplasms. Platelet counts, red cell counts, and white cell counts were followed closely in all instances. In some cases repeated observations were made of the coagulation time in siliconed tubes, clot retraction, prothrombin consumption, bleeding time, capillary fragility and bone marrow morphology. Reference has previously been made to the technics utilized.[15] The indirect method was used for counting platelets except in the animal experiments, as noted below. A decrease of approximately 50 per cent in the recipient's platelet count which persisted for from four to seven days was regarded as evidence for the presence of a circulating thrombocytopenic factor in the donor's plasma. Thrombocytopenia of greater magnitude was frequently induced.

The plasma of 31 patients was examined by an in vitro test for platelet agglutinins. The following reagents and materials were employed:

1. Silicone ("Drifilm SC-87," General Electric Chemical Division, Pittsfield, Massachusetts), diluted 1:10 with petroleum ether.
2. "Arquad 2C" (Armour Chemical Division, Chicago 9, Illinois).
3. "Parafilm" (Marathon Corporation, Menasha, Wisconsin).
4. No. 18 gauge needles.
5. Glass tubes 16 × 125 mm., 10 × 75 mm.
6. Micro test slides, depressed cell type.
7. Ethylene diamine tetraacetic acid, disodium salt ("Sequestrene, Na2," Alrose Chemical Company, Providence, Rhode Island). Five per cent solution in distilled water.
8. Citric acid, 1/3 N.
9. Whatman No. 50 filter paper.
10. Small glass funnels.
11. Large bore 1 c.c. pipettes graduated in tenths of a c.c.

TABLE I
Idiopathic Thrombocytopenic Purpura

Case No.	Patient	Age	Sex	Duration of Disease	Severity of Disease*	Therapy	Outcome	History of		Comments	Tests†		
								Trans-fusions	Preg-nancy		In Vivo	In Vitro	
												All Platelets	Some Platelets
Acute													
1	C. D.	39	M.	1 mo. 3rd episode in 10 years.	+	None	Spontaneous remission	−	−	Tests positive only during thrombocytopenia	+	+	+
2	R. S.	31	F.	10 mos. severe for 1 mo.	++	Cortisone Splenectomy	Suboptimal platelet rise. Remission	−	−		+	+	+
3	F. B.	51	F.	3 mos.	++	Cortisone	Incomplete platelet rise. Spontaneous remission	−	−	Tests positive only during thrombocytopenia	+	+	+
4	C. S.	48	F.	1½ mos. 3rd episode in 10 yrs.	++	Splenectomy	Remission	−	−	Autoagglutination demonstrated	+	−	+
5	B. P.	63	F.	5 mos.	++	Splenectomy	Remission	−	+	Transient relapse in four months	+	+	+
6	G. M.	35	F.	1 week. Relapse 5 yrs. post-splenectomy	++	Cortisone	Remission	+	+	Tests positive only during thrombocytopenia	+	0	0
7	E. T.	63	F.	6 weeks	+++	Splenectomy	Remission	−	+		+	+	+
8	L. P.	19	F.	2 weeks	+++	Cortisone Splenectomy	No response. Remission	+	+	Pregnant—baby thrombocytopenic	+	+	+

TABLE I—*Continued*

Case No.	Patient	Age	Sex	Duration of Disease	Severity of Disease*	Therapy	Outcome	History of		Comments	Tests†		
												In Vitro	
								Trans-fusions	Preg-nancy		In Vivo	All Platelets	Some Platelets
9	C. K.	6	F.	4 weeks	+++	Cortisone Splenectomy	No platelet rise. Remission	+	–	Also acquired hemolytic anemia with positive antiglobulin test	0	+	+
10	L. N.	68	F.	1 mo.	++++	Splenectomy Cortisone	No platelet rise. Remission	+	+	Also acquired hemolytic anemia with positive antiglobulin test. Autoagglutinins demonstrated	0	–	+
11	M. J.	32	F.	6 weeks	+++	Splenectomy	Remission	+	+		0	–	+
12	L. S.	59	F.	5 weeks	+++	Splenectomy	Remission	+	+	In vitro test only weakly positive after remission	0	–	+
13	F. C.	46	F.	3 mos.	++++	Splenectomy ACTH Cortisone	No change No change No change	+	–	Spontaneous though incomplete remission after 2 yrs.	+	+	+
14	M. L.	41	F.	3 mos.	++++	Splenectomy Cortisone	No change. Death, subarachnoid hemorrhage	+	+	No accessory spleen at post mortem	+	+	+
15	S. P.	17	M.	2 mos.	++++	Splenectomy	No change. Death, intracerebral hemorrhage	+	–	No accessory spleen at post mortem	+	–	+
16	M. W.	42	F.	2 weeks	+	Cortisone	Remission	–	–		–	0	0
17	W. S.	27	F.	1 mo.	+ +	ACTH	Remission	–	+		–	–	–

TABLE I—*Continued*

Case No.	Patient	Age	Sex	Duration of Disease	Severity of Disease*	Therapy	Outcome	History of		Comments	Tests†		
											In Vivo	In Vitro	
								Transfusions	Pregnancy			All Platelets	Some Platelets
18	L. J.	36	F.	1 week	+++	Splenectomy	Incomplete remission following Cesarean section and splenectomy	−	+	Infant normal	0	−	−
19	S. H.	19	F.	1 mo.	+++	ACTH Splenectomy	No effect. Remission concomitant with delivery	+	+	Infant normal	−	−	−
20	N. S.	71	F.	1 mo.	++	Splenectomy	Gradual but suboptimal platelet increase	−	+		0	−	−
21	I. B.	28	F.	1 mo.	++	ACTH Transfusion of platelet-rich blood	No response. Remission	−	+	Also moderate granulocytopenia. Normal survival of transfused platelets	−	−	−
22	V. A.	32	F.	1 week	+	Splenectomy	No response	−	−		−	0	0
							Chronic						
23	R. C.	7	M.	1 year	++	Cortisone Splenectomy	No platelet increase. Remission	−	−		+	−	+
24	B. T.	23	F.	8 years	++	Splenectomy	Remission	+	+	Gave birth to 2 thrombocytopenic infants	0	+	+

TABLE I—*Continued*

Case No.	Patient	Age	Sex	Duration of Disease	Severity of Disease*	Therapy	Outcome	History of		Comments	Tests†		
											In Vivo	In Vitro	
								Trans-fusions	Preg-nancy			All Platelets	Some Platelets
25	M. H.	34	F.	12 years	++++	Splenectomy	Suboptimal platelet increase	+	+	Gave birth to 5 thrombocytopenic infants. Auto-agglutinins demonstrated	+	–	+
26	H. S.	30	M.	10 years	+	ACTH Cortisone Splenectomy	No response No response No response	+	–		+	+	+
27	A. J.	29	F.	2 years	++++	ACTH Cortisone Splenectomy	No response. Death, subarachnoid and intracerebral hemorrhage	+	+	No accessory spleen at post mortem	+	–	+
28	D. G.	52	F.	7 years	+	None to date	Status quo	–	+	Autoagglutinins demonstrated	±	–	+
29	S. F.	8	F.	1 year	++	Cortisone Splenectomy	No response. Remission	–	–		0	–	–
30	V. G.	56	M.	9 years	+	Splenectomy	Gradual, suboptimal platelet increase	–	–		–	–	–
31	R. L.	27	F.	10 years	++	Splenectomy	No response	+	+	Intermittent granulocytopenia. No agglutinins against own platelets	–	–	+
32	J. B.	62	M.	1 year	++++	ACTH Cortisone Splenectomy	No response No response No response	+	–		–	–	–

TABLE I—*Continued*

Case No.	Patient	Age	Sex	Duration of Disease	Severity of Disease*	Therapy	Outcome	History of		Comments	Tests†		
											In Vivo	In Vitro	
								Trans-fusions	Preg-nancy			All Platelets	Some Platelets
33	M. S.	60	F.	10 years	+	ACTH Cortisone Splenectomy	No response No response No response	+	−	No agglutinins against own platelets	−	−	+
34	D. T.	38	F.	1 year	++++	ACTH Cortisone Splenectomy	No response No response No response	+	+		−	−	−
35	N. J.	2	M.	18 mos.	+++	Splenectomy	Gradual, suboptimal platelet increase	−	−		−	−	−

* Severity of disease: + = Easy bruising, few petechiae, no incapacitation or blood loss. ++ = Moderately severe purpura, moderate blood loss but no incapacitation. +++ = Severe purpura requiring transfusions to avoid incapacitation. ++++ = Severe purpura, severe blood loss, marked incapacitation.

† 0 = Tests not done. + = Positive results. − = Negative results.

Method: The citric acid, Sequestrene solution and platelet-free plasmas or sera are filtered prior to use. All glassware and needles which come into contact with platelets are siliconed. Needles may alternatively be coated with Arquad.

Ten cubic centimeters of venous blood are allowed to flow directly into a tube containing 0.3 c.c. of the Sequestrene solution. No syringe is employed, and only moderate tourniquet pressure is used. Prior to collection in the tube a few cubic centimeters of blood are allowed to flow into a gauze flat under the hub of the needle.

The tube is capped with Parafilm and inverted once to assure adequate mixing. It is then centrifuged at 200 G. for 30 minutes (1,000 RPM in an International Centrifuge Size 1, Type SB). One or 2 c.c. of supernatant platelet-rich plasma are decanted into another tube and placed in a refrigerator at 5° C. until used. This is the platelet suspension. A few hours may elapse before it is used. The remainder of the blood is centrifuged at 2,700 G (3,700 RPM) for 30 minutes. The supernatant plasma is platelet-free and is used as the source of antibody. Sterile serum may also be used 24 hours after blood has clotted at 37° C. in nonsiliconed tubes; 0.06 c.c. of the Sequestrene solution is added to each cubic centimeter of serum. The platelet-free plasma or serum is acidified with 1/3 N citric acid in a proportion of 0.1 c.c. of the acid for each 0.9 c.c. of serum or plasma.* Acidified serum or plasma should be used on the same day it is prepared.

One tenth cubic centimeter aliquots of platelet-rich (nonacidified) and platelet-free (acidified) plasma are placed in 10 mm. tubes, agitated, and either capped with Parafilm or covered with a moist towel. The tubes are then placed in a 37° C. waterbath for one hour and in a 5° C. refrigerator for two additional hours (or may be left for one more hour at 37° C.). Control studies are carried out with each platelet suspension in its own acidified serum or plasma. The tubes are then centrifuged at 200 G. for two minutes, tapped gently 10 times, and poured onto depressed-cell slides. Platelet agglutination is read microscopically under low magnification and graded 1 plus to 4 plus (figure 1). Sequestrene is anticomplementary in concentrations at least as small as four parts per thousand,† a dilution greater than that employed in this test. Therefore, lysis of agglutinated platelets would not occur if complement were necessary.

For titering purposes, 22 per cent bovine albumin to which 0.04 c.c. of the Sequestrene solution and 0.06 c.c. 1/3 N citric acid per cubic centimeter have been added is employed as the diluent. Globin, polyvinylpyrrolidone,

* The acidification procedure is a modification of the technic of Gardner,[17] in which 0.1 N HCl is employed to detect red cell panagglutinins at pH 6.5 in acquired hemolytic anemia. Citric acid has been utilized here for platelet agglutinins, because sodium chloride decreases the cataphoretic velocity of platelets and may induce spontaneous agglutination.[18] A final pH of 6.6 to 6.9 is obtained after the addition of platelet-rich plasma.

† We are indebted to Mr. Harold Ray, chief technologist, Bacteriology and Serology Laboratory, Barnes Hospital, for determining the anticomplementary activity.

Dextran and gelatin have been found to be unsatisfactory. Normal plasma and serum may be used after addition of Sequestrene and citric acid.

Slide testing anti-D serum caused prompt agglutination of D positive red cells collected in the manner described for platelets. Therefore, incomplete antibody is apparently detectable by the method outlined here and one other technic [14]; the remainder of those previously described [19, 20] were not designed for this purpose and only occasionally were performed in a manner which might detect incomplete antibody.

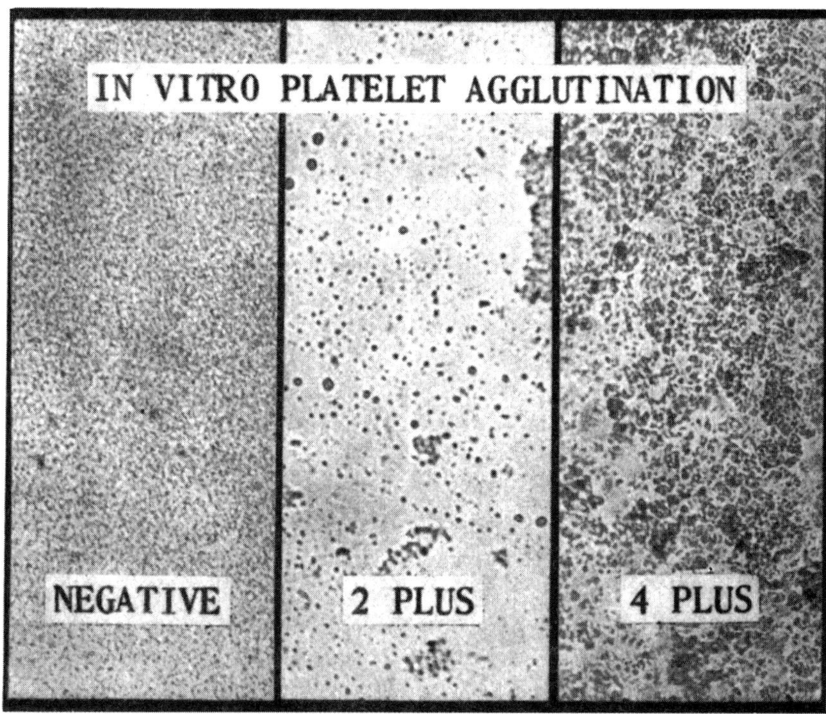

Fig. 1. Platelet agglutination as it appears at 100 × magnification. The degree of clumping is graded 1+ to 4+, as judged by both number and size of agglutinates, and number of unagglutinated platelets.

Nonspecific agglutination of platelets may be caused by unclean materials, poor or difficult venepunctures, and contaminated sera or plasmas. Rare red cells, white cells, droplets of silicone or neutral fat from lipemic plasmas do not interfere with the reading.

Other studies to be described required the preparation of anti-rat platelet serum. Blood was obtained by cardiac puncture from Wistar strain rats and pooled in 150 c.c. amounts in 3 per cent sodium citrate. The platelets were separated by differential centrifugation and washed three times in isotonic sodium chloride solution containing 0.3 per cent sodium citrate. The packed platelets were then resuspended in 6 c.c. of saline and kept refrigerated until used. One cubic centimeter of the suspensions was given intravenously at weekly intervals for five weeks to a rabbit of the New Zealand strain. Ten days following the last injection the rabbit was bled, serum was separated from the clotted blood and frozen at — 20° C. until needed. The phase microscopy technic of Brecher and Cronkite [21] was employed for platelet counts on rat tail blood.

II. Evidence for an Increased Rate of Platelet Destruction

The normal life span of circulating platelets is thought to be five to seven days,[22, 23, 24] and the "megakaryocyte ripening time" (i.e., the time required for immature megakaryocytes to mature and produce circulating platelets) is probably approximately five days.[25] Thereafter, any acute unsustained insult simultaneously affecting megakaryocytes and circulating platelets would be expected to cause a fulminant thrombocytopenia which would require approximately five days for recovery to take place.

In thrombocytopenia due to known agents [26] a "platelet crisis" [27] is induced in susceptible individuals within a few hours of administration of an offending drug, e.g., Sedormid or quinidine. In vitro studies have indicated that the low platelet level is due to an immunologic mechanism causing platelet agglutination and lysis.[28, 29, 30, 31, 32, 33] The antigen under these circumstances consists of a platelet-drug complex; the antibody is found in the patient's serum. An accelerated rate of platelet destruction is of major importance, therefore, in this variety of thrombocytopenia. Recovery usually occurs within one week following removal of the responsible agent.

Platelet agglutinins have also been demonstrated in vitro in the plasma of patients with idiopathic thrombocytopenic purpura, first by Evans [14] and later by others.[34, 35] Evans [14] specifically noted the desirability of designing his test to permit detection of incomplete antibody. In our series, plasmas from 31 patients with this disorder were studied in vitro by the technic described above. Twenty-one plasmas revealed circulating platelet agglutinins (figure 2). In addition, in vivo studies have demonstrated that most (but not all) patients with idiopathic thrombocytopenic purpura have a circulating thrombocytopenic factor.[15, 16, 36] When whole blood or plasma from patients with idiopathic thrombocytopenic purpura was transfused into normal recipients, a precipitous drop in the platelet count of the recipient occurred in 16 out of 26 instances (figure 3). At times the induced thrombocytopenia was associated with purpura and other clinical evidences of bleeding. The entire pattern of abnormal reactions of laboratory tests characteristic of thrombocytopenia was also noted: prolonged bleeding time, increased capillary fragility, decreased clot retraction, decreased prothrombin consumption, and morphologic changes in bone marrow megakaryocytes so that very little platelet formation could be seen. The depressed platelet level persisted for from four to seven days. Recovery was often characterized by a secondary thrombocytosis which lasted for several days. Red cell counts did not change unless there was blood loss. White cell counts varied, but an initial leukopenia followed in one or two days by a moderate leukocytosis was commonly observed. The platelet-depressing constituent in the donor plasma is a globulin,[16] presumably identical to the in vitro

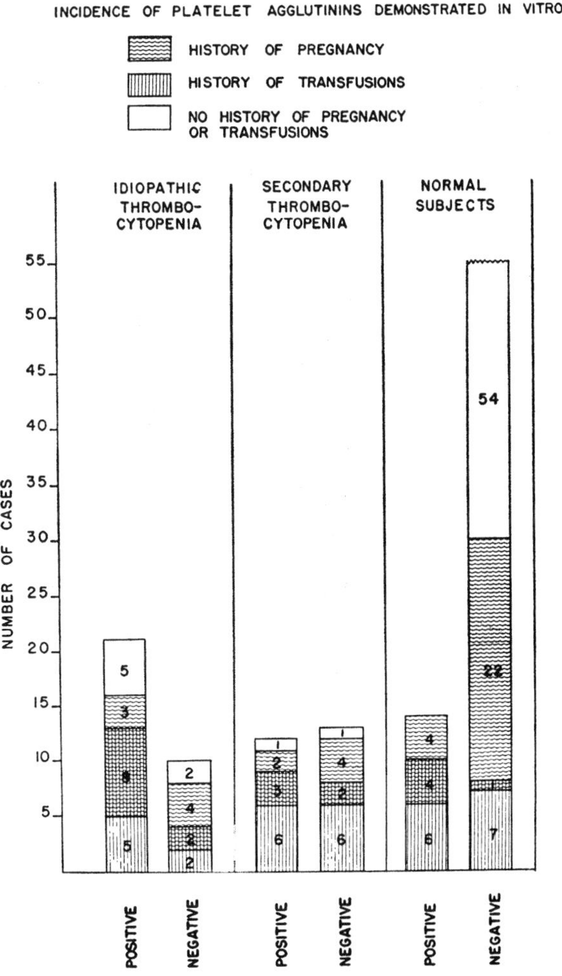

FIG. 2. The incidence of platelet agglutinins as demonstrated in vitro. Although agglutinins may develop as isoagglutinins in normal individuals following repeated transfusions or pregnancies, they may occur in idiopathic thrombocytopenia as autoagglutinins. However, many thrombocytopenic purpura patients have no agglutinins. The subjects designated as normal included a variety of disorders, e.g., refractory anemias, bleeding peptic ulcers, hereditary hemolytic syndromes, etc., in which there was no evidence of platelet disturbance.

platelet agglutinin, and presumably also capable of damaging megakaryocytes. In no instance has the in vitro test been negative when the in vivo test was positive. These in vivo observations have been corroborated [37, 38, 39, 34] and are remarkably similar to those obtained in animals by Ledingham,[40, 41]

Bedson,[42] Tocantins [43, 44, 45, 46] and others [47, 48, 49] in their classic experiments with heterologous antiplatelet sera.

A second type of in vivo evidence for a circulating thrombocytopenic factor has been obtained from observations in which the transfusions have been essentially reversed. Normal platelets transfused into patients whose

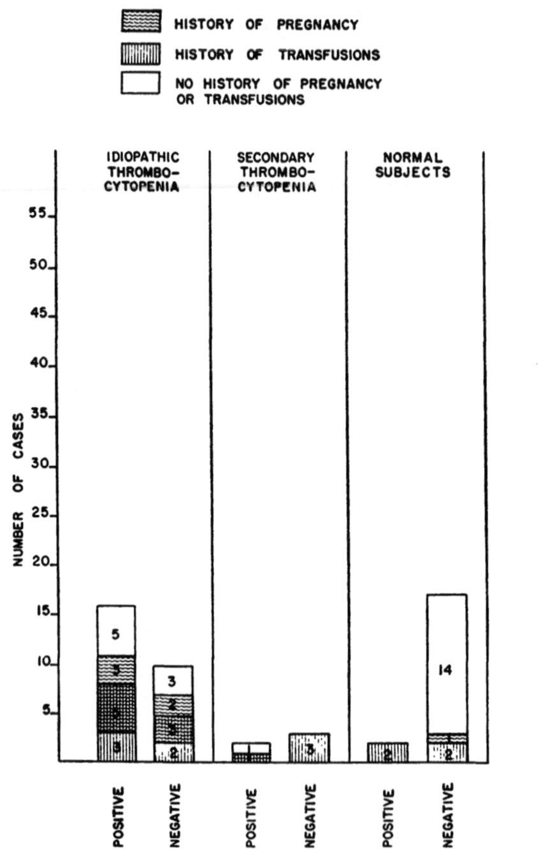

FIG. 3. The incidence of the thrombocytopenic factor as demonstrated in vivo. A low platelet count was induced in normal recipients of plasma from many patients with idiopathic thrombocytopenia, whether or not these patients had a history of pregnancy or multiple transfusions. Among normal individuals, only those who had received many transfusions had a circulating thrombocytopenic factor. The subjects designated as normal included a variety of disorders, e.g., refractory anemias, bleeding peptic ulcers, hereditary hemolytic syndromes, etc., in which there was no evidence of platelet disturbance.

thrombocytopenia was due to bone marrow aplasia remained in the circulating blood for from four to six days. However, when transfused into patients with idiopathic thrombocytopenic purpura, normal platelets could be detected for only a few hours.[50, 51, 52, 53, 36]

The following case is illustrative of the group in which a circulating thrombocytopenic factor has been demonstrated.

Case Report

Case 13. F. C., a nulliparous housewife, 46 years of age, was first admitted in August, 1950, because of petechiae, ecchymoses and epistaxes of one month's duration. Her platelet count at this time was 10,000 per mm.^{3} Splenectomy was followed by only a transient, suboptimal increase in platelets to 120,000 per mm.^{3} Within two weeks the pronounced thrombocytopenia recurred. Four transfusions of whole blood were given to her during this hospitalization. In October, 1950, transfusion of 500 c.c. of her whole blood to a normal recipient induced, within three hours, the entire clinical and laboratory syndrome of idiopathic thrombocytopenic purpura. The platelet count of the recipient was 800,000 per mm.^{3} immediately prior to the transfusion, 400,000 15 minutes later, 125,000 after one hour and 25,000 per mm.^{3} after two hours. The tourniquet test for capillary fragility was then noted to be positive, and the bone marrow, previously normal, now showed the changes seen in idiopathic thrombocytopenic purpura.[1–6, 54, 55, 56] The following day there were scattered petechiae on the lower extremities and a stool contained occult blood. An exchange transfusion of 2,000 c.c. did not alter the degree of thrombocytopenia. Recovery began on the fourth day and the platelet count attained a maximal level of 1,100,000 per mm.^{3} on the eighth day (table 2).

Table II

Effect of Whole Blood from Patient F. C. on Normal Recipient

Date	Patient F. C.		Recipient W. H. Platelets × 10^3 per mm.^{3}											
				After Transfusion of 500 c.c. of Patient's Whole Blood										
	Platelets × 10^3 per mm.^{3}	Agglutinin Titer	Before Transfusion	15 Min.	1 Hr.	2 Hrs.	1 Day	2 Days	3 Days	4 Days	5 Days	6 Days	7 Days	8 Days
10–22–50	0	1:16	800	400	125	25	. 0 .	15	35	117	260	320	675	1,100

Plasma from Patient F. C. contained agglutinins in vitro against all platelets tested.
Changes produced in the platelet count of a normal individual after transfusion of 500 c.c. of whole blood from patient F. C., whose plasma contained platelet agglutinins in a titer of 1:16 against the recipient's platelets.

These observations suggested that the thrombocytopenia in F. C. was due to an autoimmunologic mechanism. Cortisone was administered orally in a dose of 400 mg. daily for two days and 200 mg. daily for the next two weeks. A decrease in severity of her purpura was not associated with any change in her platelet count of zero, or in the effect of her plasma given intravenously to normal recipients. Furthermore, when her plasma was injected into a normal recipient who had been given ACTH (25 mg. intravenously every six hours) for one day preceding the transfusion, no inhibition of the thrombocytopenic effect was noted. Eighteen milligrams of nitrogen mustard (methyl-bis beta-chloroethyl amine hydrochloride) were given to the patient in an attempt to inhibit antibody formation,[57, 58] but an increase in severity of her bleeding manifestations developed. Transfusions of fresh, platelet rich polycythemic blood failed to increase her platelet count even momentarily[36]; also ineffective was blood from an individual who had previously been a recipient of her plasma. She was maintained for the subsequent 10 months on transfusions to replace blood continually being lost. In November, 1951, all bleeding stopped spontaneously, although her platelet count did not change significantly until June, 1952. She is now symptom-free, with a platelet count of 116,000 per mm.^{3} Thorotrast studies have not revealed any accessory splenic tissue.[59]

The evidence which indicates that a circulating thrombocytopenic factor, presumably a platelet agglutinin, is of importance in the pathogenesis of many cases of idiopathic thrombocytopenic purpura may be summarized as follows:

1. Platelet agglutinins have been demonstrated in the plasma of patients with idiopathic thrombocytopenic purpura; 21 of 31 plasmas caused agglutination of platelets in vitro (figure 2).
2. Transfusion of 500 c.c. of whole blood or its plasma equivalent from 26 patients whose thrombocytopenia was of the idiopathic variety induced a rapid and sustained decrease in the recipients' circulating platelet level in 16 instances (figure 3). When the bone marrow was also studied, changes in the morphologic appearance of megakaryocytes were observed whenever thrombocytopenia was induced.
3. The survival time of transfused platelets was markedly shortened in many cases of idiopathic thrombocytopenic purpura.

These observations support the concept that an autoantibody which damages both megakaryocytes and platelets is frequently responsible for the low platelet count.

III. Platelet Autoagglutinins, Isoagglutinins and "Types"

The incidence of autoagglutinins for platelets in the plasma of the patients studied cannot be stated for various reasons. The first of these is that all of the in vivo and most of the in vitro data were obtained by testing for isoagglutinins (i.e., agglutinins for human platelets other than those of the patient). Although the incidence of naturally occurring isoagglutinins is apparently negligible as detected by the technics herein described, immune isoagglutinins were found in the plasmas of 14 normal individuals after repeated transfusions or pregnancies (figure 2). All but nine of the patients with idiopathic thrombocytopenic purpura either had received transfusions or had been pregnant. Of these nine, five had platelet agglutinins and four did not. (Two of the four were tested only in vivo prior to the development of a satisfactory in vitro test, and accordingly are not included in figure 2.) Eight additional patients had no demonstrable platelet agglutinins, even though they had been pregnant or had been transfused. In four other instances it was possible to demonstrate autoagglutinins in the patient's plasma for his own platelets. Accordingly, it was in only these 21 patients (nine who could not have been isoimmunized, eight others with no platelet agglutinins, and four in whom autoagglutinins were demonstrated) that the presence or absence of a platelet autoagglutinin mechanism could be identified.

Secondly, platelet autoagglutinins are not always panagglutinins (i.e., are not necessarily active against all platelets, despite a strong agglutinating effect against the patient's own platelets) under the limitations of the technics herein employed. This fact was demonstrated in patients C. S., L. N., D. G. and M.H., whose plasma collected while they were thrombocytopenic agglutinated their own platelets obtained after recovery had occurred but did not agglutinate all other platelets tested (table 3).

There are also other circumstances under which platelet autoagglutinins are not panagglutinins. As pointed out previously, in purpura due to known agents a platelet-allergen complex is required for the antibody in the patient's plasma to cause agglutination. It appears likely that this mechanism is responsible for the thrombocytopenia in some cases designated as idiopathic, and that the allergen is not recognized. Under these circumstances the plasma would be expected to agglutinate only platelets similarly combined with an offending allergen. Additional evidence is obtained from the observation that transfusion of blood from a patient with purpura due to

TABLE III

Evidence That Platelet Autoagglutinins Are Not Panagglutinins

Plasmas Collected from:	Platelets from Individuals with Red Cell Group									
	ABO Rh	O +	O −	A +	A −	B +	B −	AB +	AB −	A* +*
Control subject		−	−	−	−	−	−	−	−	−
Patient L. N. during thrombocytopenia		−	−	−	+	+	+	+	+	+
Patient L. N. during remission (ACTH)		−	−	−	+	+	+	+	+	−

* L. N., platelets obtained during remission.

Data which illustrate that platelet autoagglutinins are not always panagglutinins. Plasma from patient L. N. obtained during her thrombocytopenia did not agglutinate all platelets tested, although it did agglutinate her own platelets. Her postremission plasma failed to agglutinate her own platelets, although it still agglutinated other platelets, probably as a consequence of isoimmunization from repeated transfusions.

Sedormid failed to alter the platelet count of a normal recipient who was not sensitive to Sedormid.[60]

A third reason for not being able to estimate the incidence of autoagglutinins for platelets among the patients studied is that information is only now being accumulated concerning the existence of serologically different platelet types. Patients who have frequently been transfused for anemia due to marrow aplasia sometimes have strikingly rapid disappearance of transfused platelets,[36] a phenomenon whose evolution has been noted during successive platelet transfusions.[51, 61] Immunization apparently occurs independently of ABO and Rh compatibility of red cells. Furthermore, transfusions of whole blood or plasma from donors who have repeatedly received blood for any reason can induce severe thrombocytopenia in normal recipients (figure 3).[36]

The evidence for immunologic differences in platelets from different individuals has stimulated an investigation into the feasibility of typing platelets. The "typing sera" consist of plasma obtained from patients repeatedly transfused for refractory anemia. The data obtained thus far do not permit any accurate estimate of the number or incidence of different platelet types, although eight serologically distinct ones have been identified. The approximate incidence of only one of these types (Type I, table 4) has been established by both in vitro agglutination and agglutinin-absorption technics. Among the first 110 consecutive persons tested, 18 per cent were found to have the same platelet type by both methods. Table 4 contains data obtained on 40 of these individuals collected on the basis of their availability for repeated study over a period of many months. Additional evidence for antigenic differences in platelets was obtained by immunization of a normal Type III recipient with weekly transfusions of 50 c.c. volumes of Type I whole blood collected in a siliconed syringe. After five weeks the Type III individual had definite isoagglutinins against platelets from individuals belonging to Type I.

TABLE IV

Incidence of Platelet Types

Platelets	Sera											Per Cent Incidence
	Control	1	2	3	4	5	6	7	8	9	10	
I	−	+	+	+	+	+	+	+	−	+	+	18%
II	−	−	−	−	−	−	−	−	−	−	−	20%
III	−	−	−	−	−	−	−	−	−	−	+	18%
IV	−	−	+	−	−	−	−	−	−	−	+	10%
V	−	−	+	−	+	−	−	−	−	−	+	8%
VI	−	−	+	+	−	−	−	−	+	−	+	5%
VII	−	−	−	−	−	−	−	−	+	−	+	5%
VIII	−	Five miscellaneous groups, each less than 5%										16%

The incidence of different platelet types among the 40 individuals repeatedly tested against 10 "platelet-typing sera."

Only Type I has been established by both agglutination and agglutinin absorption technics. Serum No. 8 was obtained by absorption of isoagglutinin on a Type I platelet suspension.

Figure 2 summarizes the data for platelet agglutinins demonstrated by in vitro testing. The majority of the cases of symptomatic thrombocytopenia were due to marrow replacement or aplasia. There were the following exceptions: three patients with disseminated lupus erythematosus (one positive), one infant with an extensive hemangioma of the thigh (negative), one case of postvaccinial thrombocytopenia in a child (negative), one patient with congestive splenomegaly (negative), and one man with disseminated miliary granulomas of undetermined etiology in the spleen (negative). Worthy of note are: (1) the frequency of isoagglutinins for platelets in any individual with a history of transfusions or pregnancy; of 26 parous women tested, four multiparas had strong platelet agglutinins for some platelet suspensions; (2) the absence of platelet isoagglutinins in normals who lack such a history, and (3) the spontaneous occurrence of agglutinins in patients with idiopathic thrombocytopenic purpura.

IV. Idiopathic Thrombocytopenic Purpura Without Evidence of Platelet Destruction

Fourteen patients, seven of whom were classified as having acute thrombocytopenia, had no demonstrable platelet agglutinins by the in vivo or in vitro technics employed. An increased rate of platelet destruction cannot be excluded in all these patients. In at least one instance, however (case 21), normal survival of transfused platelets was observed.[36] This observation suggests that decreased rate of formation of circulating platelets from megakaryocytes may be the sole mechanism responsible for some cases of idiopathic thrombocytopenic purpura. There are no obvious clinical features which distinguish this group of patients from that in which platelet agglutinins were identified. However, they did not seem to respond so well to splenectomy. Eleven patients in whom platelet agglutinins were not demonstrable had their spleens removed. Only one had a complete remission. Two experienced suboptimal increases in their platelet counts. One was pregnant at the time of splenectomy and developed a lasting remission only after delivery. In another pregnant patient, an incomplete remission followed combined splenectomy and Cesarean section. The remaining six were not benefited by removal of their spleens. In contrast to this, of 18 patients with platelet agglutinins who were treated by splenectomy, 11 had complete remissions, one had only a suboptimal increase in her platelet count, and six were not benefited (table 5).

Table V

Apparent Variation in Response to Splenectomy

Platelet Agglutinins	Number of Cases			
	Degree of Response			
	None	Doubtful	Incomplete	Complete
Not demonstrable	6	2*	2	1
Demonstrable	6		1	11

* Recovery probably attributable to parturition.

A tentative breakdown of the 29 cases treated by splenectomy. Because of the current limitations in detecting platelet autoagglutinins, and the numerical inadequacy of the series studied, these data can be presented as merely suggesting a variability in response to splenectomy. Patients without platelet agglutinins appear to respond less frequently than those with agglutinins.

The following case is illustrative of thrombocytopenia without circulating platelet agglutinins.

Case 32. J. B., a merchant 62 years of age, was studied in March, 1951, at which time his idiopathic thrombocytopenic purpura was of 10 months' duration. His illness was characterized by petechiae, ecchymoses and intermittent, severe gastrointestinal bleeding. Twenty-one transfusions had been required during this period, which were usually followed by a decrease in severity of bleeding manifestations for from four to six days. Transfusion of 330 c.c. of his plasma failed to alter the platelet count of a normal recipient (table 6), and agglutinins were not demonstrable in vitro against the 17 platelet suspensions tested. Cortisone given orally in a dosage of 300 mg. the first day, 200 mg. the second day and 100 mg. daily for the next 10 days produced no platelet response. Splenectomy was likewise without beneficial effect during a 12 week period of observation.

The evidence for a type of idiopathic thrombocytopenia due solely to a decrease in platelet formation from megakaryocytes is less convincing than that for thrombocytopenia due to increased platelet destruction. However, differences to be described between the newborn of mothers who have idiopathic thrombocytopenic purpura with platelet agglutinins and those who do not have the plasma factor support the concept. Also, the observation

TABLE VI

Data Illustrating the Failure of Transfusion of Plasma from a Patient without Platelet Agglutinins to Alter the Platelet Count of a Normal Recipient

Date	Patient J. B.		Recipient L. A. Platelets $\times 10^3$ per $mm.^3$				
	Platelets $\times 10^3$ per $mm.^3$	Agglutinin Titer	Before Transfusion	After Transfusion of 330 c.c. Patient's Plasma			
				1 Hour	3 Hours	1 Day	2 Days
3-11-51	8	Negative	446	441	427	392	463

Plasma from Patient J. B. contained no agglutinins in vitro against any platelets tested.

that lasting remission may follow transfusion of blood from a donor with thrombocytosis [53] suggests that in some instances deficiency of a megakaryocyte maturation factor may be responsible for the low platelet count. Patient I. B. (case 21), who had been thrombocytopenic for two months, appeared to respond to a transfusion of platelet-rich whole blood with a remission one week later.

V. The Rôle of the Spleen

There is general agreement that the spleen is somehow involved in the pathogenesis of idiopathic thrombocytopenic purpura, as the high remission rate following splenectomy is difficult to explain on any other basis. Difference of opinion exists, however, as to its exact rôle: whether it inhibits platelet production or removes circulating platelets at an excessively rapid rate. Evidence for the latter rôle has been obtained.

The first and most significant observation is that splenectomized animals are less susceptible to the action of heterologous anti-platelet serum than are paired normal litter mates. Although a sufficiently large dose of serum will cause thrombocytopenia in both normal and splenectomized rats, smaller doses will induce a rapid disappearance of circulating platelets in only the intact animal (figure 4). Previous investigators using guinea pigs and rabbits [62, 48] attributed the protective effect of splenectomy to the higher platelet count in the splenectomized animals. However, the data presented in figure 4 are representative of observations made on 14 rats splenectomized two months prior to this study, whose platelet counts had stabilized at normal levels. Under the conditions of this experiment it seems reasonable to assume that the spleen is an important site for the mechanical removal of antibody-coated platelets. A similar phenomenon was observed in several human subjects (figure 5). Transfusion of potent thrombocytopenic plasma caused fulminant, sustained thrombocytopenia in both normal and splenec-

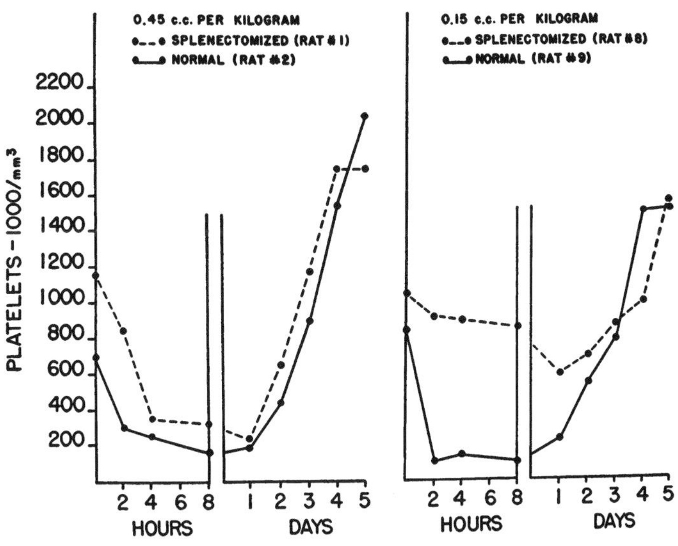

FIG. 4. Observations which indicate that splenectomized rats are less susceptible to heterologous anti-rat platelet serum than are their paired normal litter mates. Although a large dose of serum will induce similar degrees of thrombocytopenia in both groups of animals, smaller doses affect the platelet count in only the intact animals. Intravenous injections of anti-platelet serum were given at 0 time.

tomized recipients. Transfusions of relatively less potent thrombocytopenic plasma induced a low platelet count in only the recipient whose spleen had not been removed.

These observations suggest that (1) the spleen removes sensitized platelets, but (2) if the platelet antibody titer is high, platelet destruction occurs even in the absence of the spleen. They also provide a possible explanation for the failure of splenectomy to induce a remission in every patient, since high concentration of the antibody would cause continued abnormal removal of platelets even after splenectomy. Because the titer of platelet agglutinins was not being measured when most of these patients were being studied, the data are not available to determine whether therapeutic failures could be explained on the above basis. Six out of 18 patients with platelet agglutinins in their plasma failed, however, to respond to splenectomy. Platelet agglutinins persisted in the plasma of all six. When platelet agglutinins were found after splenectomy-induced remissions,[16, 36] their concentration was presumably too low to cause removal of platelets from the circulation in the absence of the unique circulatory bed of the spleen.

If the evidence is valid that the spleen is an important source of antibody,[63, 64, 65] then its removal would reduce production of platelet agglutinin

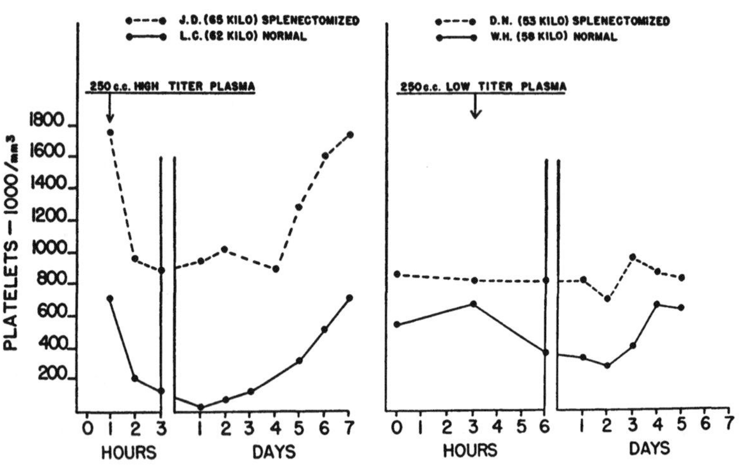

FIG. 5. The results of studies on the response of normal and splenectomized humans to transfusions of potent and relatively less potent plasma from donors with idiopathic thrombocytopenic purpura. Thrombocytopenia was induced in non-splenectomized recipients on all occasions, but in the splenectomized individuals by only the potent plasma. The scale is so constructed that the platelet count of the normal recipient of less potent plasma does not appear to have decreased significantly. The platelets decreased, however, from a pretransfusion level of 655,000 per mm.^{3} to 305,000 per mm.^{3} an unequivocal effect.

and assist in inducing a remission. The following case illustrates these effects of splenectomy in a thrombocytopenic patient with platelet agglutinins.

Case 4. C. S., a woman 46 years of age, was admitted in April, 1952, with a history of two prior episodes of purpura, one 10 years and one four months previously. There had been a recurrence seven weeks preceding admission. She had never been transfused or pregnant. Transfusion of her plasma into a normal recipient caused a significant, sustained decrease in his platelet count. Splenectomy was accomplished without administration of blood. (Five per cent glucose in water, saline, and 100 c.c. of 25 per cent serum albumin were employed.) Prompt remission occurred, although 10 days later a mild thrombocytopenic effect of her plasma was again demonstrated in the same recipient. One month later no such plasma effect was demonstrable. These data are compiled in table 7.

Lack of agreement concerning the exact rôle of the spleen has been due largely to difference in results obtained when platelet counts were performed simultaneously on splenic venous and arterial blood. Some investigators have found significantly lower levels in the venous blood,[66, 67, 68, 69, 10, 11] whereas others have been unable to confirm that observation.[69, 70, 71, 72, 73] The discrepancy may be attributable to a variable rôle of the spleen in different patients with idiopathic thrombocytopenia and also to the limitations inherent in technics of platelet sampling and counting. Significant differences in the two platelet counts would be meaningful, but since in any one circulation through the spleen only a small percentage of the total number of platelets may be removed, failure to observe a lower level in splenic venous blood would not necessarily exclude splenic sequestration of these

TABLE VII

Changes in Tests on Patient C. S. Following Splenectomy

Date	Patient C. S.		Recipient W. H. Platelets × 10³ per mm.³								
			Before Transfusions		After Transfusions of 300 c.c. of Patient's Plasma						
	Platelet × 10³ per mm.³	Agglutinin Titer	3 Hours	0 Time	3 Hours	1 Day	2 Days	3 Days	4 Days	5 Days	6 Days
4-14-52	0	1:32	680	700	465	450	240	265	720		
Splenectomy											
4-25-52	1,722	1:8	575	655	370	346	305	409	670		
5-27-52	1,251	Negative	429	455	400	693		465	493	474	585

Autoagglutinins were demonstrated for patient's platelets on April 14 and April 25 but not on May 27, 1952.

Observations on the effect in vitro and in vivo of the plasma of patient C. S. obtained prior to and 10 days and one month following splenectomy. The patient's platelet count promptly rose to supernormal levels, but both the in vitro agglutinins and the in vivo thrombocytopenic effect disappeared only gradually.

elements. Interpretations of data from studies of pulmonary removal of platelets may similarly be questioned.[74]

Among the 14 patients in whom evidence for increased platelet destruction was lacking, 11 were treated by splenectomy. Only one had a good response, and two were briefly, suboptimally benefited. The evidence is insufficient to attribute the single good response to enhancement of bone marrow function because of splenectomy or to the physiologic effects of surgical stress. As previously mentioned, two other patients improved immediately postpartum, possibly as a consequence of parturition. One of the patients had failed to obtain a lasting remission following splenectomy early in pregnancy. The other was splenectomized at term and delivered by Cesarean section.

The data available, although suggesting that the spleen functions by removing sensitized platelets, do not exclude the possibility that splenic inhibition of bone marrow megakaryocytes is of importance.[2-6] Recent physiologic studies which have demonstrated that splenectomy may be followed by increased erythrocytopoiesis[75] make more tenable the belief that thrombocytopoiesis may be similarly affected.

V. Effect of ACTH and Cortisone

In contrast to the frequent persistence of circulating platelet agglutinins after remission induced by splenectomy, remissions produced by ACTH or cortisone therapy seem to be associated with disappearance of the ag-

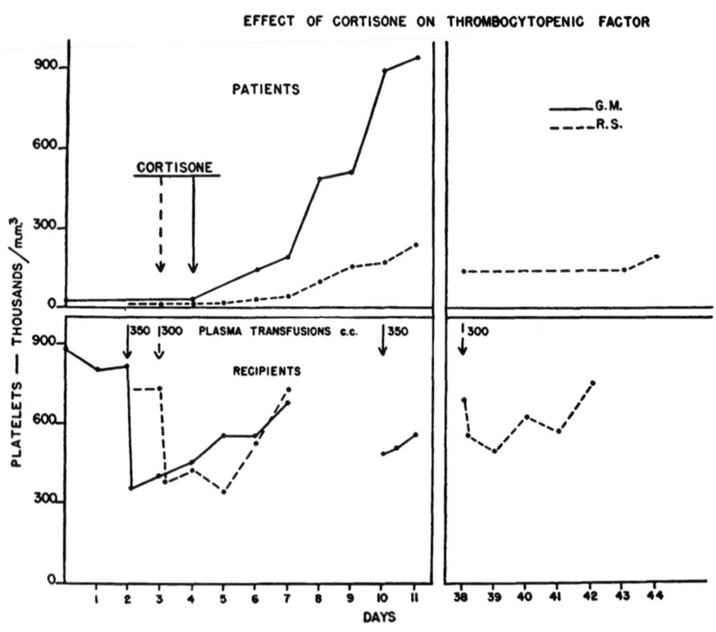

Fig. 6. Data on the effect of cortisone in two patients with idiopathic thrombocytopenia. Both received a similar daily dosage initially (200 mg.), and it was continued in 100 mg. dosage in both until the second plasma samples were obtained. The observations indicate that a complete remission from cortisone is associated with disappearance of the thrombocytopenic factor, and suggest that an incomplete remission is attended by only a partial loss of plasma potency. Patient R. S. later responded promptly to splenectomy.

glutinin.[16, 36] If it fails to disappear the platelet count persists at a low level or rises only slightly (figure 6). Collateral evidence for this rôle of adrenal cortical hormones has been obtained from animal experiments in which the administration of cortisone does not alter the thrombocytopenia induced in rats by the injection of heterologous antiplatelet serum.[76] Two patients in whose plasma platelet agglutinins could not be detected appeared to respond to adrenal cortical hormones (figure 7). Presumably the latter agents stimulated an increased rate of formation of circulating platelets. Until isotopic or other technics are available for evaluating the rate of platelet production and turnover, these effects of ACTH and cortisone cannot be established.

Decreased severity of purpura without an associated increase in platelet count [77, 78, 79] has been noted in a few instances.

VII. Mechanism of Spontaneous Remission

One patient, C. D., whose plasma contained platelet agglutinins detected by both in vivo and in vitro technics while he was thrombocytopenic, demonstrated neither phenomenon after spontaneous remission.[36] No data are

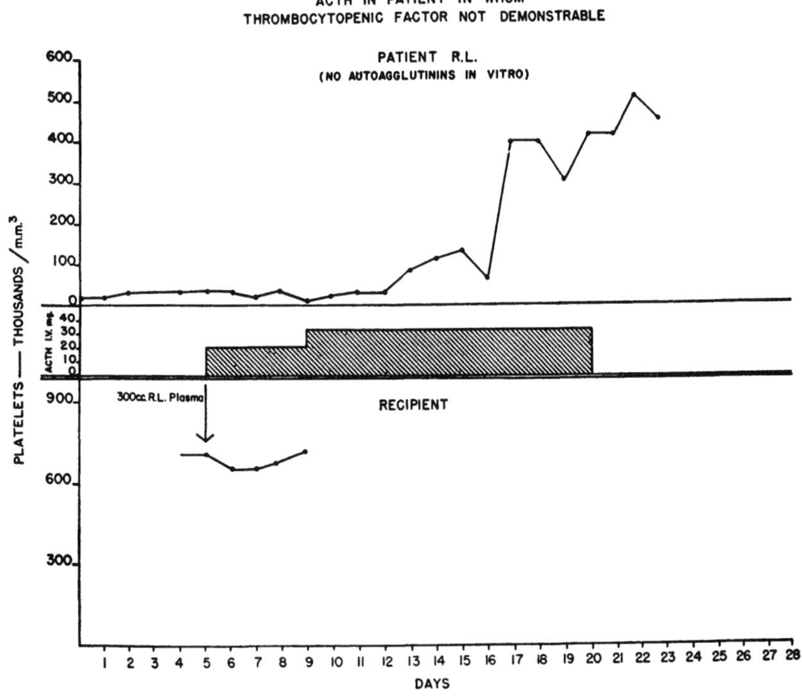

Fig. 7. A representative response to ACTH by patient R. L. On all four occasions on which she has been treated with ACTH her platelets have increased to normal levels within 10 days to two weeks. She has no autoagglutinins in vitro and no thrombocytopenic factor demonstrable by in vivo studies.

available concerning the mechanism of spontaneous remission in patients whose plasma has no platelet agglutinating effect, although one patient (R. L.), who had several spontaneous remissions, on one occasion recovered following an exploratory laparotomy, at other times seemed to respond to ACTH (figure 7).

VIII. Neonatal Thrombocytopenia

The literature on neonatal thrombocytopenia has been recently reviewed and evidence has been presented to indicate that "transplacental passage of some factor," [80] possibly an "immune body" or a "hormone," [81] is responsible for its pathogenesis. The technics described above were applied to a study of seven women who had had a combined total of 12 pregnancies in which either the mothers or the babies had purpura (table 8).

Three of the mothers had platelet agglutinins in their plasma, although two had normal platelet levels following splenectomy and the third had obtained moderate improvement from this procedure. All eight infants born to these three mothers had thrombocytopenic purpura. They illustrate one variety of neonatal thrombocytopenia.

Case 25. M. H., a housewife 31 years of age, was first hospitalized in June, 1938, with complaints of easy bruising for six years, menorrhagia for three years, recurrent epistaxes for six months, and menorrhagia for six weeks. A diagnosis of idiopathic thrombocytopenic purpura was made and splenectomy was performed, with a good initial result. Her platelet count, which had been 1,000 per mm.^{3} prior to operation, increased to 200,000 the first postoperative day and to 600,000 per mm.^{3} seven days later. Twelve transfusions were given during this hospitalization and an additional 12 during subsequent admissions. The patient was not seen again until January, 1941, at which time she was in the seventh month of her first pregnancy. In the interval since her splenectomy she had been well but for the recurrence of easy bruising. Her platelet count on the second admission was 87,000 and two months later, at the time of delivery, was 8,000 per mm.^{3} One week after delivery it had gradually increased to 490,000, only to decline to 36,000 per mm.^{3} two weeks later. On the few occasions that her platelets have been counted between pregnancies they have been in the range of 15,000 to 50,000 per mm.^{3} At term in her subsequent four pregnancies, the platelet counts have been 36,000, 7,000, 0, and 0 per mm.^{3} Purpura, of mild degree, has been present only during pregnancies. Deliveries have all been accomplished spontaneously at term, and on only one occasion (fourth pregnancy) has postpartum blood loss been excessive. In 1946 Thorotrast studies, and in 1949 abdominal arteriography, failed to reveal an accessory spleen.

Transfusion studies performed with this patient's plasma are shown in table 9. Her plasma was tested in vitro against 60 platelet suspensions and agglutinated 23 of these. In addition, autoagglutinins were demonstrable in vitro for her own platelets, and her plasma agglutinated the platelets of all four of her children so tested.

The patient has been married twice; her first husband died shortly before the birth of their first child. All five of her babies have appeared normal at birth but within a few hours have developed purpura. Pertinent data on each are given in table 8.

Once the platelets began to increase, in each case they rose from an average level of approximately 10,000 to supernormal levels in one to two weeks. Babies two and three were followed until platelet counts of 982,000 and 1,645,000 per mm.^{3} were attained.

Case 24. B. T., a housewife 23 years of age, had a diagnosis of idiopathic thrombocytopenic purpura made when she was 10 years old. Her complaints consisted of easy bruising and epistaxes for the previous four years. At the age of 16, her bleeding manifestations became milder, and during her first pregnancy two years later they were minimal. No transfusions had ever been required. In June, 1947, she delivered spontaneously at term. A platelet count during labor was 165,000 per mm.^{3} and there was no excessive postpartum blood loss. During the next five weeks her platelet count ranged from 71,000 to 149,000 per mm.^{3} Splenectomy was therefore performed in August, 1947, at which time she received 500 c.c. of whole blood. Thrombocytosis rapidly followed, her platelet count on the third and fifth postoperative days, respectively, being 1,600,000 and 2,800,000 per mm.^{3} There has been no further

TABLE VIII

Thrombocytopenia in Pregnancy and in the Newborn

Case No.	Mother								Baby									
	Name	Parity	History of Transfusions	Purpura		Tests*			Baby	Date	Sex	Platelet Count at Birth	Duration of Thrombocytopenia	Symptoms and Signs	Therapy†	Outcome	In Vitro Tests*	
				Present	Past	In Vivo	In Vitro										All Platelets	Some Platelets
							All Platelets	Some Platelets										
I. Mother and Baby Both Affected																		
25	M. H.	5	+	+	+	+	−	+	1	3- 7-41	F	zere	11 weeks	Petechiae, ecchymoses, gross and occult blood in stools.	4 transfusions	Complete recovery	0	0
									2	4-24-45	F	zero	7 weeks	Petechiae, occult blood in stools.	2 transfusions	Complete recovery	0	0
									3	8-21-46	F	zero	9 weeks	Petechiae.	5 transfusions	Complete recovery	0	0
									4	9-10-49	M	zero	12 weeks	Petechiae, ecchymoses, occult blood in stools.	5 transfusions	Complete recovery	0	0
									5	10- 4-50	F	17,000	9 weeks	Petechiae, ecchymoses, occult blood in stools.	None	Complete recovery	0	0
24	B. T.	2	+	−	+	0	+	+	1	6-27-47	F	zero	12 weeks	Petechiae, ecchymoses, hematuria.	4 transfusions	Complete recovery	0	0
									2	7-20-48	F	20,000	11 weeks	None.	None	Complete recovery	0	0
8	L. P.	1	+	−	+	+	+	+	1	10- 7-51	F	18,000	4 days	Petechiae.	None	Complete recovery	0	+

TABLE VIII—*Continued*

Case No.	Mother								Baby									
				Purpura		Tests*											In Vitro Tests*	
							In Vitro											
	Name	Parity	History of Transfusions	Present	Past	In Vivo	All Platelets	Some Platelets	Baby	Date	Sex	Platelet Count at Birth	Duration of Thrombocytopenia	Symptoms and Signs	Therapy†	Outcome	All Platelets	Some Platelets
II. Baby Alone Affected																		
36	E. M.	3	−	−	−	0	+	+	3	2-14-49	F	8,000	2 weeks	Convulsions, petechiae, ecchymoses.	None	Complete recovery	−	±
37	M. B.	2	+	−	−	0	+	+	2	3-27-52	M	Rare	8 weeks	Petechiae, ecchymoses, gastrointestinal bleeding.	Transfusions	Complete recovery	−	+
III. Mother Alone Affected																		
19	S. H.	3	+	+	+	−	−	−	3	5-17-51	M	268,000					−	−
18	L. J.	2	−	+	−	0	−	−	2	3-20-52	M	270,000					0	0

* 0 = Tests not done; + = Positive results; − = Negative results.
† Transfusions averaged 60 c.c.

Data on patients with thrombocytopenia in pregnancy or in the neonatal period. On the basis of these 12 pregnancies in seven women, it is proposed that the mother and baby may both have thrombocytopenia if there are maternal autoagglutinins for platelets, that only the infant is affected if isoagglutinins are present, and only the mother has purpura if no immunologic mechanism is demonstrable.

TABLE IX

Demonstration of a Thrombocytopenic Factor, Presumably a Platelet Agglutinin, in the Blood of Patient M. H., Mother of Five Thrombocytopenic Infants

Date	Patient M. H.		Recipient L. C. Platelets × 10³ per mm.³										
	Platelets × 10³ per mm.³	Platelet Agglutinins*	Before Transfusion		After Transfusion of 500 c.c. of Patient's Blood								
			6 Hrs.	0 Time	3 Hrs.	1 Day	2 Days	3 Days	4 Days	5 Days	6 Days	7 Days	8 Days
1-24-51	47	Not tested against L. C.	605	650	145	150	143	160	143	129	310	416	615

Autoagglutinins demonstrated in vitro for M. H. platelets.
* Positive against 23 out of 60 platelet suspensions subsequently tested.

thrombocytopenia or purpura. A platelet count done at the time of her second delivery, July 20, 1948, was 620,000, and her most recent count, in April, 1952, was 610,000 per mm.³

This woman's plasma was added to 12 different platelet suspensions and strongly agglutinated all of them. Both of her babies had neonatal thrombocytopenia. The data on these are given in table 8.

Case 8. L. P., a primipara 19 years of age, was first seen in August, 1951, at which time she was in the sixth month of pregnancy. Her complaints consisted of petechiae, hematuria and bleeding gums of two weeks' duration. ACTH intravenously, 20 mg. daily over an eight hour period, was associated with a gradual increase in the platelet level from zero, initially, to 76,000 per mm.³ after eight days. It then decreased again, however, and gastrointestinal bleeding developed. Splenectomy was followed promptly by a remission. One thousand cubic centimeters of blood were administered during the operation.

Transfusion studies were performed on the day of admission. The effect of her plasma on a normal recipient's platelet count is shown in table 10.

In vitro studies revealed platelet agglutinins against the 13 platelet suspensions with which her plasma was tested.

In October she was re-admitted and delivered of a baby girl. Petechiae were noted over the scalp and arms of the infant, whose platelet count was 18,000 per mm.³ The mother's count at this time was 1,235,000 per mm.³ Only one test could be performed with the baby's serum, which likewise revealed platelet agglutinins. Data on the baby are given in table 8.

TABLE X

Evidence for a Platelet Agglutinin in the Plasma of Patient L. P., Who Subsequently Responded to Splenectomy But Later Delivered a Thrombocytopenic Infant

Date	Patient L. P.		Recipient W. H. Platelets × 10³ per mm.³							
	Platelets × 10³ per mm.³	Platelet Agglutinins	Before Transfusion	After Transfusion of 300 c.c. of Patient's Plasma						
				5 Hrs.	1 Day	2 Days	3 Days	4 Days	5 Days	6 Days
7-27-51	2	Positive	725	410	420		425	513	586	760

It is postulated that the babies of these three mothers had neonatal thrombocytopenia because of transfer across the placenta of maternal autoagglutinins for platelets. It is true that isoimmunization to platelets could have occurred from whole blood transfusions, except for the first baby of mother B. T. Neonatal thrombocytopenic purpura is rarely seen in infants born to mothers who have never had thrombocytopenia, despite the frequency of pregnancy in women who have been transfused. Therefore, it seems more reasonable to attribute the low platelet counts at birth in these eight babies to the postulated mechanism of placental transmission of maternal autoagglutinins. The duration of the thrombocytopenia in the infants of M. H. and B. T. is of interest because of the much shorter course of the thrombocytopenia induced in normal adults in the in vivo studies previously described. This may be attributable to persistence of platelet agglutinins for many weeks in the plasma of the newborn, as has been established for red cell agglutinins in hemolytic disease of the newborn due to Rh incompatibility.[82, 83] Lozner, who for many years has been interested in the problem of congenital thrombocytopenia, is particularly impressed with the persistence of a low platelet count for an extended period of time in most cases of this disorder.[84]

An unusual variety of idiopathic thrombocytopenia of the newborn, which has been designated "primary thrombocytopenia,"[85] occurs without concomitant maternal thrombocytopenia or without a prior episode of this disorder which had been treated by splenectomy. In this variety, mothers who are in an apparently perfect state of health may occasionally give birth to infants with thrombocytopenic purpura. It is suggested that this syndrome may develop because of placental transfer of maternal isoagglutinins for platelets developed as a consequence of prior pregnancies with fetal and maternal platelet incompatibilities. Data to support the hypothesis have been obtained in two instances.

Case 36. J. M.,* a white female infant, appeared normal at birth in February, 1949. She had a convulsion the following day, however, and petechiae and ecchymoses were then noted. She was seen at this time by Dr. William C. Moloney, who established the diagnosis of neonatal thrombocytopenia. There was no evidence of any infection or metabolic disease to account for the low platelet count. Pertinent data on the baby are shown in table 8.

The mother was 38 years of age and in good health. Three previous pregnancies had been uneventful, and her current delivery had been accomplished without difficulty but for midforceps instrumentation. She had never been given any transfusions and did not have thrombocytopenia. Both the mother and baby had the same red cell type: O, Rh positive. There was no agglutination of the infant's red cells in albumin when tested against her mother's serum.

The mother's plasma caused agglutination of her baby's and of all six other platelet suspensions to which it was added, but caused no agglutination of her own platelets. Only equivocal agglutination of one platelet suspension was caused by the child's plasma when studied in February, 1952.

* Arrangements to study this patient and her mother were kindly made by Dr. William C. Moloney, The Boston City Hospital, Boston, Massachusetts.

Case 37. M. B.,* a white male infant, was first noted to have thrombocytopenia 14 hours after birth. There was no evidence of sepsis, syphilis or metabolic disease to account for the low platelet count. Two bone marrow examinations showed an adequate cellularity, with many megakaryocytes. Only a rare, abnormal platelet could be seen in the peripheral blood. Recovery occurred after two months.

This had been the mother's second pregnancy, the first having been in 1948. Both deliveries were accomplished by Cesarean section because of cephalopelvic disproportion. During the first of these the mother had received two transfusions. She did not have thrombocytopenia.

The red cell phenotypes of M. B. and his father were identical: Group B, CDe, MN. His mother's red cells were Group O, CDe, N.

Sera from the patient and both of his parents were added to 13 different platelet suspensions (table 8). The mother had platelet agglutinins for all of these, the baby for seven and the father for two. It was not possible to test either the mother's serum or the patient's serum from the thrombocytopenic phase against his platelets after remission.

It appears certain that both of these mothers were isoimmunized to platelets through pregnancy alone in one instance, and pregnancy or transfusions in the other. Reference has already been made to the evidence that such isoimmunization can occur by either means. Isoagglutinins in the maternal serum for the child's platelets were demonstrated in one case. Although it has not been possible to perform the critical experiment, to demonstrate agglutinins in an infant's pre-remission serum for his post-remission platelets, nevertheless the presence of isoagglutinins in the sera of both newborn infants makes it likely that they were there as a consequence of maternal transmission and were active against the newborn's platelets. In addition to the obvious similarities between this mechanism and that which is well established for hemolytic disease of the newborn due to Rh incompatibility, it should be pointed out that thrombocytopenia has been noted in some cases of the latter.[86] Concomitant red cell and platelet isoimmunization may therefore occur.

Further evidence in support of the theory that a variety of neonatal thrombocytopenia may be caused by maternal isoimmunization to fetal platelets is derived from the observations of Goldstein,[87] who studied the blood of fraternal twins born to a mother with no history of purpura. One infant had thrombocytopenic purpura with a platelet count of 63,000. His sister had a platelet count of 158,000 per mm.^{3} and no evidence of bleeding tendency. The mother had 182,400 platelets per mm.^{3} probably a normal postpartum value, although the author considered it subnormal.

An attempt was made to reproduce in rats the phenomenon of neonatal thrombocytopenia. Rabbit anti-rat platelet serum was administered to pregnant female rats a few hours before delivery. This was unsuccessful; despite severe purpura in the mothers, the offspring were normal. Apparently the heterologous platelet antibody did not pass the placental barrier.

Another experiment was then carried out. Platelets from six Wistar

* Permission to refer to this case was kindly given by Dr. Nathan Smith, St. Christopher's Hospital for Children, Philadelphia, by whom the sera were supplied for this study.

strain albino rats and six black hooded rats were pooled separately. Three females of each strain were then injected intramuscularly with the pooled platelets obtained from the other strain. Injections were given twice weekly for three weeks. The black hooded females were then mated with an albino male, and the albino females were mated with a black hooded male. No significant differences were noted in the platelet counts of the newborn of either species, though they suckled "immunized" mothers. However, no platelet isoagglutinins were demonstrable in the maternal circulation. No further attempts have yet been made to reproduce in animals the syndrome of neonatal thrombocytopenia due to maternal isoagglutinins for fetal platelets, although further studies along these lines are warranted because of the studies of Young et al.,[88] who were able to produce hemolytic disease of the newborn in pups, provided they suckled an immunized dam.

Two mothers had severe thrombocytopenic purpura at the time of delivery but had no platelet agglutinins in their plasma. The infants in both instances were normal.

TABLE XI

Data Which Illustrate the Lack of Effect on a Recipient's Platelets of 500 c.c. of Plasma from Patient S. H., Whose Thrombocytopenia Was Apparently Not Associated with Circulating Platelet Agglutinins. Although Purpuric Herself, She Subsequently Delivered a Normal Infant

Date	Patient S. H.		Recipient E. B. Platelets $\times 10^3$ per mm.^{3}				
	Platelets $\times 10^3$ per mm.^{3}	Platelet Agglutinins	Before Transfusion		After Transfusion of 500 c.c. of Patient's Plasma		
			2 Days	0 Time	2 Hours	1 Day	4 Days
3-19-51	4	Negative	1,485	1,551	1,330	1,400	1,255

Case 19. S. H., a gravida three housewife 19 years of age, was admitted in March, 1951, because of gastrointestinal, vaginal and nasal bleeding of one month's duration. She was in the sixth month of her third pregnancy at this time. Her platelet count of 2,000 per mm.^{3} was not altered by six transfusions. Transfusion of 500 c.c. of her plasma failed to alter the platelet count of a normal recipient (table 11).

Splenectomy was followed by a one week period during which there was no response, and eight additional transfusions of whole blood were required, after which her platelets gradually increased to 221,000 per mm.^{3} over the following seven days. She was not seen again until she entered the hospital for delivery two months later. She had experienced recurrent bleeding for several days, and her platelet count was 30,000 per mm.^{3} Cortisone therapy was instituted but the delivery took place a few hours later. Her platelets promptly rose to normal thereafter. The baby showed no purpura and had a platelet count of 268,000 at birth and 400,000 per mm.^{3} three weeks later (table 8).

Case 18. L. J.,* a gravida three housewife 36 years of age, was admitted in March, 1952, in her ninth month of pregnancy. She gave a history of epistaxes, petechiae and ecchymoses of two weeks' duration. Blood obtained on entry showed

* We are indebted to Dr. Harry Agress, for permitting us to study this patient's serum. The surgery was performed by Dr. Sam Schneider and Dr. Seymour Monat.

no platelet agglutinins in vitro against the six platelet suspensions with which it was tested. Her treatment consisted of simultaneous Cesarean section and splenectomy. Excessive oozing and bleeding were encountered during the procedure, but her hospital course thereafter was uneventful. Her initial platelet count was 89,000 per mm.^{3} A suboptimal rise occurred following splenectomy, and although she has remained symptom-free a platelet count in June was still sub-normal at 143,000 per mm.^{3}

The baby was entirely normal, and at no time showed any evidence of a bleeding tendency. His platelet count was 270,000 per mm.^{3}, and no thrombocytopenia developed during his first week of life, the period for which he was observed (table 8).

These two cases are considered to represent examples of maternal thrombocytopenia in which platelet agglutinins have played no rôle in pathogenesis, and as a consequence, the infants' platelets were normal.

On the basis of the few cases of thrombocytopenia in pregnancy and the newborn which have been studied, it would not be reasonable to imply that other mechanisms are not at times responsible and may not be of even greater importance than those postulated above. The data available at present do, however, suggest that:

1. If the mother has a sufficiently high titer of an autoagglutinin for platelets, so that the agglutinin passes the placental barrier, the baby should have purpura.
2. If she has an isoagglutinin for the baby's platelets, presumably developed in a manner similar to Rh isoimmunization and probably an incomplete antibody, the baby should have purpura.
3. The mother may have extensive purpura, but if it is not due to a circulating platelet agglutinin the baby should be normal.

Comment

The divergence of opinions about the pathogenesis of idiopathic thrombocytopenic purpura has already been discussed. Evidence summarized in this presentation suggests that the disease may not be a specific entity, but a syndrome which may develop as a consequence of more than one abnormal mechanism.[89, 9, 90, 91] It seems reasonable to believe that ultimately one may be able to attribute the disorder in some instances to a deficiency of a factor or factors necessary for platelet formation; in others, to suppression of platelet production by metabolic or splenic dysfunctions; and in others, to excessively rapid platelet destruction. Before such differentiation can become possible, better methods for studying rates of platelet formation and destruction must be devised.

A beginning, however, can be made. The thrombocytopenic factor which has been demonstrated in the plasma of many patients with idiopathic thrombocytopenic purpura probably causes accelerated breakdown of platelets. The evidence for this is two-fold: (a) the rapidity with which plasma containing the factor causes thrombocytopenia when it is transfused into normal recipients, and (b) the fast rate at which transfused platelets disappear from the circulation of patients known to have the factor. The thrombocytopenic substance may be a platelet antibody, since its presence seems to be associated with a platelet agglutinin. It is therefore presumably an immune body which might be expected to alter megakaryocytes as well as platelets, and thereby cause a decrease in platelet formation. Observations on the bone marrow of normal recipients who have been given plasma containing the factor tend to support that conclusion.[15, 16, 36] It is therefore suggested that the thrombocytopenia which occurs in association with the thrombocytopenic factor is caused both by abnormal destruction and by deficient production of platelets. On the other hand, in those patients with thrombocytopenia who develop their disease in the absence of a platelet antibody, there seemed to be only inadequate formation of platelets. Their plasma does not cause a lowering of the platelet count in normal recipients, and platelets transfused into them seem to survive normally.

The possibility that an increased potential for platelet production is induced in normal recipients of plasma from patients with idiopathic thrombocytopenia is suggested by the observation that supernormal platelet levels commonly followed the thrombocytopenic phase in the recipients. The nature of the vascular abnormality in idiopathic thrombocytopenic purpura needs further clarification. There is general agreement that capillary function is altered,[42, 77, 78, 92, 93, 94] but its relationship to the low platelet level has not been precisely defined.

Although the management of idiopathic thrombocytopenia has been facilitated by the use of adrenal cortical hormones,[95, 77, 96, 78, 79, 97, 98, 99, 100, 101, 102] many patients fail to respond either to this therapy or to splenectomy.[103, 104, 105] The suggestion is made that in some patients therapeutic failures from splenectomy result when a high concentration of platelet agglutinins persists after the operation so that rapid destruction continues in the absence of the spleen, and megakaryocytes continue to be affected by the antibody. In addition, it appears likely that the spleen is of less importance in the pathogenesis of the disease when platelet antibodies are not demonstrable. Methods for physiologically correcting the low platelet count are limited because of deficiencies in current knowledge concerning the processes which regulate normal formation, delivery and destruction of platelets. Furthermore, there is little likelihood that platelet transfusions [23, 106, 36, 107] will prove to be of value in the long-term management of most cases of idiopathic thrombocytopenia, even after platelet typing and cross-matching technics are more fully developed.

Summary

Evidence has been presented to indicate that an immunologic mechanism is responsible for the low platelet count in many cases of idiopathic thrombocytopenic purpura:

1. Platelet agglutinins have been demonstrated in vitro in the plasma of many patients whose thrombocytopenia was of the idiopathic variety.
2. A factor presumably identical to this platelet agglutinin is capable of inducing thrombocytopenic purpura and altering megakaryocytes in normal recipients of this plasma.

Remission following splenectomy is not necessarily accompanied by disappearance of the thrombocytopenic factor from the patient's plasma, a correlation which is seen in spontaneous remissions and those induced by ACTH or cortisone.

The spleen probably serves at least two functions in the pathogenesis of idiopathic thrombocytopenic purpura: that of removal of sensitized platelets, and that of producing some of the platelet agglutinin.

The lack of evidence for increased platelet destruction in some patients indicates that idiopathic thrombocytopenic purpura probably is a syndrome which may also arise solely from failure of megakaryocytes to produce circulating platelets.

Reference was made to the existence of serologically different platelet types.

Neonatal thrombocytopenia may develop as a result of transmission across the placenta of maternal autoagglutinins for platelets, or it may be due to development of isoagglutinins because of fetal and maternal platelet incompatibilities.

BIBLIOGRAPHY

1. Frank, E.: Die essentielle Thrombopenie. (Konstitionelle Purpura Pseudo-Hämophilie) I. Klinisches Bild., Berl. klin. Wchnschr. **52**: 454, 1915. II. Pathogenese, *Ibid.* **52**: 490, 1915.
2. Frank, E.: Die hämorrhagischen Diathesen, *in* Schittenhelm, A.: Handbuch der Krankheiten des Blutes und der Blutbildenden Organe, 1925, Julius Springer, Berlin, vol. 2, p. 289.
3. Seeliger, S.: Über Organbefunde und ihre Bedeutung für die Pathogenese bei essentieller Thrombopenie und Aleukie, Klin. Wchnschr. **3**: 731, 1924.
4. Limarzi, L. R., and Schleicher, E. M.: The reaction of peripheral blood and bone marrow in chronic hemorrhage and in essential thrombopenic purpura, J. A. M. A. **114**: 12, 1940.
5. Dameshek, W., and Miller, E. B.: The megakaryocytes in idiopathic thrombocytopenic purpura, a form of hypersplenism, Blood **1**: 27, 1946.
6. Dameshek, W., and Estren, S.: The spleen and hypersplenism, 1947, Grune and Stratton, New York.
7. Kaznelson, P.: Verschwinden der hämorrhagischen Diathese bei einem Falle von "essentieller Thrombopenie" (Frank) nach Milzextirpation. Splenogene thrombolytische Purpura, Wien. klin. Wchnschr. **29**: 1451, 1916.
8. Kaznelson, P.: Thrombolytische Purpura, Ztschr. f. klin. Med. **87**: 133, 1919.
9. Doan, C. A., Curtis, G. M., and Wiseman, B. K.: The hemolytopoietic equilibrium and emergency splenectomy, J. A. M. A. **105**: 1567, 1935.

10. Wiseman, B. K., Doan, C. A., and Wilson, S. J.: The present status of thrombocytopenic purpura with special reference to diagnosis and treatment, J. A. M. A. **115**: 8, 1940.
11. Wright, C-S., Doan, C. A., Bouroncle, B. A., and Zollinger, R. M.: Direct splenic arterial and venous blood studies in the hypersplenic syndromes before and after epinephrine, Blood **6**: 195, 1951.
12. Riveros, M., Torres, C. M., and Máas, L. C.: Lesões microscopicas do baço na purpura trombocitopenica idiopatica, Mem. Inst. Oswaldo Cruz **45**: 591, 1947.
13. Evans, R. S., and Duane, R. T.: Acquired hemolytic anemia. I. The relation of erythrocyte antibody production to activity of the disease. II. The significance of thrombocytopenia and leukopenia, Blood **4**: 1196, 1949.
14. Evans, R. S., Takahashi, K., Duane, A. B., Payne, R., and Lui, C.: Primary thrombocytopenic purpura and acquired hemolytic anemia; evidence for a common etiology, Arch. Int. Med. **87**: 48, 1951.
15. Harrington, W. J., Hollingsworth, J. W., Minnich, V., and Moore, C. V.: Demonstration of a thrombocytopenic factor in the blood of patients with idiopathic thrombocytopenic purpura, J. Clin. Investigation **30**: 646, 1951 (abstract).
16. Harrington, W. J., Minnich, V., Hollingsworth, J. W., and Moore, C. V.: Demonstration of a thrombocytopenic factor in the blood of patients with thrombocytopenic purpura, J. Lab. and Clin. Med. **38**: 1, 1951.
17. Gardner, F. H.: Transfer to normal red cells of an agglutinin demonstrable in the the acidified sera of patients with acquired hemolytic jaundice, J. Clin. Investigation **28**: 783, 1949 (abstract).
18. Starlinger, W., and Sametnik, S.: Über die Entstehungsbedingungen der spontanen Venenthrombose, Klin. Wchnschr. **6**: 1269, 1927.
19. Toda, T.: The relationship of the blood platelet and red corpuscles: an attempt to group human platelets with red-cell grouping sera, J. Path. and Bact. **26**: 303, 1923.
20. Stefanini, M., and Silverberg, J. H.: Studies on platelets. I. The relationship of platelet agglutination to the mechanism of blood coagulation, Am. J. Clin. Path. **21**: 1030, 1951.
21. Brecher, G., and Cronkite, E. P.: Morphology and enumeration of human blood platelets, J. Appl. Physiol. **3**: 365, 1950.
22. Lawrence, J. S., and Valentine, W. N.: The blood platelets. The rate of their utilization in the cat, Blood **2**: 40, 1947.
23. Hirsch, E. O., Favre-Gilly, J., and Dameshek, W.: Thrombopathic thrombocytopenia: successful transfusion of blood platelets, Blood **5**: 568, 1950.
24. Favre-Gilly, J., Hirsch, E. O., Dameshek, W., and Pratt, J.: Succès d'une transfusion de sang par seringue siliconée dans une cas de thrombocytopathie hémorrhagique. Intérêt du silicone pour la survie des plaquettes après transfusion, Sang **21**: 681, 1950.
25. Moeschlin, S.: Personal communication.
26. Madison, F. W.: The role of allergy in the pathogenesis of purpura and thrombocytopenia, Blood **3**: 1083, 1948.
27. Smith, C. M.: Severe bleeding and purpura following the administration of neoarsphenamin, Arch. Dermat. and Syph. **11**: 237, 1925.
28. Grandjean, L. C.: A case of purpura haemorrhagica after administration of quinine with specific thrombocytolysis demonstrated *in vitro,* Acta med. Scandinav. (supp. 213) **131**: 165, 1948.
29. Ackroyd, J. F.: The pathogenesis of thrombocytopenic purpura due to hypersensitivity to Sedormid, Clin. Sc. **7**: 249, 1949.
30. Graudal, H.: Thrombopeni efter allymid (aetyl-allyl-acetyl-karbamid), Ugesk. f. læger **111**: 958, 1949.
31. Ackroyd, J. F.: The role of complement in Sedormid purpura, Clin. Sc. **10**: 185, 1951.
32. Ackroyd, J. F.: Sedormid purpura: an immunologic study of a form of drug hypersensitivity, Prog. in Allergy **3**: 531, 1952.

33. Bigelow, F. S., and Desforges, J. F.: Platelet agglutination by an abnormal plasma factor in thrombocytopenic purpura associated with quinidine ingestion, Am. J. M. Sc. **224**: 274, 1952.

34. Stefanini, M., Chatterjea, J. B., and Adelson, E.: Immunologic aspects of idiopathic thrombocytopenic purpura, J. Clin. Investigation **31**: 665, 1952 (abstract).

35. Dausset, J., Delafontaine, P., and Fleuriot, Y.: Agglutination et destruction "in vitro" des plaquettes normales par le sérum d'une malade atteinte de purpura thrombopénique aigu. Inhibition par ce sérum de la rétraction du caillot normal, Sang **23**: 373, 1952.

36. Sprague, C. C., Harrington, W. J., Lange, R. D., and Shapleigh, J. B.: Platelet transfusions and the pathogenesis of idiopathic thrombocytopenic purpura, J. A. M. A. **150**: 1193, 1952.

37. Jamra, M.: Personal communication.

38. Kissmeyer-Nielsen, F.: Personal communication.

39. Diamond, L. K.: Personal communication.

40. Ledingham, J. C. G.: The experimental production of purpura in animals, Lancet **1**: 1673, 1914.

41. Ledingham, J. C. G., and Bedson, S. P.: Experimental purpura, Lancet **1**: 311, 1915.

42. Bedson, S. P.: Blood platelet anti-serum, its specificity and role in the experimental production of purpura, J. Path. and Bact. **25**: 94, 1922.

43. Tocantins, L. M.: Experimental thrombopenic purpura in the dog, Arch. Path. **21**: 69, 1936.

44. Tocantins, L. M.: Experimental thrombopenic purpura; cytological and physical changes in the blood, Ann. Int. Med. **9**: 838, 1936.

45. Tocantins, L. M.: The mammalian blood platelet in health and disease, Medicine **17**: 155, 1938.

46. Tocantins, L. M., and Stewart, H. L.: Pathological anatomy of experimental thrombopenic purpura in the dog, Am. J. Path. **15**: 1, 1939.

47. Lee, R. I., and Robertson, O. H.: The effect of antiplatelet serum on blood platelets and the experimental production of purpura hemorrhagica, J. M. Research **33**: 323, 1916.

48. Elliott, R. H. E., Jr., and Whipple, M. A.: Observations on the interrelationship of capillary, platelet, and splenic factors in thrombocytopenic purpura, J. Lab. and Clin. Med. **26**: 489, 1940.

49. Leonard, M. E., and Falconer, E. H.: Experimental thrombocytopenic purpura in the guinea pig, J. Lab. and Clin. Med. **26**: 648, 1941.

50. Hirsch, E. O., and Gardner, F. H.: The life span of transfused human blood platelets, J. Clin. Investigation **30**: 649, 1951 (abstract).

51. Hirsch, E. O., and Gardner, F. H.: The transfusion of human blood platelets, J. Lab. and Clin. Med. **39**: 556, 1952.

52. Stefanini, M., and Chatterjea, J. B.: Rate of platelet survival in thrombocytopenia, J. Clin. Investigation **30**: 676, 1951 (abstract).

53. Stefanini, M., Chatterjea, J. B., Dameshek, W., Zannos, L., and Perez Santiago, E.: Studies on platelets. II. The effect of transfusion of platelet-rich polycythemic blood on the platelets and hemostatic function in "idiopathic" and "secondary" thrombocytopenic purpura, Blood **7**: 53, 1952.

54. Diggs, L. W., and Hewlett, J. S.: A study of the bone marrow from thirty-six patients with idiopathic hemorrhagic (thrombopenic) purpura, Blood **3**: 1090, 1948.

55. de la Fuente, V.: Megakaryocytes in normal and in thrombocytopenic individuals, Blood **4**: 614, 1949.

56. Kissmeyer-Nielsen, F.: A study of the thrombopoiesis in various thrombopenic states. II. Idiopathic thrombopenic purpura, Acta med. Scandinav. **141**: 205, 1951.

57. Bukantz, S. C., Dammin, G. J., Wilson, K. S., and Johnson, M. C.: The inhibitory effect of nitrogen mustard (bis beta-chloroethyl amine) on the development of

humoral antibodies, cutaneous hypersensitiveness, and vascular lesions in rabbits following injections of horse serum (abstract), J. Lab. and Clin. Med. **33**: 1463, 1948.

58. Dameshek, W., Rosenthal, M. C., and Schwartz, L. I.: The treatment of acquired hemolytic anemia with adrenocorticotrophic hormone (ACTH), New England J. Med. **244**: 117, 1951.
59. Loeb, V., Jr., Seaman, W. B., and Moore, C. V.: The use of thorium dioxide sol (thorotrast) in the roentgenologic demonstration of accessory spleens, Blood **7**: 904, 1952.
60. Moeschlin, S.: Die Sedormid—Thrombozytopenie anhand von Sternalpunktaten, Belastungs und Transfusionsversuchen, Schweiz. med. Wchnschr. **72**: 119, 1942.
61. Stefanini, M., Dameshek, W., and Adelson, E.: Platelets. VII. Shortened "platelet survival time" and development of platelet agglutinins following multiple platelet transfusions, Proc. Soc. Exper. Biol. and Med. **80**: 230, 1952.
62. Bedson, S. P.: The effect of splenectomy on the production of experimental purpura, Lancet **2**: 1117, 1924.
63. Wagley, P. F., Shen, S. C., Gardner, F. H., and Castle, W. B.: Studies on the destruction of red blood cells. VI. The spleen as a source of a substance causing agglutination of the red blood cells of certain patients with acquired hemolytic jaundice by an antihuman serum rabbit serum (Coomb's serum), J. Lab. and Clin. Med. **33**: 1197, 1948.
64. Rowley, D. A.: The effect of splenectomy on the formation of circulating antibody in the adult male albino rat, J. Immunol. **64**: 289, 1950.
65. Rowley, D. A.: The formation of circulating antibody in the splenectomized human being following intravenous injection of heterologous erythrocytes, J. Immunol. **65**: 515, 1950.
66. Cori, G.: Zur Klinik und Therapie (Splenektomie) der essentiellen Thrombopenie, Ztschr. f. klin. Med. **94**: 356, 1922.
67. Myers, B., Maingot, R., and Gordon, A. K.: Three cases of splenectomy for essential thrombocytopenic purpura haemorrhagica, Proc. Roy. Soc. Med. **19**: 37 (March 12) 1926.
68. Howell, W. H., and Donahue, D. D.: Production of blood platelets in the lungs, J. Exper. Med. **65**: 177, 1937.
69. Holloway, J. K., and Blackford, L. M.: Comparison of the blood-platelet count in splenic arterial and venous blood, Am. J. M. Sc. **168**: 723, 1924.
70. Tsunashima, Y.: Cited by Tocantins.[45]
71. König, W.: Experimentelle Untersuchungen über die Entstehung der Thrombose. Ein Beitrag zur Lehre von den Blutplättchen, Arch. f. klin. Chir. **171**: 447, 1932.
72. Cumings, J. N.: A method for the enumeration of blood-platelets, Lancet **1**: 1230, 1933.
73. Stefanini, M., Chatterjea, J. B., Dameshek, W., Welch, C. S., and Swenson, O.: Studies on platelets. III. The absence of "selective sequestration" and destruction of platelets by the spleen in "idiopathic" thrombocytopenic purpura, Blood **7**: 289, 1952.
74. Stefanini, M., Chatterjea, J. B., and Dameshek, W.: Studies on platelets. V. Observations on the removal by the pulmonary circulation of platelets injected into patients with idiopathic thrombocytopenic purpura, J. Lab. and Clin. Med. **39**: 865, 1952.
75. Loeb, V., Jr., Moore, C. V., and Dubach, R.: The physiologic evaluation and management of chronic bone marrow failure, Am. J. Med., in press.
76. Spaet, T. H., and Mednicoff, I.: The effect of cortisone on artificially induced thrombocytopenic purpura in rats, Bull. New England M. Center **13**: 201, 1951.
77. Robson, H. N., and Duthie, J. J. R.: Capillary resistance and adrenocortical activity, Brit. M. J. **2**: 971, 1950.
78. Faloon, W. W., Greene, R. W., and Lozner, E. L.: The hemostatic defect in thrombocytopenia as studied by the use of ACTH and cortisone, Am. J. Med. **13**: 12, 1952.
79. Evans, R. S., and Lui, C. K.: Effect of corticotrophin on chronic severe primary thrombocytopenic purpura, Arch. Int. Med. **88**: 503, 1951.

80. Robson, H. N., and Davidson, L. S. P.: Purpura in pregnancy with special reference to idiopathic thrombocytopenic purpura, Lancet **2**: 164, 1950.
81. Epstein, R. D., Lozner, E. L., Coffey, T. S., and Davidson, C. S.: Congenital thrombocytopenic purpura. Purpura hemorrhagica in pregnancy and in the newborn, Am. J. Med. **9**: 44, 1950.
82. Wiener, A. S.: Rh factor in immunological reactions, Ann. Allergy **6**: 293, 1948.
83. Mollison, P. L., and Cutbush, M.: Haemolytic disease of the newborn: criteria of severity, Brit. M. J. **1**: 123, 1949.
84. Lozner, E. L.: Personal communication.
85. La Driere, R. J.: Thrombocytopenia of the newborn, South. M. J. **44**: 355, 1951.
86. Blackfan, K. D., and Diamond, L. K.: Atlas of the blood in children, 1944, The Commonwealth Fund, New York, p. 90.
87. Goldstein, L. S.: Congenital essential thrombopenic purpura. Report of condition in fraternal twins, Am. J. Dis. Child. **73**: 575, 1947.
88. Young, L. E., Christian, R. M., Ervin, D. M., Davis, R. W., O'Brien, W. A., Swisher, S. N., and Yuile, C. L.: Hemolytic disease in newborn dogs, Blood **6**: 291, 1951.
89. Minot, G. R.: Diminished blood platelets and marrow insufficiency, Arch. Int. Med. **19**: 1062, 1917.
90. Moore, C. V.: Discussion of paper of Limarzi and Schleicher.[4]
91. Dameshek, W.: The "humors" and idiopathic thrombocytopenic purpura, Blood **6**: 954, 1951.
92. Macfarlane, R. G.: Critical review: The mechanism of haemostasis, Quart. J. Med. **10**: 1, 1941.
93. Humble, J. G.: The mechanism of petechial hemorrhage formation, Blood **4**: 69, 1949.
94. Robson, H. N.: Idiopathic thrombocytopenic purpura, Quart. J. Med. **18**: 279, 1949.
95. Meyers, M. C., Miller, S., and Bethell, F. H.: Administration of ACTH in hypersplenic syndromes, J. Lab. and Clin. Med. **36**: 965, 1950 (abstract).
96. Wintrobe, M. M., Cartwright, G. E., Kuhns, W. J., Palmer, J. G., and Lahey, M. E.: The effects of ACTH on the hematopoietic system, Blood Club Proceedings, Blood **5**: 789, 1950.
97. Bethell, F. H., Miller, S., and Meyers, M. C.: Administration of ACTH and cortisone in hypersplenic syndromes, Proceedings of the Second Clinical ACTH Conference, New York, 1951, The Blakiston Co., Philadelphia, vol. 2, p. 173.
98. Jacobson, B. M., and Sohier, W. D.: The effects of ACTH and of cortisone on the platelets in idiopathic thrombopenic purpura, New England J. Med. **246**: 247, 1952.
99. Editorial: ACTH and cortisone in hypersplenic syndromes, J. A. M. A. **149**: 485, 1952.
100. Stefanini, M., Perez Santiago, E., Chatterjea, J. B., Dameshek, W., and Salomon, L.: Corticotropin and cortisone in idiopathic thrombocytopenic purpura, J. A. M. A. **149**: 647, 1952.
101. Meyers, M. C., Miller, S., Linman, J. W., and Bethell, F. H.: The use of ACTH and cortisone in idiopathic thrombocytopenic purpura and idiopathic acquired hemolytic anemia, Ann. Int. Med. **37**: 352, 1952.
102. Wilson, S. J., and Eisemann, J.: The effect of corticotropin (ACTH) and cortisone on idiopathic thrombocytopenic purpura, Am. J. Med. **13**: 21, 1952.
103. Wintrobe, M. M.: Clinical hematology, 3d Ed., 1951, Lea & Febiger, Philadelphia, pp. 752–753.
104. Elliott, R. H. E., Jr., and Turner, J. C.: Splenectomy for purpura hemorrhagica, Surg., Gynec. and Obst. **92**: 539, 1951.
105. Leading article: Ideas on primary purpura, Lancet **2**: 574, 1951.
106. Dillard, G. H. L., Brecher, G., and Cronkite, E. P.: Separation, concentration, and transfusion of platelets, Proc. Soc. Exper. Biol. and Med. **78**: 796, 1951.
107. Minor, A. H., and Burnett, L.: A method for separating and concentrating platelets from normal human blood, Blood **7**: 693, 1952.

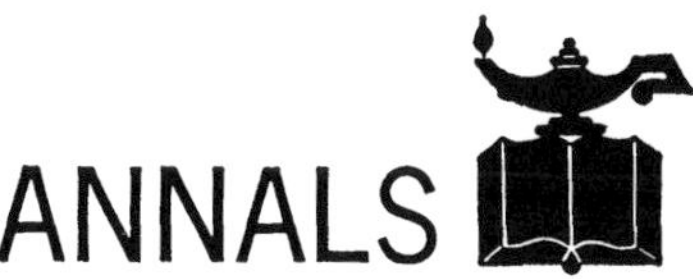

# of Internal Medicine

DECEMBER 1970 · VOLUME 73 · NUMBER 6

Published Monthly by the American College of Physicians

Combination Chemotherapy in the Treatment of Advanced Hodgkin's Disease

VINCENT T. DEVITA, JR., M.D., F.A.C.P., ARTHUR A. SERPICK, M.D., F.A.C.P., and PAUL P. CARBONE, M.D., Bethesda and Baltimore, Maryland

Forty-three patients with advanced, primarily untreated Hodgkin's disease were treated with a combination of vincristine sulfate, nitrogen mustard (or cyclophosphamide), procarbazine hydrochloride, and prednisone, given in cyclical fashion for 6 months. The limiting toxicity was primarily bone marrow suppression and, although occasionally severe, was generally tolerable. Other toxicity such as alopecia and neurotoxicity were troublesome but reversible. The response rate was superior to that previously reported with the use of single drugs with 35 of 43, or 81% of the patients achieving a complete remission, defined as the complete disappearance of all tumor and return to normal performance status. The duration of these responses after all therapy was discontinued was gratifyingly long, with a median of not less than 29 and not more than 42 months. Seventeen of 35 patients continue free of their disease, and 28 of these 35 are still alive. The median survival of the responding group is greater than 42 months, and life table analysis of the results indicates that of those complete responders at risk for 4 years, 77% remain alive and 47% are continuously free of their disease. The surviving fraction of the entire group at risk 4 years is 63%. It appears that combinations of effective drugs that act by different mechanisms and manifest different toxicities can be used effectively to increase the response rate and probably the survival of patients with sensitive tumors such as Hodgkin's disease.

► From the Solid Tumor Service, Medicine Branch, National Cancer Institute, National Institutes of Health, Bethesda, Md.; and the Baltimore Cancer Research Center, National Cancer Institute, Baltimore, Md.

Annals of Internal Medicine 73:881-895, 1970

HODGKIN'S DISEASE is a malignant tumor with a pleomorphic histologic picture and protean clinical manifestations. Understanding of its variability has increased in the past decade with the development of improved methods of diagnosis, staging, and treatment. Radiotherapy is probably curative in the early stages (1). Many patients with advanced disease respond to drug treatment, and there is evidence that responders are benefited by living longer than nonresponders (2). A number of different classes of independently active antitumor agents have been developed that have significant antitumor effect in Hodgkin's disease (3). Among the most effective are the alkylating agents (4); the vinca alkaloids (5-10); the methylhydrazine deriva-

Table 1. Clinical Features and Response to Therapy

Patient¶	Age at Onset of Treatment	Sex	Stage	Symptoms*	Node Areas Involved†	Organs Involved‡
	yr					
S.G.	16	F	IIIA	—	C,M,R	—
M.D.	48	F	IIIA	—	C,Su,A,R	—
C.S.	26	M	IIIA	—	C,A,R	—
M.S. (C)	25	M	IIIB	S,W	C,Su,M,A,R	—
F.B. (C)	20	M	IIIB	S,F,W	Su,A,R	—
J.F. (C)	16	M	IIIB	F,S	C,M,R	—
E.S.	43	M	IIIB	F,S,W	C,M,A,R,I	—
J.H.	28	M	IIIB	F,S	C,A,Sp	—
G.C.	20	F	IVA	—	A,R,Sp	Lung mass with necrosis
D.C. (C)	46	F	IVA	—	R	Pancreas‡, liver
N.H.	23	F	IVA	—	M	Marrow‡
C.R.	61	M	IVA	—	Su,A	Bone‡
R.A. (C)	40	F	IVB	S,F,W	Su,A,R	Pleura‡
G.Ba.	21	M	IVB	F	M	Bone‡
C.Bw.	47	F	IVB	F,S,W,P	M,A,R,I	Lung, liver, marrow‡
S.B. (C)	19	F	IVB	S,F,W	R,Sp	Bone, liver
C.B. (C)	13	M	IVB	F,P,W	C,Su,M,A	Lung mass with effusion
J.B.	21	M	IVB	S,W	C,M,A	Lung
W.B.	20	M	IVB	F,S,W	C,Su,M,A,R, Sp,I	Bone
R.Cs.	48	M	IVB	F	C,Su,M,R	Liver
R.Ct.	19	M	IVB	F,S,W	M,Sp	Liver, marrow‡
C.C.	32	M	IVB	F,W	Su,M,E,R	Liver
J.D.	38	F	IVB	F,S,P	C,M,A,I	Liver, pleural effusion
M.G.	50	F	IVB	S,W	A,Sp	Jejunum‡, liver
L.L.	14	F	IVB	F,P,W	C,Su,M	Lung‡
A.L.	65	F	IVB	F,S,W	C,Su,M,R	Liver
J.M.	17	M	IVB	F,S,W	A,R	Liver
J.N.	49	M	IVB	F,S	C,Su,A,R,Sp	Liver‡
N.P.	12	F	IVB	F,S,W	C,M.A	Lung‡, liver
D.P. (C)	38	F	IVB	F,S,P,W	Su,A,R,I	Lung, bone
G.P.	23	M	IVB	F	Sp	Liver‡
H.Q.	69	F	IVB	P,W	—	Lung, duodenum‡
J.Ra.	45	M	IVB	F,W	C,Su,M,A, R,I	Marrow‡
T.R.	49	M	IVB	F,S,W	C,A,Sp	Liver‡
D.S.	24	F	IVB	F,P	C,Su,M,A	Bone‡
A.S.	30	M	IVB	F,W	C,M,A,R,I	Marrow‡, bone‡
R.Se. (C)	20	M	IVB	F,S,P,M	C,Su,M,A,R, I	Bone, liver, pleural mass
J.S. (C)	18	F	IVB	F,S,P	C,Su,M	Liver, bone
M.Sm.	26	F	IVB	F,S,P,W	C,Su,M,A,R, I,Sp	Lung
M.S. (C)	22	F	IVB	F,S,W	C,M,A	Lung, pleura
R.St.	38	M	IVB	F,S,W	Su,M,Sp	Lung‡
B.T.	24	M	IVB	F,S,W	M	Lung‡, liver
L.Z. (C)	16	F	IVB	F,S,W	Su,M	Liver, bone

¶ Patients marked (C) given cyclophosphamide.
* F = fever; S = sweats; W = weight loss > 10%; P = pruritis.
† C = cervical; A = axillary; R = retroperitoneal; I = inguinal; Sp = spleen; M = mediastinum; E = epitrochlear; Su = supraclavicular.
‡ Biopsy proved.

Table 1. (Continued)

Histology§	Prior Therapy	Response to Therapy‖	Duration of First Remission‖ (from Last Therapy)	Survival from Onset of Treatment‖	Delayed Hypersensitivity** Pre-treatment	Delayed Hypersensitivity** Post-treatment
			months			
MC	None	CR	46+	53+	NT	NT
LD	None	CR	16	19E	NT	NT
MC	Local X ray	CR	52+	57+	NT	R
MC	None	CR	11	33+	A	NT
NS (LD)	None	CR	11	35+	A	A
LD	None	CR	29+	35+	R	R
MC	None	CR	35+	44+	R	R
MC	Single dose nitrogen mustard	CR	42	71+	NT	R
NS (LP)	Local X ray	CR	37+	42+	A	A
MC	Local X ray	CR	27+	35+	A	A
MC	None	CR	43+	51+	NT	NT
LD	None	CR	49+	54+	R	R
MC	Local X ray	CR	29+	34+	A	R
NS (MC)	Steroid course	CR	15	52+	NT	R
NS (MC)	Local X ray	CR	9	24E	A	NT
MC	None	CR	11	35+	R	NT
NS (LD)	None	IF	—	10E	A	NT
LD	None	CR	38+	43+	R	R
MC	Local X ray	CR	30	55+	A	NT
MC	None	CR	11	30E	A	NT
LD	None	IF	—	14E	NT	NT
NS (MC)	None	CR	9	54+	A	NT
NS (MC)	Local X ray	CR	3	31E	NT	NT
U	None	CR	15	22E	A	NT
LD	None	IF	—	27E	R	NT
MC	None	CR	48+	54+	A	R
MC	Local X ray	CR	40+	45+	A	R
LD	Splenectomy	CR	42	55+	NT	NT
LP	None	CR	18	59+	A	R
NS (LD)	None	IF	—	36+	R	NT
U	None	CR	6	31E	NT	R
LD	None	IF	—	5E	A	NT
LD	None	CR	41+	47+	NT	R
LP	None	CR	10	20E	R	NT
LD	Local X ray; steroid	CR	42+	49+	R	R
LD	None	CR	43+	49+	NT	R
MC	None	IF	—	0.5E	A	NT
NS (MC)	None	CR	3	39+	R	NT
NS (MC)	None	IF	—	38E	A	NT
NS (MC)	None	CR	32+	38+	A	R
NS (LD)	None	IF	—	1.0E	R	NT
NS (LD)	None	CR	2	22E	NT	R
NS (MC)	None	CR	34+	40+	R	NT

§ Histology (Lukes-Butler Classification); MC = mixed cellularity; LD = lymphocyte depleted; NS = nodular sclerosis; LP = lymphocyte predominant; U = unclassified.

‖ CR = complete remission; IF = remission induction failure; + = first remission or survival continues; E = expired.

** A = anergic; R = at least one skin test positive; NT = not tested.

tive, procarbazine (11-15); and the corticoids (16-18). Used singly these agents have certain features in common. They usually produce significant tumor shrinkage; uncommonly, there is complete disappearance of tumor masses. The responses are generally short-lived, but patients who develop resistance to one type of drug will often respond in a similar fashion to a drug from a different class. There is also evidence that the durability of the responses is related to the completeness of tumor regression (19).

Studies in drug-sensitive experimental animal tumor systems have indicated a relationship between dose of an effective drug and survival (20). Manipulation of doses and schedules and the use of effective drugs in combination increase the therapeutic index by increasing tumor cell kill or by preventing the development of drug resistance (21). In the early 1960's these principles were first applied to the treatment of acute lymphocytic leukemia of childhood, resulting in an increased remission rate and duration of unmaintained remissions (22-24). Hodgkin's disease can also be considered a sensitive human tumor. In 1963 a pilot study was instituted at the Solid Tumor Service of the National Cancer Institute (NCI), National Institutes of Health, to explore combination chemotherapy in the treatment of Hodgkin's disease (25-27). This study used 4 drugs: vincristine sulfate, cyclophosphamide, methotrexate, and prednisone (combination 1). A remission rate higher than that with single drugs was achieved. The folic acid antagonists were known to have only marginal activity in the treatment of lymphomas (28), and as information became available on the use of the new methylhydrazine derivative, procarbazine, this drug was substituted for methotrexate (combination 2). The present study with the latter combination of drugs was conducted between 1964 and July 1967 (29, 30). The primary goals were to increase the complete remission rate and study the duration of unmaintained remission. The results of treatment of the first 43 patients, all entered on study before July 1967, are the subject of this report.

Materials and Methods

From January 1964 to July 1967, 44 consecutive patients were entered on study. Patients were admitted to the hospital for initial workup and classified as to the extent of disease according to what was agreed on in 1966 as the Rye classification (31).

PATIENT SELECTION

Patients with Hodgkin's disease were referred to the Solid Tumor Service and Baltimore Cancer Research Center of the National Cancer Institute from a wide segment of the country. Those who had received significant amounts of prior therapy were not accepted for this study. Demonstrated resistance to one or more of the agents to be used was considered a significant reason for exclusion. A patient who had a single course of one of the drugs was admitted to the study. Patients who had received local X irradiation (one or two fields) in the past and now had relapsed because of extension into an organ system were considered stage IV and were entered on study. Nine patients had received such local X-ray therapy before referral to the NCI. In addition, one patient had received a single dose of alkylating agent and two, a short course of corticoids before admission to the NCI (Table 1). These patients thus represented 37 consecutive suitable patients, as defined above, referred to the Solid Tumor Service, and 6 such patients referred to the Baltimore Cancer Research Center of the National Cancer Institute.

PATHOLOGIC MATERIAL

In all patients the histologic material was confirmed as Hodgkin's disease by the pathologist of record at the two institutions. After completion of treatment pathologic material was once more reviewed and patients classified in the Lukes and Butler classification (32, 33). This classification was modified to include subcategories of the nodular sclerosis group as lymphocyte predominant, mixed cellularity, or lymphocyte depleted.

STAGING

In addition to taking a history, a physical examination, complete blood counts, liver function tests, and extensive radiologic evaluation were performed. This included a posteroanterior and lateral chest roentgenogram with whole chest tomography when mediastinal disease was present, metastatic bone series, intravenous pyelography, inferior venocavography, and lymphangiography. Bone marrow biopsies were performed routinely with a modified Vim-Silverman marrow biopsy needle. Stronium-85 bone scans were performed on patients who either had systemic symptoms or evidence suggestive of bone involvement, such as bone pain, hypercalcemia, or unexplained elevation of serum alkaline phosphatase. Lymphangiograms were reviewed by a single radiologist with one of the authors to avoid observer variation. It is the policy at the NCI for all patients with equivocally positive lymphangiograms to have an exploratory laparotomy for a definitive pathologic examination of the lymph nodes involved. This was not required for any patient in the present study.

DIAGNOSTIC CRITERIA FOR ORGAN INVOLVEMENT

The criteria listed below were used in the present study.

Liver: A standardized approach was used to determine liver involvement. Liver function studies performed routinely included serum alkaline phosphatase and transaminases, bilirubin, and 45-min sulfobromophthalein (Bromsulphalein®) (BSP) retention. Isotopic scanning of the liver with technetium sulphur colloid or ^{131}I rose bengal was performed if any liver function test was abnormal or if hepatomegaly was present with or without abnormal liver function studies. Needle biopsies of the liver were performed in all patients who had at least one abnormal liver function test, hepatomegaly, or both, or an abnormal liver scan. If, in the case of a normal liver size and only one abnormal liver function test, the biopsy was normal, no further diagnostic tests were performed. If two abnormal liver function tests were present and a needle biopsy was normal, open surgical exploration and biopsy of the liver were done to determine if the liver was involved with tumor. These criteria for diagnosis of Hodgkin's disease in the liver evolved over time, and patients treated earlier in the study were diagnosed as having liver involvement on the basis of two abnormal liver function tests (increased alkaline phosphatase and abnormal BSP retention) and hepatomegaly, without the benefit of a biopsy procedure.

Lung: Parenchymal lung involvement was usually suspected from routine chest roentgenograms and confirmed by whole chest tomography. Our past experience indicated that when patients with suspected lung involvement were explored surgically, the lesions were invariably positive; thus, routine histological conformation of Hodgkin's disease of the lung was not required if, in the opinion of the radiologist, the chest tomograms indicated parenchymal lung involvement. In those patients with lung lesions not confirmed histologically before treatment, the rapid improvement with treatment, using only antitumor agents, tended to serve as confirmation of the diagnosis.

Bone: In a patient with known Hodgkin's disease X-ray evidence of erosion of bone, confirmed by bone scanning with strontrium-85, or a positive bone scan alone was considered sufficient evidence for bone involvement, although bone biopsies of positive areas on scan were performed when possible.

Bone Marrow: Bone marrow biopsies with a modified Vim-Silverman needle were performed in the posterior iliac crest on all patients. Bone marrow involvement was diagnosed only when clearly identifiable Reed-Sternberg cells were seen. Other abnormalities frequently seen in Hodgkin's disease such as erythroid, myeloid, and eosinophilic hyperplasia were not considered sufficient evidence of involvement of the marrow with tumor.

IMMUNOLOGIC STATUS

Thirteen of the 43 patients did not have pretreatment skin testing. The remaining 30 patients had careful evaluation of their delayed hypersensitivity. Twenty-four were sensitized with dinitrochlorobenzene (DNCB) by a method previously described (34) and, in addition, had at least four intradermal skin tests (purified protein derivative of tuberculin, coccidioidin, candidin, and histoplasmin) and often five skin tests (the preceding four plus mumps). The additional six patients tested had the skin tests but were not sensitized to DNCB.

Patients were retested, if possible, once all therapy had been discontinued for a significant period of time. Thirteen of the 30 patients previously tested were thus restudied. In addition, 6 of the 13 patients not skin-tested before therapy were challenged with skin tests and DNCB sensitization after therapy.

TREATMENT PROGRAM

The drugs used were selected to avoid overlapping and dose-limiting toxicity of the bone marrow as much as possible. A significant number of varied and troublesome side effects were nevertheless expected and discussed in advance with each patient before obtaining consent for treatment. These side effects included risks of bone marrow suppression, the acute side effects, the expected alopecia, and neurotoxicity. The possible effects of these drugs on children conceived during or after treatment and the future ability to reproduce were also considered important parts of pretreatment discussions since the population was often made up of young people.

Therapy consisted of the intermittent administration of four drugs—vincristine sulfate (Oncovin®) procarbazine hydrochloride, nitrogen mustard (Mustargen®) and prednisone (combination 2, MOPP). In 12 patients (indicated by C in Table 1) cyclophosphamide was substituted for nitrogen mustard. The treatment was administered in monthly cycles for a total of six treatments. Figure 1 illustrates a single cycle of therapy. Vincristine and nitrogen mustard (or cyclophosphamide) were given as a rapid injection into the tubing of an intravenous infusion on days 1 and 8 of each cycle. Each dose of vincristine totaled 1.4 mg/m² of body surface area. For nitrogen mustard a dose of 6 mg/m² was given at each injection. When cyclophosphamide was substituted for nitrogen mustard it was given in a dose of 650 mg/m² of body surface area. From days 1 through 14 oral procarbazine was given in a single dose of 100 mg/m² of body surface area daily. Prednisone was administered only during cycles 1 and 4 and given orally at a dose of 40 mg/m² per day for 14 days. After each 14-day treatment period patients were given no other therapy for an additional 14 days, and then, blood counts permitting, the next cycle was reinstituted. Each treatment cycle took approximately 1 month. Although patients were staged in the hospital, they were generally discharged to receive the chemotherapy as outpatients. Premedication for nausea and vomiting was used at the discretion of the physician in charge of each patient. Areas of disease involvement, liver, and renal function studies were monitored by appropriate studies before the institution of each cycle of therapy.

The treatment itself was regulated by the results of weekly WBC and platelet counts and hemoglobin values. A sliding scale was used (Table 2) for reduction of the dosage of each drug for the next cycle if the WBC and platelet counts had not returned to acceptable levels. In general, if a patient's blood cell counts were near levels that would allow full dosage

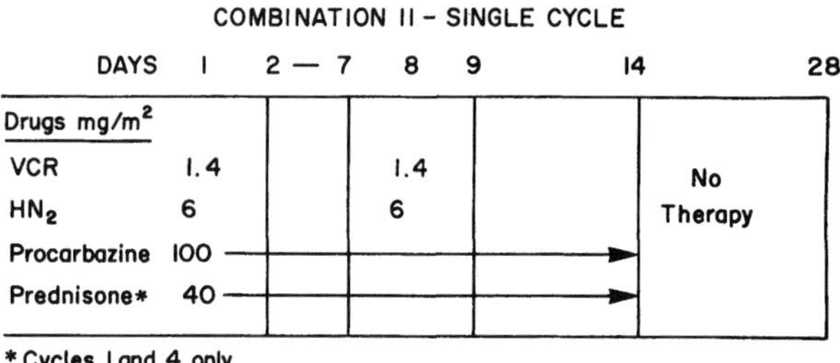

Figure 1. A single cycle of therapy with drug combination **2.** VCR = vincristine sulfate; HN_2 = nitrogen mustard.

on day 28, extra time was allowed, usually a few days and not more than 1 week, to allow recovery to protocol levels and thus delivery of a full cycle of treatment. If recovery was not satisfactory after 1 extra week, therapy was reinstituted at reduced dose levels, as calculated from the sliding scale.

RESPONSE TO TREATMENT

Patients were evaluated as to the status of their disease at the end of six cycles. If any evidence of disease was present, the patients were considered a remission induction failure and were transferred to other treatment programs. If at the termination of the sixth cycle the patient had no evidence of Hodgkin's disease, he was considered in a state of complete remission, and no further therapy was given; patients were then followed at approximately monthly intervals in the Clinic. For the sake of consistency durations of all remissions reported refer to the length of time free of tumor from the last day of drug treatment; the time each patient took to reach a complete remission was also noted.

To achieve a complete remission, the patient's complaints, physical examination, performance status, and laboratory and roentgenographic studies had to return to normal. Areas of known involvement before therapy were reexamined posttreatment. For example, dye in a positive lymphangiogram was followed with repeated abdominal films. With elution of dye, lymphangiograms were repeated to document the status of retroperitoneal nodes. If possible, patients having long responses were readmitted yearly for restaging by lymphangiography if dye elution had occurred and if this study was positive in the past. Similarly, whole chest tomography was used to monitor chest lesions. Appropriate biopsies were performed in accessible areas previously involved. The magnitude of the decrease in all tumor volume was noted for all patients considered induction failures.

DIAGNOSIS AND MANAGEMENT OF A DISEASE RELAPSE

Evidence of disease relapse in lymph nodes was confirmed by biopsy in all cases. When other studies became positive, even if in an area previously involved, biopsy confirmation was generally attempted. If biopsy was not possible and disease recurrence suspected, the patient was considered to have relapsed at that point. Patients who came for their monthly clinic visit with symptoms that ultimately proved to be due to disease recurrence had their time of relapse dated back to the point of the first appearance of the symptoms.

Induction failures were given vinblastine as their next form of treatment, followed by BCNU (1, 3-Bis(2-chloroethyl)-1-nitrosourea) (35). After BCNU therapy, treatment was variable and depended on the patient's condition and the availability of new drugs. Patients who relapsed after having achieved a complete remission were retreated with the same combination of drugs in the same fashion. The achieved response was then maintained with intermittent exposure to two cycles of chemotherapy, both containing steroids, separated by 3-month intervals. If the patients failed on this program, they were treated in a fashion similar to that described for the primary remission induction failures. Survival for all patients was tabulated from the beginning of combination chemotherapy.

Table 2. Dosage Attenuation Schedule for Bone Marrow Depression

If WBC count before starting new course was	Then dosage was adjusted to
>4,000	100% of all drugs
3,999-3,000	100% of vincristine, 50% nitrogen mustard and procarbazine
2,999-2,000	100% of vincristine, 25% nitrogen mustard and procarbazine
1,999-1,000	50% vincristine, 25% nitrogen mustard and procarbazine
999-0	No drug
If platelet count before starting new course was	**Then dosage was adjusted to**
>100,000	100% of all drugs
50,000-1,000,000	100% vincristine, 25% nitrogen mustard and procarbazine
>50,000	No drug

Results

Forty-four patients were entered into the study program and treated; one was excluded from the study after six cycles of treatment because on review of her biopsy material the diagnosis was changed to lymphosarcoma. This patient had a year-long remission, relapsed, and is alive on other therapy at this time. No other patient entered on this study has been excluded. The details of the patient population are shown in Table 1. All patients had a histologic diagnosis of Hodgkin's disease, and 41 of the 43 patients could be subclassified in the Lukes and Butler classification. Only two patients had the lymphocyte predominant histology. The rest were divided among the mixed cellularity (14 patients), lymphocyte depleted (11 patients), and nodular sclerosis varieties (14 patients). The subclassification of the 14 patients in the nodular sclerosis group into the various subcategories showed that 1 had lymphocyte predominant; 5, lymphocyte depleted; and 8, mixed cellularity nodular sclerosis.

The characteristics of the patient population are shown in Table 3. The mean age was 31 years, and sex distribution was fairly equal. The median time from diagnosis to treatment was 2 months. All but seven patients were staged as IV A or B, with a significant number having multiple organ systems involved. Seven patients were called stage IV on the basis of liver involvement only. Three of these patients had histologic proof of Hodgkin's disease in the liver. The rest had at least two significantly abnormal liver function tests, hepatomegaly, and a normal closed liver biopsy specimen as the basis

Table 3. Characteristics of Study Patients

Sex	20 females, 23 males
Mean age	31 (12-69 years)
Median time from diagnosis to treatment	2 months
Stage IIIA patients	2
III B patients	5
Stage IVA patients	4
IV B patients	31
Multiple organs involved	13
Lung alone	8
Liver alone	7
Bone alone	4
Bone marrow alone	2
GI tract alone	1

for diagnosing liver involvement; two patients had no biopsy procedure at all. Eight patients were staged as IV on the basis of lung involvement only; three of these were confirmed histologically before treatment. In the other five, whole chest tomography showed parenchymal lung involvement, and the response to antitumor drugs alone provided additional confirmation of the diagnosis. Only four patients were classified as stage IV on the basis of bone involvement alone. Three had histologic confirmation, and the fourth was diagnosed by a positive bone scan only. Two patients had bone marrow as the only extranodal site of involvement. The diagnosis was not made in the marrow aspiration specimen obtained at the same time as the marrow biopsy. Of the 13 patients with multiple organ systems involved, 7 had biopsy confirmation of Hodgkin's disease of at least 1 organ.

ACUTE TOXICITY

Nausea and vomiting were invariably present to some degree in all patients treated and tended to be worse on days 1 and 8 of therapy with nitrogen mustard. Administration of sedatives in the evening after afternoon drug administration seemed to serve as the best control of these acute side effects. Some patients tolerated each cycle increasingly well, whereas others tended to develop more severe vomiting with each exposure. The fact that therapy would end in a finite period of time seemed to serve as incentive for patients to undergo continued drug administration. In many of the symptomatic patients the rapid disappearance of symptoms and regression of tumor, coupled with improvement in their performance status, tended to outweigh the side effects produced by drug administration.

Bone marrow suppression was the dose-limiting toxicity in spite of the attempt to reduce this side effect by the selection of vincristine over the alternative and favored vinca alkaloid, vinblastine. The dosage of all drugs except the corticoids was reduced progressively with each cycle. By protocol, 6 months would be required for therapy; in actuality, therapy was given over an average period of 5.8 months. The projected full dosage of each drug is shown in Table 4 along with the dose reduction that was necessary for each drug in each cycle. An average of 92% of the projected dose of vincristine was actually given. Likewise, 83% of the projected dose of the alkylating agent, either nitrogen mustard or cyclophosphamide, and 75% of the dose of procarbazine were actually given to the patients. Acute toxicity was not significantly different in either of the groups receiving nitrogen mustard or cyclophosphamide.

Two patients died after the initial cycle of chemotherapy, Patients R. Se. and R. St. (Table 1)—both died as a result of rapid necrosis of tumor masses. Patient R. Se., a young man with extensive Hodgkin's disease, had undiagnosed bowel involvement. One week after the first half of the first cycle he abruptly went into shock and died. Blood cultures showed clostridial species, and autopsy disclosed multiple perforations of the small bowel caused by tumorous involvement. Patient R. St. had an extremely large mass of tumor in his lung that necrosed after the first cycle of treatment. He developed a pseudomonas lung abscess and died 1 month after the first cycle from pseudomonas septicemia, with no further chemotherapy. Patient R. St. was not leukopenic, and patient R. Se. had a WBC count of 2,400/mm^3 at the time of death. These patients were considered to have drug-related deaths but, in spite of their short exposure to therapy, were included in the evaluation of overall response and survival. Another patient developed staphylococcal septicemia associated with a bone marrow biopsy-site infection. This patient was leukopenic at the time and had bone marrow involvement with Hodgkin's disease (Patient G. Bv.). She recovered uneventfully on antibiotics. No other episodes of sepsis were noted during chemotherapy in this group.

Leukopenia, although occasionally severe, was quite tolerable; the mean nadir WBC counts and the

Table 4. Average of Projected Dose* Given per Cycle

Drugs	Cycle						Average Total Course
	1	2	3	4	5	6	
	←			%			→
Vincristine	99	98	94	92	82	84	92
Alkylating agent	95	87	78	88	73	72	83
Procarbazine	93	79	79	79	63	61	75
Total average	96	88	83	86	73	72	83

* Projected full dose/m^2 body surface area: vincristine, 16.8 mg; nitrogen mustard, 72.0 mg; cyclophosphamide, 7.8 g; procarbazine, 8.4 g.

Table 5. White Blood Cell Count Suppression

Cycle	Mean Nadir WBC Count	Patients with WBC Counts			
		<1,000/mm³	<2,000/mm³	<3,000/mm³	<5,000/mm³
		%			
1	7,800	2	20	37	63
2	3,300	0	27	46	88
3	3,900	3	18	49	82
4	4,000	0	9	49	77
5	3,000	3	26	62	97
6	3,000	3	21	53	91

percentage of patients with WBC counts at each level are illustrated in Table 5. Almost all patients developed some degree of leukopenia, but relatively few developed WBC counts below 2,000/mm³ and even fewer below 1,000/mm³. A significant tendency for the same patients to develop severe leukopenia with each cycle was noted. Leukopenia generally became more severe with each cycle, and a greater dose reduction was required as the treatment progressed (Table 4). There was no significant difference in the degree of leukopenia noted between the group treated with nitrogen mustard and those treated with cyclophosphamide.

Significant thrombocytopenia was uncommon (Table 6). A trend toward less thrombocytopenia in the cyclophosphamide-treated group compared with the group treated with nitrogen mustard was noted but was not statistically significant. Hemorrhage caused by thrombocytopenia was not encountered, and platelet transfusions were not required. A trend toward recurrence of more severe thrombocytopenia in the same patients with each cycle was again noted. Thrombocytopenia was uncommonly the reason for dose reduction since a platelet level of 100,000/mm³ was considered adequate for full dosage. Patients with bone marrow involvement who presented with leukopenia and thrombocytopenia tended to have improvement in their peripheral blood counts, rather than suppression, with the first cycle of therapy.

Table 6. Peripheral Platelet Count Suppression

Cycle	Mean Nadir Platelet Count × 10³	Patients with Platelet Counts	
		<50,000	<100,000
		%	
1	234	5	15
2	182	2	15
3	165	0	18
4	170	3	22
5	148	8	19
6	160	3	18

CHRONIC TOXICITY

Anemia related to drug administration was not a common problem. Seven patients (17%), however, appeared particularly sensitive to the drug combination and developed a normochronic normocytic anemia with an average drop in hemoglobin of 34% by the fourth and fifth cycle. Cessation of treatment was associated with prompt recovery to normal in the five patients (R.C., G.C., D.G., N.P., and C.S.) who achieved a complete remission. The two patients categorized as induction failures (C.B. and H.Q.) remained anemic until their death; none of the patients had bone marrow involvement with tumor.

Liver toxicity was not dose limiting; there were five mild, transient, and otherwise unexplained elevations of serum alkaline phosphatase and three minor transient increases in serum glutamic oxalacetic transaminase during treatment. Two patients developed a clinical picture of viral hepatitis after therapy, unassociated with the transfusion of blood products. Needle biopsy specimens of the liver in each case were compatible with this diagnosis, and although one patient appears to have recovered completely, the other (Patient N.H.) has persistent biopsy evidence of smoldering viral hepatitis. This latter patient feels entirely well and has no clinical evidence of Hodgkin's disease. There were seven cases of a minor transient increase in blood urea nitrogen during therapy. One patient developed proteinuria during the fourth cycle of treatment. Hemorrhagic cystitis, attributed to cyclophosphamide, was noted in only one patient.

The combination of vincristine and cyclophosphamide produced severe hair loss. All patients receiving cyclophosphamide instead of nitrogen mustard developed severe alopecia. Only 30% of those receiving vincristine and nitrogen mustard experienced noticeable alopecia, which was always reversible. The high prevalence of alopecia and the failure to reduce bone marrow toxicity, when cyclophosphamide was substituted for nitrogen mustard, were the major reasons for reversion to the original use of the latter drug. Neurotoxicity, secondary to vincristine, was common. All patients lost their deep tendon reflexes by the third cycle of therapy, and hyperesthesia of the fingers and toes was always present. No patient in this study developed foot drop, although weakness and easy fatigability of the leg muscles were common complaints. Once deep tendon reflexes were lost, patients did not seem to have increasing severe neurotoxicity at the dose schedule used in spite of continued drug administration. Although, according to protocol, vincristine dosage could have been reduced at the discretion of the physician, this was done infrequently as is illustrated by the minor reduction in the dose of vincristine in each cycle (Table 4). Recovery to normal always occurred in those patients achieving a complete remission. Although constipation was encountered, anticipatory treatment with laxatives and stool softeners tended to alleviate this problem. All the side effects attributed to vincristine were more severe in the older patients.

ANTITUMOR EFFECT

Remission Induction: Details of the response to treatment and the duration of remissions are summarized in Table 7. As previously mentioned, two patients died after their first cycle of therapy. In addition, 6 patients, indicated in Table 1 by IF in the Response column, responded with a greater than 50% reduction of tumor masses but failed to achieve complete disappearance of tumor. Failure in five of these six patients was caused by persistence of lung lesions after six cycles. In only two patients (H.Q. and C.B.) was regrowth of lesions apparent during therapy.

Thirty-five patients (81%) had complete disappearance of all evidence of Hodgkin's disease and returned to a normal status after six cycles of treatment. The average time for a patient to achieve a complete remission was 3 months. Peripheral adenopathy tended to clear more rapidly than other areas of tumor, and the last evidence of lymph node tumor was frequently noted in the retroperitoneal area on lymphangiography. Lung lesions tended to clear slowly, even in those patients who achieved a complete response.

Table 7. Response to (Combination Chemotherapy) Treatment

Mean duration of treatment	5.8 months
Deaths during treatment	2
Responded but failed to achieve a complete remission	6
Achieved a complete remission	35 (81%)
Mean time to complete remission	3 months
Median duration of complete remission (from the cessation of all therapy)	29-42 months
Number who have relapsed	18 (51%)
Median time to relapse	11 months

Duration of Remissions: The last data in this study have been tabulated up to 1 March 1970. Because patients have not been entered on this phase of the study since July 1967, the minimum follow-up time is 32 months. The duration of each remission was calculated from the last day of all treatment in those patients entering complete remission. As of 1 March 1970, 18 of 31 patients have relapsed with a median time to reappearance of disease of 11 months. Although 51% of the patients have relapsed, the median duration of remission is indeterminate and will not be less than 29 months or greater than 42 months. Relapses occurred from as early as 2 months to as late as 42 months after treatment. The longest continuing remission, as of 1 March 1970, is 52 months. Of the 17 patients still in remission, 9 are female and 8 male.

Clinical Response Related to Initial Stage: Response and present status by initial stage of disease is shown in Table 8. All the induction failures and deaths during induction treatment occurred in patients with stage IVB disease, but 23 of the 29 patients (79%) with stage IVB disease who completed six cycles achieved a complete remission, and 39% of these patients are still in their first remission. None of the patients in the other stages failed to obtain a complete remission. None of the stage IVA patients have relapsed. The one IIIA patient who expired died of cerebral toxoplasmosis after 16 months in remission; autopsy showed retroperitoneal Hodgkin's disease. All three IIIB patients who relapsed did so in lymph node areas previously involved, have responded again to treatment, and remain alive.

STATUS BY HISTOLOGIC CLASSIFICATION

Table 9 illustrates the response to treatment and the present status of patients as related to the initial histologic classification in the Lukes and Butler scheme. Fourteen patients were subclassified as nodular sclerosis. Although the numbers are small, the usual favorable prognosis imparted to patients classified in the nodular sclerosis category was not apparent in this study (36). One of two deaths during induction and three of six induction failures occurred in patients who had a histologic picture of nodular sclerosis. Although 10 of 14 patients in this category achieved a complete remission, only 3 of these remain in their first remission, and 5 of the 14 deaths were diagnosed as nodular sclerosing Hodgkin's disease. Patients in the other two histo-

Table 8. Results of Combination Chemotherapy-Response and Status by Stage of Disease

Stage	Total Number of Patients	Induction Failures	Complete Remissions	First Remission Continuing	Deaths
IVB	31	8*	23	9	13*
IVA	4	0	4	4	0
IIIB	5	0	5	2	0
IIIA	3	0	3	2	1

* Includes both deaths after initial cycle of treatment.

Table 9. Results of Combination Chemotherapy: Status by Histology

Histology	Total Number of Patients	Induction Failure	Complete Remission	First Remission Continues	Deaths
Lymphocyte predominant	2	0	2	0	1
Mixed cellularity	14	1*	13	8	2*
Lymphocyte depleted	11	3	8	6	4
Nodular sclerosis (5LD, 7MC, 2LP)†	14	4*	10	3	5*
Unclassified	2	0	2	0	2
Totals	43	8*	35	17	14

* Includes deaths after first cycle.
† LD = lymphocyte depleted; MC = mixed cellularity; LP = lymphocyte predominant.

logic categories making up most of the rest of the group—mixed cellularity and lymphocyte depleted —appeared about equal in regard to durability of response. Patients previously diagnosed as having Hodgkin's sarcoma, long considered the histologic subgroup with the worst prognosis, are, however, included in the lymphocyte-depleted variety and could have been expected to have less favorable results; this was not apparent.

RESULTS RELATED TO PRETREATMENT IMMUNOLOGIC STATUS AND REPEAT SKIN TESTING

Results of skin testing in each patient are shown in Table 1. Of the 30 patients who had skin tests before treatment, 18 (60%) were anergic. Thirteen of these 18 anergic patients had been tested with the intradermal skin tests and by dinitrochlorobenzene (DNCB) sensitization. Five had only the intradermal skin tests. Twelve of the 30 tested patients were not anergic and reacted to at least one skin test or DNCB. Only one of these patients was not exposed to DNCB. Of the 11 responsive patients tested with both DNCB and the intradermal skin tests, 5 responded only to DNCB sensitization, and in none was the reaction greater than 2+. Three of these 11 patients responded to at least one intradermal skin test but could not be sensitized to DNCB. Seventy-seven percent of the patients would have been unreactive and considered anergic by routine skin testing with a battery of antigens that ordinarily produce a positive response in 95% of a normal population (37). If one considered DNCB only, sensitization was attempted in 24 patients and 16 (66%) were unresponsive. By any standard a large portion of the population tested was anergic.

An attempt was made to reapply both intradermal skin tests and a challenging dose of 50 and 100 μg of DNCB to patients in remission. The minimum time in remission for those previously anergic patients so tested was 10 months. Eight of 18 previously anergic patients were retested; and 5 of 8 (63%) responded to one or more intradermal skin tests, but none responded to challenge doses of 50 and 100 μg of DNCB. Before treatment all these patients had been exposed to a 2,000-μg sensitizing dose of DNCB and had also failed to respond to a challenge dose later applied. Only 5 of the 12 patients previously responsive to an intradermal skin test were retested posttreatment, and all 5 remained responsive to the same test while in remission. Of the 13 patients not skin tested before treatment, 6 were tested with the intradermal skin tests while in remission, and 5 of them responded to at least one. Two of these patients were sensitized at this time with a 1,000-μg dose of DNCB and responded normally to a challenge dose 14 days later. When patients were compared by their skin test category, there were essentially three groups; those anergic, those skin-test responsive, and those not tested before therapy. The complete remission rates in these groups were 78, 75, and 92%, respectively. Of the 17 patients still in remission, 6 were anergic, 6 were skin-test responsive, and 5 had not been tested before treatment. There were no significant differences in duration of unmaintained remission and survival among the three groups. As of 1 March 1970 a larger fraction of skin-test responsive patients (0.67) remain in remission than those previously anergic (0.50). The group not previously skin-tested represents the patients first entered on study and has the longest follow-up; the fraction of this group still in remission is 0.58. These differences are not statistically significant.

SURVIVAL

Survival data are summarized in Table 10. Five of the six induction failures have died, with a median survival of 20 months. The survivor is alive on drug therapy with active tumor at 36 months.

The median survival of the 35 patients achieving a complete remission has not been reached with 28 patients still living. The median will be greater than 42 months.

Seventeen of those 28 living patients from the group achieving complete remissions remain in their first remission. Figure 2 shows a life table analysis of survival for the entire group and the 35 patients achieving a complete remission. The surviving fraction for the total group at risk 4 years is 0.63. For the group entering complete remission and at risk for 4 years, the surviving fraction is 0.77. Figure 3 illustrates a life table analysis of the rate of relapse from the first remission. The highest risk of relapse is in the first 18 months from the end of treatment, after which the relapse rate appears to level off. For those patients at risk for 4 years the fraction remaining in their first remission is 0.47. There was no difference in survival in regard to sex.

When the 11 patients at risk 4 years are examined in a different fashion, 5 of the 11 remain free of disease in their first remission; 3 of the 11 are free of disease, having had a remission reinduced with the same combination of drugs; 2 are alive with active disease on other single drugs; and 1 is dead. Thus, 8 of the 11 at risk for 4 years (73%) are alive and free of their disease as a result of treatment with the four drugs in combination.

There was no apparent difference in the amount of drug given to patients who had six cycles but failed to have a complete response or to patients who achieved a complete response but have now

Table 10. Effect of Combination Chemotherapy on Survival

Effect	Total Patients	Patients Still in Complete Remission	Living	Median Survival
				months
Deaths during therapy	2	—	—	—
Remission induction failures	6	—	1	20
Complete remissions	35	17	28	42+
Total	43			

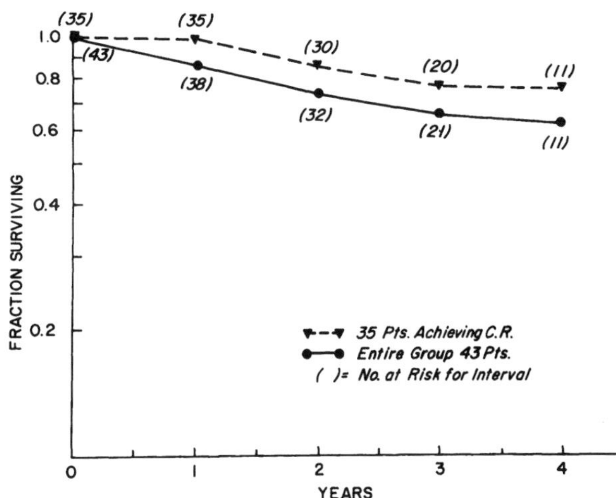

Figure 2. Life table analysis of survival for entire group of 43 patients (*solid line*) and the 35 patients achieving a complete remission (*C.R.*) (*dotted line*). Figures in parentheses next to each point indicate the number of patients at risk for that interval.

relapsed when compared with those still in complete remission. Since cyclophosphamide was substituted for nitrogen mustard, starting in late 1966 and extending through most of 1967, the follow-up of patients so treated is shorter than average. When this group of 12 patients was analyzed separately with regard to response and durability of remissions, however, no differences were apparent. There was one death during induction treatment and two induction failures in this group. Nine of 12 (75%) achieved a complete remission, and 5 of 9 (55%) remain in complete remission. The median time to relapse was 11 months, and the median duration of complete remission will be greater than 27 months in this group. All are at risk for 2½ years, and 83% are alive at that interval.

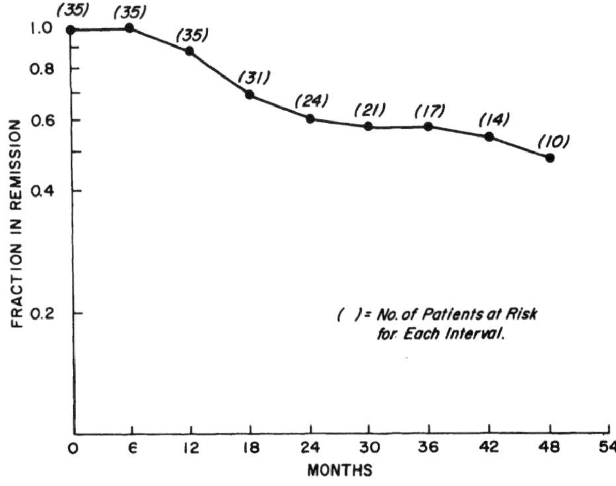

Figure 3. Life table analysis of the rate of relapse from the first admission.

Discussion

The reasons for using intensive treatment in sensitive tumor systems—either large doses of single drugs or, in the case of the present study, combinations of drugs—stem, in part, from the work of Skipper, Shabel, and Wilcox (20) and are based on the cell-kill hypothesis derived in the sensitive murine leukemia L1210. Survival in such tumor-bearing animals is related to the number of cells the animal is inoculated with and the number that remain after therapy. When an effective drug is used in the treatment of this sensitive tumor, a clear dose-response relationship is noted between dose and survival (20, 21). Skipper, Shabel, and Wilcox (38) also emphasized that a constant fraction, rather than an absolute number, of cells was destroyed with a given dose of drug. If the dose of the effective drug could be increased enough or treatment begun when the cell population was small enough, either the tumor population could be reduced to zero or the small residual of cells could be controlled by the host's own defense mechanism. At least in the L1210 system, however, one leukemia cell can lead to the death of the animal (38, 39). Drugs with a low therapeutic index present some difficulty since the limiting toxicity may prevent the use of an optimal dose. Using combinations of drugs with differing mechanisms of action and various dose-limiting toxicities could presumably overcome this problem and does so in the animal system (21), provided each drug has some independent salutory effect. Leukemia L1210 differs from most human tumors in its cell-cycle characteristics and rate of growth, as well as its sensitivity to drugs (40). The difficulty in exploiting these principles derived from models of tumors in mice is not in the lack of appreciation of these differences but in the lack of knowledge of the biology of human tumors that is necessary to make the adjustments from mouse to man. These principles can be tested in man, provided the tumor in question is sensitive to several drugs that may be used effectively in large doses or safely in combination to increase their therapeutic index. Such treatment seems even more justified in those tumors considered drug sensitive than those considered resistant. The occurrence of frequent partial responses with an ultimately poor outcome resulting from the modest use of a single drug should suggest the possibility of improving the results with more intensive treatment. Such an approach with resistant tumors—that is, those that rarely regress with single drug treatment—awaits either the development of more tumor-specific drugs or a better understanding of the biology of these tumors. In resistant tumors such combinations may lead to increased toxicity with little gain in therapeutic effect.

Hodgkin's disease is considered to be a drug-responsive human tumor. A review of the literature shows a certain sameness to the therapeutic data regardless of the drug used. The overall response rate to the alkylating agents, the vinca alkaloids, procarbazine, and steroids ranges from 40 to 75% for both complete and partial responses (3). When complete responses are dealt with separately, however, it is apparent that few patients achieve such a response—usually from 10 to 30% (19). The proportion of complete responses is affected by the prior treatment status of the patient. Prior therapy appears to compromise the ability of single drugs to induce remission (19). The duration of the remission also appears to be a function of the completeness of the antitumor response. Thus, complete remissions last longer than partial remissions if no maintenance therapy is given. The median duration of unmaintained partial remissions is very short—4 to 6 weeks (3). Although complete remissions last longer, they rarely exceed 12 to 16 weeks (19).

One difficulty in interpreting such data is the duration of induction therapy. Such treatment is usually given for a finite period of time, usually 4 to 6 weeks, and then the patient's status is evaluated for the completeness of response. This approach assumes that the rate of improvement is similar in all patients and that an incomplete response at 6 weeks will not become complete if induction therapy is continued for 12 or 24 weeks. It is of interest that in our own study, in spite of the intensity of the treatment, the median time to complete remission was 3 months. This fact opens to question the adequacy of the usual 6-week protocol induction period. The duration of remissions, complete or partial, has been shown to be prolonged with some form of drug maintenance program (3, 19, 41). The average duration of remission for all types of responders, while on maintenance treatment, is 8 to 10 months, but the median duration of remission in complete responders after maintenance therapy has been reported to be as long as 13 months in one study (19). Although maintenance therapy seems beneficial, survival of patients with Hodgkin's disease is not affected whether maintenance treatment is continual or patients are allowed to relapse and then retreated periodically (19). Maintenance treatment may, in fact, be a form of continued induction therapy. Such data also suggest that long-term, more intensive treatment programs as the initial form of therapy might improve the initial response rate and the magnitude and duration of the responses achieved.

The results of the present study suggest that to some degree this is true. The patients had not received a significant amount of prior therapy, and the therapeutic effect of the drug combination appears superior to that of previous studies using single drugs, including our own (19). Eighty-one percent of the patients treated achieved a complete remission. The designation "complete remission" was made only after careful posttreatment evaluation, and the durability of these responses in most of these patients suggests the criteria for complete remissions were meaningful. Although patients achieving a complete remission received no further treatment, the median duration of their responses was surprisingly long and will be between 29 and 42 months.

A high remission induction rate was also noted in the prior pilot study performed at the National Cancer Institute (26) with similar combination chemotherapy, using methotrexate instead of procarbazine. The duration of treatment in that study was only 2½ months. In the pilot study, as in the present one, some patients ending the prescribed protocol treatment period were continuing to respond but had not achieved complete remission. The results in the earlier study led to the expansion of the treatment period to 6 months in the present one. Since July 1967 our approach has been slightly different; patients have been treated for a minimum of six cycles, but those with residual disease who are continuing to respond are given further therapy. The maximum number of cycles given to induce a complete remission, thus far, is 11. Lacher and Durant (42) also reported on the use of combination chemotherapy in Hodgkin's disease using vinblastine and chlorambucil. In spite of modest doses of each drug and prior radiotherapy of the patients, the complete remission rate was 40%, which was superior to that previously reported with single agents.

The drugs in the present study were used in full doses. The total projected dose of vincristine in the combination is equivalent to a 12-week course of this drug at 0.033 mg/kg body weight per week. For nitrogen mustard an equivalent dose used in a standard fashion would be a monthly dose of 0.4 mg/kg body weight for 6 months. The equivalent single dose of procarbazine would be 100 mg/m^2 of body surface area per day for 3 months. Prednisone was used only in the first and fourth cycle to avoid the well-known side effects of corticoids. In retrospect, prednisone could probably have been used with each cycle since its side effects were negligible in the present study.

The treatment itself, although more complicated than the use of single drugs, was not overly difficult to administer in a cancer clinic. The acute toxicity—nausea and vomiting—was slightly more severe than one would expect using full intravenous doses of nitrogen mustard alone. Therapy was administered in the outpatient clinic in most cases. Most of the patients continued to work during therapy, usually losing only 2 days of work for each cycle. Some patients, unable to work before treatment, were able to return to work while on treatment because of rapid improvement in their performance status. Once patients achieved a complete remission, they uniformly returned to their former occupation. Although the 6 months of treatment was rigorous, the long disease-free interval with no repeated medication and with only monthly visits to the Clinic appears to be a decided advantage over the use of single agents. Because hair loss was unpredictable, wigs were routinely provided and accepted by female patients but rarely necessary for men.

Leukopenia, as expected, was the dose-limiting toxicity. It was expected that progressive dose reduction would be required, and almost all patients did require some reduction in doses, especially later in the treatment course. Two deaths were drug-related but largely caused by rapid necrosis of tumor, an effect that may be difficult to avoid. We have now treated over 125 patients with Hodgkin's disease in this fashion, and these remain the only 2 deaths that can be related to combination drug treatment. The other side effects, although troublesome, were not difficult to regulate. The most severe problem in addition to leukopenia and thrombocytopenia was the anemia that developed in 17% of the patients. This process required red-blood-cell transfusion for support, but it promptly and dramatically reversed within 1 month of cessation of therapy. The mechanism is unknown but appears to be a drug-induced red cell aplasia and not a hemolytic process.

Most patients skin tested before therapy were anergic, and reversion of skin tests to positive was common in those tested while in remission. This finding indicates that intensive treatment with immunosuppressive drugs does not impair the ability to recover responsiveness to delayed hypersensitivity antigens. As a further indication of a residual intact immunologic status, those known to be positive for intradermal skin tests before treatment remained so after treatment. The return of the delayed hypersensitivity response after treatment, after a minimum of 10 months in remission, was consistent with the continued general good health of these patients. The initial response, duration of remissions, and survival, however, do not appear to have been affected by the immunologic status before treatment.

Staging of patients with Hodgkin's disease has been and continues to be progressively more complex. The great controversy centers on diagnosing early involvement of the liver. While this phase of the study was in progress, we accepted two abnormal liver function studies in the face of normal needle, or open biopsy of liver, or both, as evidence that Hodgkin's disease, and not some other form of diffuse liver disease, was the cause of the liver function abnormality. Thus, it could be argued that some of our patients diagnosed as Stage IVB liver, on this basis, might actually be Stage IIIB. Even at the present time no solution to this dilemma exists, and patients with hepatomegaly and significantly abnormal liver function tests are difficult to treat with radiotherapy alone. Since most of our patients had other laboratory and clinical evidence of abnormalities of the liver, we still consider the possibility of liver tumor quite high in those five patients in question.

The ultimate test of therapeutic results is improvement in survival of the population in question. Survival data in the literature are difficult to interpret but have generally indicated that the median survival of patients with advanced Hodgkin's disease is less than 2 years (2, 3, 43-46). One recent study recording the lifespan of patients from the time they first received chemotherapy to death reported a median survival of 24 months (47). The results of another large controlled clinical trial of the management of patients with lymphoma were similar (19). Most studies lack separate data on the survival of patients who achieve a complete response, although the improved survival of responders in general has been noted (2). The median survival of the entire group and of the complete responders in the present study has not been reached but in the latter case will be in excess of 42 months. Twenty-eight of the 35 complete responders are still living, and 17 remain in their first complete unmaintained remission. The median survival of the group of six patients who responded but failed to achieve a complete remission is comparable to the average survival reported in the literature, 20 months, with only one patient remaining alive. With a minimum follow-up time of 32 months, 29 of the 43, or 67% of the entire population, remain alive.

Our patients and the patient populations reported in the literature are quite heterogeneous in regard to prior treatment, histologic categories, immunologic status, and pretreatment staging. Because of this and the lack of suitable internal controls, comparisons between these data should be interpreted with caution. Examination of all the above measures, which are known to influence prognosis in Hodgkin's disease, in our patients, however, failed to disclose a high degree of selection of a favorable group. That is, the histology was generally advanced, as was the clinical stage, and most patients tested were anergic. Most, however, had received no significant prior therapy that could be expected to exert a favorable influence. Results using single drugs in patients with no prior therapy are available for comparison (19). The results of the present study compare favorably.

Hodgkin's disease has a variable and complex natural history, and although our understanding of factors that influence prognosis has improved in recent years, it is apparent that some patients with advanced disease and an apparently poor prognosis survive for long periods of time. What is equally apparent is that this is not a common occurence (48). These long-surviving patients generally have easily identifiable areas of disease and require some form of repeated therapy. The most unusual aspect of the present study is the long-term, disease-free interval after successful treatment; 47% of those patients at risk for 4 years have been continuously free of their disease in the face of continued detailed reexamination. Although the survival of patients treated in this fashion seems superior to those treated with single drugs, these results require confirmation in controlled clinical trials with comparably staged patients of equivalent histologic classification. Nonetheless, the use of combinations of effective drugs as the initial form of therapy in the treatment of sensitive tumors appears to have therapeutic efficacy.

ACKNOWLEDGMENTS: The authors express their sincere gratitute to the many clinical associates who participated in the care of these patients. The cooperation and assistance of Drs. Costan Berard, Louis Thomas, and Jean Herdt have been invaluable. The authors are grateful to Dr. Emil Frei, III, for his continued interest in this study and to Miss Myra Stull for preparation and editing of the manuscript.

Received 10 June 1970; revision accepted 5 August 1970.

► Requests for reprints should be addressed to Vincent T. De Vita, M.D., National Cancer Institute, Bldg. 10, Room 12N226, Bethesda, Md. 20014

References

1. KAPLAN HS: The radical radiotherapy of regionally localized Hodgkin's disease. *Radiology* 78:553-561, 1960
2. ULTMANN JE, CUNNINGHAM JK, GELLHORN A: The clinical picture of Hodgkin's disease. *Cancer Res* 26:1047-1061, 1966
3. ULTMANN JE, NIXON DD: The therapy of lymphoma. *Seminars Hemat* 6:376-403, 1969
4. GOODMAN LS, GILMAN A: *The Pharmacologic Basis of Therapeutics*, 3rd ed. New York, The MacMillan Co., 1965, p. 1345
5. FREI E III, CARBONE PP, SHNIDER BI, et al: A study of vinblastine in the treatment of patients with neoplastic disease. *Arch Intern Med (Chicago)* 117:846-952, 1965
6. FROST JW, GOLDWEIN MI, BRYAN JA: Clinical experience with vinca leukoblastine in far advanced Hodgkin's disease and various malignant states. *Ann Intern Med* 56:854-859, 1962

7. Wright TL, Hurley J, Korst DR, et al: Vinblastine in neoplastic diseases. *Cancer Res* 23:169-179, 1963
8. Bleehan NM, Jelleffe A: Vinblastine sulphate in the treatment of malignant disease. *Brit J Cancer* 19:268-273, 1963
9. Bohanan R, Miller D, Diamond H: Vincristine in the treatment of the lymphomas and leukemia. *Cancer Res* 23: 613-621, 1963
10. Carbone PP, Bono V, Frei E III, et al: Clinical studies with vincristine. *Blood* 21:640-647, 1963
11. Bruner KW, Young CW: A methylhydrazine derivative in Hodgkin's disease and other malignant neoplasms. *Ann Intern Med* 63:69-86, 1965
12. DeVita VT, Serpick A, Carbone PP: Preliminary clinical studies with Ibenzmethyzin. *Clin Pharmacol Ther* 7:542-546, 1966
13. Todd IDH: Natulan in management of late Hodgkin's disease, other lymphoreticular neoplasms, and malignant melanomas. *Brit Med J* 5435:628-631, 1965
14. Bollag W, Grunberg E: Tumor inhibitory effects of a new class of cytotoxic agents: methylhydrazine derivatives. *Experientia* 19:130-131, 1963
15. Mathé G, Schweisguth O, Schneider M, et al: Methylhydrazine in the treatment of Hodgkin's disease. *Lancet* 2: 1077-1080, 1963
16. Freyman JG, Vander JB, Marler EA, et al: Prolonged corticosteroid therapy of chronic lymphocytic leukemia and the closely allied malignant lymphomas. *Brit J Haemat* 6: 303-323, 1960
17. Kofman J, Perla CP, Boesen E, et al: Role of corticosteroids in treatment of malignant lymphomas. *Cancer* 15: 338-345, 1962
18. Hall TC, Choi GS, Abadi A, et al: High dose corticoid therapy in Hodgkin's disease and other lymphomas. *Ann Intern Med* 60:1144-1153, 1967
19. Carbone PP, Spurr C: Management of patients with malignant lymphoma. A comparative study with cyclophosphamide and vinca alkaloids. *Cancer Res* 28:811-822, 1968
20. Skipper HE, Shabel FM Jr, Wilcox WS: Experimental evaluation of potential anticancer agents XIII on the criteria and kinetics associated with "curability" of experimental leukemia. *Cancer Chemother Rep* 35:1-111, 1964
21. Venditti JM, Goldin A: Drug synergism in antineoplastic chemotherapy, in *Advances in Chemotherapy,* edited by Goldin A and Hawkins S. New York, Academic Press, Inc., Publishers, 1964, p. 397
22. Frei E III: For leukemia group B: the effectiveness of combination of antileukemia agents in inducing and maintaining remission in children with acute leukemia. *Blood* 26: 642-656, 1965
23. Freireich EJ, Karon M, Frei E III: Quadruple combination therapy (VAMP) for acute lymphocytic leukemia of childhood. *Proc Amer Ass Cancer Res* 5:20, 1964
24. Freireich EJ, Henderson ES, Karon MR, et al: The treatment of acute leukemia considered with respect to cell population kinetics, in *The Proliferation and Spread of Neoplastic Cells.* Baltimore, The Williams & Wilkins Co., 1968, pp. 441-452
25. DeVita VT, Moxley JH III, Brace K, et al: Intensive combination chemotherapy and X-irradiation in the treatment of Hodgkin's disease. *Proc Amer Ass Cancer Res* 6: 15, 1965
26. Moxley JH III, DeVita VT, Brace K, et al: Intensive combination chemotherapy and X-irradiation in Hodgkin's disease. *Cancer Res* 27:1258-1263, 1967
27. Frei E III, DeVita VT, Moxley JH III, et al: Approaches to improving the chemotherapy of Hodgkin's disease. *Cancer Res* 26:1284-1289, 1966
28. Frei E III, Spurr CL, Brindley CO, et al: Clinical studies of dichloromethotrexate. *Clin Pharmacol Ther* 6:160-171, 1965
29. DeVita VT, Serpick A: Combination chemotherapy in the treatment of advanced Hodgkin's disease. *Proc Amer Ass Cancer Res* 8:13, 1967
30. DeVita VT, Serpick A, Carbone PP: Combination chemotherapy of advanced Hodgkin's disease: the NCI program a progress report. *Proc Amer Ass Cancer Res* 10:19, 1969
31. Rosenberg SA: Report of the committee on the staging of Hodgkin's disease. *Cancer Res* 26:1310, 1966
32. Lukes RJ, Butler JJ: The pathology and nomenclature of Hodgkin's disease. *Ibid.,* pp. 1063-1083
33. Lukes RJ: Report of the nomenclature committee. *Ibid.,* p. 1311
34. Brown RS, Haynes HA, Foley HT, et al: Hodgkin's disease—immunologic, clinical, and histologic features of 50 untreated patients. *Ann Intern Med* 67:291-303, 1967
35. Lessner HE: For the Southeastern Cancer Chemotherapy Cooperative Study Group, BCNU (1,3,Bis(2-chloroethyl)-1-nitrosourea) effects on advanced Hodgkin's disease and other neoplasia. *Cancer* 22:451-456, 1968
36. Keller AR, Kaplan HS, Lukes RJ, et al: Correlation of histopathology with other prognostic indicators in Hodgkin's disease. *Ibid.,* pp. 487-499
37. Waldorf DS, Sheagren JN, Trautman JR, et al: Impaired delayed hypersensitivity in patients with lepromatous leprosy. *Lancet* 2:773-776, 1966
38. Skipper H, Schabel F, Wilcox WS: Experimental evaluation of potential anticancer agents XIV, further study of certain basic concepts underlying chemotherapy of leukemia. *Cancer Chemother Rep* 45:5-28, 1965
39. Furth J, Kahn NC: The transmission of leukemia of mice with a single cell. *Amer J Cancer* 31:276-282, 1937
40. Yankee RA, DeVita VT, Perry S: The cell cycle of leukemia L1210 cell *in vivo. Cancer Res* 27:2381-2385, 1967
41. Scott JL: The effect of nitrogen mustard and maintenance chlorambucil in treatment of advanced Hodgkin's disease. *Cancer Chemother Rep* 27:27-32, 1963
42. Lacher MJ, Durant JR: Combined vinblastine and chlorambucil therapy of Hodgkin's disease. *Ann Intern Med* 62: 468-476, 1965
43. Jacobs FM, Peters FC, Luce JK, et al: Mechlorethamine HCl and cyclophosphamide in the treatment of Hodgkin's disease and lymphomas. *JAMA* 203:392-398, 1968
44. Ezdinli EA, Stutzman L: Vinblastine vs. nitrogen mustard therapy of Hodgkin's disease. *Cancer* 22:473-479, 1968
45. Gellhorn A: End results in lymphosarcoma and Hodgkin's disease, in *Proceedings of the Third National Cancer Conference.* Philadelphia, J. B. Lippincott Co., 1957, pp. 862-869
46. Sohier WD Jr, Wong RKL, Aisenberg AC: Vinblastine in the treatment of advanced Hodgkin's disease. *Cancer* 22: 467-472, 1968
47. Rapoport A, Cole P, Mason J: Correlation of survival after initiation of chemotherapy in 142 cases of Hodgkin's disease. *Cancer* 23:377-381, 1969
48. Lacher M: Long survival in Hodgkin's disease. *Ann Intern Med* 70:7-19, 1969

Section VII

Infectious Diseases

Pneumococcal bacteremia with especial reference to bacteremic pneumococcal pneumonia.

Austrian R, Gold J. Ann Intern Med. 1964;60:759-776.

Not long after Louis Pasteur's 1881 discovery of the pneumococcus, epidemic pneumococcal pneumonia was recognized among men recruited to work in South African gold mines. Mortality was 35%, and in 1904, striking miners demanded action. Mine owners responded by encouraging and supporting efforts to develop a vaccine. A candidate vaccine was developed as early as 1914, and clinical trials of others were carried out over the next few decades. In 1944, a randomized, placebo-controlled trial demonstrated safety and efficacy of a tetravalent polysaccharide vaccine; the U.S. Food and Drug Administration approved and licensed it in 1946. The vaccine became available at a time when most physicians thought it was no longer needed: Penicillin had become available in 1945 and was widely believed to be a "magic bullet." Penicillin sales thrived; vaccine use waned; and, for financial reasons, vaccine production was discontinued in 1951.

Robert Austrian, drawing on his personal experiences at Kings County Hospital in Brooklyn, did not agree with the widely held view that penicillin had made the devastation of pneumococcal pneumonia a thing of the past. The 1964 article that he co-authored with Jerome Gold showed unequivocally that, despite antibiotic use, pneumococcal pneumonia and bacteremia remained a serious and often fatal problem. They documented approximately 2000 cases of pneumococcal pneumonia and 529 instances of pneumococcal bacteremia over 10 years on a 225-bed medical service. Mortality in treated bacteremic patients was 17%. Their study also provided evidence that a few pneumococcal serotypes were responsible for most cases of the disease. Figure 6 from their article tells the most important tale: Although treatments dramatically improved survival, the death rate during the first 5 days was the same among those who received no treatment compared with those who received serum therapy or antibiotic. Austrian and Gold concluded that "antimicrobial therapy has little or no effect upon the outcome of infection among those destined, at the onset of illness, to die within 5 days." They suggested that vaccine prophylaxis offered "the best available means of lowering the morbidity and mortality resulting from pneumococcal infection."

Austrian remained a vaccine advocate after publication of this important article, and in 1972, he initiated a 4-year placebo-controlled vaccine trial in South African gold miners that demonstrated 79% efficacy in preventing infections due to vaccine-included strains. This finding led the FDA to license a 14-valent vaccine in 1977 for people 50 years of age or older and those with chronic illness. The children and adults who benefit from the pneumococcal vaccines in widespread use today are indebted to Austrian and Gold's study.

Quantitative relationships between circulating leukocytes and infection in patients with acute leukemia.

Bodey GP, Buckley M, Sathe YS, Freireich EJ. Ann Intern Med. 1966; 64:328-40.

The advent of aggressive cytotoxic chemotherapy for hematologic malignancies resulted in remissions and cures for illnesses that previously had been uniformly and rapidly fatal. However, chemotherapy led to an increase in infections that often became the cause of death. A long-standing principle of treatment of infectious diseases had been to withhold the use of antimicrobials until there was clear evidence of infection. But, in cancer patients receiving chemotherapy, fever in the absence of any other clinical manifestations of infection sometimes heralded life-threatening bacteremia. In such patients, withholding antibiotics while waiting a day or two for a positive blood culture might result in death from an otherwise treatable infection.

In 52 patients with acute leukemia admitted to the Clinical Center of the National Institutes of Health, Bodey and colleagues showed a clear relationship between the number of circulating neutrophils and the presence of infection. In their own words, "The presence of infection in patients with acute leukemia is related to the level of circulating granulocytes" and "Furthermore, the lower the level of these leukocytes, the more likelihood that infection will be present." Their study established neutropenia as the most important risk factor for infection among patients with leukemia and showed that when fever occurs in this setting, the degree and duration of neutropenia are important determinants of the presence of infection. When the neutrophil count decreases to less than 1000 cells/mm^3, increased susceptibility to infection is expected. The infection risk rises considerably when the counts drop from 1000 cells/ mm^3 to less than 500 cells/mm^3. At least one fifth of febrile patients with neutrophil counts of 100 cells/mm^3 or less have bacteremia. The finding that infection was more common during relapse than remission for any given neutrophil count suggested that abnormalities of leukocyte function or other immune deficits may further increase the risk of infection in a neutropenic patient.

The observations reported in this seminal article resulted in a new approach to fever in the neutropenic patient. Management algorithms were developed that included the immediate administration of broad-spectrum antimicrobials to a febrile neutropenic patient when the neutrophil count is less than 500 cells/mm^3, regardless of the cause of neutropenia. This approach has been the standard of care for more than three decades and has saved many lives.

Plasma viral load and CD4+ lymphocytes as prognostic markers of HIV-1 infection.

Mellors JW, Muñoz A, Giorgi JV, et al. Ann Intern Med. 1997;126: 946-954.

The disease we now call the acquired immunodeficiency syndrome (AIDS) first came to attention in the summer of 1981 as a few barely noticed case reports, It has since grown into a catastrophic global pandemic that ranks as one of the most devastating microbial scourges in history.

Once it became possible to diagnose infection with HIV-1—the causative virus—it became evident that the clinical course differed greatly among infected persons. Some individuals developed AIDS and died within a year or two of diagnosis, whereas others appeared to remain free of disease for many years. A relationship was noted between decreasing circulating CD4$^+$ lymphocyte counts and progression to AIDS. In the mid-1990s, new techniques permitted accurate quantification of the amount of circulating virus, measured as the plasma concentration of HIV-1 RNA (viral load).

In their crucial article, Mellors and colleagues prospectively studied the prognostic value of plasma viral load compared with clinical, serologic, and cellular markers in more than 1600 HIV-infected men and demonstrated that plasma viral load was the single best predictor of progression to AIDS and death. The proportion of patients who died of AIDS within 6 years was 0.9% when initial viral loads were 500 copies/mL or less, 18.1% when they were 3001 to 10,000 copies/mL, and 69.5% when they were more than 30,000 copies/mL. The amount of virus in the blood, as defined by plasma HIV-1 RNA concentration, discriminated the risks for progression to AIDS and death at all levels of CD4$^+$ lymphocyte count and predicted the subsequent rate of decline of these cells. A combined measurement of viral load and CD4$^+$ lymphocyte count was even more accurate in predicting disease progression.

This study provided strong evidence that viremia is central to the pathogenesis of HIV-1 disease and defined the prognostic power of viral load measurement. It led to the routine and widespread use of combined viral load and CD4$^+$ lymphocyte count to decide when to begin treatment and how to monitor response to therapy, and these criteria serve as surrogate markers for disease response in clinical trials of new antiretroviral agents.

Pneumococcal Bacteremia with Especial Reference to Bacteremic Pneumococcal Pneumonia

ROBERT AUSTRIAN, M.D., and JEROME GOLD, M.D.

Philadelphia, Pennsylvania

TWENTY-FIVE YEARS have elapsed since the subject of pneumococcal bacteremia has been reviewed (1, 2). In that period many changes have taken place both in the treatment of this disorder and in the attitude of the medical profession toward it. The introduction of a series of antimicrobial drugs effective against all capsular types of pneumococcus has led to widespread abandonment of the more precise bacteriologic techniques designed for the recognition of this organism and secondarily to the impression that pneumococcal disease no longer constitutes a serious medical problem. To determine the validity of these practices and attitudes, established techniques for the isolation and identification of pneumococcus were reintroduced as routine procedures in 1952, into the clinical research bacteriologic laboratory of the Department of Medicine, State University of New York Downstate Medical Center, at Kings County Hospital, Brooklyn, N. Y. In the decade after this step was taken, approximately 2,000 cases of pneumococcal pneumonia and 529 instances of pneumococcal bacteremia were recognized on the medical wards served by this laboratory. A study of the patients with pneumococcal bacteremia follows and suggests that highly effective antimicrobial drugs must be supplemented by other measures, both prophylactic and therapeutic, if the significant mortality resulting still from pneumococcal infection is to be reduced.

In analyzing the results of antimicrobial therapy, the data will be contrasted where relevant with those reported by Tilghman and Finland (1), who described a similar group of 480 patients with bacteremic pneumococcal pneumonia treated symptomatically at the Boston City Hospital between 1929 and 1935. Though the latter group cannot be considered a control in the strict sense of the term, its use for comparative purposes is dictated by the inadmissibility of withholding antipneumococcal therapy during the present investigation.

MATERIALS AND METHODS

The patients included in this study were all admitted to the 225-bed Division B Medical Service of Kings County Hospital, Brooklyn, N. Y., between September 1, 1952, and August 31, 1962. All were over 12 years of age. In every instance blood was obtained for culture before the administration of antimicrobial drugs because of the presence of fever, signs of respiratory infection, an altered state of consciousness, and/or acute pulmonary edema. Twenty ml of blood were drawn from an antecubital vein, 15 ml of which were inoculated into 50 ml of trypticase soy broth, 2 ml into 20 ml of thioglycolate broth, and 3 ml into citrate solution to prevent clotting. Pour plates were made by inoculating agar with unclotted

Received December 2, 1963; accepted for publication January 7, 1964.

From the Department of Medicine, State University of New York Downstate Medical Center, the Medical Service of Kings County Hospital, Brooklyn, New York, and the Department of Research Medicine, the University of Pennsylvania School of Medicine, Philadelphia, Pennsylvania.

These data were presented in part at the 76th Session of the Association of American Physicians, April 30, 1963.

Requests for reprints should be addressed to Robert Austrian, M.D., Hospital of the University of Pennsylvania, Philadelphia 4, Pennsylvania.

TABLE 1. Incidence of Pneumococcal Types in Bacteremic Infections Associated with Pneumonia, with Pneumonia Complicated by an Extrapulmonary Focus of Pneumococcal Infection and with Nonpulmonary Infection

Type of Pneumococcus	Type of Infection									Total		
	Pneumonia			Pneumonia with Extrapulmonary Focus			Nonpulmonary Infection					
	All Cases	Fatal Cases		All Cases	Fatal Cases		All Cases	Fatal Cases		All Cases	Fatal Cases	
	no.	*no.*	%	*no.*	*no.*	%	*no.*	*no.*	%	*no.*	*no.*	%
I	78	6	8	2	0	0	0	0	0	80	6	7.5
II	8	1	13	2	0	0	0	0	0	10	1	10
III	35	18	51	8	3	38	6	6	100	49	27	55
IV	43	8	19	1	1	100	1	1	100	45	10	22
V	23	2	9	2	2	100	0	0	0	25	4	16
VI	10	3	30	1	1	100	0	0	0	11	4	35
VII	61	7	11	3	2	67	1	1	100	65	10	15
VIII	54	8	15	9	4	44	1	1	100	64	13	20
IX	6	2	33	0	0	0	1	1	100	7	3	43
X	1	0	0	1	1	100	0	0	0	2	1	50
XI	1	0	0	0	0	0	0	0	0	1	0	0
XII	32	7	22	3	1	33	3	2	67	38	10	26
XIII	1	0	0	1	1	100	0	0	0	2	1	50
XIV	14	1	7	3	2	67	2	1	50	19	4	21
XV	3	1	33	0	0	0	1	0	0	4	1	25
XVI	3	2	67	0	0	0	2	0	0	5	2	40
XVII	4	1	25	1	1	100	0	0	0	5	2	40
XVIII	11	2	18	1	0	0	2	1	50	14	3	21
XIX	14	6	43	0	0	0	2	2	100	16	8	50
XX	12	5	42	1	0	0	1	0	0	14	5	35
XXI	0	0	0	1	1	100	0	0	0	1	1	100
XXII	6	1	17	0	0	0	0	0	0	6	1	17
XXIII	6	3	0	1	1	100	0	0	0	7	3	43
XXIV	1	0	0	0	0	0	1	1	100	2	1	50
XXV	7	1	14	0	0	0	1	0	0	8	1	12
XXVIII	1	0	0	0	0	0	0	0	0	1	0	0
XXIX	1	0	0	1	1	100	0	0	0	2	1	50
XXX, LIV	1	0	0	0	0	0	0	0	0	1	0	0
XXXI	2	0	0	0	0	0	0	0	0	2	0	0
XXXIII	7	2	29	1	0	0	0	0	0	8	2	25
XLIV, LV, LVI	2	1	50	2	2	100	0	0	0	4	3	75

TABLE 1. (Continued)

Type of Pneumococcus	Type of Infection											
	Pneumonia			Pneumonia with Extrapulmonary Focus			Nonpulmonary Infection			Total		
	All Cases	Fatal Cases		All Cases	Fatal Cases		All Cases	Fatal Cases		All Cases	Fatal Cases	
	no.	*no.*	%	*no.*	*no.*	%	*no.*	*no.*	%	*no.*	*no.*	%
XLVIII, L, LI	1	0	0	0	0	0	0	0	0	1	0	0
LIII	1	0	0	0	0	0	0	0	0	1	0	0
LVII, LVIII, LIX	2	0	0	0	0	0	0	0	0	2	0	0
LXXII	1	1	100	0	0	0	0	0	0	1	1	100
Untyped	2	0	0	2	1	50	2	0	0	6	1	17
Total	455	89	19.5	47	25	53.2	27	17	63	529	131	24.8

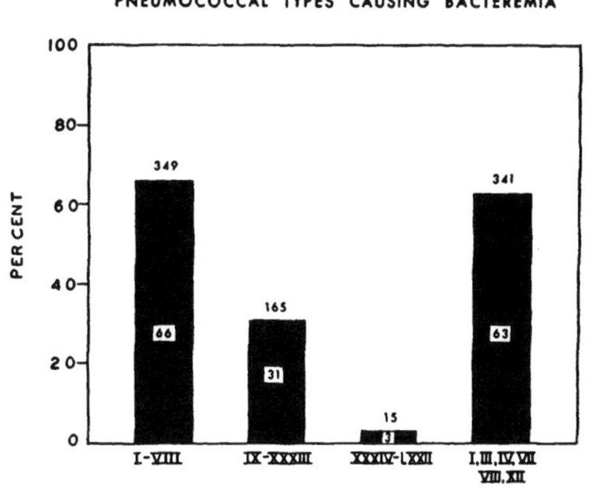

FIGURE 1. Number within bar represents per cent of total cases. Number above bar indicates number of cases.

blood routinely, but bacterial counts were not analyzed because blood drawn at night was frequently incubated several hours before the plates were poured. All cultures were performed during the life of the patient, and positive confirmatory cultures were obtained at postmortem examination only from patients who received no antimicrobial therapy prior to death.

Pneumococci were identified by use of the Gram stain and the capsular swelling reaction, by their solubility in sodium desoxycholate, and by their ability to produce fatal infection in mice (3). Capsular typing serums for Types I

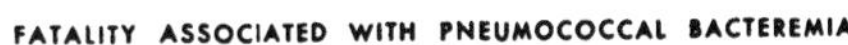

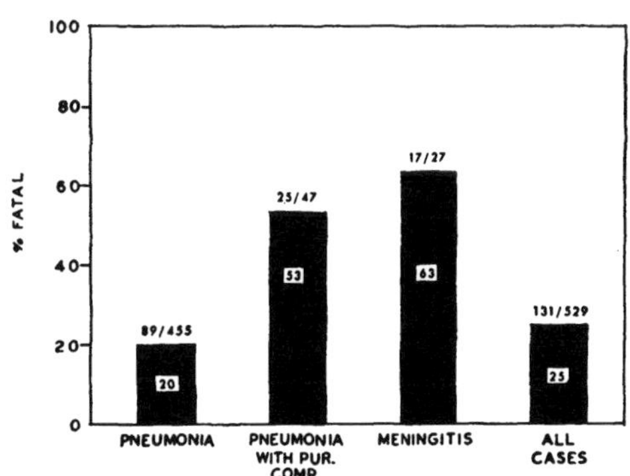

FIGURE 2. Denominator of fraction above bar indicates number of cases, numerator number of fatal cases. Number within bar indicates per cent of fatal cases. "Pur. comp." includes cases of bacteremic pneumococcal pneumonia with an extrapulmonary focus of pneumococcal infection. The bar for meningitis includes only those cases not secondary to pneumonia.

Table 2. Incidence of Bacteremia and Mortality in Pneumonia Caused by Pneumococci of Several Capsular Types

Type of Pneumo-coccus	Bacteremic			Nonbacteremic			All Cases			% Bacteremic	
	All Cases	Fatal Cases		All Cases	Fatal Cases		All Cases	Fatal Cases		All Cases	Fatal Cases
	no.	*no.*	%	*no.*	*no.*	%	*no.*	*no.*	%	%	%
I	80(2)*	6	8	134	1	1	214	7	3	37	86
II	10(2)*	1	10	9	0	0	19	1	5	52	100
III	43(8)*	21(3)*	19	230	41	18	273	62	22	16	34
IV	44(1)*	9(1)*	21	109	10	9	153	19	13	29	47
VII	64(3)*	9(2)*	14	142	10	7	206	19	9	31	47
VIII	63(9)*	12(4)*	18	120	10	8	183	22	12	33	54
XII	35(3)*	8(1)*	23	47	4	9	82	12	14	42	67
Total	339(28)*	66(11)*	19	791	76	10	1130	142	13	30	46

* Numbers in parentheses designate number of bacteremic cases with an extrapulmonary focus of pneumococcal infection.

to XXXIV * were used throughout the period of the study. Serums for the identification of types higher than XXXIV † became available in January, 1957, and all strains of pneumococcus recovered from the blood thereafter were identified by capsular typing. The six untyped strains included in the study possessed all the other biologic attributes of pneumococcus.

Results

The distribution of pneumococcal capsular types causing bacteremia together with the fatality rate associated with each type is recorded in Table 1. The table is subdivided further to delineate bacteremia associated with pneumonia, bacteremia associated with pneumonia and an extrapulmonary focus of pneumococcal infection, and bacteremia secondary to pneumococcal infection unaccompanied by pneumonia.

With few exceptions, the distribution of capsular types (Figure 1) causing infection was similar to that noted in earlier studies, and the first eight capsular types accounted for two thirds of the cases of pneumococcal disease with bacteremia. Types XII, XIV, XVIII, XIX, and XX were also recovered with relative frequency from the blood. Infection with numerical types higher than XXXIII was followed rarely by bacteremia, only 3 per cent of the positive blood cultures being accounted for by these types. Mortality was least when bacteremia was associated only with pneumonia and was two to three times as great when an extrapulmonary focus of pneumococcal infection was present (Figure 2).

The mortality from infection with different capsular types showed considerable variation. The fatality rate for Type I pneumococcal bacteremia was 8 per cent

* Capsular typing serums were made available through the courtesy of Dr. H. D. Piersma, Lederle Laboratories Division, American Cyanimid Company, and of Dr. E. F. Roberts, Wyeth Laboratories, American Home Products Corporation.

† Statens Seruminstitut, Amagar Boulevard 80, Copenhagen S., Denmark. Serums for all capsular types are available at a cost of approximately $2.25 per ml.

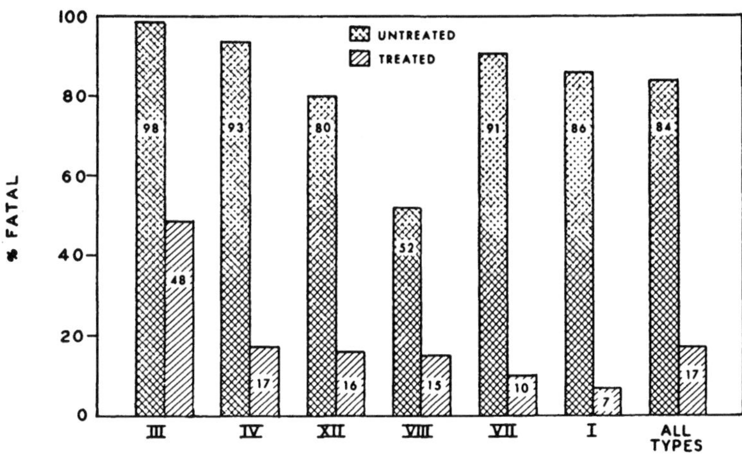

FIGURE 3. Number within bar indicates per cent of fatal cases. Data for untreated cases from Tilghman and Finland (1).

for all cases whereas that for Type III infection was 55 per cent. Mortality from infection with other capsular types seen in significant numbers was in the range of 15 to 25 per cent. Figure 3 depicts these differences, contrasting the outcome in untreated and penicillin-treated patients with bacteremic pneumococcal pneumonia. It is noteworthy that the prognosis for Type III pneumococcal infections has been improved significantly less than that for infections caused by other capsular types. As will be noted subsequently, other factors, such as the age distribution of patients with infection caused by different capsular types, account probably in part for the more striking differences in mortality.

Table 2 records the incidence of bacteremia in pneumonic infection caused by the six capsular types responsible most often for invasion of the circulation and by pneumococcus Type II. With the exception of Type III, these findings bear close resemblance to those of the earlier study of Tilghman and Finland (1). Type III pneumococcus was recovered from the respiratory tract of 350 nonbacteremic patients during the present investigation. Of these, 230 had unequivocal evidence of pneumonia, 76 had questionable involvement of the lungs, and the remainder were clearly carriers. The incidence of bacteremia in Type III pneumococcal pneumonia was distinctly lower than that associated with infection by the other six capsular types analyzed. This fact notwithstanding, both bacteremic and nonbacteremic infections with Type III pneumococcus were followed

TABLE 3. Mortality According to Age and Sex in Pneumococcal Bacteremia, All Cases

Age	All Cases	Fatal Cases	
yr	*no.*	*no.*	%
12–19	11	0	0
20–29	40	4	10
30–39	95	5	5
40–49	110	19	17
50–59	99	18	18
60–69	80	34	43
70–79	58	28	48
80–89	30	18	60
90+	6	5	83
Total	529	131	24.8
Males	384	90	23.4
Females	145	41	28.3

Table 4. Bacteremia and Mortality According to Age in Pneumococcal Pneumonia Uncomplicated by an Extrapulmonary Focus of Infection

Type of Pneumococcus	12–29 Years Blood Culture							30–49 Years Blood Culture							50 Years or Older Blood Culture						
	Positive				Negative			Positive				Negative			Positive				Negative		
	No. of Cases	Fatal Cases	Fatal Cases	% Positive	No. of Cases	Fatal Cases	Fatal Cases	No. of Cases	Fatal Cases	Fatal Cases	% Positive	No. of Cases	Fatal Cases	Fatal Cases	No. of Cases	Fatal Cases	Fatal Cases	% Positive	No. of Cases	Fatal Cases	Fatal Cases
		no.	%			*no.*	%		*no.*	%			*no.*	%		*no.*	%			*no.*	%
I	15	1	6	23	51	0	0	29	0	0	40	44	0	0	34	5	15	48	37	1	3
III	1	0	0	5	19	0	0	6	2	33	9	61	3	5	28	16	57	16	149	38	26
IV	5	1	20	16	27	0	0	12	1	9	22	42	0	0	26	6	23	39	40	10	25
VII	7	0	0	15	39	1	3	30	2	6	33	60	2	3	24	5	21	60	40	6	15
VIII	4	0	0	15	22	0	0	23	2	9	32	49	2	4	27	6	22	38	44	7	16
XII	5	1	20	29	12	0	0	14	2	14	45	17	0	0	13	4	31	42	18	4	22
Total 6 types	37	3	8	13	170	1	1	114	9	8	29	273	7	3	152	42	28	32	328	66	20
Other	11	1	9	—	—	—	—	64	7	11	—	—	—	—	77	27	35	—	—	—	—
Total	48	4	8	—	—	—	—	178	16	9	—	—	—	—	229	69	30	—	—	—	—

by a higher mortality than that accompanying infection with any other capsular type seen in significant numbers. Because of its former prominence, infection with pneumococcus Type II merits comment. In all, only 19 infections with this organism were observed, 10 of which were bacteremic. Despite its infrequence during the period of the study, it continued to manifest the invasiveness shown in the era when it was more commonly observed.

In Table 3 are recorded the fatality rates for all cases of pneumococcal bacteremia by age in decades and the mortality in the two sexes. Mortality rises sharply in the seventh decade and remains high thereafter. Although pneumococcal bacteremia was detected three times more often in men than in women, no significant difference in mortality is observed between the two sexes.

Table 4 describes the age adjusted mortality for pneumonia with and without bacteremia uncomplicated by an extrapulmonary focus of infection and caused by the six capsular types invading the circulation most frequently. Similar data for bacteremic pneumonia caused by all other capsular types are included also. The differences in age distribution and in mortality between infections engendered by Type I and Type III are striking. Whereas little more than a third of infections caused by the former type were found in persons 50 years of age or older, two thirds of all infections with pneumococcus Type III were detected in this age group. Even when adjustments for age are made, the mortality after infection with pneumococcus Type III was several-fold than that caused by pneumococcus Type I and higher than that associated with any other pneumococcal type. In accord with earlier studies, the bacteremia rate tends to rise with advancing age, and the difference between the fatalities associated with bacteremic and nonbacteremic infections narrows in similar fashion.

As anticipated, prognosis in this series of patients was influenced by the extent of pulmonary consolidation, the mortality after involvement of two lobes being twice that when only a single lobe was affected (Table 5). Multilobar consolidation, however, was observed much less frequently in patients treated with antimicrobial drugs than in those under care at a time when these agents were unavailable. Whereas three fifths of the patients reported by Tilghman and Finland (1), whether untreated or treated with serum, had involvement of two or more lobes, fewer than one third of the patients in the present series had pneumonia involving more than a single lobe. Lesions were limited not in-

Table 5. Mortality According to Number of Pulmonary Lobes Involved in Bacteremic Pneumococcal Pneumonia Uncomplicated by an Extrapulmonary Focus of Infection

Lobes	All Cases	Incidence	Fatal Cases	
no.	*no.*	%	*no.*	%
1	308	68	38	12
2	99	22	24	24
3	16	3	10	63
4	1	—	1	100
Unknown	31	7	16	52
Total	455	100	89	19.5

Table 6. Relation of Leukocyte Count on Admission to Prognosis in Bacteremic Pneumococcal Pneumonia Uncomplicated by an Extrapulmonary Focus of Infection

Leukocyte Count in Thousands	All Cases		Fatal Cases	
	no.	%	*no.*	%
Less than 5	34	7	13	38
5 to 9	78	17	19	24
10 to 14	126	28	17	14
15 to 24	139	30	18	13
25 to 34	53	12	10	19
35 and over	9	2	2	22
Unknown	16	4	10	60
Total	455	100	89	19.5

frequently to a single pulmonary segment.

The leukocyte count at the time of hospitalization (Table 6) had the same predictive value regarding the likelihood of recovery in patients who were treated with antimicrobial drugs as in those who were not. A total leukocyte count of 10,000 to 25,000 per mm^3 appeared most favorable.

In agreement with the aforementioned authors, the presence or absence of alcoholism, acute or chronic, seemed of little prognostic import. Unless alcoholism were associated with leukopenia or with hepatic insufficiency, patients with this disorder acquiring pneumococcal pneumonia with bacteremia fared no worse than nonalcoholics. Fever, however, was observed to be of longer duration in patients whose infection was complicated by delirium tremens.

Comparable in importance to age in its influence on prognosis was the presence or absence of complicating pre-existing illness. In one form or another, significant systemic disease was present in 56 per cent of those afflicted with pneumococcal pneumonia and bacteremia. The various types of complicating illness are recorded in Table 7. No predilection for infection by any specific pneumococcal capsular type was observed. The difference in mortality between those patients with and those without complicating illness was striking, however, being four times greater in the former. If patients receiving no antimicrobial therapy are removed from consideration, the ratio is reduced but slightly. Figure 4 contrasts the outcome of illness among the untreated patients of Tighman and Finland and among those in the present study treated with antibiotics. Improvement in outlook has been less marked for those with pre-existing illness than for those who lacked it.

When deaths are analyzed with regard to the pneumococcal type responsible for infection, age, and the presence or absence of complicating illness (Table 8), several facts become evident. Forty-three per cent

TABLE 7. Effect of Pre-existing Complicating Illness on Mortality in Bactermic Pneumococcal Pneumonia Uncomplicated by an Extrapulmonary Focus of Infection

Complicating Illness	All Cases	Fatal Cases	
	no.	*no.*	%
Cardiac disease	55(3)*	27(3)*	49
Pregnancy	1	0	0
Delirium tremens	36	5	14
Postoperative	1	0	0
Cerebral accident	5	1	20
Carcinoma	10(1)*	7(1)*	70
Nephritis and uremia	8	5	63
Blood dyscrasia	13(3)*	4(3)*	31
Pulmonary tuberculosis	18(1)*	3	17
Bronchial asthma	10	0	0
Cirrhosis of liver	22(4)*	9(4)*	41
Diabetes	18	3	17
Diabetic acidosis	3(1)*	3(1)*	100
Infection, nonpneumococcal	13	1	8
Miscellaneous (trauma, morphine addiction, bronchiectasis, emphysema, peptic ulcer, etc.)	35(1)*	7	20
With pre-existing illness	248(14)*	75(12)*	30
Without pre-existing illness	207(3)*	14(2)*	7

* Numbers in parentheses indicate number of patients receiving no antimicrobial therapy.

TABLE 8. Deaths in Bacteremic Pneumococcal Pneumonia Uncomplicated by an Extrapulmonary Focus of Infection Caused by Types I, III, IV, VII, VIII, and XII in Different Age Groups and in the Presence or Absence of Pre-existing Illness

Type of Pneumococcus	Under 50 years		50 years and older	
	No. of Deaths	No. of Deaths in Cases with Pre-existing Illness	No. of Deaths	No. of Deaths in Cases with Pre-existing Illness
I	1	1	5	5
III	2	0	16	13
IV	2	2	6	6
VII	2	2	5	5
VIII	2	2	6	5
XII	3	1	4	4
Total	12	8	42	38
% of all deaths	13	9	47	43

of the fatal illnesses resulted from infection with one of the pneumococcal Types I, III, IV, VII, VIII, or XII in persons 50 years of age or older with complicating illness. The same six capsular types were responsible for an additional 4 per cent of the total deaths in patients in the same age group without complicating illness and, in patients under 50 with complicating illness, for 9 per cent of the total deaths. Nearly three fifths of all deaths from pneumococcal pneumonia and bacteremia in the absence of an extrapulmonary focus of infection, therefore, resulted from infection with one of six capsular types, of persons who had complicating systemic disease, had lived 50 years or more, or both.

With regard to complicating illness, several additional observations seem noteworthy. Eighteen patients admitted to the hospital for other disorders developed pneumococcal disease on the ward and of these, nine succumbed. In several instances, the time between the initial signs of infection and death was less than 24 hours, and some received no specific antimicrobial therapy. Eleven patients developed pneumococcal infection as a complication of heart disease and pulmonary edema. Signs of infection in these patients were often obscure, and several had no fever. Mortality was unusually high, however, death being the outcome in nine of the eleven. Six patients receiving adrenocorticosteroids or their analogues developed pneumococcal bacteremia. Of these, two died. Only one of five patients with disease of the reticuloendothelial system who were similarly infected failed to recover. Pneumococcal bacteremia occurred as a complication of pulmonary tuberculosis in 18 persons, 10 of whom had active disease. Three deaths occurred in patients in this group, one of whom had active tuberculosis.

Mixed acute infection (Table 9) with multple types of pneumococcus or with pneumococcus and klebsiella was recognized with certainty in four patients, and its possible occurrence was noted in ten other instances. On one occasion, two strains of pneumococcus (Types III and XXX or LIV) were recovered from the same blood culture; and, in two other patients, pneumococcus Type I or V and klebsiella Type 2 (Friedländer's bacillus Type B) were cultured simultaneously or sequentially within 24 hours from the blood. In a fourth patient, klebsiella Type 1 (Friedländer's bacillus Type A) was present in the blood and pneumococcus Type IX, in the pleural

TABLE 9. Multiple Types of Pneumococci and Simultaneous Infection with Klebsiellas in Cases of Pneumococcal Infection

Case	Termination*	Type of Pneumococcus or Klebsiella†	
		Blood	Sputum
1	S	I	Untyped Pnc.
2	S	I	XI
3	S	I, K1.2	K1.2 (urine)
4	S	I	I, K1.4
5	D	III, XXX or LIV	III, XXX or LIV
6	S	III	III, XIII
7	D	III	III, and XXXIX, XL, XLII, or LXX
8	S	IV	IV, K1.1
9	D	V, K1.2	V, K1.2
10	D	K1.1	IX (pleura)
11	S	XI	VI
12	D	XXI	XVII
13	S	XXVII	XXVII, IX
14	D	XLIV, LV or LVI	XLIV, LV or LVI (ascitic fluid), K1.1 (sputum)

* S indicates survival; D, death.
† Roman numeral indicates pneumococcal type; K1. and Arabic numeral designate klebsiella type.

exudate. The presence at the same time of more than one potential respiratory pathogen in the sputum of a patient with pneumonia makes determination of the cause of infection impossible in the absence of other data. The fact that mixed infection may occur, however, makes careful examination of the respiratory flora an im-

TABLE 10. Therapy in Bacteremic Pneumococcal Pneumonia Uncomplicated by an Extrapulmonary Focus of Infection

Treatment	All Cases	Fatal Cases		Cases Surviving ≤ 24 hr	Fatal Cases Surviving > 24 hr
	no.	*no.*	%	%	%
Penicillin	338	57	17	19	12
Tetracyclines	55	10	18	5	10
Erythromycin	7	0	0	0	0
Chloramphenicol and streptomycin	7	2	29	1	17
Mixed	30	6	20	2	14
None	17	14	82	11	50
Total	454*	89	19.5	38	12.2

* Treatment of one surviving patient unknown.

TABLE 11. Outcome of Bacteremic Pneumococcal Pneumonia Uncomplicated by an Extrapulmonary Focus of Infection in Different Age Groups after Symptomatic, Serum, and Penicillin Therapy

Age	Symptomatic Therapy*		Serum Therapy†		Penicillin Therapy	
	D/T‡	Fatal	D/T‡	Fatal	D/T‡	Fatal
		%		%		%
12–29	79/120	66	8/31	26	2/36	6
30–49	292/391	75	23/47	49	11/142	8
50+	322/345	93	14/22	64	44/160	28
Total	693/856	80	45/100	45	57/338	17

* Data from references 1 and 2.
† Data from reference 1, pneumococcal Types I and II only.
‡ D/T indicates died/total.

portant prerequisite for the proper determination of therapy.

Treatment of pneumococcal infection during the period being reviewed differed markedly from that employed prior to 1940 and was subject also to variation between 1952 and 1962, during which time several controlled therapeutic studies were carried out. In Table 10 are recorded the various types of treatment received by 454 patients with pneumococcal pneumonia and bacteremia. No striking differences in the outcome are discernible among the several types of therapy employed, and penicillin and tetracyclines appear to be equally efficacious in the treatment of pneumococcal pneumonia with bacteremia. The fatality rate for all patients, irrespective of therapy, was 19.5 per cent. If those patients receiving no therapy are eliminated from consideration, the fatality rate is 17 per cent. Of perhaps greater significance is the fact that 43 per cent of all deaths (36 per cent of all deaths in treated patients) occurred within 24 hours of the patients' admission to the hospital, an indication either of fulminant infection or of undue delay in seeking medical attention. If deaths during this period are eliminated from consideration, the mortality rate becomes 12.2 per cent.

In Table 11 and in Figure 5 the age-adjusted mortality from pneumococcal pneumonia and bacteremia in two series of patients treated before antimicrobial drugs were available is contrasted with similar figures from the present study. The greatest reduction in mortality has taken place in the patients in the youngest age group and has been progressively less with advancing years.

In the light of the foregoing data, it is pertinent to inquire whether or not all patients treated with antibiotics are benefitted significantly by such therapy. To answer this question, the proportion of survivors on each day of illness in three

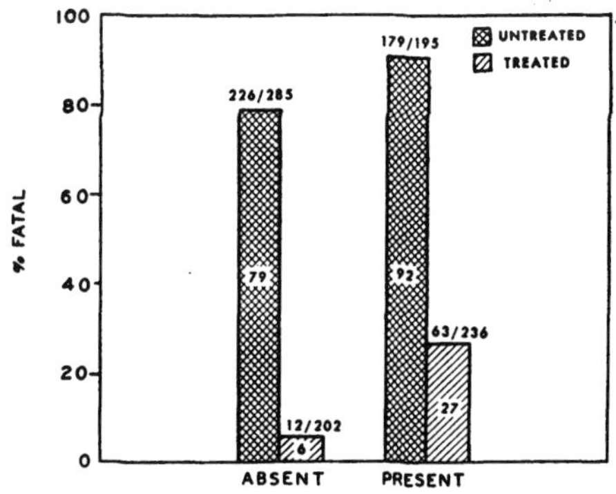

FIGURE 4. For significance of fractions above and numbers within bars, see Figure 2. The fractions 12/202 and 63/236 should read 12/204 and 63/234, respectively.

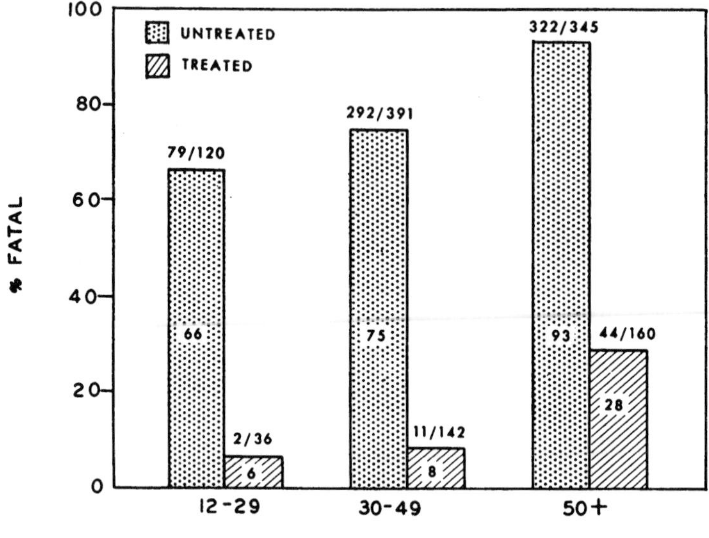

FIGURE 5. For significance of fractions above and numbers within bars, see Figure 2. Data for untreated cases include those of Tilghman and Finland (1) and those of Bullowa (2).

TABLE 12. Relation of Survival to Duration of Illness in Bacteremic Pneumococcal Pneumonia Uncomplicated by an Extrapulmonary Focus of Infection Treated Symptomatically, with Serum, with Penicillin or with Tetracyclines

Day of Illness	Therapy							
	Symptomatic (384)*†		Serum (93)*†		Penicillin (298)†		Tetracyclines (49)†	
	Survivors		Survivors		Survivors		Survivors	
	no.	%	*no.*	%	*no.*	%	*no.*	%
1	382	99	93	100	296	99	49	100
2	378	98	92	99	292	98	46	94
3	372	97	91	98	280	94	43	88
4	350	91	89	96	272	91	43	88
5	331	86	81	87	270	91	43	88
6	305	79	76	82	268	90	43	88
7	260	68	73	79	261	88	43	88
8	227	59	65	70	261	88	43	88
9	192	50	62	67	260	87	43	88
10	162	42	60	65	257	86	43	88
11	137	36	57	61	255	86	42	86
12	122	32	56	60	254	85	42	86
13–15	100	26	53	57	254	85	42	86
16–20	83	22	53	57	253	85	42	86
20+	65	17	49	53	253	85	42	86

* Data from reference 1. Serum-treated cases include only pneumococcal Types I and II.
† Numbers in parentheses indicate number of patients.

groups of patients with bacteremic pneumococcal pneumonia has been determined: in those treated symptomatically, in those treated with serum, and in those treated with penicillin. The results are given in Table 12 and Figure 6. Although the three curves in the figure diverge widely after the fifth day of illness, they are strikingly similar prior to that time. Results of treatment of fewer patients with tetracyclines are superimposable on those obtained with penicillin. The data suggest that antimicrobial therapy has little or no effect upon the outcome of infection among those destined, at the onset of illness, to die within 5 days. It is noteworthy that 60 percent of all deaths among patients treated with penicillin occurred in this 5-day period and that exitus may be the outcome even when treatment is initiated on the first or second day of illness (Table 13 and Figure 7). If treatment is delayed until or after the fourth day of disease, some improvement in prognosis is discernible and

TABLE 13. Outcome in Bacteremic Pneumococcal Pneumonia Uncomplicated by an Extrapulmonary Focus of Infection Related to Day of Illness on Which Treatment with Penicillin was Initiated

Day of Illness Treatment Begun	All Cases	Fatal Cases	
	no.	*no.*	%
1	40	5	12.5
2	64	11	17.2
3	49	11	22.4
4	65	9	13.8
5	31	3	9.7
6	13	1	7.7
7	22	3	13.6

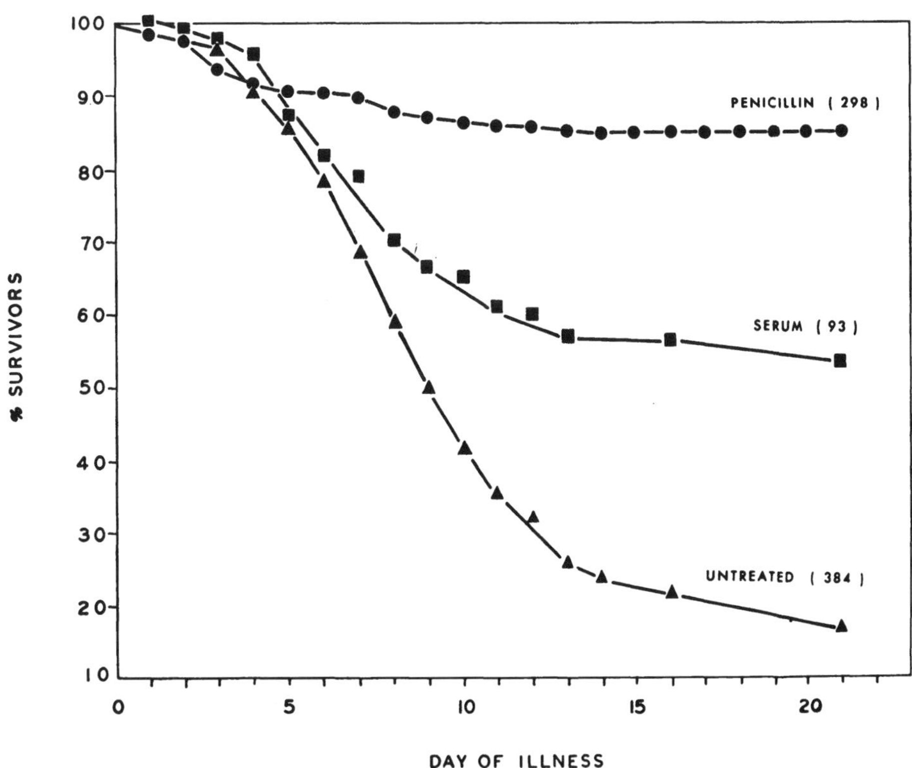

FIGURE 6. Numbers in parentheses indicate size of each group of patients. Data for untreated and serum-treated patients (capsular Types I and II only) from Tilghman and Finland (1).

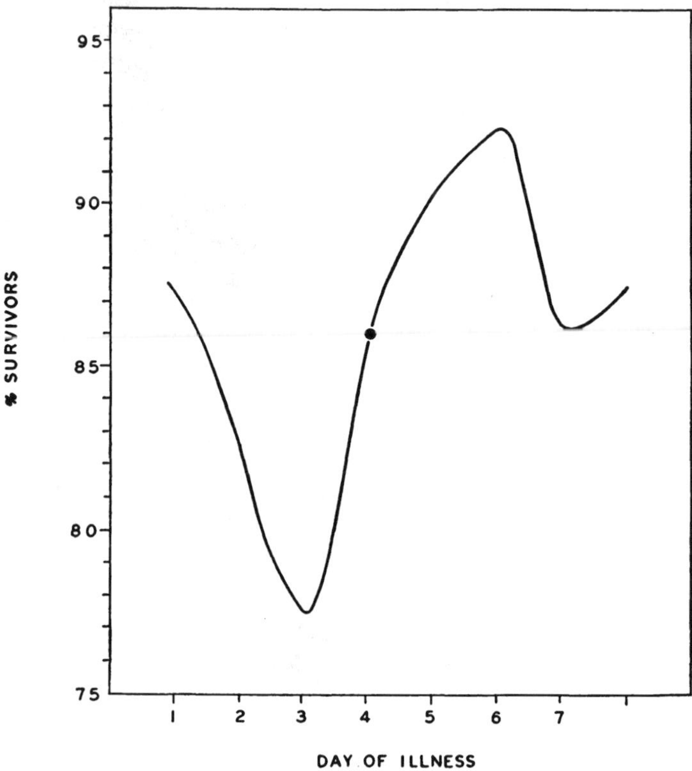

FIGURE 7. For numbers of patients, see Table 13.

TABLE 14. Complications of Bacteremic Pneumococcal Pneumonia

	All Cases	Fatal Cases	
	no.	*no.*	%
Suppurative Complications			
Meningitis	21	17	81
Empyema	18	4	22
Endocarditis	9	5	56
Arthritis	3	1	33
Peritonitis	2	2	100
Nonsuppurative Complications			
Delayed resolution	26	1	4
Sterile effusion	15	3	20
Pulmonary embolus	4	4	100
Thromboplebitis	2	0	0
Drug reaction	8	1	13
Spontaneous pneumothroax	1	0	0

may be related to the development of specific anticapsular antibody.

Fifty-three instances of an extrapulmonary focus of pneumococcal infection were seen in 47 patients admitted to the hospital with primary pulmonary infection and bacteremia. Of these, 55 per cent were caused by capsular Types I, III, IV, VII, VIII, and XII. In no case was there evidence indicative of the development of an extrapulmonary focus of pneumococcal infection after the initiation of antimicrobial therapy. Table 14 records the various complications seen. Meningitis was the most common followed by pleural empyema and endocarditis. The infrequent occurrence of empyema (3.6 per cent) when contrasted with the observed incidence of 7.5 per cent accompanying pneumococcal bacteremia when antimicrobial drugs were not available represents a considerable advance. As noted in Table 1, the presence of an extrapulmonary focus of pneumococcal infection has a strongly unfavorable effect on the outlook for recovery.

Nonsuppurative complications of infection are included also in Table 14. Of these, delay in the resolution of the pneumonic process beyond 3 weeks was observed 26 times and led to segmental pulmonary resection or lobectomy in several instances. The single death in this group followed an anaphylactic reaction to topical anaethesia administered for bronchoscopy. Sterile pleural effusion was detected in 15 patients, 1 of whom had congestive heart failure and 3 of whom died. Other complications were infrequent. Reactions to penicillin were described in 8 patients, 1 of whom died, and 13 others with a history of hypersensitivity to penicillin were treated with other drugs.

Pneumococcal meningitis secondary to infection of the upper respiratory tract was seen in 40 patients during the period of the study. In these the patients, the relationship of bacteremia to survival was significant. Of the 27 patients with bacteremia, 17 succumbed, whereas no deaths were noted among the 13 patients whose blood cultures were sterile.

Discussion

Pneumonia remains one of the major causes of morbidity and mortality in the United States today and, together with influenza, ranks sixth among the ten leading causes of death in this country (4). Despite recent interest in respiratory infections caused by staphylococci and enterobacteria, pneumococcus is still the most common cause of acute bacterial pneumonia and accounts probably for more than 80 per cent of such infections. The widespread lack of appreciation of this fact has resulted from the abandonment of well-established bacteriologic techniques for the isolation and identification of pneumococcus. Failure routinely to obtain blood cultures before treatment, to inoculate sputum intraperitoneally into mice, and to employ the efficient serologic methods for capsular typing have been followed by less frequent recognition of this organism and by a consequent tendency on the part of many to regard pneumococcal pneumonia as a rarity. That such is not the case has been readily demonstrable whenever suitable bacteriologic techniques have been reintroduced. Until these techniques are used routinely once again and until capsular typing serums are made generally available, it is likely that misconceptions concerning the prevalence and seriousness of pneumococcal infection will continue to be held by many.

In the absence of more exact epidemiologic data, it is difficult to assess precisely the magnitude of the problem of pneumococcal infection in the United States today. From the studies of Dingle and his associates (5) and from the material presented by Reimann (6), it may be estimated conservatively that there are 150,000 to 300,000 cases of pneumococcal pneumonia per annum, a fourth to a third of which are accompanied by bacteremia. If half these illnesses are caused by Types I, III, IV, VII, VIII, and XII, as suggested by the information available, then it may be estimated further that between 9,000 and 18,000 deaths a year result from infection by these pneumococcal types. These figures are compatible with the report of 55,000 deaths from pneumonia and influenza in the United States in 1961 (7), a year in which influenza was not epidemic.

It is questionable that a more effective antipneumococcal drug than penicillin can be developed. It is bactericidal in very low concentrations, and no well-documented case of therapeutic failure as a result of pneumococcal resistance to penicillin has ever been reported. In addition, for those sensitive to penicillin, equally effective antimicrobial drugs are available among the tetracyclines. Death from pneumococcal infection appears to result from failure of the host's defensive mechanisms prior to the institution of antimicrobial treatment. The patient may die, therefore, either as a result of failure to receive a specific antipneumococcal drug or as a result of having passed the physiologic "point of no return" before such therapy was instituted. It is not known at present what factors determine the difference in outcome between recovery and death. Some information, however, is available. Natural recovery from pneumococcal infection depends upon phagocytosis of the organism in both the absence and presence of type-specific anticapsular antibody. The resistance of pneumococcus Type III to surface phagocytosis accounts in part, at least, for the lesser improvement in prognosis for those infected with this organism (8, 9). The fatality in bacteremic Type III pneumococcal pneumonia is 51 per cent, a figure which contrasts strikingly with that of 8 per cent after comparable infection with pneumococcus Type I and one which approaches the mortality seen in Friedländer's pneumonia. Despite the striking rise in mortality with increasing age, the data available suggest that aged persons are not deficient in the ability to produce antibody (10) and that their leukocytes are as actively phagocytic in vitro as those of younger persons (11). Additional aspects of leukocytic function and the role of serologic factors other than anticapsular antibody (12), however, may be important to recovery and require investigation. Until more is learned about the mechanisms that are responsible for recovery or death from infection, it is unlikely that improvement in the outlook for recovery from pneumococcal pneumonia can be achieved by therapeutic measures.

In the light of the foregoing facts, prophylaxis, which has been suggested by others since the introduction of antibiotics (13), would appear to offer the best available means of lowering the morbidity and mortality resulting from pneumococcal infection. Although the large number of pneumococcal capsular types precludes, on practical grounds, the preparation of a vaccine for immunizing against infection by all pneumococcal types, the fact that the preponderance of serious infections caused by this organism is engendered by a limited number of such types makes immunization a potentially feasible procedure.

A sizeable body of data has been developed which points to the efficacy of vaccination with pneumococcal capsular polysaccharides as a means of preventing pneumococcal infection. One of the more recent and convincing of such studies is that of MacLeod, Hodges, Heidelberger, and Bernhard (14) carried out during World War II at an Air Force base where pneumococcal pneumonia caused by organisms of several capsular types was epidemic. By immunizing against infection with certain of the epidemic types and by using other epidemic types as controls, these investigators were able to provide a clear demonstration of the efficacy of vaccination with purified capsular polysaccharides as means of preventing infection with pneumococcal Types I, II, V, and VII. That elderly persons as well as those of military age are protected has been shown by the studies of Kaufman (15). In 5,750 individuals, 98.5 per cent of whom were 50 years or older, immunized against infection with pneumococcus Types I, II, and III, there were three cases of pneumonia, one with bacteremia, caused by organisms of these three types. In an unvaccinated control group of 5,153 subjects, 96.1 per cent of whom were 50 years or older, there were 33 cases of pneumonia, 12 accompanied by bacteremia and caused by the same pneumococcal types.

In the light of present knowledge, it would seem reasonable to vaccinate persons at high risk of fatal pneumococcal disease against those pneumococcal types shown to be responsible for the preponderance of infection. Pneumococcal infection is the cause at present of far more illness and of many more deaths than is poliomyelitis; yet little is being done prophylactically with regard to the former disease. If it is reasonable to vaccinate against viral influenza those persons at high risk of fatal infection, then it seems equally reasonable to vaccinate against those types of pneumococci responsible for the preponderance of infections the individuals most likely to succumb to them. Pneumococcal polysaccharides are effective antigens and half maximal amounts of circulating antibody have been shown to be present as long as 5 years after a single injection of polysaccharide (16). In addition, it has been demonstrated that the antibody response to each of six pneumococcal polysaccharides administered in a single preparation is comparable to that when each is administered separately when vaccines containing polysaccharide Types I, II, III, V, VII, and VIII or Types I, IV, VI, XIV, XVIII, and XIX are employed (17). Vaccines of this kind were available commercially after World War II but were not used widely because of misconceptions about pneumococcal infections resulting from failure to study them adequately. As a consequence, they were withdrawn from the market. The evidence now available suggests that a vaccine containing the capsular polysaccharides of pneumococcal Types I, III, IV, VII, VIII, and XII should be effective and its production is advocated. If given to persons with systemic illness, to those 50 years of age or older, or to both, it should bring about a significant reduction in the mortality from pneumococcal disease among those most likely to die of such infection.

It is obvious that, for a program of the type proposed to succeed, it is essential that continuous surveillance of the prevalence of pneumococcal types be carried out over a wide geographical area. To do so requires that pneumococcal typing serums be made readily available and be far more widely employed than they are at the present time. By the use of established bacteriologic and prophylactic methods, there is every reason to believe that a further significant reduction can be made in the morbidity and mortality resulting from pneumococcal disease. If this reduction is to be brought about, however, it will be necessary for the medical profession to show greater awareness of the problem of pneumococcal infection than it has manifested in the past two decades.

Summary and Conclusions

The biology of infections caused by the several pneumococcal types varies and the dissimilarities are reflected by differences in invasiveness and mortality in both untreated and treated infections.

Some persons are at higher risk of death from pneumococcal infections than others and cannot be prevented from dying either by antimicrobial therapy or by measures now available to correct the physiologic derangements of infection.

Evidence extant suggests strongly that the morbidity and mortality from pneumococcal infection can be reduced significantly by prophylactic vaccination of persons at high risk with a preparation of six pneumococcal capsular polysaccharides.

Pneumococcal infection constitutes a serious illness and merits the same careful bacteriologic study afforded many other infectious diseases. There is need for the reinstitution of capsular typing and of other bacteriologic techniques employed formerly if better understanding and control of one of the most important bacterial infections in the United States today are to be achieved.

Acknowledgments

The technical assistance of the following persons is gratefully acknowledged: Dorothy Hirsch, Erna Constantinoff, Helena Laitenen, Edna Lindsey, Geraldine Mendelsohn, Diane Sussman, Onnely Bauer, Anne

Shustek, Edna Rosenthal, Naomi Karsh, Ruth Lawson, and Harold Resnick.

Invaluable assistance was rendered by Miss Irene Cambridge and her associates in the Record Library, Kings County Hospital.

Figures 3 through 6 are reprinted from the *Transactions* of the Association of American Physicians and are reproduced with the permission of the Association.

Summario in Interlingua

Le biologia de infectiones causate per diverse typos pneumococcal varia, e le differentias es reflectite in dissimilitudes del invasivitate e del mortalitate in casos de infection tanto tractate como etiam non-tractate.

Certe subjectos curre un plus alte risco de morir ab infectiones pneumococcal que alteres e non pote esser salvate ab le morte per therapias antimicrobial e non per le nunc disponibile mesuras pro le correction del disturbationes physiologic del infection.

Le existente evidentia suggere fortemente que le morbiditate e le mortalitate ab infection pneumococcal pote esser reducite significativemente per le vaccination prophylactic de subjectos in alte risco con un preparato de sex capsular polysaccharidas pneumococcal.

Infection pneumococcal constitue un serie morbo e merita le mesme meticulose studio bacteriologic que es accordate a multe altere morbos infectiose. Il existe un urgente desiderato pro le reinstitution de typage capsular e altere previemente empleate technicas si on vole effectuar un meliorate comprension e un meliorate combattimento de un del plus importante infectiones bacterial in le Statos Unite.

References

1. Tilghman, R. C., Finland, M.: Clinical significance of bacteremia in pneumococcal pneumonia. *Arch. Intern. Med.* (*Chicago*) 59: 602, 1937.
2. Bullowa, J. G. M.: *The Management of the Pneumonias*, Oxford University Press, New York, 1937.
3. MacLeod, C. M., Austrian, R., Finland, M.: Pneumococcus, in *Diagnostic Procedures and Reagents*, American Public Health Association, New York, 1963, pp. 222–30.
4. *Statistical Abstract of the United States, 1958, 79th Annual Edition:* U. S. Department of Commerce, Bureau of the Census, U. S. Government Printing Office, Washington, D. C., 1958, p. 6.
5. Dingle, J. H., Badger, G. F., Feller, A. E., Hodges, R. G., Jordan, W. S., Jr., Rammelkamp, C. H., Jr.: A study of illness in a group of Cleveland families. I. Plan of study and certain general observations. *Amer. J. Hyg.* 58: 16, 1953.
6. Reimann, H. A.: Current problems of the pneumonias. *Ann. Intern. Med.* 56: 144, 1962.
7. *Advance Report, Vital Statistics of the United States, 1961. Final Natality and Mortality Statistics:* National Vital Statistics Division, Department of Health, Education, and Welfare, United States Public Health Service, Nov., 1962.
8. Wood, W. B., Jr., Smith, M. R.: The inhibition of surface phagocytosis by the capsular "slime layer" of pneumococcus Type III. *J. Exp. Med.* 90: 85, 1949.
9. Wood, W. B., Jr., Smith, M. R.: Host-parasite relationships in experimental pneumonia due to pneumococcus Type III. *J. Exp. Med.* 92: 85, 1950.
10. Balch, H. H.: Relation of nutritional deficiency in man to antibody production. *J. Immun.* 64: 397, 1950.
11. Balch, H. H., Spencer, M. T.: Phagocytosis by human leukocytes. II. Relation of nutritional deficiency in man to phagocytosis. *J. Clin. Invest.* 33: 1321, 1954.
12. Jeter, W. S., McKee, A. P., Mason, R. J.: Inhibition of immune phagocytosis of *Diplococcus pneumoniae* by human neutrophiles with antibody against complement. *J. Immun.* 86: 386, 1961.
13. Dowling, H. F., Lepper, M. H.: The effect of antibiotics (Penicillin, Aureomycin, and Terramycin) on the fatality rate and incidence of complications in pneumococcic pneumonia. *Amer. J. Med. Sci.* 222: 396, 1951.
14. MacLeod, C. M., Hodges, R. G., Heidelberger, M., Bernhard, W. G.: Prevention of pneumococcal pneumonia by immunization with specific capsular polysaccharides. *J. Exp. Med.* 82: 445, 1945.
15. Kaufman, P.: Pneumonia in old age. *Arch. Intern. Med.* (*Chicago*) 79: 518, 1947.
16. Heidelberger, M.: Persistence of antibodies in man after immunization, in *The Nature and Significance of the Antibody Response*, edited by Pappenheimer, A. M., Jr., Columbia University Press, New York, 1953, pp. 90–101.
17. Heidelberger, M., MacLeod, C. M., Di Lapi, M.: The human antibody response to simultaneous injection of six specific polysaccharides of pneumococcus. *J. Exp. Med.* 88: 369, 1948.

Quantitative Relationships Between Circulating Leukocytes and Infection in Patients with Acute Leukemia

GERALD P. BODEY, M.D., MONICA BUCKLEY, B.A., Y. S. SATHE, PH.D. and EMIL J FREIREICH, M.D.

Bethesda, Maryland

INFECTION IS CURRENTLY the major fatal complication of acute leukemia (1). Previous studies have indicated a relationship between leukopenia and the presence of infection in patients with acute leukemia (2–4) and various types of agranulocytosis (5–7). Chemotherapeutic agents with bone marrow toxicity are being used with increasing frequency in malignant and other chronic diseases. Also, a high incidence of infection has accompanied the use of these agents as immunosuppressive therapy in patients receiving organ transplantation (8). The present study examines the quantitative relationships between the presence of infection and the degree and duration of leukopenia in patients with acute leukemia. The effect of changes in the level of circulating leukocytes on the occurrence, type and outcome of infections is also considered.

METHODS

The 52 patients selected for this study were first admitted to the Clinical Center of the National Institutes of Health during the period from August, 1959, to April, 1963.

Received July 28, 1965; accepted for publication October 14, 1965.

From the Medicine Branch, Leukemia Service, and the Mathematical and Statistics and Applied Mathematical Section, National Cancer Institute, National Institutes of Health, Bethesda, Md.

Requests for reprints should be addressed to Gerald P. Bodey, M.D., Building 10, Room 2B45, National Institutes of Health, Bethesda, Md. 20014.

The diagnosis of acute leukemia was confirmed by bone marrow examination in every patient. Thirty-four patients received similar initial antileukemic therapy consisting of 6-mercaptopurine and prednisone according to protocol of a study of the Leukemia Co-operative Study Group B (Protocol V) (9). The remaining patients received treatment with methyl glyoxal bis-(guanylhydrazone) (Methyl GAG) (10).

The clinical record of every patient was examined and all determinations of granulocytes, lymphocytes, and abnormal cells were tabulated. When the leukemic process was active, blood counts were obtained three times a week. When the leukemia was in remission, and the patients were otherwise healthy, the blood counts were recorded every 1 to 4 weeks. On days when no blood counts were available, the values were assumed to be the same as those next recorded. Patients were followed from initial admission at the onset of leukemia to death or until July 31, 1964.

White blood cell counts were determined by the Coulter counter technique. Twenty lambda of blood were diluted with 10 ml normal saline 1% saponin solution. The standard error for the procedure is 7.56% with a 1 to 2% error in the machine (11). Differentials were obtained by counting 100 cells, unless the white blood cell count was les than 1,000/mm^3 blood, when only 25 or 50 cells were counted. Absolute levels of these blood cells were calculated from the white blood cell count and differential.

The absolute values of granulocytes and lymphocytes were grouped as: less than 100 cells/mm^3 blood, 100 to 500 cells, 500 to 1,000 cells, 1,000 to 1,500 cells, 1,500 to 2,000 cells, and greater than 2,000 cells. Granulocytopenia and lymphopenia, when used in this paper, include all values less than 1,000 cells/mm^3.

Severe granulocytopenia and severe lymphopenia indicate values less than 100 cells/mm³ blood.

The clinical history and other laboratory data were carefully examined to determine the type, onset and duration of infection. This information was obtained independent of the hematological data to prevent any bias in dating onset and duration of infection. Infections were classified as: no infection; fevers without proven infection—this category includes fevers of unknown origin, fever which may have been due to the leukemic process itself, viral upper respiratory infections, and a few episodes of childhood exanthems; local infections—bacterial or fungal pharyngitis, tracheobronchitis, otitis media, skin abscess, and cellulitis are included in this category; organ infections—this category includes pneumonia of any type, pulmonary and brain abscesses, and urinary tract infections; disseminated infections—septicemia, disseminated fungal, and disseminated viral infections (herpes simplex, cytomegalic inclusion disease) were included in this category. The term severe infection, when used herein, refers to the combination of organ and disseminated infections. Identified infection includes all types of proven infection.

Results

Thirty-four patients with acute lymphocytic leukemia and 18 patients with acute myelogenous leukemia were included in the study.

The patients' ages varied from 1 to 77 years. The total time considered was 17,743 patient days. Survival ranged from 6 to 791 days (average, 329 days). Patients with acute myelogenous leukemia had a shorter survival time (average, 227 days) than patients with acute lymphocytic leukemia (average, 402 days). Five patients with acute lymphocytic leukemia were still living at the end of the study (July, 1964), having an average survival time of 426 days.

During 38% of the time studied (6,768 patient days) the patients had active acute leukemia as evidenced by a bone marrow category of A2 or A3 according to the criteria of the Acute Leukemia Co-operative Study Group (12). The patients were in bone marrow remission during the remaining 62% of the time. The patients with acute myelogenous leukemia spent less time in remission (43%) than the patients with acute lymphocytic leukemia (68%). Ten patients with acute mylogenous leukemia and four patients with acute lymphocytic leukemia never achieved a remission.

The patients spent approximately 50% of the time with granulocyte and lymphocyte levels less than 1,500/mm³. Severe granulocytopenia (less than 100/mm³) occurred more frequently than severe lymphopenia. Granulocytopenia occurred much more frequently during relapse than during remission. Granulocyte levels greater than 2,000/mm³ were more common during remission but still were present less than one half of the time. The distribution of lymphocyte levels was very similar during relapse and remission.

Leukocyte Distribution

The patients with acute myelogenous leukemia had a different distribution of leukocytes than the patients with acute lymphocytic leukemia. Granulocytopenia (less than 1,000/mm³) occurred more often in the patients with acute myelogenous leukemia, during both relapse and remission. Patients with acute lymphocytic leukemia spent much more time with granulocyte levels greater than 2,000/mm³, but this difference was present only during remission. Lymphopenia was more prevalent in patients with acute myelogenous leukemia during remission and in patients with acute lymphocytic leukemia during relapse. During remission, lymphocyte levels greater than 2,000/mm³ occurred three times more frequently in patients with acute lymphocytic leukemia.

Granulocytes and Infection

The effect of granulocyte levels on the presence of infection is illustrated in Figure 1. Since the relationship was similar for all types of proven infection, they have been combined. However, fever without proven infection was not closely related to the level of granulocytes. At less than 100 granulocytes/mm³, 53% of the patient days were spent with identified infection. The

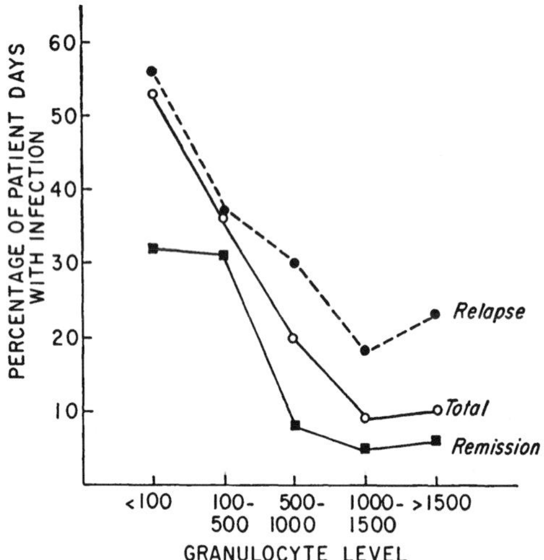

Figure 1. The effect of granulocyte level on the presence of identified infection. The percentage of days spent with infection is plotted at each level of circulating granulocytes. This percentage decreased with increasing granulocyte level and was always higher during relapse than during remission.

percentage of time spent with identified infection then decreased sharply with increasing granulocyte levels. However, there was no further reduction at granulocyte levels above 1,500/mm³. This relationship was similar during relapse and remission but the proportion of time spent with infection was always greater during relapse.

The risk of developing severe infection at a given granulocyte level was determined from the number of severe infectious episodes occurring per 1,000 days at each granulocyte level (Figure 2). Since infection influenced subsequent granulocyte levels (see below), granulocyte data during periods of infection were not included in these calculations. When severe granulocytopenia was present, 43 episodes of severe infection were observed per 1,000 days. This incidence dropped sharply with increasing granulocyte levels, but no further reduction occurred at granulocyte levels above 1,500/mm³. The incidence of severe infection was always higher during relapse than during remission. This difference was most pronounced in the absence of granulocytopenia.

LYMPHOCYTES AND INFECTION

The effect of lymphocyte levels on the presence of identified infection is illustrated in Figure 3. This figure is very similar to the figure of granulocyte levels (Figure 1). As with granulocytes, fever without proven infection was not related to lymphocyte levels. The proportion of time spent with identified infection of all types decreased with increasing lymphocyte levels. However, identified infection continued to decrease with increasing lymphocyte levels above 1,500/mm³, which was not true for granulocyte levels. Infection was always present more frequently in relapse than in remission at any given level of lymphocytes. This difference was even greater for lymphocytes than for granulocytes at every level.

The risk of infection at various lymphocyte levels was also examined (Figure 4). Severe lymphopenia (less than 100/mm³) was not considered separately since the figures were unreliable, being based on only a few days (138 days for the entire study). The risk of developing severe in-

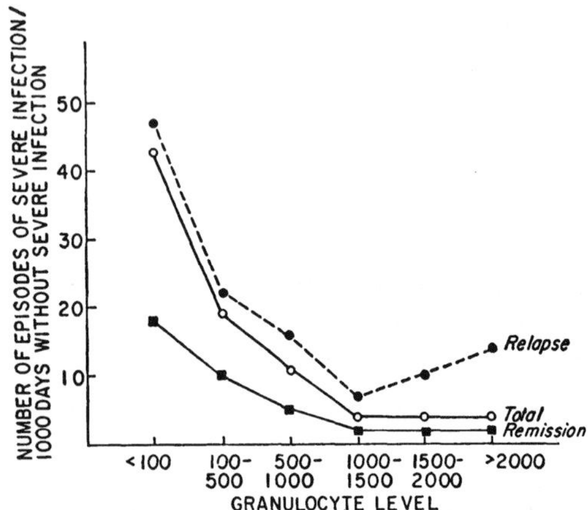

Figure 2. The frequency of infectious episodes related to the granulocyte level. The number of episodes of severe infection/1,000 days without severe infection is plotted for each granulocyte level. The risk of developing severe infection decreases with increasing granulocyte level. However, no further reduction occurs above a granulocyte level of 1,500/mm³. The risk is greater in relapse than in remission for every granulocyte level.

fection decreased with increasing lymphocyte levels, but the decrease was more gradual than it was for granulocytes (Figure 2). Again, severe infectious episodes occurred more frequently during relapse than during remission at every lymphocyte level.

LEUKOCYTE LEVELS DURING INFECTIONS

The granulocyte levels recorded during infectious episodes were examined next. The proportion of time spent with low

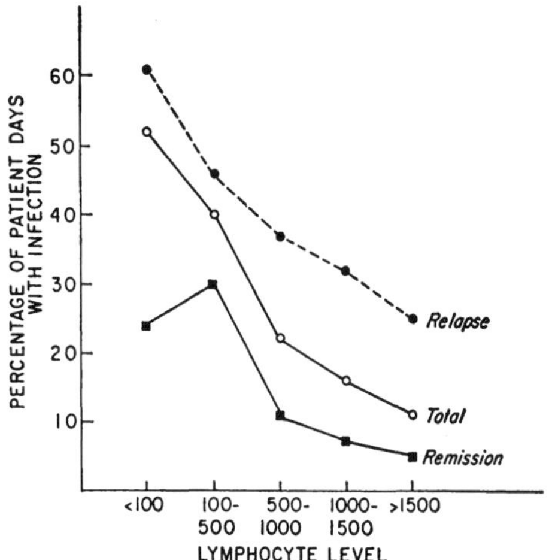

FIGURE 3. The effect of the lymphocyte level on the presence of identified infection. The percentage of days spent with infection is plotted at each level of circulating lymphocytes. This percentage decreased with increasing lymphocyte level and was always higher during relapse than during remission.

granulocyte levels (less than 500/mm³) increased with increasingly severe types of infection. Conversely, the proportion of time spent with higher granulocyte levels (greater than 1,500/mm³) decreased with increasingly severe types of infection. Figure 5 illustrates this relationship for low granulocyte levels. During remission, the proportion of time spent with low granulocyte levels was relatively constant for all types of identified infection.

A similar analysis was made for lymphocyte levels. While the same general patterns existed for lymphocytes as were

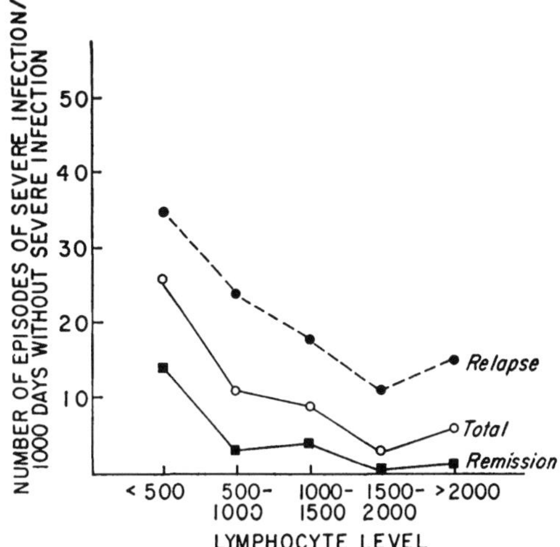

FIGURE 4. The frequency of infectious episodes related to the lymphocyte level. The number of episodes of severe infection/1,000 days without severe infection is plotted for each lymphocyte level. The figures for < 100 lymphocytes/mm³ and 100 to 500 lymphocytes/mm³ are combined. The incidence figures for lymphocyte levels < 100/mm³ were not statistically reliable because there were only a few days when such low lymphocyte levels were observed. The risk of developing infection decreased with increasing levels of circulating lymphocytes.

present for granulocytes, the relationships were less striking. Figure 6 illustrates the frequency of low lymphocyte levels (less

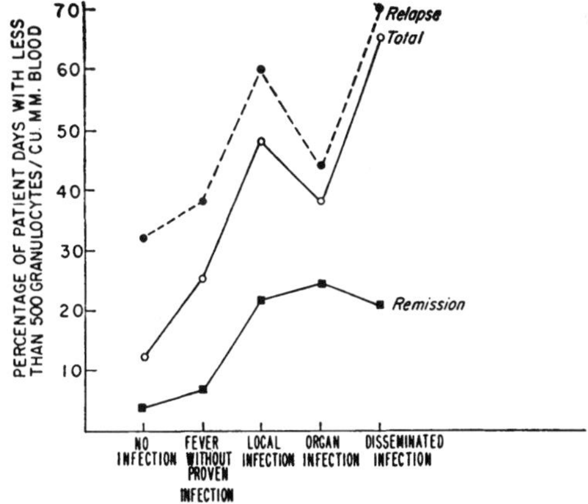

FIGURE 5. The frequency of granulocytopenia (< 500 granulocytes/mm³ blood) during infection. The percentage of days with granulocyte levels less than 500/mm³ is plotted for each type of infection. In general, the more severe the infection, the greater the proportion of time spent with granulocytopenia. However, this relationship did not apply during remission.

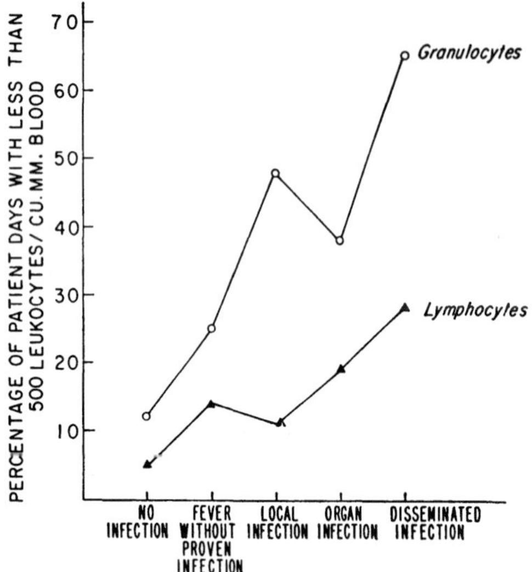

FIGURE 6. The frequency of lymphopenia (< 500 lymphocytes/mm³ blood) during infection. The percentage of days with lymphocytes less than 500/mm³ is plotted for each type of infection. The same curve for granulocytes (obtained from Figure 3) is included for comparison. The more severe the infection, the greater the proportion of time spent with lymphopenia. However, this relationship is not as pronounced for lymphocytes as for granulocytes. Since the figures were similar for lymphocytes during relapse and remission, they are not included.

than 500/mm³) during infection. The curve for granulocytes from Figure 5 is included for comparison. Since the differences between relapse and remission were only minor for lymphocytes, these curves are not included in the figure.

Patients with acute lymphocytic leukemia had no infection during 82% of the time compared with 63% for patients with

TABLE 1. Time Spent with Severe Infections*

Granulocytes	Acute Myelogenous Leukemia	Acute Lymphocytic Leukemia
/mm³	%	%
Total time		
<1,500	19	14
>1,500	16	4
Time in relapse		
<1,500	25	22
>1,500	27	12
Time in remission		
<1,500	8	6
>1,500	7	3

* Expressed as percentage of patient days.

acute myelogenous leukemia. Each type of infection occurred more often in patients with acute myelogenous leukemia and this was true both during relapse and remission. Table 1 compares the time spent with severe (organ and disseminated) infections in patients with acute myelogenous and acute lymphocytic leukemia. While severe infection was much more prevalent at low levels of granulocytes (less than 1,500/mm³) in patients with acute lymphocytic leukemia, this was not true for patients with acute myelogenous leukemia. Furthermore, this finding applied for both relapse and remission.

TABLE 2. Relationship Between Granulocytes and Lymphocytes During Severe Infection

Group	Granulocytes	Lymphocytes	Total Incidence*	Incidence During Relapse*	Incidence During Remission*
	/mm³	*/mm³*			
1	<1,000	<1,000	28	37	10
2	<1,000	>1,000	14	19	6
3	>1,000	<1,000	6	13	3
4	>1,000	>1,000	3	10	1

* Expressed as number/1,000 days without severe infection.

RISK OF INFECTION (GRANULOCYTES VERSUS LYMPHOCYTES)

Table 2 indicates the relative importance of granulocytopenia and lymphopenia in the risk of developing severe infection. When both granulocytopenia and lymphopenia (Group 1) were present, the incidence of severe infection was highest. When granulocytopenia was present alone (Group 2), the incidence of severe infection was greater than when lymphopenia was present alone (Group 3). The lowest incidence of infection was observed when both granulocytopenia and lymphopenia were absent (Group 4). These relationships were very similar during relapse and remission, but again, the incidence of severe infection was always higher during relapse.

GRANULOCYTE FLUCTUATIONS RELATED TO INFECTION

The fluctuations in granulocyte levels during the week preceding severe infection were also examined (Table 3). This information was available in 115 of the 129 episodes of severe infection. Thirty-six per cent of the episodes were preceded by a fall in granulocyte level and in one half of these episodes the fall was greater than 500/mm³. In one half of the episodes of severe infection, the granulocyte level either rose or remained greater than 1,000/mm³.

TABLE 3. Changes in Granulocyte Level During the Week Prior to Onset of Severe Infection

Granulocyte Level		Episodes	
Initial	Change		
	/mm³	*no.*	%
Any level	Any fall	41	36
Any level	Fall of >500	19	17
>1,000	<1,000	16	14
Any level	Rise	26	23
>1,000	None	28	24
	Total	115	

Table 4 indicates the relationship between episodes of falling granulocytes and the occurrence of severe infection. The granulocyte level fell during 331 1-week periods. This does not include the episodes of falling granulocyte levels that occurred during severe infections. Twelve per cent of all episodes of falling granulocyte levels terminated in severe infection. The incidence was slightly higher if the granulocyte count fell more than 500/mm³. When granulocytopenia was already present, any further reduction in the granulocyte count resulted in a 28% incidence of infection.

TABLE 4. Episodes of Falling Granulocytes During 1-Week Periods

Granulocyte Level		Total Occurrences	Severe Infectious Episodes	Percentage Associated with Severe Infection
Initial	Change			
	/mm³	*no.*		%
Any level	Any fall	331	41	12
Any level	Fall of greater than 500	117	19	16
Any level	Fall of greater than 1,000	58	10	17
>1,000	Fall, but remained greater than 1,000	139	5	4
>1,000	Fall to less than 1,000	117	16	14
<1,000	Any fall	75	21	28
Any level	Fall to 2,000	66	1	2
Any level	Fall to 1,500	73	4	5
Any level	Fall to 1,000	70	7	10
Any level	Fall to 500	75	14	19
Any level	Fall to <100	47	13	28

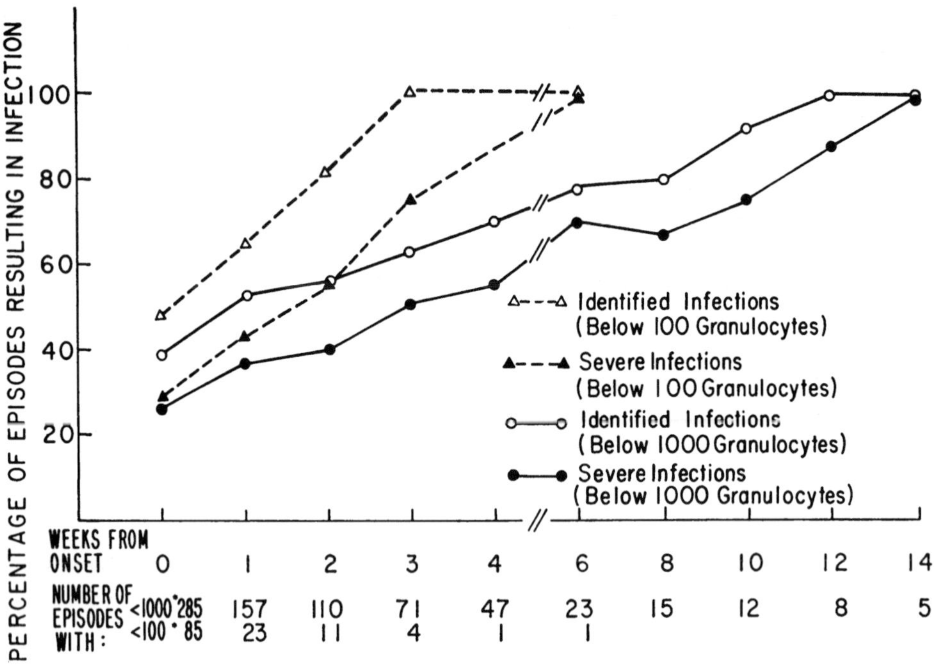

*Granulocyte levels/mm^3 blood

FIGURE 7. The effect of duration of granulocytopenia on the frequency of infection. The duration of granulocytopenia is plotted against the percentage of episodes resulting in infection. Along the abscissa are recorded the number of episodes of granulocytopenia (< 1,000/mm^3) and severe granulocytopenia (< 100/mm^3) for each time interval. The curves illustrate the percentage of episodes at both granulocyte levels resulting in any infection and in severe infection. The risk of developing infection increases the longer granulocytopenia is present and this risk is consistently greater at the lower granulocyte level.

If the granulocyte count was greater than 1,000/mm^3 at the beginning of the week and subsequently fell to less than 1,000/mm^3, there was a 14% incidence of severe infection. Very few severe infections occurred if the granulocyte count fell but remained greater than 1,000/mm^3. The final granulocyte count was the best index of the risk of developing severe infection. Regardless of the magnitude of the fall, the risk of developing infection increased as the final granulocyte count decreased. One of every four episodes during which the granulocyte count fell to less than 100/mm^3 terminated in severe infection. When these events were compared during relapse and remission, only a few differences were apparent. Although the risk of developing infection with any fall in granulocyte count was greater during relapse (16% versus 8%), if the fall exceeded 500 granulocytes/mm^3 the risk was the same for relapse and remission. If the granulocyte count fell to less than 100/mm^3 severe infection occurred in 24% of the episodes during relapse and 60% during remission.

Figure 7 depicts the risk of developing infection with increasing duration of granulocytopenia. Any episode of granulocytopenia, regardless of its duration, had a 39% chance of resulting in identified infection. As the duration of granulocytopenia lengthened the risk increased. Persistent granulocytopenia of 12 weeks' duration resulted in identified infection 100% of the time. The curve for severe infection was similar but at any given time, the risk of developing severe infection was less. When only episodes of severe granulocytopenia (less than 100/mm³) were considered, the risk of developing infection was always greater and the slope of the curve was steeper. One hundred per cent of the episodes of severe granulocytopenia lasting 3 weeks or more were accompanied by identified infection.

RESPONSE TO INFECTION

The granulocytic response to severe infection was then analyzed. The changes in granulocyte level during the first week of the 129 episodes of severe infection are listed in Table 5. The granulocyte level fell or remained in the same category as often as it rose. When the granulocyte level changed in response to infection, the rise or fall was greater than 500/mm³ in one half of the episodes. There was no difference in the granulocytic response to infection when relapse and remission were compared.

The fatality rate of severe infection was related to changes in the granulocyte level during the first week of infection (Table 6). The fatality rate was highest for patients who had persistent severe granulocytopenia (less than 100/mm³). When the granulocyte count fell to less than 100/mm³ regardless of the initial level, the fatality rate was 72%. Patients had a lower

TABLE 5. Changes in Granulocyte Levels During First Week of Severe Infection

Change in Granulocyte Level	Total Episodes			
/mm³	no.		%	
Any fall	40		31	
Fall >500		19		15
Any rise	44		34	
Rise >500		27		21
No change	45		35	
Total	129			

TABLE 6. Fatality Rate of Severe Infections Related to Change in Granulocyte Level During First Week of Infection

Granulocyte Level: Initial	Granulocyte Level: Change	Episodes: Total	Episodes: Fatal
	/mm³	no.	%
<100	None	15	80
<1,000	None or fall	44	59
<1,000	Rise, but still <1,000	15	40
<1,000	Rise to >1,000	26	27
>1,000	Rise	44	32

fatality rate if the granulocyte level rose regardless of the final level. The fatality rate was only approximately 30% if the final granulocyte level was greater than 1,000/mm³, regardless of the initial level. In general, these relationships applied both during relapse and remission.

TYPES OF INFECTION

The severe infections considered above included 45 episodes of urinary tract infection, 43 of pneumonia, 27 of septicemia, and 10 of disseminated fungus. The fatality rate for all of the 129 episodes of severe infections was 41%; during relapse it was 47% and during remission 23%. Eighty per cent of disseminated fungus infections were fatal, 63% of septicemia, 35% of pneumonia, and 20% of urinary tract infection. The fatality rate was similar during relapse and remission for all types of infection except pneumonia (47% versus 13%). The mean duration of infection was similar for fatal and nonfatal episodes. However, if pneumonia persisted beyond 2 weeks, the fatality rate increased to 78%.

Ninety per cent of disseminated fungus infections and 78% of septicemia arose when the granulocyte level was less than 500/mm³. However, only 15% of septicemia and 10% of disseminated fungus occurred when the granulocyte count was greater than 2,000/mm³. Forty per cent of pneumonia and 38% of urinary tract infection occurred in the absence of granulocytopenia. As might be expected, septicemia and disseminated fungus accounted for 58% of severe infections associated with severe granulocytopenia (less than 100/mm^3), and for only 25% of severe infections associated with a granulocyte level greater than 2,000/mm^3. Thirty-five per cent of pneumonia occurred during remission, accounting for 56% of all severe infections in remission. Only 18% of urinary tract infection, 10% of disseminated fungus infection, and 7% of septicemia occurred during remission.

Discussion

The presence of infection in patients with acute leukemia is related to the level of circulating granulocytes and lymphocytes. All types of infection, ranging from a localized cellulitis at a venipuncture site to a disseminated fungus infection, are more likely to be present when the levels of granulocytes and lymphocytes are low. Furthermore, the lower the level of these leukocytes, the more likelihood that infection will be present.

Not only is infection more likely to be present at low levels of granulocytes and lymphocytes, but when severe infection is present the leukocyte level will usually be low. Conversely, when infection is minimal or absent, the leukocyte level is more apt to be high. The great frequency of leukopenia with severe infection is not surprising, since it has been demonstrated that overwhelming infection may cause leukopenia (13). Leukopenia occurring during infection has been reported in alcoholics (14). Furthermore, one third of all severe infectious episodes in this study were accompanied by a fall in granulocyte count. Other observers have noted an even higher incidence of falling granulocyte levels associated with infection occurring in patients with acute leukemia (15, 16).

Infection was present more often during relapse at every leukocyte level. This suggests that other factors play a role in predisposing to infection. Patients are apt to receive higher doses of antileukemic agents during relapse, and steroids are seldom administered as maintenance therapy during remission. Hersh, Carbone, Wong, and Freireich (17) have demonstrated that antileukemic agents depress antibody response to primary antigens. These agents are often toxic to the gastrointestinal tract, thus allowing infection to develop at sites of tissue damage. Methyl GAG frequently causes phlebitis, conjunctivitis, balanitis, and otitis media and these complications often predispose to bacterial infections. This may be one of the factors responsible for the higher incidence of infection in patients with acute myelogenous leukemia, irrespective of the granulocyte level. Other factors must also be involved since infection was more common in these patients with acute myelogenous leukemia during remission as well, at a time when Methyl GAG was not being administered.

The proportion of time spent with infection at higher granulocyte levels during relapse could be affected by patients having large numbers of circulating abnormal cells. Under these circumstances there may be a spuriously high absolute granulocyte count, since small errors in the differential, in the presence of a very high leukocyte count, would result in large errors in the absolute granulocyte count. In this study, very high numbers of circulating abnormal cells were seldom encountered, and had a negligible effect on any of these results.

Since the level of circulating leukocytes may be altered by the presence of infection, their effect on the risk of developing infection is best assessed by eliminating those days when infection is present. When this was done in the current study, the risk of developing identified infection was found to decrease with increasing levels of granulocytes and lymphocytes. It is interesting that no further reduction in the incidence of infection occurred above the level of 1,500 granulocytes/mm^3. Very low levels of circulating granulocytes probably reflect complete absence of granulocyte reserves since there is such a striking decrease in the incidence of infection when the granulocyte level increases from less than 100 to greater than 500 granulocytes/mm^3. These relationships were similar when the first, second, third, and fourth episodes of infection per patient were considered separately. Consequently, it can be concluded that the risk of developing infection is not influenced by preceding episodes of infection, if they have been completely eradicated.

Other investigators have also found a high incidence of infection associated with leukopenia in patients with leukemia. Boggs, Winthrop, and Maxwell (15) found that patients with low granulocyte levels on admission had a higher incidence of infection. However, this analysis failed to consider the intervening changes in granulocyte levels. The experience of this study indicates that leukocyte levels may fluctuate greatly from day to day, especially when patients are receiving antileukemic therapy. Miller and Shanbrom (2) found a high incidence of granulocytopenia associated with the onset of infection in patients with leukemia and lymphomas. A similar relationship was reported by Baker (5) in an autopsy series of disseminated fungus infection in acute leukemia.

The reason for this relationship between leukocyte level and occurrence of infection may be found in studies of the inflammatory response of patients with leukemia. Jaffe (18) concluded from an autopsy study that if granulopoiesis is completely exhausted, there is no defense reaction to infection. If some myeloid tissue capable of maturation remains, the patient with leukemia can react normally to infection. Braude, Feltes, and Brooks (19) discovered from phagocytic studies that the extreme susceptibility of patients with acute leukemia to bacterial infection is due to the marked decrease in total number of mature granulocytes rather than to a decrease in function of these mature granulocytes. Several studies using the skin window technique in patients with leukemia have demonstrated a deficiency of granulocytes in the inflammatory exudates if the number of granulocytes in the peripheral blood is reduced (20–22). Page and Good (23) found similar results in a patient with cyclic neutropenia and also in rabbits made granulocytopenic with nitrogen mustard.

Not only is the incidence of infection related to the granulocyte level, but also the outcome. The highest percentage of deaths occurred among patients with persistent severe granulocytopenia (less than 100/mm^3). Those patients having initial granulocytopenia (less that 1,000/mm^3) who experience a further fall in granulocyte level, also had a high fatality rate. Patients who could respond with any increment in granulocyte level had a more favorable prognosis. This experience differs from that of Raab, Hoeprich, Wintrobe, and Cartwright (24) who concluded that the outcome of infection was not related to granulocyte level. Obviously, the outcome of infection is influenced by the type of organism involved. Fungus infections are usually fatal, due to the inefficacy of currently available antifungal agents against *Candida* and *Aspergillus* species. On the other hand, staphylococcal infections are seldom fatal since the semisynthetic penicillins have become available (1).

While the onset of infection is related to the presence of lymphopenia, it is clear that granulocytes are of more importance. It is possible that the level of circulating lymphocytes does not reflect accurately the lymphocyte reserve. However, when there are few circulating granulocytes, the bone marrow is also usually deficient in granulocytes. Another possible explanation for the lesser importance of lymphocytes may be found in the experiments of Page and Good (23). They discovered that lymphocytes did not appear in inflammatory exudates unless granulocytes were first present. Therefore, if the granulocyte level is low perhaps neither cell type will function adequately, but if the lymphocyte level is low, the granulocytes will still perform their functions.

Several aspects of granulocyte dynamics in patients with acute leukemia are useful in predicting risk of infection. A fall in granulocyte level carries a 12% risk of infection. Regardless of the magnitude of the fall, the risk is greater the lower the final granulocyte level. These results differ somewhat from those obtained by Silver, Beal, Schneiderman, and McCullough (3). They found that the median granulocyte count during periods without infection could not be correlated with the frequency of infection. However, 17 of 18 episodes of bacterial infection were preceded by a fall in granulocyte count. Since the time intervals are not mentioned, it is not possible to relate the results of thir study to the present one. The most important factor in predicting risk of infection is the duration of granulocytopenia. There is a 60% risk of developing infection if granulocytopenia persists for 3 weeks. If the level of granulocytes is less than 100/mm^3, the risk increases to 100%. This fact must be taken into consideration when patients are undergoing cancer chemotherapy with agents that are able to depress the circulating granulocyte level.

Of course, the level of circulating granulocytes and lymphocytes is not the only factor predisposing to infection. As previously mentioned, antileukemic therapy may damage organs such as those of the gastrointestinal tract and allow infection to develop. The level of immune globulins and the ability to form antibodies are also very important. Furthermore, the reticuloendothelial system plays a crucial role in the body's response to infection (25, 26). Nevertheless, a knowledge of these relationships between leukocyte levels and infection may be very useful in understanding the infectious complications of acute leukemia and related hematological disorders.

Summary

Granulocytopenia and lymphopenia occurred frequently in patients with acute leukemia, even during remission. The presence of infection was related to the level of circulating granulocytes and lymphocytes. The prevalence of all types of identified infection decreased with increasing levels of these leukocytes. However, fever without proven infection was not related to leukocyte levels. Furthermore, the proportion of time spent with granulocyte and lymphocyte levels less than 500/mm^3 increased with increasing severity of infection.

The incidence of infectious episodes also decreased with increasing levels of granulocytes and lymphocytes. A critical level existed for granulocytes (1,500/mm^3), above which level there was no further decrease in the incidence of infection. At every level of granulocytes and lymphocytes, the frequency of infectious episodes was greater during relapse. Infection occurred most commonly when both granulocytopenia and lymphopenia were present. However, the incidence of infection was greater in the presence of granulocytopenia alone than in the presence of lymphopenia alone.

Only 36% of severe infectious episodes were preceded by a fall in granulocyte level. Twelve per cent of all episodes of falling granulocyte levels terminated in severe infection. However, if granulocytopenia was already present, a further fall in granulocyte level resulted in a 28% incidence of infection. The best indicator of the risk of infection was not the magnitude of the fall in granulocyte level, but rather the final granulocyte count. The risk of developing infection increased with increasing duration of granulocytopenia.

Although there was no characteristic granulocytic response during infection, the fatality rate for infection was related to the granulocyte level. The highest rate occurred among patients with persistent severe granulocytopenia, but those patients with low granulocyte levels who were able to respond to infection with an increment in granulocyte level had a more favorable prognosis.

Acknowledgment

The authors wish to express thanks to Mrs. Grace Ensminger for assistance in preparing this manuscript.

Summario in Interlingua

Le nivellos de granulocytos e de lymphocytos de 52 patientes con leucemia acute esseva tabulate durante le complete curso de lor morbo. Esseva includite in le studio un total de 17.743 dies/patiente. Le patientes se trovava in remission osseo-medullari de lor leucemia acute durante 62 pro cento del tempore. Granulocytopenia (minus que 1000 per mm^3) e lymphopenia occurreva frequentemente, mesmo durante periodos de remission. Le procentage del tempore durante le qual le patiente habeva un identificate infection declinava con le altiamento del nivellos de granulocytos. Iste relation valeva tanto durante recidivas como durante periodos de remission, sed le proportion del tempore associate con infection a omne nivello de granulocytos esseva plus grande durante recidivas. Simile relationes existeva pro lymphocytos. Le proportion del tempore con basse nivellos de granulocytos o de lymphocytos (minus que 500 per mm^3) cresceva con le crescimento del severitate del infectiones.

Ben que le risco de contraher infectiones esseva relationate tanto con le nivellos del granulocytos como etiam con illos del lymphocytos, le nivellos de granulocytos esseva clarmente plus importante. Infectiones occurreva plus frequentemente in granulocytopenia sol que in lymphopenia sol.

Trenta-sex pro cento del episodios de infection sever (pneumonia, infection del vias urinari, septicemia, infection fungal constitutional, etc.) esseva associate con un declino del nivello de granulocytos durante le septimana anterior. Dece-duo pro cento de omne episodios de descendente nivellos de granulocytos observate individualmente pro le varie septimanas se terminava in infection sever. Omne episodio de granulocytopenia, sin reguardo a su duration, habeva un probabilitate de 39 pro cento de resultar in un infection identificabile. Como le duration del granulocytopenia se prolongava, assi le risco se elevava.

Infection sever causava un declino subsequente in le nivello de granulocytos tanto frequentemente como illo causava un augmento de ille nivello. Le responsa granulocytic a infection esseva simile durante recidevas e periodos de remission. Le mortalitate in consequentia de infection sever esseva plus alte inter patientes qui habeva nivellos granulocytic persistentemente infra 100 cellulas per mm^3. Le mortalitate esseva plus basse pro patientes respondente a infection con un augmento de lor nivellos granulocytic.

References

1. Hersh, E. M., Bodey, G. P., Nies, B. A., Freireich, E. J: The causes of death in acute leukemia. A study of 414 patients from 1954–1963. *JAMA* 193: 105, 1965.
2. Miller, S. P., Shanbrom, E.: Infectious syndromes of leukemias and lymphomas. *Amer. J. Med. Sci.* 246: 420, 1963.
3. Silver, R. T., Beal, G. A., Schneiderman, M. A., McCullough, N. B.: The role of the mature neutrophil in bacterial infections in acute leukemia. *Blood* 12: 814, 1957.
4. Baker, R. D.: Leukopenia and therapy in leukemia as factors predisposing to fatal mycoses. Mucormycosis, aspergillosis, and cryptococcosis. *Amer. J. Clin. Path.* 37: 358, 1962.
5. Browne, E. A., Marcus, A. J.: Chronic idiopathic neutropenia. *New Eng. J. Med.* 262: 795, 1960.
6. Kostmann, R.: Infantile genetic agranulocytosis. *Acta Paediat.* (*Stockholm*) (Supplement 105) 45: 1, 1956.
7. Spaet, T. H., Dameshek, W.: Chronic hypoplastic neutropenia. *Amer. J. Med.* 13: 35, 1952.
8. Hill, J., Rolla B., Rowlands, D. T., Jr., Rifkind, D.: Infectious pulmonary disease in patients receiving immunosuppressive therapy for organ transplantation. *New Eng. J. Med.* 271: 1021, 1964.
9. Frei, E., III, Karon, M., Levin, R. H., Freireich, E. J, Taylor, R. J., Hananian, J., Selawry, O., Holland, J. F., Hoogstraten, B., Wolman, I. J., Abir, E., Sawitsky, A., Lee, S., Mills, S. D., Burgert, E. O., Jr., Spurr, C. L., Patterson, R. B., Ebaugh, F. G., James, G. W. III, Moon, J. H.: Effectiveness of combinations of antileukemic agents in inducing and maintaining remission in children with acute leukemia. In press.
10. Levin, R. H., Henderson, E., Karon, M., Freireich, E. J: Treatment of acute leukemia with methylglyoxal-bis-guanylhydrazone (Methyl GAG). *Clin. Pharmacol. Ther.* 6: 31, 1965.

11. Richar, W. J., Breakell, E. S.: Evaluation of an electronic particle counter for the counting of white blood cells. *Amer. J. Clin. Path.* 31: 384, 1959.

12. Bisel, H. F.: Criteria for the evaluation of response to treatment in acute leukemia. *Blood* 11: 676, 1956.

13. Wintrobe, M. M.: *Clinical Hematology*, 5th ed. Lea & Febiger, Philadelphia, 1961, p. 254.

14. McFarland, W., Lebre, E. P.: Abnormal leukocyte response in alcoholism. *Ann. Intern. Med.* 59: 865, 1963.

15. Boggs, D. R., Wintrobe, M., Cartwright, G. E.: The acute leukemias. Analysis of 322 cases and review of the literature. *Medicine (Balt.)* 41: 163, 1962.

16. Boggs, D. R., Frei, E., III: Clinical studies of fever and infection in cancer. *Cancer* 13: 1240, 1960.

17. Hersh, E. M., Carbone, P. P., Wong, V. G., Freireich, E. J: Inhibition of the primary immune response in man by antimetabolites. *Cancer Res.* In press.

18. Jaffe, R. H.: Morphology of the inflammatory defense reactions in leukemia. *Arch. Path. (Chicago)* 14: 177, 1932.

19. Braude, A. I., Feltes, J., Brooks, M.: Differences between the activities of mature granulocytes in leukemic and normal blood. *J. Clin. Invest.* 33: 1036, 1954.

20. Boggs, D. R.: The cellular composition of inflammatory exudates in human leukemias. *Blood* 15: 466, 1960.

21. Perillie, P. E., Finch, C.: The local exudative cellular response in leukemia. *J. Clin. Invest.* 39: 1353, 1960.

22. Perillie, P. E., Finch, S. C.: Quantitative studies of the local exudative cellular reaction in acute leukemia. *J. Clin. Invest.* 43: 425, 1964.

23. Page, A. R., Good, R. A.: A clinical and experimental study of the function of neutrophils in the inflammatory response. *Amer. J. Path.* 34: 645, 1958.

24. Raab, S. O., Hoeprich, P. D., Wintrobe, M. M., Cartwright, G. E.: The clinical significance of fever in acute leukemia. *Blood* 16: 1609, 1960.

25. Miller, C. P.: The effect of irradiation on natural resistance to infection. *Ann. N. Y. Acad. Sci.* 66: 280, 1956.

26. Derby, B. M., Rogers, D. E.: Studies on bacteremia. V. The effect of simultaneous leukopenia and reticuloendothelial blockade on the early blood stream clearance of staphylococci and Escherichia coli. *J. Exp. Med.* 113: 1053, 1961.

Plasma Viral Load and CD4$^+$ Lymphocytes as Prognostic Markers of HIV-1 Infection

John W. Mellors, MD; Alvaro Muñoz, PhD; Janis V. Giorgi, PhD; Joseph B. Margolick, MD, PhD; Charles J. Tassoni, PhD; Phalguni Gupta, PhD; Lawrence A. Kingsley, DrPH; John A. Todd, PhD; Alfred J. Saah, MD; Roger Detels, MD; John P. Phair, MD; and Charles R. Rinaldo Jr., PhD

Background: The rate of disease progression among persons infected with human immunodeficiency virus type 1 (HIV-1) varies widely, and the relative prognostic value of markers of disease activity has not been defined.

Objective: To compare clinical, serologic, cellular, and virologic markers for their ability to predict progression to the acquired immunodeficiency syndrome (AIDS) and death during a 10-year period.

Design: Prospective, multicenter cohort study.

Setting: Four university-based clinical centers participating in the Multicenter AIDS Cohort Study.

Patients: 1604 men infected with HIV-1.

Measurements: The markers compared were oral candidiasis (thrush) or fever; serum neopterin levels; serum β_2-microglobulin levels; number and percentage of CD3$^+$, CD4$^+$, and CD8$^+$ lymphocytes; and plasma viral load, which was measured as the concentration of HIV-1 RNA found using a sensitive branched-DNA signal-amplification assay.

Results: Plasma viral load was the single best predictor of progression to AIDS and death, followed (in order of predictive strength) by CD4$^+$ lymphocyte count and serum neopterin levels, serum β_2-microglobulin levels, and thrush or fever. Plasma viral load discriminated risk at all levels of CD4$^+$ lymphocyte counts and predicted their subsequent rate of decline. Five risk categories were defined by plasma HIV-1 RNA concentrations: 500 copies/mL or less, 501 to 3000 copies/mL, 3001 to 10 000 copies/mL, 10 001 to 30 000 copies/mL, and more than 30 000 copies/mL. Highly significant ($P < 0.001$) differences in the percentages of participants who progressed to AIDS within 6 years were seen in the five risk categories: 5.4%, 16.6%, 31.7%, 55.2%, and 80.0%, respectively. Highly significant ($P < 0.001$) differences in the percentages of participants who died of AIDS within 6 years were also seen in the five risk categories: 0.9%, 6.3%, 18.1%, 34.9%, and 69.5%, respectively. A regression tree incorporating both HIV-1 RNA measurements and CD4$^+$ lymphocyte counts provided better discrimination of outcome than did either marker alone; use of both variables defined categories of risk for AIDS within 6 years that ranged from less than 2% to 98%.

Conclusions: Plasma viral load strongly predicts the rate of decrease in CD4$^+$ lymphocyte count and progression to AIDS and death, but the prognosis of HIV-infected persons is more accurately defined by combined measurement of plasma HIV-1 RNA and CD4$^+$ lymphocytes.

Ann Intern Med. 1997;126:946-954.

For author affiliations and current author addresses, see end of text.

The rate of disease progression among persons infected with human immunodeficiency virus type 1 (HIV-1) varies greatly. Approximately 5% of infected persons (1, 2) develop the acquired immunodeficiency syndrome (AIDS) within 3 years of infection. By contrast, approximately 12% of infected persons are expected to remain free of AIDS for more than 20 years (1, 3). The variable course of HIV-1 infection causes uncertainty for the infected person and complicates decisions about when antiretroviral therapy should begin.

Many clinical and laboratory measures have been used to assess prognosis in HIV-1 infection (4). In a previous comparative study of eight cellular and serologic markers (5), the single best predictor of progression to AIDS was the percentage or absolute number of circulating CD4$^+$ lymphocytes. Since that report was published, new methods have been developed to reproducibly quantify plasma viral load, measured as the concentration of HIV-1 RNA (6–8). Previous studies have shown that the HIV-1 RNA concentration in plasma after acute HIV-1 infection (seroconversion) provides prognostic information that is independent of the CD4$^+$ lymphocyte count (9–12). In a recent study (13), plasma viral load was found to be a better indicator of prognosis than the CD4$^+$ lymphocyte count; this study, however, had a small cohort and did not assess the value of other predictive markers or combinations of markers. In the present study, we compared the prognostic value of plasma viral load with that of clinical, serologic, and cellular markers in a large cohort of HIV-infected men. We have incorporated the two most predictive markers—plasma viral load and CD4$^+$ lymphocyte count—into a regression tree that is useful for assessing the prognosis of individual patients.

See related articles on pp 929-938 and 939-945 and editorial comment on pp 983-985.

Methods

Study Sample

Between March 1984 and April 1985, the Multicenter AIDS Cohort Study (MACS) enrolled a cohort of 4954 homosexual men who were 18 years of age or older and were free of clinical AIDS (according to the Centers for Disease Control and Prevention 1987 definition). Other details about the recruitment and characteristics of the MACS cohort have been reported elsewhere (14). Participants in MACS returned for follow-up visits at 6-month intervals. All participants gave written informed consent, and the study was approved by the internal review boards of each clinical center.

The baseline visit for the current study was either the third or fourth MACS follow-up visit (these visits occurred 1.0 or 1.5 years after enrollment). These later visits were selected to minimize the inherent variability in collecting and processing blood samples in the start-up phase of cohort studies. The eligible study sample consisted of HIV-1–infected persons who were free of AIDS at the baseline visit for this study and were either seropositive at enrollment into MACS (n = 1813) or had seroconverted before the baseline visit for this study (n = 169). All study participants were required to have a baseline $CD4^+$ lymphocyte count (measured at the third or fourth MACS follow-up visit), to have plasma samples available in the repository for measurement of HIV-1 RNA concentration, and to have had follow-up after the baseline visit for this study. A total of 1639 of 1982 eligible men (83%) met these criteria; HIV-1 RNA concentration was measured in 1604 of these men.

Measurement of Plasma HIV-1 RNA Concentrations

Heparinized plasma samples were stored at −70 °C until testing was done. The average interval between collection of blood and freezing of plasma samples is estimated to have been approximately 6 hours, but times were not always recorded. A sensitive branched-DNA (bDNA) assay (Chiron Corp., Emeryville, California) was used to quantify HIV-1 RNA in duplicate 1.0-mL samples. This assay has a lower quantification limit of 500 copies/mL and is linear to concentrations as high as 1.6×10^6 copies/mL (one copy of HIV-1 RNA is equal to one molecule of HIV-1 RNA). Additional details about the bDNA assay and its performance characteristics are reported elsewhere (15). The mean coefficient of variation between the 1604 duplicate results was 10.3%.

Measurement of T-Lymphocyte Subsets, Serum Levels of β_2-Microglobulin, and Serum Levels of Neopterin

T-lymphocyte subsets were measured in ficoll–hypaque purified peripheral blood mononuclear cells (done in the centers in Baltimore and Pittsburgh) or EDTA-anticoagulated whole blood (done in the centers in Chicago and Los Angeles) by staining with fluorescent dye–conjugated monoclonal antibodies that were specific for $CD3^+$, $CD4^+$, and $CD8^+$ lymphocytes (Becton Dickinson, Mountain View, California), as reported previously (16). Serum levels of β_2-microglobulin (Kabi Pharmacia, Uppsala, Sweden) and neopterin (Henning, Berlin, Germany) were measured by using commercial radioimmunoassays in comparison with standards provided by the manufacturers.

Study Variables

We analyzed plasma HIV-1 RNA concentrations; the number and percentage of $CD3^+$, $CD4^+$, and $CD8^+$ lymphocytes at the baseline visit; and participants' reports of either oral candidiasis (thrush) or fever of no less than 2 weeks' duration. Neopterin and β_2-microglobulin levels were measured at the baseline visit; if no baseline levels were available, we used levels obtained during visits that occurred within 1 year before the baseline visit.

Two time intervals were used in analyses of disease progression: the time to development of AIDS (according to the 1987 definition from the Centers for Disease Control and Prevention) and the time to AIDS-related death. Censoring strategies have been reported elsewhere (1). The date of analysis for this study was 1 July 1995. For participants in whom two or more $CD4^+$ lymphocyte counts were available after the baseline visit (1531 of 1604 participants [95%]), we determined the rate of decline of $CD4^+$ lymphocyte counts as an alternate outcome measure.

Statistical Analysis

To assess the relative prognostic power of each marker, a variant of q-q plots (17) (Splus software: q-q plot function [Statistical Sciences, Inc., Seattle, Washington]) was used to compare the percentile values of each marker in the group that developed AIDS with the percentile values in the group that remained AIDS-free. We calculated the natural logarithms of the ratios of the percentile values because these ratios have no units and will approximate zero if the distribution of the marker values does not differ between groups.

We divided the study sample into four groups of approximately the same size according to the baseline HIV-1 RNA concentration (that is, quartiles), with breakpoint values of 3000, 10 000, and 30 000 copies/mL. To separate participants whose HIV-1 RNA concentrations were below the quantification limit of the bDNA assay, we subdivided the first group at 500 copies/mL. This produced five categories (I through V) of HIV-1 RNA concentrations: 500 copies/mL or less; 501 to 3000 copies/mL; 3001 to 10 000 copies/mL; 10 001 to 30 000 copies/mL, and more than 30 000 copies/mL. Kaplan–Meier curves (18) and log-rank tests for the HIV-1 RNA categories were calculated for the entire study sample and for the subgroups that either subsequently received antiretroviral therapy or never received such therapy.

We used a proportional hazards model with risk-set stratification (18) to estimate and test the statistical significance of the values of relative risks for AIDS and death among persons in HIV-1 RNA categories I through V (PROC PHREG software, SAS Institute, Cary, North Carolina). Strata were defined by five categories (I through V) of $CD4^+$ lymphocyte count (with breakpoint values at 200, 350, 500, and 750 cells/mm^3), two categories of neopterin levels (with a breakpoint value equal to the median of 11.5 nmol/L), and two categories of symptoms (the presence of thrush or fever or the absence of both thrush and fever). The breakpoint $CD4^+$ lymphocyte values of 350, 500, and 750 cells/mm^3 correspond to the approximate quartile values. The first quartile was divided into two categories ($\leq$200 and 201 to 350 cells/mm^3) because persons who have 200 $CD4^+$ lymphocytes/mm^3 have a higher risk for AIDS (19).

To determine the predictive value of combining the baseline HIV-1 RNA concentration with $CD4^+$ lymphocyte counts, we constructed a regression tree using all five categories for both HIV-1 RNA concentrations and $CD4^+$ lymphocyte counts. To define the first five nodes of the tree, we compared the results of two Cox regression analyses using the five categories of the two variables and selected the variable with the highest likelihood ratio statistic. For each of the first five nodes, we then used recursive partitioning (20) to determine which categories of the second variable defined significantly different risks for AIDS (that is, likelihood ratio test of Cox regression for a binary split significant at the 5% level). We summarize the effect of the second variable by providing the *P* value that corresponded to the likelihood ratio statistic for each group of secondary nodes of the tree. Estimates of the probability of AIDS by 3, 6, and 9 years were derived from Kaplan–Meier curves for each group defined by the terminal nodes of the tree. The percentile method was applied to 500 bootstrap samples in order to provide 95% CIs for the estimates (21).

Funding Source

The MACS investigators analyzed and interpreted all data; analysis was not influenced by the funding source (National Institute of Allergy and Infectious Diseases) or the manufacturer of the bDNA assay (Chiron Corp.).

Table. Baseline Values of Prognostic Markers*

Prognostic Marker	All Participants (*n* = 1604)	Participants with AIDS (*n* = 998)	Participants without AIDS (*n* = 606)	Participants Who Died of AIDS (*n* = 855)	Participants Who Are Alive or Died of Cause Other Than AIDS (*n* = 749)†	Correlation with HIV-1 RNA (95% CI)‡
HIV-1 RNA, *copies/mL*§	10 825 (3392–33 370)	19 145 (7153–52 900)	3636 (1111–10 340)	24 200 (8918–61 740)	4426 (1308–11 460)	
$CD4^+$ lymphocyte count, *cells/mm^3*§	527 (376–716)	466 (332–633)	636 (467–836)	454 (314–608)	630 (450–815)	−0.42 (−0.46 to −0.38)
$CD4^+$ lymphocytes, %§	30 (24–37)	28 (21–35)	34 (28–39)	27 (20–33)	34 (28–39)	−0.43 (−0.47 to −0.39)
$CD8^+$ lymphocyte count, *cells/mm^3*§	748 (531–981)	751 (532–990)	747 (527–959)	757 (539–1007)	736 (525–950)	0.05 (0.00 to 0.10)
$CD8^+$ lymphocytes, %§	43 (35–50)	45 (37–53)	40 (32–46)	46 (37–54)	40 (33–47)	0.30 (0.25 to 0.34)
$CD3^+$ lymphocyte count, *cells/mm^3*§	1352 (1044–1719)	1303 (1006–1662)	1433 (1128–1825)	1299 (1003–1671)	1402 (1115–1780)	−0.15 (−0.20 to −0.10)
$CD3^+$ lymphocytes, %§	77 (71–83)	77 (71–82)	77 (70–83)	77 (71–82)	77 (71–83)	−0.01 (−0.06 to 0.04)
Neopterin level, *nmol/L*§‖	11.49 (8.60–16.24)	12.74 (9.57–17.80)	9.88 (7.43–13.52)	13.03 (9.70–18.30)	10.11 (7.65–13.90)	0.29 (0.24 to 0.34)
β_2-microglobulin level, *μg/L*§¶	2.26 (1.76–3.00)	2.41 (1.84–3.07)	2.04 (1.64–2.86)	2.44 (1.89–3.16)	2.06 (1.62–2.84)	0.20 (0.15 to 0.25)
Thrush or fever, %	6.4	8.5	3.0	9.3	3.2	NA

* AIDS = acquired immunodeficiency syndrome; HIV-1 = human immunodeficiency virus type 1; NA = not applicable.
† Includes 60 participants who died of causes other than AIDS.
‡ Pearson correlation with HIV-1 RNA in log base 10.
§ Values in the second through the fifth columns are the median (interquartile range: 25th percentile–75th percentile).
‖ Neopterin values were missing for 184 participants.
¶ β_2-microglobulin values were missing for 170 participants.

Results

Study Sample and Comparison of Prognostic Markers

Of the 1604 study participants, 998 had developed AIDS and 855 had died of AIDS by 1 July 1995. Median follow-up of AIDS-free participants was 9.6 years. The **Table** provides descriptive statistics for the prognostic markers at baseline. Comparison of the natural logarithms of the ratios of the quartile values in the AIDS group and AIDS-free group for each prognostic marker indicated that HIV-1 RNA concentrations were the strongest predictive marker, followed by $CD4^+$ lymphocyte counts, neopterin levels, and β_2-microglobulin levels; $CD4^+$ lymphocyte counts were only slightly more predictive than neopterin levels. The superiority of the HIV-1 RNA concentration as a predictive marker was a consistent finding when we separately analyzed data from each of the four MACS centers. The **Table** also shows that HIV-1 RNA concentrations were significantly correlated (95% CI excludes zero) with $CD4^+$ lymphocyte count, percentage of $CD4^+$ lymphocytes, percentage of $CD8^+$ lymphocytes, $CD3^+$ lymphocyte count, and levels of neopterin and β_2-microglobulin.

Antiretroviral therapy was not available at the time of the baseline visit for this study (most baseline visits occurred in September 1985). Subsequently, 1006 of the 1604 participants (63%) received antiretroviral treatment, primarily monotherapy with zidovudine, didanosine, zalcitabine, or stavudine. The median values of the prognostic markers were not different in the subgroups that did or did not receive antiretroviral therapy during follow-up ($P >$ 0.05; data not shown).

Outcome Discrimination by HIV-1 RNA

To assess the effect of baseline plasma concentration of HIV-1 RNA on subsequent decline in $CD4^+$ lymphocyte count, we used a random-effects linear model (22) to compute change in $CD4^+$ lymphocyte counts over time, allowing the intercept and slope to vary among participants (PROC MIXED, SAS Institute). **Figure 1** shows a monotonic relation between HIV-1 RNA concentrations and decline in $CD4^+$ lymphocyte counts—the higher the HIV-1 RNA concentration, the greater the rate of decline in $CD4^+$ lymphocyte count.

The percentages of participants in HIV-1 RNA categories I through V who developed AIDS within 6 years were 5.4%, 16.6%, 31.7%, 55.2%, and 80.0%, respectively ($P <$ 0.001). The percentages of participants who died of AIDS within 6 years were 0.9%, 6.3%, 18.1%, 34.9%, and 69.5%, respectively ($P <$ 0.001). Risk discrimination by baseline HIV-1 RNA concentration was independent of subsequent antiretroviral therapy or prophylaxis against *Pneumocystis carinii* pneumonia (data not shown).

To determine the prognostic value of HIV-1 RNA at different $CD4^+$ lymphocyte counts, Kaplan–Meier curves for AIDS by HIV-1 RNA category were calculated among participants with $CD4^+$ lymphocyte counts of 200 cells/mm^3 or less, 201 to 350 cells/mm^3, 351 to 500 cells/mm^3, or more than 500 cells/mm^3 (**Figure 2**). Within each $CD4^+$ lymphocyte category, HIV-1 RNA provided significant discrimination of time without AIDS ($P <$ 0.001) and duration of survival ($P <$ 0.001; data not shown). A similar analysis of HIV-1 RNA among categories defined by percentage of $CD4^+$ lymphocytes (0 to 14%, >14% to 24%, >24% to 29%, and >29%) also showed highly significant ($P <$ 0.001) discrimination of time without AIDS and duration of survival (data not shown).

To determine the prognostic information provided by the baseline HIV-1 RNA concentration after controlling for the other markers that were correlated with it, we used a proportional hazards regression procedure in which the underlying hazard was allowed to differ in strata defined by the five categories of $CD4^+$ lymphocyte count, two categories of neopterin level (breakpoint of 11.5 nmol/L), and the presence or absence of thrush or fever.

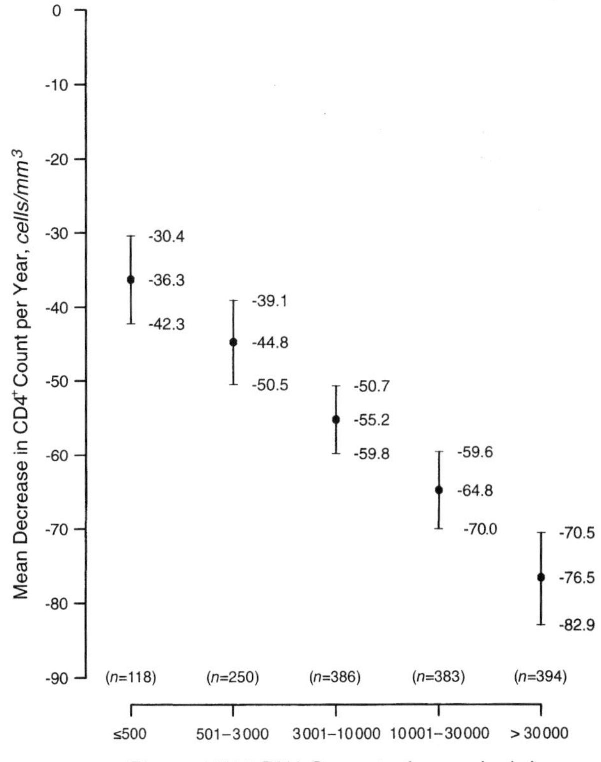

Figure 1. Estimated slopes of $CD4^+$ lymphocyte counts by human immunodeficiency virus type 1 (*HIV-1*) RNA category. Vertical bars represent 95% CIs.

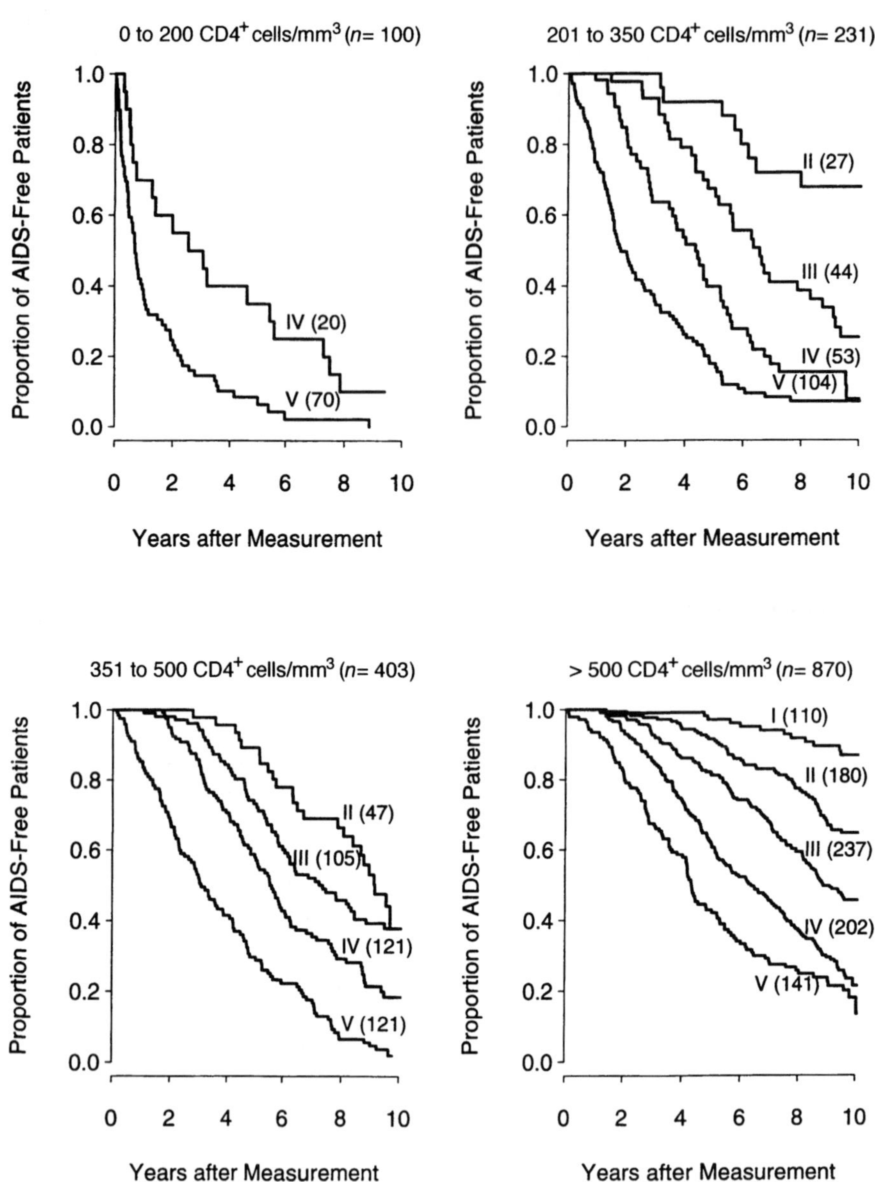

Figure 2. Kaplan–Meier curves showing acquired immunodeficiency syndrome (*AIDS*)–free survival by human immunodeficiency virus type 1 (HIV-1) RNA category among groups with different baseline CD4⁺ lymphocyte counts. The five categories of HIV-1 RNA were the following: I, 500 copies/mL or less; II, 501 to 3000 copies/mL; III, 3001 to 10 000 copies/mL; IV, 10 001 to 30 000 copies/mL; and V, more than 30 000 copies/mL. Numbers in parentheses are the sample sizes of the groups at baseline. Groups that were too small to provide estimates were omitted. The following table lists the numbers of participants in each group after 3, 6, and 9 years:

HIV-1 RNA Category	3 Years	6 Years	9 Years
0–200 CD4⁺ cells/mm³			
IV	10	5	2
V	10	1	0
201–500 CD4⁺ cells/mm³			
II	25	20	16
III	40	23	12
IV	33	14	6
V	35	9	6
351–500 CD4⁺ cells/mm³			
II	45	35	19
III	95	60	33
IV	101	48	19
V	60	24	6
>500 CD4⁺ cells/mm³			
I	103	90	77
II	173	146	100
III	218	167	100
IV	169	101	50
V	93	40	20

Data on all four variables were available for 1416 (88.3%) of the 1604 participants. The adjusted relative risks for AIDS or death from AIDS differed significantly ($P < 0.001$) among the five categories of HIV-1 RNA concentrations; the higher the baseline HIV-1 RNA concentration, the higher the relative risk for AIDS and death from AIDS. Specifically, the adjusted relative risks for AIDS with HIV-1 RNA categories II through V compared with category I were 2.4 (95% CI, 1.4 to 4.1), 4.3 (CI, 2.5 to 7.3), 7.5 (CI, 4.4 to 12.7), and 12.8 (CI, 7.5 to 21.8), respectively. The adjusted relative risks for AIDS-related death with HIV-1 RNA categories II through V compared with category I were 2.8 (CI, 1.4 to 5.6), 5.0 (CI, 2.5 to 9.8), 9.8 (CI, 4.9 to 19.1), and 18.1 (CI, 9.2 to 35.7), respectively. The reciprocal analyses—relative risk for AIDS and AIDS-related death according to $CD4^+$ lymphocyte category after controlling for HIV-1 RNA concentration, neopterin level, and thrush or fever—showed that the adjusted relative risks differed significantly among the $CD4^+$ lymphocyte categories but that the magnitude of the relative risks was much lower. For example, the adjusted relative risks for AIDS with $CD4^+$ lymphocyte categories I through IV relative to category V were 1.5 (CI, 1.2 to 1.8), 1.8 (CI, 1.5 to 2.3), 2.4 (CI, 1.9 to 3.1), and 4.0 (CI, 3.0 to 5.5), respectively. Use of five categories of percentage of $CD4^+$ lymphocytes (breakpoint values of 14%, 24%, 29%, and 34%) rather than absolute $CD4^+$ lymphocyte count did not change the magnitude or significance of the adjusted relative risks. The adjusted relative risks also remained the same when age and race were included in each stratified regression analysis.

Regression Tree Analysis

The final regression tree shown in **Figure 3** contains 12 distinct risk categories and provides excellent discrimination of risk for AIDS. To illustrate, among participants in the lowest risk category (HIV-1 RNA concentration ≤500 copies/mL and $CD4^+$ lymphocyte count >750 cells/mm^3), only 1.7% developed AIDS within 6 years. By contrast, 97.9% of participants in the highest risk category (HIV-1 RNA concentration >30 000 copies/mL and $CD4^+$ lymphocyte count ≤200 cells/mm^3) developed AIDS within 6 years. The overall association with AIDS development was stronger for HIV-1 RNA than for $CD4^+$ lymphocytes; in some instances, however, participants with higher HIV-1 RNA concentrations and higher $CD4^+$ lymphocyte counts had a better prognosis than did those with lower HIV-1 RNA concentrations and lower $CD4^+$ lymphocyte counts. For each of the 12 risk categories, we determined whether additional prognostic information was provided by levels of neopterin or β_2-microglobulin. Neopterin levels that exceeded the median of 11.5 nmol/L were associated with significantly higher risk for AIDS ($P < 0.05$; likelihood ratio test) in only 2 of the 12 risk categories. Levels of β_2-microglobulin did not provide additional prognostic information. Because older age at seroconversion is associated with shorter time to AIDS (1, 23), we examined the effect of a 10-year difference in age on the risk for AIDS. The adjusted relative risk for AIDS was significantly higher than 1.0 ($P <$ 0.05) only in participants with HIV-1 RNA concentrations of 10 000 copies/mL or less.

Discussion

Our study compared the prognostic value of viral load, measured as the concentration of HIV-1 RNA in plasma, with that of other traditional markers of risk for AIDS in a large, well-characterized cohort of men infected with HIV-1. Plasma viral load was the single best predictor of clinical outcome, followed (in order of predictive value) by $CD4^+$ lymphocyte counts and neopterin levels, β_2-microglobulin levels, and thrush or fever. We observed a strong association between viral load and the subsequent rate of decline in $CD4^+$ lymphocyte counts; this relation has not been shown previously. Plasma viral load also provided important prognostic information in all commonly used strata of $CD4^+$ lymphocyte counts (**Figure 2**). Although our analyses showed that HIV-1 RNA concentrations are a better predictor than $CD4^+$ lymphocytes, incorporation of both markers into a regression tree provided more prognostic information than did either marker alone (**Figure 3**). A limitation of our study, however, is the absence of women or children in the cohort and the underrepresentation of members of ethnic and racial minority groups (12.2%).

The third or fourth MACS follow-up visit was used as the baseline for this study to allow time for better standardization of sample collection and laboratory methods among the four sites. For each MACS center, HIV-1 RNA concentrations and $CD4^+$ lymphocyte counts measured at the third visit showed significant ($P < 0.05$) dose–response relations with AIDS or death from AIDS. A previous study (13) that used $CD4^+$ lymphocyte counts from the first MACS visit at one center failed to show a dose–response relation between $CD4^+$ lymphocyte counts and outcome. This was probably due to imprecision in measurement of $CD4^+$ lymphocyte counts because measurements from the first visit at the other three MACS centers confirmed the dose–response relation (5, 16).

Baseline HIV-1 RNA concentrations were highly predictive of the rate of decline of $CD4^+$ lympho-

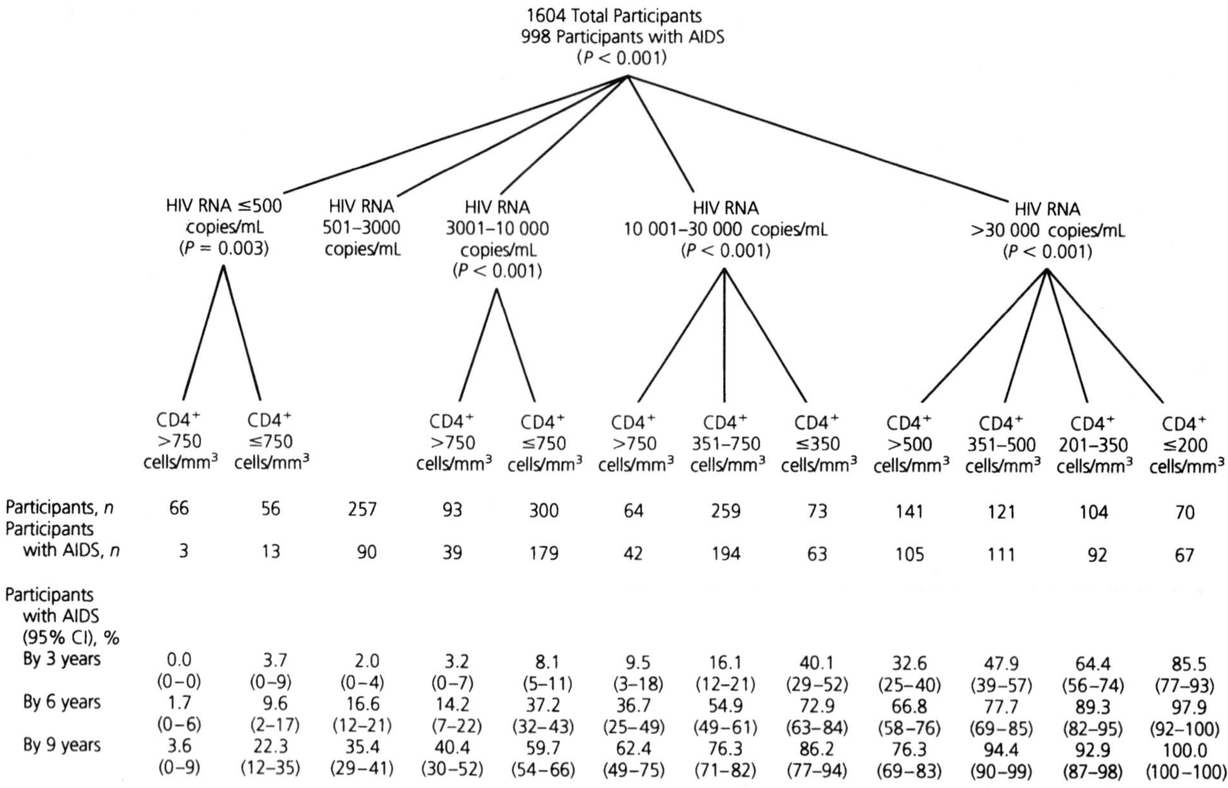

Figure 3. Probability of developing the acquired immunodeficiency syndrome (*AIDS*) according to human immunodeficiency virus type 1 (*HIV-1*) concentration and CD4+ lymphocyte count. The *P* values are derived from the likelihood ratio test using Cox regression. Mean 95% CIs were derived from 500 bootstrap samples using the percentile method.

cyte counts, of AIDS development, and of death over a 10-year span. The strong link between plasma viral load and clinical outcome provides solid evidence that viremia is central to the pathogenesis of HIV-1 disease. Recent studies (24–26) indicate that viremia in HIV-1 infection is sustained by continuous, rapid viral replication, with approximately 10^{10} virions produced per day (range, 0.4 to 32.0×10^{10} virions per day). In addition, plasma viral load is a direct indicator of the total number of virus-producing cells in an infected person (26). Patients with higher plasma viral loads may develop AIDS in a shorter time because greater virus production more quickly exhausts the host's capacity to replenish destroyed $CD4^+$ lymphocytes. The specific mechanisms responsible for the destruction of $CD4^+$ lymphocytes and the critical factors that control the level of virus production are still largely undefined.

Studies on the degradation of HIV-1 RNA in blood samples indicate that the type of anticoagulant agent used and the time interval between collection and freezing of plasma influence the number of HIV-1 RNA molecules detected. To minimize HIV-1 RNA degradation, it is recommended that blood be collected in tubes that contain EDTA as the anticoagulant and that the blood be processed within 4 hours of collection (27). The plasma samples used in our study were separated from heparinized blood and stored at −70 °C after an average delay of 6 hours. Studies that have compared blood samples collected in heparin or EDTA indicate that the HIV-1 RNA concentration measured by the bDNA assay in heparinized plasma is approximately 65% of that in EDTA-anticoagulated plasma after a processing delay of as long as 2 hours and approximately 45% of that in EDTA-anticoagulated plasma after a delay of 30 hours (27). This suggests that the plasma HIV-1 RNA values in our study are likely to be approximately 50% to 60% of those that would have been obtained if samples had been collected in EDTA, processed within 4 hours, and tested by the bDNA assay. This important difference should be considered when the results of this study are incorporated into clinical practice.

We used a sensitive bDNA signal-amplification assay to measure plasma HIV-1 RNA concentrations. Plasma HIV-1 RNA can be quantified with other methods, including reverse transcriptase–initiated polymerase chain reaction (RT-PCR) and nucleic acid sequence–based amplification (7, 8). An RT-PCR technique has recently been approved for clinical use by the U.S. Food and Drug Administration (FDA). We assayed a subset of 400 of the 1604 samples from this study by using the FDA-approved RT-PCR assay; the assay was performed after heparinase was added to destroy heparin in the samples because heparin inhibits RT-PCR. The correlation coefficient for the results obtained with the two assays was 0.93 ($P < 0.001$). Concentrations of HIV-1 RNA obtained with RT-PCR were approximately two times higher than those obtained with the bDNA assay; however, the magnitude of the difference varied across the range of values. To illustrate, samples that were found to contain 3000, 10 000, and 30 000 HIV-1 RNA copies/mL when the bDNA assay was used had 6911, 20 442, and 54 894 copies/mL, respectively, according to RT-PCR (differences of 2.30-, 2.04-, and 1.83-fold, respectively). The relation between the results of the two assays is summarized by the following formulas: 1) RT-PCR (copies/mL) = 5.13 × (bDNA copies/mL)$^{0.9}$ and, conversely, 2) bDNA value (copies/mL) = 0.2 × (RT-PCR copies/mL)$^{1.1}$.

Our study establishes HIV-1 RNA as an important prognostic marker before antiretroviral therapy has been initiated. Our analyses were not confounded by antiretroviral therapy because baseline HIV-1 RNA values did not differ between the subgroups that did and did not receive therapy during follow-up and because HIV-1 RNA concentrations predicted highly significant differences in time without AIDS and duration of survival independent of subsequent therapy.

In summary, measurement of HIV-1 RNA concentrations and $CD4^+$ lymphocyte counts at one time point provides excellent discrimination of the risk for AIDS and death from AIDS. Risk for disease progression exists on a continuum that increases directly with the plasma HIV-1 RNA concentration and inversely with the $CD4^+$ lymphocyte count. Combined use of these prognostic markers should prove useful in individual patient management and in the design and evaluation of therapeutic trials. Such trials are needed to define the optimal time to initiate antiretroviral therapy on the basis of individual risk for disease progression.

Appendix

The following are investigators in the Multicenter AIDS Cohort Study.

Baltimore, Maryland: The Johns Hopkins University School of Public Health: Alfred J. Saah (*Principal Investigator*), Haroutune Armenian, Homayoon Farzadegan, Donald Hoover, Nancy Kass, Joseph Margolick, and Ellen Taylor.

Chicago, Illinois: Howard Brown Health Center and Northwestern University Medical School: John P. Phair (*Principal Investigator*), Joan S. Chmiel, Bruce Cohen, Maurice O'Gorman, Daina Variakojis, Jerry Wesch, and Steven M. Wolinsky.

Los Angeles, California: University of California, Los Angeles, Schools of Public Health and Medicine: Roger Detels (*Principal Investigator*), Barbara R. Visscher, Janice P. Dudley, John L. Fahey, Janis V. Giorgi, Andrew Kaplan, Oto Martinez-Maza, Eric N. Miller, Hal Morgenstern, Parunag Nishanian, John Oishi, Jeremy Taylor, and Harry Vinters.

Pittsburgh, Pennsylvania: University of Pittsburgh, Graduate School of Public Health: Charles R. Rinaldo (*Principal Investigator*), James Becker, Phalguni Gupta, Monto Ho, Lawrence Kingsley, John Mellors, Oliver Ndimbie, Sharon Riddler, and Anthony Silvestre.

Data Coordinating Center: The Johns Hopkins University School of Hygiene and Public Health, Baltimore, Maryland: Alvaro Muñoz (*Principal Investigator*), Cheryl Enger, Stephen Gange, Lisa P. Jacobson, Cindy Kleeberger, Robert Lyles, Steven Piantadosi, Charles Tassoni, and Sol Su.

National Institutes of Health: National Institute of Allergy and Infectious Diseases, Bethesda, Maryland: Lewis Schrager (*Project Officer*); National Cancer Institute, Bethesda, Maryland: Sandra Melnik.

From the University of Pittsburgh and Veterans Affairs Medical Center, Pittsburgh, Pennsylvania; The Johns Hopkins School of Public Health, Baltimore, Maryland; University of California, Los Angeles, Schools ofMedicine and Public Health, Los Angeles, California; Chiron Corp., Emeryville, California; and Northwestern University School of Medicine, Chicago, Illinois.

Acknowledgment: The authors thank the MACS participants and staff for their dedication.

Grant Support: By the National Institute of Allergy and Infectious Diseases with supplemental support grants U01-AI-35042, 5-MO1-RR-00722 (GCRC), UO1-AI-35043, UO1-AI-37984, UO1-AI-35039, UO1-AI-35040, UO1-AI-37613, UO1-AI-35041 from the National Cancer Institute.

Requests for Reprints: John W. Mellors, MD, Graduate of School of Public Health, 603 Parran Hall, 130 DeSoto Street, University of Pittsburgh, Pittsburgh, PA 15261.

Current Author Addresses: Dr. Mellors: University of Pittsburgh, Graduate School of Public Health, 603 Parran Hall, 130 DeSoto Street, Pittsburgh, PA 15261.
Dr. Muñoz: Department of Epidemiology, Johns Hopkins School of Public Health, Room E-7008, 615 North Wolfe Street, Baltimore, MD 21205.
Dr. Giorgi: University of California, Los Angeles, School of Medicine, Department of Medicine, Factor Building, 650 Circle Drive South, Los Angeles, CA 90095-1745.
Dr. Margolick: Molecular Microbiology and Immunology, Johns Hopkins School of Public Health, Room E-4014, 615 North Wolfe Street, Baltimore, MD 21205.
Dr. Tassoni: Department of Epidemiology, Johns Hopkins School of Public Health, Room E-7009, 615 North Wolfe Street, Baltimore, MD 21205.
Dr. Gupta: University of Pittsburgh, Graduate School of Public Health, A448 Crabtree Hall, 130 DeSoto Street, Pittsburgh, PA 15261.
Dr. Kingsley: University of Pittsburgh, Graduate School of Public Health, 402 Parkvale Building, 130 DeSoto Street, Pittsburgh, PA 15261.
Dr. Todd: Chiron Corp., 4560 Horton Street, Emeryville, CA 94608-2916.
Dr. Saah: Department of Epidemiology, Johns Hopkins School of Public Health, Room E-6008, 615 North Wolfe Street, Baltimore, MD 21205.
Dr. Detels: University of California, Los Angeles, School of Public Health, Department of Epidemiology, Center for the Health Sciences, Room 71-267, 10833 Le Conte Avenue, Los Angeles, CA 90095-1772.

Dr. Phair: Northwestern University Medical School, Comprehensive AIDS Center, 680 North Lake Shore Drive, Suite 1106, Chicago, IL 60611-4402.

Dr. Rinaldo: University of Pittsburgh, Graduate School of Public Health, 448 Crabtree Hall, 130 DeSoto Street, Pittsburgh, PA 15261.

References

1. **Muñoz A, Xu J.** Models for the incubation of AIDS and variations according to age and period. Stat Med. 1996;15:2459-73.
2. **Phair J, Jacobson L, Detels R, Rinaldo C, Saah A, Schrager L, et al.** Acquired immune deficiency syndrome occurring within 5 years of infection with human immunodeficiency virus type-1: the Multicenter AIDS Cohort Study. J Acquir Immune Defic Syndr. 1992;5:490-6.
3. **Sheppard HW, Lang W, Ascher MS, Vittinghoff E, Winkelstein W.** The characterization of non-progressors: long-term HIV-1 infection with stable CD4+ T-cell levels. AIDS. 1993;7:1159-66.
4. **Tsoukas CM, Bernard NF.** Markers predicting progression of human immunodeficiency virus-related disease. Clin Microbiol Rev. 1994;7:14-28.
5. **Fahey JL, Taylor JM, Detels R, Hofmann B, Melmed R, Nishanian P, et al.** The prognostic value of cellular and serologic markers in infection with human immunodeficiency virus type 1. N Engl J Med. 1990;322:166-72.
6. **Pachl C, Todd JA, Kern DG, Sheridan PJ, Fong SJ, Stempien M, et al.** Rapid and precise quantification of HIV-1 RNA in plasma using a branched DNA (bDNA) signal amplification assay. J Acquir Immune Defic Syndr Hum Retrovirol. 1995;8:446-54.
7. **Mulder J, McKinney N, Christopherson C, Sninsky J, Greenfield L, Kwok S.** Rapid and simple PCR assay for quantitation of human immunodeficiency virus type 1 RNA in plasma: application to acute retroviral infection. J Clin Microbiol. 1994;32:292-300.
8. **Kievits T, van Gemen B, van Strijp D, Schukkink R, Dircks M, Adriaanse H, et al.** NASBA isothermal enzymatic in vitro nucleic acid amplification optimized for the diagnosis of HIV-1 infection. J Virol Methods. 1991;35:273-86.
9. **Jurriaans S, Van Gemen B, Weverling GJ, Van Strijp D, Nara P, Coutinho R, et al.** The natural history of HIV-1 infection: virus load and virus phenotype independent determinants of clinical course? Virology. 1994;204:223-33.
10. **Henrard DR, Philips JF, Muenz LR, Blattner WA, Wiesner D, Eyster ME, et al.** Natural history of HIV-1 cell-free viremia. JAMA. 1995;274:554-8.
11. **Mellors JW, Kingsley LA, Rinaldo CR Jr, Todd JA, Hoo BS, Kokka RP, et al.** Quantitation of HIV-1 RNA in plasma predicts outcome after seroconversion. Ann Intern Med. 1995;122:573-9.
12. **O'Brien TR, Blattner WA, Waters D, Eyster E, Hilgartner MW, Cohen AR, et al.** Serum HIV-1 RNA levels and time to development of AIDS in the Multicenter Hemophilia Cohort Study. JAMA. 1996;276:105-10.
13. **Mellors JW, Rinaldo CR Jr, Gupta P, White RM, Todd JA, Kingsley LA.** Prognosis in HIV-1 infection predicted by the quantity of virus in plasma. Science. 1996;272:1167-70.
14. **Kaslow RA, Ostrow DG, Detels R, Phair JP, Polk BF, Rinaldo CR Jr.** The Multicenter AIDS Cohort Study: rationale, organization, and selected characteristics of the participants. Am J Epidemiol. 1987;126:310-8.
15. **Todd J, Pachl C, White R, Yeghiazarian T, Johnson P, Taylor B, et al.** Performance characteristics for the quantitation of plasma HIV-1 RNA using branched DNA signal amplification technology. J Acquir Immune Defic Syndr Hum Retrovirol. 1995;10(Suppl 2):S35-44.
16. **Giorgi JV, Cheng HL, Margolick JB, Bauer KD, Ferbas J, Waxdal M, et al.** Quality control in the flow cytometric measurement of T-lymphocyte subsets: The Multicenter AIDS Cohort Study Experience. Clin Immunol Immunopathol. 1990;55:173-86.
17. **Chambers JM, Cleveland WS, Kleiner B, Tukey PA.** Graphical Methods for Data Analysis. Belmont, CA: Wadsworth; 1983:48-57.
18. **Kalbfleisch JD, Prentice RL.** The Statistical Analysis of Failure Time Data. New York: Wiley; 1980:10-9, 87-9.
19. **Phair J, Muñoz A, Detels R, Kaslow R, Rinaldo C, Saah A.** The risk of *Pneumocystis carinii* pneumonia among men infected with human immunodeficiency virus type 1. Multicenter AIDS Cohort Study Group. N Engl J Med. 1990;322:161-5.
20. **Ciampi A, Lawless JF, McKinney SM, Singhal K.** Regression and recursive partition strategies in the analysis of survival data. J Clin Epidemiol. 1988;41:737-48.
21. **Efron B, Tibshirani R.** An Introduction to the Bootstrap. New York: Chapman and Hall; 1993:170-4.
22. **Diggle PJ, Liang KY, Zeger SL.** Analysis of Longitudinal Data. Oxford: Oxford Univ Pr; 1994:79-90, 133-5.
23. **Pezzotti P, Phillips AN, Dorrucci M, Cozzi Lepri A, Galai N, Vlahov D, et al.** Category of exposure to HIV and age in the progression to AIDS: longitudinal study of 1199 people with known dates of seroconversion. HIV Italian Seroconversion Study Group. Br Med J. 1996;313:583-6.
24. **Ho DD, Neumann AU, Perelson AS, Chen W, Leonard JM, Markowitz M.** Rapid turnover of plasma virions and CD4 lymphocytes in HIV-1 infection. Nature. 1995;373:123-6.
25. **Wei X, Ghosh SK, Taylor ME, Johnson VA, Emini EA, Deutsch P, et al.** Viral dynamics in human immunodeficiency virus type 1 infection. Nature. 1995;373:117-26.
26. **Perelson AS, Neumann AU, Markowitz M, Leonard JM, Ho DD.** HIV-1 dynamics in vivo: virion clearance rate, infected cell life-span, and viral generation time. Science. 1996;271:1582-6.
27. **Holodniy M, Mole L, Yen-Lieberman B, Margolis D, Starkey C, Carroll R, et al.** Comparative stabilities of quantitative human immunodeficiency virus RNA in plasma from samples collected in VACUTAINER CPT, VACUTAINER PPT, and standard VACUTAINER tubes. J Clin Microbiol. 1995;33:1562-6.

Vex not his ghost; O, let him pass!
He hates him
That would upon the rack of this tough world
Stretch him out longer.

William Shakespeare
King Lear

Submitted by:
Karen J. Fahey
Rogue Medical Group
Grants Pass, OR 97526

Submissions from readers are welcomed. If the quotation is published, the sender's name will be acknowledged. Please include a complete citation, as done for any reference.—*The Editor*

Section VIII

Nephrology

The effects of shock on the kidney.

Van Slyke DD. Ann Intern Med. 1948;28:701-722.

Several of the major advances in our current understanding of medicine relate to the major principles in physiology that evolved in the first half of the past century. William Harvey (1578–1657), who described, quantified, and demonstrated the functional significance of the heart and circulation in 1628, is considered a founder of the new physiologic approach to medicine. However, the role of the circulation in the function of other organs was not elucidated until the turn of the 20th century, when Ernest Starling (1866–1927) reported his studies on microvascular permeability and fluid distribution between the blood and tissues, in which he identified the central role of the kidney in maintaining fluid balance and homeostasis. The physiologist Walter B. Cannon (1871–1945) studied the challenges of maintaining homeostasis after trauma, a major issue for soldiers in World War I; he published his studies in 1923 under the title *Traumatic Shock* and went on to popularize the concept of homeostatsis in *The Wisdom of the Body* (1932). Thereafter, the study of kidney function in acutely altered hemodynamic states attracted increasing attention, and the clinical course and pathology of acute loss of kidney function in varied conditions was described under disparate names (such as "renal inadequacy," "necrotizing nephrosis," "acute uremia," and "traumatic nephritis") in the publications of disciplines ranging from medicine to surgery, pathology, and gastroenterology. Interest in kidney function after trauma was rekindled in 1941, when crush victims during the London bombings were reported to develop impaired renal function. Reports of similar cases from the battlefields of World War II prompted a concerted effort to study the functional and structural changes of the kidney after trauma, and their treatment.

Donald W. Van Slyke's prescient article is an eloquent summary of those studies. The introduction of the term "acute renal failure" shortly thereafter by Homer Smith (1895–1992) in 1951 served as a unifying banner around which all subsequent reports of the entity would rally. Van Slyke (1883–1971) was a chemist who had undertaken the study of kidney physiology in the 1930s. The first part of his article is a clinical description of the entity. Anticipating future developments, Van Slyke emphasizes the reversible nature of kidney function in the first phase of shock and refers to this state as "injury" rather than "necrosis." As he may have foreseen, the term "acute tubular necrosis" that was introduced in the 1950s has been shown to be a misnomer, and a major move is now under way to replace it with the term "acute kidney injury." The second part summarizes the experimental studies that provide the physiologic basis of the clinical description of the entity and its treatment. Van Slyke's article is a perfect example of translational research that was being performed long before the concept was introduced.

The nephrotic syndrome in adults: a common disorder with many causes.

Kark RM, Pirani CL, Pollack VE, Muehrcke C, Blainey JD. Ann Intern Med. 1958;49:751-774.

The nephrotic syndrome as a well-defined clinical entity is barely a century old, but its roots lie deep in antiquity at the very origins of medical observations. As an illness with external manifestations, swelling of the body was long recognized as a disease that came to be termed "hydrops," "hydropsy," and ultimately "dropsy." The association of frothy urine with kidney disease and dropsy, and of certain dropsies with diseases of the "flanks and loins," has been traced to Hippocrates (ca. 460-370 BCE) and with "hardened kidneys" to Rufus of Ephesus (ca. 1st to 2nd century CE). In fact, much of the reference to kidney disease in the medical literature throughout the 19th century relates it to what was known then as "dropsy." The differentiation between dropsy due to kidney disease and dropsy from other causes began with the medical case reports of Richard Bright (1789-1858), who showed that some of his dropsical patients with albumin in the urine had striking changes in their kidneys at autopsy. The decades that followed described the varied clinical manifestations and abnormalities of patients with Bright's disease, not all of whom died. Nevertheless, examination of the kidney remained limited to the fatal cases that came to autopsy.

Beginning in 1950, Robert M. Kark (1911–2002) and colleagues pioneered kidney biopsy and launched the systematic study of the renal tissue obtained under the microscope. Kark and colleagues' 1958 article joins two technological advances that were instrumental in the clarification of Bright's disease and the emergence of nephrology as a discipline: the microscope, introduced in the 1840s, and the kidney biopsy, introduced in the 1930s. Bright had described the gross appearance of three forms of the diseased kidneys, one of which he characterized as large, swollen, and yellowish in appearance. Subsequent microscopic examination of such cases revealed "degeneration" of the tubules without marked glomerular changes in the absence of the inflammatory changes of "nephritis" that were termed "nephroses" in 1905. As chemical analyses and protein fractionation became available in the 1920s, the clinical and laboratory features of these cases came to be identified as edema, albuminuria, hypoalbuminemia, hyperlipidemia, and fatty casts in the urine. The frequent coincidence of these four features led to the term "nephrotic syndrome," and the term for its pathologic characteristics became "lipoid nephrosis." These two entities were considered one disease well into the 1950s. From the outset, however, dissonant voices argued that the nephrotic syndrome was a phase of glomerulonephritis; a test of that concept had to await antemortem kidney biopsy in nephrotic patients.

Kark and colleagues' article in *Annals of Internal Medicine* summarizes their experience and clearly establishes the multiple causes of the nephrotic syndrome. Technical advances and refinements in the microscopic examination of kidney biopsy samples and subsequent experimental studies have established that the nephrotic syndrome arises from increased permeability of the glomerular capillary ultrafiltration barrier in various forms of glomerular diseases, independent of the gross appearance of the kidneys.

A more accurate method to estimate glomerular filtration rate from serum creatinine: a new prediction equation.

Levey AS, Bosch JP, Lewis JB, Greene T, Rogers N, Roth D, for the Modification of Diet in Renal Disease Study Group. Ann Intern Med. 1999;130:461-470.

Progress in medicine can be traced to changes in the focus of research (1). One such change occurred with the gradual shift from structural to physiologic studies that began at the end of the 19th century and peaked in the first half of the 20th century. Such physiologists as Homer W. Smith (1895–1962), A. Newton Richards (1895–1962), and James A. Shannon (1904–1994) used intact animal and micropuncture studies to establish the excretory functions of the kidney and introduce the mathematical concept of clearance, which led to use of the glomerular filtration rate (GFR) as the best measure of kidney function in health and disease. The GFR cannot be measured directly; it must be calculated and is at best an estimate. The quest for a metabolically inert substance that is filtered at the glomerulus and neither absorbed nor secreted downstream in the tubules led to identification of inulin as the ideal substance to determine GFR. However, inulin clearance requires intravenous infusion and several timed urine collections, which made it inconvenient to measure in the clinical setting and impossible to use for large-scale population studies of renal disease. Alternative methods for measuring GFR used various radioactive substances, such as iothalamate, and remained cumbersome and costly. Use of exogenous creatinine clearance as an alternative to inulin for calculating GFR in dogs provided the basis for the subsequent use of endogenous creatinine in man as a measure of kidney function, and the 24-hour creatinine clearance emerged as the most widely used measure of GFR in clinical practice. Difficulties in obtaining an accurate collection of urine for 24 hours led to the introduction of prediction formulas to estimate GFR from the serum creatinine concentration.

The Modification of Diet in Renal Disease (MDRD) Study was a randomized, controlled clinical trial designed to evaluate the effect of dietary protein restriction and strict blood pressure control on the progression of chronic kidney disease (CKD). The study incorporated several measures of kidney function, including iothalamate clearance as a measure of GFR. Levey and colleagues reported on the refined prediction equation developed by applying multivariate statistical techniques to find the best clinical predictions of the baseline measurements of GFR in the MDRD Study. Com-pared with other prediction equations, the proposed MDRD formula estimates GFR more accurately than does the 24-hour creatinine clearance or other formulas. Other studies have validated the applicability of the MDRD formula, but the methods to assure standardization of creatinine measurement in all clinical laboratories vary, an issue that is now being addressed at the international level. In addition, the validity of the equation when the GFR is greater than 60 mL/min/1.73 m^{2fv} remains to be established.

These limitations notwithstanding, data derived from population studies using the MDRD equation for estimated GFR led to an established classification and stratification of CKD, whose application worldwide has documented the epidemic prevalence of CKD, and the identification of CKD as a multiplier of the risk of other co-existent chronic diseases, such as diabetes, hypertension, and cardiovascular disease.

ANNALS OF INTERNAL MEDICINE

VOLUME 28 APRIL, 1948 NUMBER 4

THE EFFECTS OF SHOCK ON THE KIDNEY *

By DONALD D. VAN SLYKE, *New York, N. Y.*

THE type of "shock" here discussed is the condition, caused by hemorrhage, burns, trauma, dehydration, or other injury, in which there is an inadequate volume of blood to fill the vascular bed. The visible effects in man, prostration, cold perspiration, bloodless or cyanotic skin, etc., are familiar. It appears that similar renal effects can result from a period of peripheral circulatory failure due, not to decreased blood volume, but to cardiac failure, or to pooling of blood in part of the vascular bed; but the present discussion is limited to conditions of shock in which decreased volume of the circulating blood, resulting from loss of blood or plasma or from dehydration, is the primary cause.

The immediate and later effects of shock on the kidney, indicated by available data, will first be outlined. Experiments illustrating these effects will then be presented.

The First, or Ischemic, Phase of Shock Kidney. The immediate effects of shock on the kidney are circulatory. Renal blood flow is diminished, and with it renal excretory function.[1, 2, 3] The decrease may be so great that complete anuria results. However, if the renal ischemia is not too complete and prolonged, the kidney cells are not injured, and restoration of normal general circulation is followed by recovery of normal renal function within a short time. A lag period of an hour or more may intervene, due perhaps to continued constriction of renal vessels, after the general circulation is restored before renal function recovers, but then normal excretion is resumed.

The initial shutdown of the renal circulation appears to be part of a defense reaction of the organism to loss of circulating blood volume; the vascular bed is contracted by peripheral constriction so that the diminished volume of available blood will be adequate to supply the vital organs, such as the brain, whose function must be maintained to avoid immediate death. If

* From an address given at the Twenty-Eighth Annual Session of the American College of Physicians, Chicago, April 30, 1947.

From The Hospital of The Rockefeller Institute for Medical Research, New York 19, New York.

blood loss is severe, the kidneys are included in the constricted periphery; the necessity for this inclusion is obvious from the fact that the kidneys in the resting subject normally receive about 20 per cent of the blood.

Fall in blood pressure below 40 to 60 mm. systolic is in itself sufficient to cause anuria because the pressure is insufficient to maintain glomerular filtration.* In shock, however, failure of renal function often occurs before blood pressure falls to such levels (see figure 5, this paper). It appears that renal failure during shock usually owes its onset to renal vasoconstriction,† and that, even in cases where the blood pressure falls below 60 mm., constriction of the renal vessels occurs before the falling blood pressure reaches this level.

With regard to the solicitude with which their blood supply is maintained in time of deficit, the kidneys appear to stand intermediate between the skin and skeletal muscles,[5] which can survive long periods of ischemia, and the central nervous system, which can survive almost none. If the deficit of circulating blood volume is sufficiently severe and prolonged, the kidneys are sacrificed in the apparent attempt to maintain circulation through heart, lungs, and brain.

The Second, or Renal Damage, Phase of Shock Kidney. If shock is severe and prolonged, restoration of the general circulation and recovery from the circulatory symptoms of the shock may not be accompanied by resumption of normal renal excretion. Anuria or oliguria may persist, or urine of low specific gravity may be excreted; urea clearance is low. This period of complete or partial renal failure may last until fatal uremia develops in a period that may vary from two to 20 days.[6] Or gradual return of function may occur, so that within the days of grace allowed, excretion

* Literature on the relation between arterial blood pressure and glomerular filtration is reviewed by Lassen and Husfeldt (Jr. Clin. Invest., 1934, xiii, 263) together with observations on subjects in whom blood pressure was lowered by spinal anesthesia.

† Trueta[4] and his collaborators offer a different explanation for renal failure during acute shock. They have demonstrated, in a series of brilliant experiments with rabbits, that application of a tourniquet for a number of hours to the left hind leg of a rabbit caused a withdrawal of blood from the *left* renal cortex, while the total blood flow through the kidney was increased, as evidenced by the observations, that time required for blood to traverse the kidney was halved, that the blood issuing from the renal vein changed partially or wholly to arterial red color, and that the renal vein was swollen and showed pulsation of arterial type. These, and other data, indicated that the condition was caused by dilation of vascular channels through the medulla, causing the renal blood to rush through them, and to by-pass completely its channels through the cortex. It was suggested that this phenomenon, of apparently neurogenic origin, might, "by preventing blood from reaching the filter of the kidney in the cortex" cause the cessation of renal function "in hemorrhage or conditions with decreased blood volume." However, measurements by other investigators of renal blood flow during acute hemorrhagic and traumatic shock (for example see figure 5 of this paper) show that the total renal blood flow is not accelerated, as in the condition studied by Trueta, but is greatly diminished, and that in severe shock the renal blood flow approaches zero. Also the fact, illustrated in figure 1, that during acute hemorrhagic or traumatic shock, sufficiently severe to lower renal blood flow to a small fraction of normal, the kidneys continue to extract 85 to 90 per cent of para-amino hippurate from the plasma indicates that such blood as continued to perfuse the kidneys was supplying nephrons of normal excretory capacity. The phenomena observed by Trueta and his collaborators appear to be quite different from those that accompany shock from hemorrhage, dehydration, or trauma other than pressure on the legs.

becomes sufficiently restored to prevent uremia, and ultimate recovery of the kidneys may be complete.

Whereas, in its initial phase during acute shock, renal failure is a quickly reversible functional affair, renal failure persisting after recovery from shock is attributable to organic injury, and is reversible slowly and sometimes not at all. There is no sharp dividing line between the two phases: the purely functional failure due to lack of renal circulation passes during prolonged shock gradually into a condition of increasing organic damage.

Of anuria observed during acute shock the interpretation is different from that of anuria or depressed renal function persisting after recovery from shock. Anuria during shock indicates that the kidneys are subject to ischemia, which in a few hours in man may cause irreversible injury. After recovery from shock, persisting anuria or depressed function indicates that organic damage has occurred, but not necessarily that it is progressing. There is at least a partial resumption of renal blood flow, and repair of the damage may proceed, so that even several days of post-shock renal depression may be followed by recovery. In some cases, it is true, renal function partially recovered after shock may fail again, indicating progress of the lesion.

The Degree of Shock That Is Followed by Uremia. Uremia can develop from shock only when the latter is within a certain limited zone of severity and duration. The shock must be severe and prolonged in order to cause irreversible damage to the kidneys. But if it is too severe it causes death, usually from circulatory failure, before the patient has time to develop uremia. Presumably because the zone is narrow, renal failure is a cause of death in only a small percentage of the cases that survive shock. But the inability to stop the progress of uremia in such cases was a cause of major concern to surgeons in the late war. Thus, a letter from Dr. E. D. Churchill stated: "By excellent forward surgery and the liberal use of whole blood transfusion as well as plasma we are saving lives, but also keeping certain men alive temporarily only to display later kidney damage. There has been either complete anuria with death, or in one case a fall of urinary output to 200 c.c. with ultimate recovery of kidney function. This phenomenon is not unique to the 'crush syndrome,' but may occur in any wounded man who experiences a long period of greatly reduced volume flow."

Renal Lesions Caused by Shock. Lucké[6] has examined kidneys from 538 army cases showing what he terms "lower nephron nephrosis." Although the original injuries were various, the histological kidney pictures were all similar: glomeruli and proximal tubules practically undamaged, distal convoluted tubules and thick tubules of Henle degenerated or showing actual necrosis. Of the 538 cases 403 were from subjects who had suffered the type of injury that produces shock, viz. battle wounds, crushing injuries, abdominal operations, burns, heat stroke (dehydration), while 67 were from cases of poisoning (sulfonamides, arsenicals, carbon tetrachloride, etc.).

Mallory[7] has studied the lesions in some 260 cases of battle injury, and is able to draw conclusions concerning the time of appearance of the successive stages of the lesions: (1) Within 24 hours after injury, lipid vacuolization of the ascending limb of the loop of Henle; (2) twenty-four to 72 hours after injury precipitation of myoglobin or hemoglobin in the distal convoluted and collecting tubules; (3) sometimes on the third day, regularly on the fourth and fifth, necrosis and regeneration of epithelium in the ascending limbs and distal tubules. "Renal insufficiency was found to antedate all structural changes, but was never progressive in the absence of a definite pigment nephropathy." Mallory's observation, that visible lesions do not appear until a day or more after the original injury, indicates that the lesions are after-effects of damage, not histologically demonstrable, suffered by the tubular cells during shock. Mallory did not find the tubular lesions caused by temporary clamping of the renal artery in animals identical with those observed in human cases of post-shock renal damage, but Badenoch and Darmady[8] found that the lesions produced in rabbits by such clamping resembled those observed in human cases.

The Cause of Organic Renal Damage. The renal ischemia that has been found to occur during severe shock[1, 2, 3] appears to be the inciting cause of the changes that lead to the development of organic damage.[1, 6] When approximately complete renal ischemia is produced in dogs by clamping the renal artery for two hours transitory partial renal failure results (figure 6), and such ischemia continued for three to four hours is followed by death in uremia[1] (figure 7). The duration of ischemia required to produce these effects is of the order of that required by severe shock to cause similar effects in man. The view that the primary cause of renal injury is probably ischemia suffered by the kidneys during shock has been adopted as the result of clinical observation by Darmady et al.[9] and Maegraith.[10]

Corcoran and Page[11] and Mallory[7] consider that deposits of hemoglobin products, forming in damaged tubules after the first to third day following injury,[7] contribute to further progress of the tubular lesions that have been initiated by ischemia. That the tubular lesions typical of post-shock uremia can occur in man without the deposits, however, appears from the observation of Lucké,[6] that in some of his cases the deposits were scanty or absent.

Mechanism of Renal Failure Persisting After Recovery from Shock. The similarity of the histological picture in the post-shock kidney to that caused by nephrotoxic poisons leads Lucké[6] to consider that the mechanism of the anuria in both conditions is probably the same. The effects of nephrotoxic poisons had been observed by Richards[12] in the nephrons of frogs poisoned by mercuric chloride and other nephrotoxic substances. Filtration in the glomeruli of these frogs went on with normal rapidity, but *the entire filtrate was reabsorbed from the tubules,* so that no urine entered the bladder. In such a condition the cells of the tubular epithelium lose their normal power of selected reabsorption. By this power the normal kidney tubules return from the glomerular filtrate to the blood the solids whose retention is essential to the organism (glucose, amino acids, salts, etc.), together with the amount of water required to maintain normal hydration, while they bar the way to return of waste products, such as urea, uric acid, creatinine, and superfluous water and electrolytes. In contrast to this selective reabsorption by the normal tubular wall, the tubular walls devitalized by poison in Richards' experiments appeared to approach dead membranes in their behavior, and to permit all the glomerular filtrate, both water and solids, to pass indiscriminately back into the blood of the tubular capillaries, presumably drawn by the osmotic attraction of the plasma proteins for the filtrate water, with anuria as the result.

Lucké's explanation of persistent post-shock renal failure is consistent with the observation (figure 1) that after experimental renal ischemia continued for two hours the tubules of dogs' kidneys lose most or all of their ability to extract para-amino hippurate from the renal blood plasma, indicating severe injury to tubular function. Another functional evidence of tubular injury is the commonly observed fact, that the kidney damaged by shock loses much or all of its ability to concentrate the glomerular filtrate. It appears that renal ischemia, such as occurs in man during shock, may be one of many nephrotoxic factors that produce "lower nephron nephrosis," with renal failure from tubular reabsorption.

Reabsorption must be considered as a tentative, rather than a demonstrated, explanation of post-shock renal failure, because total tubular reabsorption, such as was observed by Richards in the tubules of poisoned frogs, has not been demonstrated by such direct observation in the post-shock kidney. But the weight of evidence in favor of tubular reabsorption appears to be strong.

Some investigators have considered that post-shock uremia might be due to mechanical blockage of the tubular lumina by detritus staining like hemoglobin or a heme derivative. This explanation is rejected by Lucké[6] because of frequent absence of upper tubular and capsular dilatation that would result from such obstruction, and because in many cases he found heme casts scanty or absent. Also the fact that in shock oliguria the urine gravity is low, despite the small volume, indicates that the renal injury is general, rather than localized to blocked nephrons. Mechanical obstruction as the cause of renal failure is also rejected by Bywaters,[13] although both he and Corcoran and Page[11] and Mallory[7] consider that the detritus forming in damaged tubules may contribute to the progress of the lesions initiated by ischemia.

Historical Resumé. Present concepts concerning the effects of shock on the kidney have developed from the studies of many investigators. The following resumé necessarily omits many of importance.

That the renal failure (first stage of shock kidney) accompanying hemorrhage, dehydration, and other conditions that have in common the peripheral circulatory signs of shock, could be due to decreased renal blood flow, was deduced by Fishberg[14] from the fact that the urea clearance, which falls low in these conditions, had been experimentally observed[15] to parallel physiological changes in renal blood flow. Fishberg suggested that the extraordinary ischemia and vasoconstriction observed in the skin and limbs during shock might be shared by the kidneys.

The accuracy of Fishberg's deduction was confirmed when the Rockefeller Hospital group [1, 3] measured the renal blood flow in hemorrhagic and traumatic shock (figure 5), and found it depressed in proportion to the severity of the shock. Lauson, Bradley, and Cournand [2] at the same time observed in human subjects in shock similar depression of the para-amino hippurate clearance, which has been found (figure 2) to parallel the renal blood flow in shock, provided the shock has not lasted long enough to cause organic renal damage.

That renal function can remain depressed after recovery from shock ("second stage" of shock kidney), so that death in uremia occurs some days later, was observed by Rogers [16] over 30 years ago, in his classic studies of cholera, where shock is caused by dehydration. That similar uremia can occur after recovery from shock caused by trauma was noted by Bywaters [13] in his description of the "crush syndrome" early in World War II. It is probably due to Bywaters' description of the crush syndrome that post-shock uremia was soon recognized as a not infrequent after-effect of severe battle injuries.

The facts, (1) that renal ischemia occurs during shock,[1, 2, 3] (2) that renal ischemia caused by temporary occlusion of renal arteries in animals is followed by renal failure, either transitory or fatal depending on the duration of the ischemia,[1, 17, 18, 19, 20] and (3) that similar periods of severe shock in man are followed by similar transitory or fatal renal failure, were presented by Van Slyke, Phillips, and their collaborators [1] as support for the hypothesis that renal failure persisting after shock is due to organic injury initiated during shock by ischemia.

Histological studies of Bywaters and his colleagues,[13] Lucké,[6] Mallory [7] and others have revealed severe damage to the renal tubules, chiefly the distal tubule and loop of Henle, with little or no glomerular damage, as a constant finding in post-shock uremia. Observations by Mallory [7] and by Corcoran and Page [11] indicate that debris of heme derivatives, forming in the tubules one or more days after onset of renal failure,[7] may contribute to progress of tubular damage initiated by ischemia.

The identity of the tubular lesions with those caused by various nephrotoxic agents led Lucké to suggest that the cause of post-shock uremia may be, not failure of filtration in the glomeruli, but the same indiscriminate tubular reabsorption of glomerular filtrate and its excretory constituents that was noted by Richards [12] in the kidneys of frogs made anuric by nephrotoxic poisons. The probable validity of Lucké's explanation is supported by functional evidence of tubular damage, viz. the commonly observed inability of the kidneys in post-shock renal failure to excrete concentrated urine, and their decreased ability to extract para-amino hippurate from the renal blood.[19]

A series of renal circulatory phenomena, of quite different nature from those summarized above, but also leading to renal failure, has been recently described by Trueta and his collaborators [4] in animals following periods of pressure on the legs, and due apparently to pressure on the nerves. The renal blood flow is accelerated rather than retarded, but the blood courses through dilated medullary vessels and by-passes the renal cortex and its glomeruli. It appears that this phenomenon may account for some cases of renal failure in the "crush syndrome," but not for the renal effects of shock caused by hemorrhage, dehydration, circulatory failure, or trauma other than that of pressure on the limbs.

Experiments Illustrating Effects of Shock and Renal Ischemia on the Kidneys

Following are examples of experimental observations from our laboratory illustrating the immediate and later effects of shock and renal ischemia. The examples are taken from experiments carried out during the war by Drs. Phillips, Dole, Hamilton, Hiller, Emerson, and Archibald,[1, 3, 19, 20] with support of the Committee of Medical Research of the Office of Scientific Research and Development, in the United States Naval Research Unit of the Hospital of The Rockefeller Institute.

The Immediate Effects of Hemorrhage and Traumatic Shock, and the After Effects of Renal Ischemia, on Tubular Function Measured by the Completeness with Which the Kidneys Extract Para-amino Hippurate from the Blood Plasma. While all evidence is to the effect that (in the kidneys of man and the dog) the normal excretory products, such as urea, creatinine, salts, etc., are removed from the renal blood by filtration of about 20 to 30 per cent of the plasma water and its crystalloid solutes in the glomeruli,[21] certain foreign substances when injected into the blood stream evoke the additional aid of excretion by the tubules to obtain a more rapid clearance of these substances from the blood. Such substances are phenol red, diodrast, and para-amino hippurate. Of the para-amino hippurate [8] entering the kidneys in the plasma of the renal artery, an average of about 87 per cent is removed by the kidneys of the normal dog * and of man.[22] Since only about 20 per cent is normally filtered in the glomeruli,[21] it is evident that the greater part must be excreted by the tubules.

Figure 1 shows that in acute hemorrhagic or traumatic shock the kidneys continued to extract the PAH with this same degree of completeness, until the shock was so severe that the renal blood flow was decreased below 5 per cent of normal, an effect that was reached in these experiments only after shock was maintained during several hours by repeated hemorrhage or trauma. Until this extreme stage was reached the tubular cells retained their vitality and continued to excrete 85 to 90 per cent of the PAH from the plasma that perfused the kidney.

When, without hemorrhage or shock, the kidneys were submitted to two hours of ischemia [1, 20] by clamping of the renal arteries, subsequent restoration of the renal blood flow was followed by a period during which only

* Para-amino hippurate will be designated by the symbol PAH.

10 to 20 per cent of the hippurate was extracted from the plasma (see solid circles, figure 1). If the clamp was left on for as long as four hours, anuria followed, with death in uremia four to eight days later,[1, 20] as in human cases that fail to recover renal function after prolonged shock.

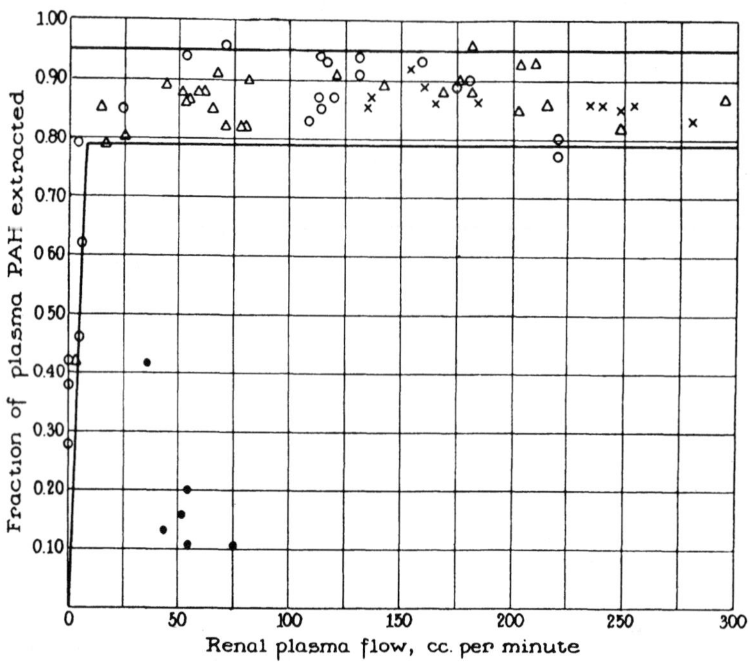

FIG. 1. Percentages of para-amino hippurate extracted from the plasma of the renal blood by the kidneys of dogs, in which the renal blood flow was either normal or diminished by conditions indicated by symbols as follows:

× Normal dogs.

△ Dogs immediately after loss of varying amounts of blood.

○ Dogs during traumatic shock of varying degrees.

● Dogs immediately after clamping the renal artery for two hours and then removing the clamp.

In each dog one kidney had previously been removed, and the observations were made on the functions of the remaining kidney. Renal plasma flows are not estimated from clearances, but are measured values calculated as (PAH excreted per minute)/(PAH extracted from 1 c.c. of renal plasma).

The results show that hemorrhagic or traumatic shock did not decrease the completeness with which the kidneys extracted PAH from the renal plasma until shock became so severe that the renal plasma (and blood) flow fell below 5 per cent of normal.

After temporary renal ischemia caused by clamping the renal artery for two hours, although removal of the clamp was at once followed by restoration of blood flow to about 50 per cent of pre-operative, the PAH extraction was only 10 to 20 per cent, about as much as would be filtered in the glomeruli, indicating that the tubules had nearly or quite ceased extracting PAH from the renal plasma. (Reprinted by permission from the American Journal of Physiology.)

The completeness of PAH extraction in the acute first phase of hemorrhagic shock (upper part of figure 1) can be explained by assuming that when the renal blood flow is decreased by hemorrhage or trauma the flow is completely shut off from part of the nephrons, while those that continue to be perfused continue to function in a normal way.

This assumption also could explain the observation[23] that during this phase of shock there is no significant decrease in the oxygen saturation of the renal venous blood. In contrast, in the body as a whole when the circulation rate is decreased the tissues compensate for the retarded blood flow by extracting a larger part of the oxygen from the blood, so that the venous blood, from the right heart, becomes dark and shows an increased degree of oxygen unsaturation.[23] In the kidneys, on the contrary, the blood flow can be reduced by hemorrhagic or traumatic shock without causing the renal venous blood to lose its normal, nearly arterial degree of redness or lower its oxygen content.[23] This also would be explainable if the diminished volume of renal blood passes through a proportionally diminished area of renal tissue at a normal rate, the rest of the kidney receiving relatively little blood.

After the kidney has suffered prolonged ischemia and reached the second phase of shock kidney, where restoration of the general circulation does not restore normal renal function, the incompleteness with which hippurate is extracted (points marked ● in figure 1) indicates decreased efficiency of the tubule. A possible explanation of this phase is that suggested by Trueta,[4]

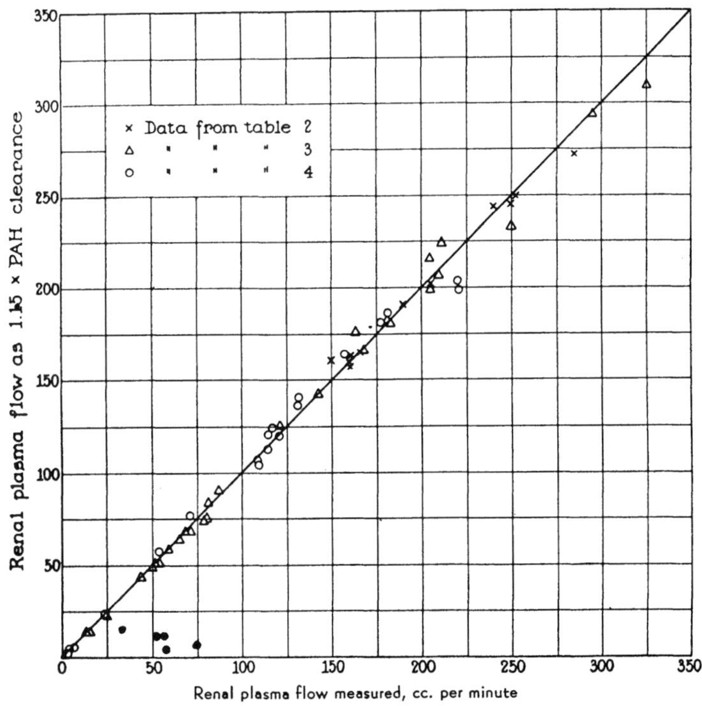

Fig. 2. Relation of renal plasma flows estimated as 1.15 times PAH plasma clearance to actual renal plasma flows measured as (PAH excreted per minute)/(PAH extracted from 1 c.c. of renal plasma). Symbols same as in figure 1.

The results show that in acute hemorrhagic or traumatic shock the PAH clearance serves as a measure of the renal blood flow, but that after the kidneys are injured by ischemia from 2 hour clamping of the renal artery the PAH clearance does not serve as a measure of the renal blood flow. (Reprinted by permission from the American Journal of Physiology.)

that the renal blood flow is diverted from the cortex to the medulla, where the nephrons apparently function less efficiently. But the explanation that seems at present more probable is that, as believed by Lucké, the tubular cells of the nephrons are damaged by the ischemia.

The data of figure 1, in addition to their significance concerning the effect of shock on the kidney, indicate that during the acute first phase of shock kidney, the plasma clearance of para-amino hippurate serves as a measure of the volume of blood plasma that perfuses the kidneys per minute. (The PAH clearance is the volume of plasma, the PAH content of which is excreted per minute. It is calculated as (PAH excreted per minute)/(PAH in 1 c.c. of arterial plasma).) If extraction of PAH were 100 per cent complete, the PAH clearance would exactly equal the renal plasma flow. When the extraction is 87 per cent complete, the renal plasma flow is the clearance multiplied by 1/0.87, or 1.15.

When, however, the kidneys have suffered a period of ischemia so severe and prolonged that the tubules are damaged (second phase of shock kidney) the PAH plasma clearance no longer serves as a measure of renal plasma flow. The close relation of PAH clearance to renal plasma flow in the first

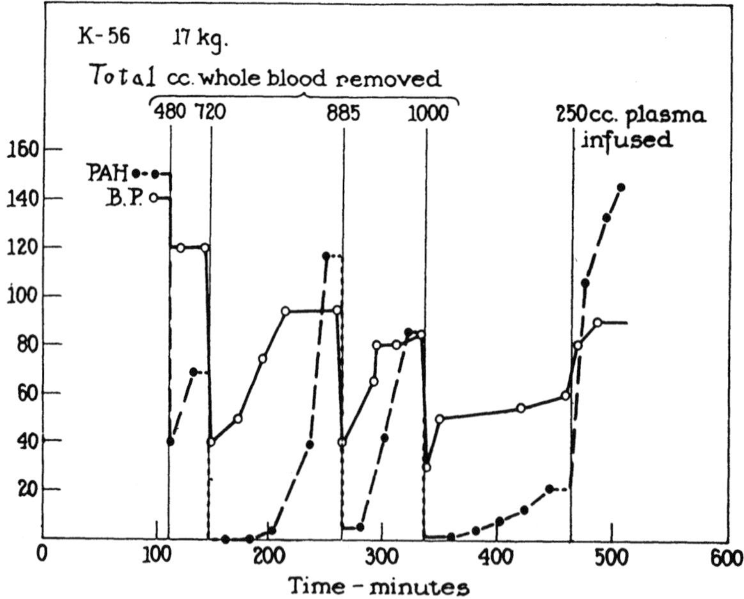

Fig. 3. Reversible shock. The effects of four successive hemorrhages on the blood pressure and the para-amino hippurate plasma clearance (PAH curve). Under the conditions of this experiment the PAH clearance serves as a measure of the renal plasma flow (figures 1 and 2).

The results show repeated recovery of blood pressure and renal blood flow (PAH curve) after repeated hemorrhages, the recoveries being attributable to shrinkage of the extra-renal vascular bed by peripheral constriction. The effectiveness of the relatively small plasma infusion in restoring general blood pressure and renal blood flow at the end of the experiment appears attributable to the continued maintenance of peripheral constriction. The shock had not become irreversible. (Reprinted by permission from the American Journal of Physiology.)

phase of shock kidney, and the absence of relation in the second phase, are indicated by figure 2.

Acute Hemorrhagic Shock Reversible with Respect to Both Renal Function and Circulation. In figure 3 are shown the effects of four successive quick hemorrhages during three hours on the arterial blood pressure and on the para-amino hippurate clearance of a dog. (Since the condition is acute reversible shock, PAH clearance may be assumed to indicate approximately renal plasma flow.) Each hemorrhage caused an immediate reduction in both blood pressure and hippurate clearance (PAH curve), but after each of the first three bleedings there quickly followed a rise both in arterial blood pressure and in the PAH clearance (renal plasma flow). After a fourth hemorrhage restoration of the PAH clearance was incomplete, but infusion of a volume of plasma equal to only one-fourth of the blood that had been withdrawn restored the clearance to practically normal.

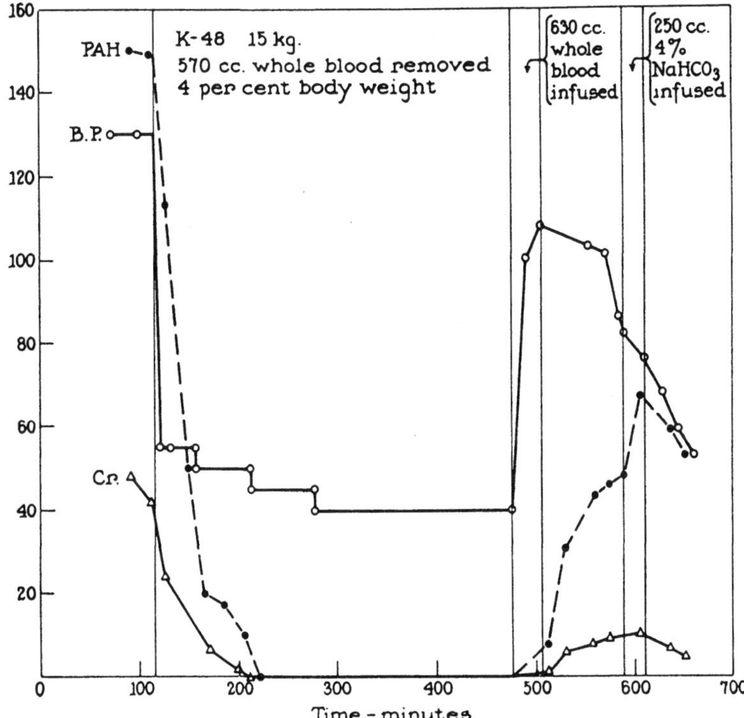

Fig. 4. Acute hemorrhagic shock reversible with respect to renal function but irreversible with respect to general circulation. *PAH* indicates para-amino hippurate clearance, *B. P.* blood pressure, *Cr* creatinine clearance (glomerular filtration rate in c.c. per minute). Although the blood withdrawn was less than in the experiment of figure 3, restoration of even more than the volume of whole blood withdrawn caused in this case only a temporary rise in blood pressure and in renal function. It appears that peripheral constriction had been replaced by dilation before the blood infusion was given. From [3]. The quick transitory rise in PAH and creatinine clearances after the infusion indicates that the kidneys were still capable of functioning.

The apparent explanation of these phenomena is that immediately after a sudden hemorrhage the kidney shares with the peripheral circulation a decrease in blood flow, but that within a period, which may be only a few minutes, constriction of the extra-renal peripheral circulation sets in, blood pressure rises, and the circulation of the kidney is more or less completely restored. Presumably this peripheral constriction is caused by a vasoconstrictor substance shown to be present in the blood during shock [24, 25, 26, 27, 28, 29, 30, 31]; apparently either the vasoconstrictor substance or its precursor is formed in the kidney.

Acute Hemorrhagic Shock Reversible with Respect to Renal Function but Irreversible with Respect to General Circulation. Figure 4 shows an experiment in which successive bleedings followed each other so rapidly that the effects of compensatory peripheral constriction in restoring renal function, seen in figure 1, did not appear. After five hours in severe shock, with mean arterial blood pressure at 40 mm., infusion of a volume of blood equal to that withdrawn caused only temporary rise in blood pressure, followed by a rapid decline. It is apparent that this animal had reached the stage of shock in which peripheral vasoconstriction is replaced by vasodilation [28, 29, 30, 31] and circulatory death can no longer be prevented by transfusions. The fact that during the temporary rise of blood pressure following the transfusion a partial restoration of renal function at once occurred, as shown by the hippurate and creatinine clearances, indicates that the nephrons were not yet too severely damaged to recover.

Analysis of the Effects of Acute Hemorrhagic Shock on Renal Function. In figure 5 are data which permit an analysis of the immediate effects of hemorrhage on different parts of the renal function. Blood was withdrawn from the dog in successive portions as indicated by the curve at the bottom of the figure. The renal plasma flow in c.c. per minute was determined by dividing the amount of para-amino hippurate excreted in the urine per minute by the amount removed from 1 c.c. of plasma during passage of the kidney, as measured by simultaneous analyses of the plasma of arterial and renal venous blood. Creatinine clearances were determined and interpreted as measures of the filtration rate in terms of volume of glomerular filtrate formed per minute, since such interpretation appears valid during the first phase of shock. Dividing the filtration rate by the plasma flow gives the fraction of water in the plasma that is filtered during passage of the glomerulus. This "filtered fraction" is normally about 20 ± 5 per cent of the plasma water.[21]

Renal plasma flow underwent a progressive fall after withdrawal of the first 25 c.c. of blood per kilo. (Total blood volume in the dog is about 90 to 100 c.c. per kilo.) The arterial blood pressure, however, was maintained until the withdrawal exceeded 40 c.c. per kilo; it is evident that during this period peripheral constriction served to keep up the general arterial blood pressure. The fall in renal plasma flow after 25 c.c. of blood per kilo were withdrawn showed that from this point vascular constriction included the kidney as well as peripheral tissues. A compensatory effect in maintaining renal excretory function is seen in the marked increase in the percentage of plasma water filtered in the glomerulus. This rose from 26 per cent to 38 per cent during the first four hours of the experiment. After this period

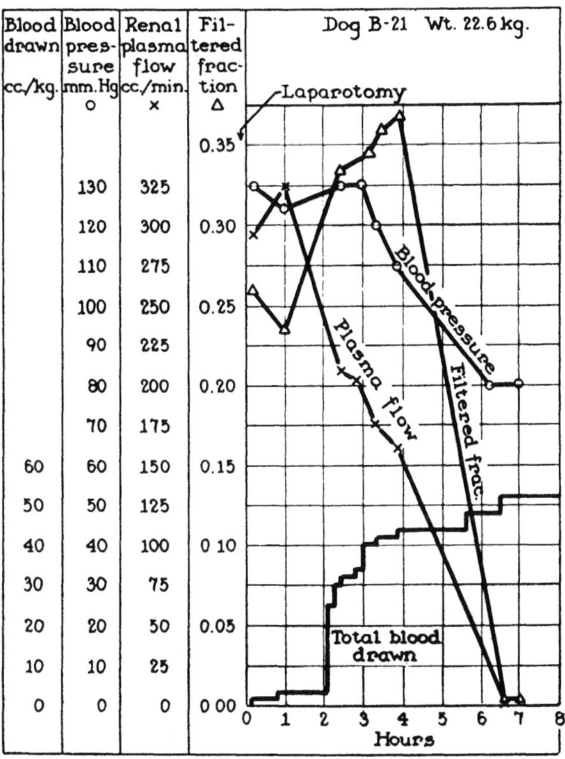

FIG. 5. Effects of gradual blood withdrawal on blood pressure, renal plasma flow, and the fraction of plasma water filtered in the glomeruli. The renal plasma flow fell steadily as amounts of blood over 25 c.c. per kilo were withdrawn, but the effect of the retarded flow on creatinine excretion was for three hours partly compensated by the increase in the filtered fraction of the plasma, presumably achieved by constriction of the efferent renal arterioles. When the volume of blood withdrawn exceeded 48 c.c. per kilo, renal blood flow and renal excretion fell to nearly zero. Since blood pressure in the femoral artery was still 80 mm., it appears that the final shutdown of the kidneys was attributable to constriction of the renal artery or its branches. The renal plasma flows were measured as (PAH excreted per minute)/(PAH extracted·from 1 c.c. of renal plasma). The "PAH extracted from 1 c.c. of renal plasma" was measured directly by analyses of PAH in arterial plasma and in plasma of renal venous blood, the difference being the amount extracted from the plasma by the kidneys. This method of measuring renal plasma flow does not depend on any assumptions concerning the completeness of PAH extraction, or the mechanism by which PAH is excreted. (Reprinted by permission from the American Journal of Physiology.)

there was a rapid fall in both renal plasma flow and in the filtered fraction, so that the excretory function of the kidney fell almost to zero. This debacle of the kidney occurred despite the fact that the general blood pressure (femoral artery) was still maintained at 80 mm.; cessation of renal blood flow and function was therefore apparently due chiefly to constriction of the renal artery or its branches.

The terminal stage of the experiment of figure 5 illustrates the manner in which, when loss of blood volume is sufficiently severe to demand a maximal peripheral constriction in order to maintain blood pressure and blood flow through the heart and brain, the blood flow to the kidney is shut off along with the flow to the skin and skeletal muscles, and the function of the kidney is suppressed.

After-effects of Renal Ischemia Produced by Temporary Clamping of the Renal Artery. The kidneys of the dog have been shown to stand complete occlusion of the renal artery by clamping it for as long as three, and sometimes four, hours without irreversible damage.[20] After ischemia exceeding four hours, however, the damage was practically always irreversible and the animal died later in uremia without return of renal function.[20] In figure 6 is shown the slow recovery of renal function, as measured by the urea clearance, after two hours' clamping of the renal artery. Figure 7 shows the effects of ischemia prolonged for three hours; renal function, although not entirely abolished, did not recover sufficiently to prevent ultimate uremia.

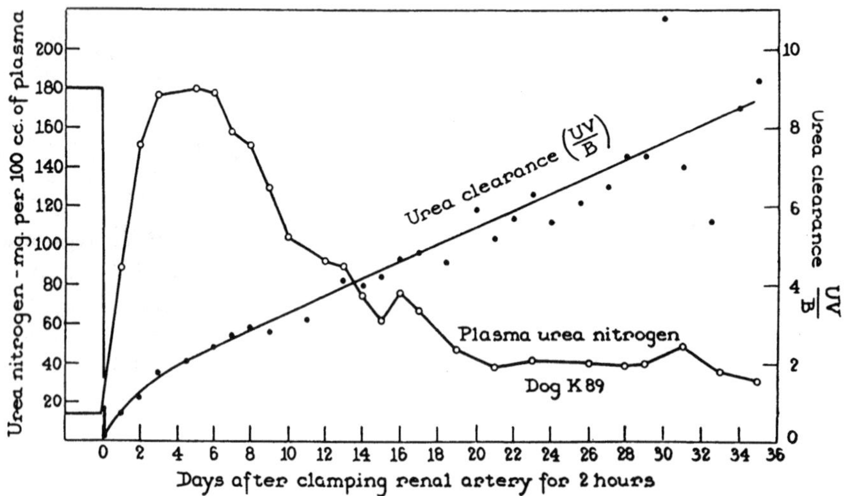

FIG. 6. Slow recovery from the effects of clamping the renal artery of the left kidney of a dog for two hours, the right kidney having previously been excised. After 34 days the plasma urea clearance reached its pre-operative level of 8 to 9 c.c. per minute. It will be noted that during the first four days urea was accumulating in the blood plasma, although the renal function, indicated by the urea clearance, was improving. It was only after the clearance had passed 2 c.c. per minute that the blood urea reached a plateau and then began to fall. (Reprinted by permission from the American Journal of Physiology.)

The renal damage caused by clamping the renal artery was more severe in the dog than the effect of hemorrhage sufficient to reduce the renal blood flow for the same length of time to so slow a rate that it could not be measured by the method employed. It was possible, as shown in figure 3, to depress the renal blood flow to nearly zero by hemorrhage for as long as three hours, and then obtain almost immediate return of function by restoration of the lost blood. It is probable that during the depression caused by hemorrhage some small trickle of blood continued to get through the kidneys, so that the nephrons were not damaged as rapidly as by complete closure of the renal artery. It appears to be more difficult to produce post-shock uremia in the dog than in man. The apparent reason is that in the dog the kidneys, relatively to the circulatory system or other vital organs, are more resistant

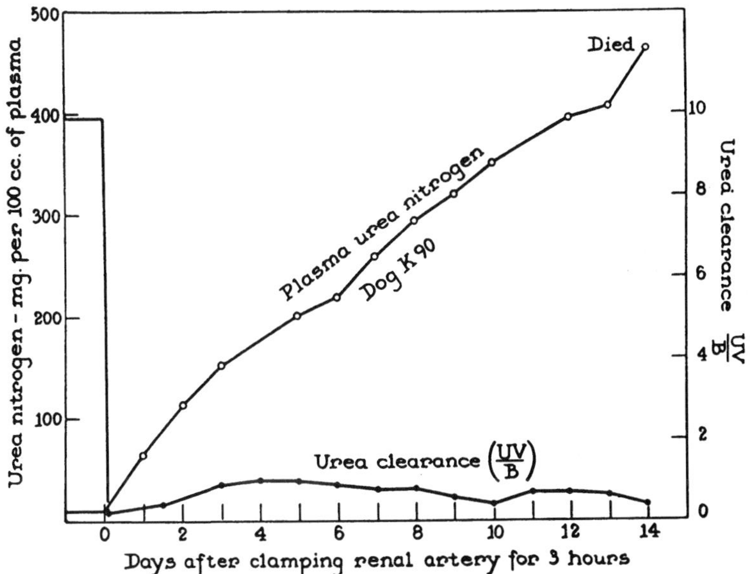

FIG. 7. Irreversible effects of renal ischemia caused by clamping the left renal artery of a dog for three hours, the right kidney having previously been excised. The slight increase in urea clearance observed during the first three days was not maintained, and was afterwards followed by a decrease, with death in uremia 14 days after the clamping. (Reprinted by permission from the American Journal of Physiology.)

than in man. Attempts to employ traumatic or hemorrhagic shock sufficiently severe and prolonged to cause irreversible renal failure in the dog caused acute death from circulatory failure (e.g. figure 4).

TREATMENT DURING SHOCK TO PREVENT RENAL DAMAGE

During acute shock, the renal damage caused by ischemia increases with its duration. Hence *the first move to forestall subsequent uremia is to cut the period of shock as short as possible by restoration of blood volume by rapid infusions, of saline solution in dehydration, or of saline, plasma or whole blood as needed after dehydration, burns, trauma, hemorrhage,* etc.* Restoration of a flow of 1 c.c. of urine per minute containing 2 gm. or more of NaCl per liter serves as one indication of adequate fluid infusion [32, 33] provided the renal damage phase of shock kidney has not been reached.

However, the practice of continuing infusion until a normal flow of urine is reëstablished can not be blindly followed. When the renal damage phase

* However, when signs of shock are due primarily, not to factors causing loss of blood or fluid, but to cardiac failure, fluid infusion is obviously not indicated.

of shock kidney has been reached, anuria or oliguria may continue even after the patient is overhydrated, because the kidneys are incapable of resuming excretion. *Continuance of the infusion can then cause fatal cardiac or pulmonary embarrassment. Overadministration of fluids can be as dangerous as shock.* Criteria other than urine flow must be used, in cases with kidneys already damaged by shock, to indicate when enough fluid has been infused. Onset of pulmonary or subcutaneous edema warns that infusion has been overdone. Observations of the blood composition before and during infusion help to forestall such over-administration. When the cause of shock is dehydration, as in cholera, or loss of plasma, as in burns, blood specific gravity is high, and its return to normal during infusion of saline solution or plasma serves as a criterion of adequate infusion. Use of the blood specific gravity as a criterion was applied in Rogers'[16] classic work on cholera, and in Reimann's[34] modern treatment. The easily handled copper sulfate method[35] for blood and plasma specific gravity, which permits estimating the concentrations of both the plasma protein and the blood hemoglobin in a few minutes, has proved particularly practical in shock treatment.

When acidosis is present (as it is in most forms of severe shock except that caused by loss of gastric juice), the work of Sellards[36] and Rogers[16] with cholera shows that administration of adequate amounts of bicarbonate can diminish the incidence of post-shock uremia.* The presence of severe acidosis appears either to accelerate renal damage during shock, or to retard subsequent repair of the damage. The amounts of bicarbonate required for correction of acidosis, according to the plasma CO_2 and the size of the subject are indicated by the line chart of figure 8.† For alkali therapy during acute shock, sodium bicarbonate is preferable to sodium lactate. The lactate does not act as alkali until the lactate anion is burned, and oxidation is likely to be retarded in shock, so that lactic acid is not oxidized; in fact the acidosis of acute shock appears to be partly due to failure to oxidize the endogenous lactic acid produced by the body. In prolonged post-shock renal failure, acidosis may develop, as in nephritis, from failure to form ammonia and to excrete acid products.

Correction of acidosis, besides its effect in decreasing the incidence of post-shock uremia,[16] appears to have an immediately beneficial effect on renal

* That acidosis also plays a part in the damage, presumably extra-renal, that causes death in acute shock, and that alkali therapy can decrease the mortality is shown by Wiggers and Ingraham.[37]

† The line chart is calculated from data of Palmer and Van Slyke.[38]

Bywaters[13] recommends as first step in treatment of crush injury, giving $NaHCO_3$ 4 gm. per hour, by mouth if the subject is not nauseated, otherwise by vein, until the urine is alkaline, and giving about 30 gm. per day for the next two days to keep the urine alkaline. Such a procedure, based on urinary pH, may be followed when it is not feasible to determine plasma CO_2. However, administering alkali until the urine turns alkaline may lead to over-administration. Darmady[9] found that shock falls within the group of conditions, usually marked by dehydration and salt deficit, in which the urine may fail to turn alkaline when plasma bicarbonate exceeds the normal limits. Experimental studies of this paradoxical concurrence of internal alkalosis and acid urine under conditions of dehydration and salt deficit in dogs and men have recently been published by K. K. Van Slyke and E. I. Evans.[32] Darmady[9] found that determinations of plasma chloride as well as CO_2 were essential in guiding fluid replacement in shock since chloride depletion was frequent.

function. We have seen anuria, persisting after adequate saline infusion, relieved at once when sufficient bicarbonate was infused to relieve the acidosis.

When shock is due to dehydration with loss of body salts, as in diabetes and cholera, and great volumes of saline infusion are required, it

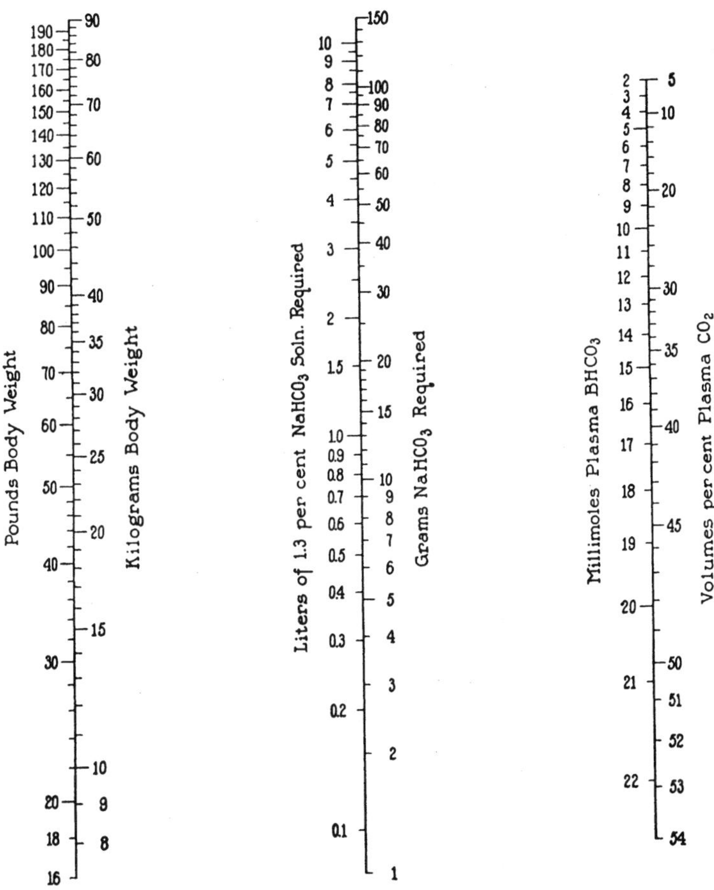

FIG. 8. Line-chart showing amounts of sodium bicarbonate required to overcome acidosis of varying degree. A straight line drawn from the point on the right hand scale indicating the subject's plasma CO_2 or HCO_3 content to the point on the left scale indicating his body weight cuts the middle scale at a point showing the amount of $NaHCO_3$ required to restore the plasma CO_2 to a normal value of 60 volumes per cent or 27 millimoles per liter. The chart is based on the finding of Palmer and Van Slyke [38] that 0.026 gm. of $NaHCO_3$ per kilo body weight is required to raise the plasma CO_2 by 1 volume per cent.

appears safer to include K, Ca, and Mg in the infusions, rather than only NaCl and $NaHCO_3$. One cannot use Ca and $NaHCO_3$ in the same solution, as the slight amount of Na_2CO_3 that is formed, in the equilibria, $H_2CO_3 \leftrightarrows NaHCO \rightleftharpoons Na_2CO_3$, suffices to precipitate $CaCO_3$. Calcium can be infused separately as $CaCl_2$, as was done by Rogers [16] in treating cholera, or as gluconate. That plasma potassium deficit may become sufficient to cause dangerous symptoms in patients treated for diabetic acidosis has been shown by Martin and Werkman.[39] Van Slyke and Evans [32, 33] found marked decrease of plasma potassium also in dogs that were dehydrated by loss of gastric juice, and then rapidly rehydrated by NaCl infusions. Hartmann [40] uses a balanced solution containing, per liter, 6 gm. of NaCl, 4 gm. of sodium lactate, 0.4 gm. of KCl, 0.2 gm. of $MgCl_2 \cdot 6H_2O$, and 0.2 gm. of $CaCl_2 \cdot 2H_2O$. This does not contain enough alkali (lactate) to treat severe acidosis, but appears safer than "physiological" 0.9 per cent NaCl solution, which is really unphysiological, for routine infusion.

Treatment after Shock to Prevent Uremia

When, after recovery from the general effects of shock, anuria persists, or the urine specific gravity remains low in comparison with the volume output and blood urea shows a steady rise, one has to deal with persisting renal damage. The objects of treatment during this stage are (1) to provide optimal conditions for renal recovery, and (2) to minimize the accumulation of excretory products, in order that onset of uremia may be retarded, and that thereby life may be prolonged to give the kidneys as much time as possible to recover. Recovery of renal function may occur after several days of anuria in this stage.

Maintenance of normal plasma bicarbonate and chloride concentrations appears to favor recovery of the kidneys. A high-calorie diet consisting chiefly of fats and carbohydrates, and low in protein,[41] minimizes the formation of nitrogenous products of catabolism, and also the acid products, phosphoric and sulfuric acids. A diet of rice and butter has been found satisfactory.[41] It also provides an intake low in potassium, the accumulation of which in the blood may reach a toxic level in renal failure. The low protein diet is indicated only as long as deficient renal function persists. The depletion of blood and tissue proteins, which frequently accompanies or follows the conditions that produce shock, indicates change to a generous protein diet as soon as renal function is restored.

Kolff [42, 43] has shown that the accumulation of toxic products, either organic or inorganic, during renal failure can be prevented by vividialysis with the "artificial kidney," which was devised by Abel [44] and developed for clinical application by Kolff.[42, 43] Blood from an artery is passed through a long cellophane tube bathed in a solution containing NaCl, $NaHCO_3$, KCl, and glucose, and then returned to a vein. Kolff [41] has seen recovery of normal kidney function in a case that had suffered post-shock anuria for two weeks, during which uremia was prevented by vividiffusion. Experiments by Fine, Frank, and Seligman [45] indicate that similar results may be obtainable by peritoneal irrigation, although the danger of peritonitis appears serious.

Throughout the post-shock period of depressed renal action, it is essential to guard against overhydration, since the ability of the kidneys to excrete salt and water may be limited. Observing blood and plasma protein concentrations by such means as specific gravity measurements[35] assists in detecting overhydration before its unfavorable effects become serious.

Summary

An immediate effect of shock from hemorrhage, trauma, or dehydration is a decrease in renal blood flow and function, which may lead to complete anuria. Compensatory constriction of non-renal peripheral vessels follows, and if the loss of circulating blood volume has not been too severe, renal blood flow and function may be quickly restored.

If shock is sufficiently severe, the kidney is included in the peripheral constriction. Renal constriction and anuria in this phase may continue even when the arterial blood pressure is as high as 100 millimeters.

The above phenomena accompany the first, or circulatory, phase of the shock kidney. If renal ischemia does not continue too long even severe shock does not damage the renal cells, and restoration of renal function quickly follows restoration of the general circulation.

If, however, severe renal ischemia continues for a sufficient number of hours, the second, or renal damage phase, of shock kidney develops. The kidneys are damaged, so that restoration of the general circulation no longer causes rapid restoration of renal function. The most obvious visible damage is located in the cells of the loop of Henle and the distal tubules, and tubular reabsorption of excretory products from the glomerular filtrate appears to be the most probable cause of renal failure in this phase.

If the renal damage is not too severe gradual recovery of the kidneys may occur, so that even after several days of post-shock anuria the renal function may improve sufficiently to prevent uremia, and recovery may eventually become complete. In fatal cases anuria or inadequate excretion persists, and death in uremia occurs in a period that may vary from two to 20 days.

To diminish the danger of death from post-shock uremia, certain precautions appear to be indicated: (1) Cut the duration of shock as short as possible by quick restoration of blood volume through adequate replacement of lost blood, plasma, or saline solution. (2) If acidosis is present, either during or after shock, administer adequate amounts of bicarbonate. (3) While administration of large amounts of fluid may be necessary to obtain normal blood volume and hydration, overadministration is to be avoided both during and after shock, or circulatory embarrassment may be caused. Measuring blood and plasma specific gravities is of practical assistance in planning and guiding fluid administration. (4) When, after recovery from acute shock, anuria or excretion of urine of low volume and specific gravity persists, and blood urea continues to mount, give a diet high in carbohydrates and fat, and low in protein, to retard accumulation of catabolic products. (5) It appears also that vividiffusion or peritoneal irrigation may retard onset of uremia and increase the opportunity for recovery of renal function.

BIBLIOGRAPHY

1. Van Slyke, D. D., Phillips, R. A., Hamilton, P. B., Archibald, R. M., Dole, V. P., Emerson, K., Jr., with the technical assistance of Stanley, E. G., Becker, W. H., and Osserman, F.: Effect of shock on the kidney, Trans. Assoc. Am. Phys., 1944, lviii, 119.
2. Lauson, H. D., Bradley, S. E., and Cournand, A.: The renal circulation in shock, Jr. Clin. Invest., 1944, xxiii, 381.
3. Phillips, R. A., Dole, V. P., Hamilton, P. B., Emerson, K., Jr., Archibald, R. M., and Van Slyke, D. D.: Effects of acute hemorrhagic and traumatic shock on renal function of dogs, Am. Jr. Physiol., 1946, cxlv, 314.
4. Trueta, J., Barclay, A. E., Daniel, P. M., Franklin, K. J., and Prichard, M. L.: Renal pathology in the light of recent neurovascular studies, Lancet, 1946, ii, 237; Studies of the renal circulation, 1947, Blackwell Scientific Publications, Oxford, England.
5. Green, H. D., Cosby, R. S., and Lewis, R. N.: Modification of blood flow in skin and muscle of dogs in hemorrhagic shock, Fed. Proc., 1942, Part II, i, 32.
6. Lucké, B.: Lower nephron nephrosis, Mil. Surg., 1946, xcix, 371.
7. Mallory, T. B.: Hemoglobinuric nephrosis in traumatic shock, Am. Jr. Clin. Path., 1947, xvii, 427.
8. Badenoch, W. W., and Darmady, E. M.: The effects of temporary occlusion of the renal artery in rabbits and its relationship to traumatic uraemia, Jr. Path. and Bact., 1947, lix, 79.
9. Darmady, E. M., Siddons, A. H. M., Corson, T. C., Langton, C. D., Vitek, Z., Badenoch, A. W, and Scott, J. C.: Traumatic uremia. Report on 8 cases, Lancet, 1944, ii, 809.

   Darmady, E. M.: Renal anoxia and the traumatic uraemia syndrome, British Jr. Surg., 1947, xxxiv, 262.
10. Maegraith, B. G., Adelaide, M. B., Havard, R. E., and Parsons, D. S.: Renal syndrome of wide distribution induced possibly by renal anoxia, Lancet, 1945, ii, 293.
11. Corcoran, A. C., and Page, I. H.: Genesis of crush syndrome, Jr. Lab. and Clin. Med., 1945, xxx, 351.
12. Richards, A. N.: Direct observations of change in function of the renal tubule caused by certain poisons, Trans. Assoc. Am. Phys., 1929, xliv, 64.
13. Bywaters, E. G. L.: Ischemic muscle necroses. Crushing injury, traumatic edema, the crush syndrome, traumatic anuria, compression syndrome: a type of injury seen in air raid casualties following burial beneath debris, Jr. Am. Med. Assoc., 1944, cxxiv, 1103. (This review provides references to earlier work of Bywaters and his collaborators.)
14. Fishberg, A. M.: Hypertension and nephritis, 4th Ed., 1939, p. 55 et seq., Lea and Febiger, Philadelphia.
15. Van Slyke, D. D., Rhoads, C. P., Hiller, A., and Alving, A.: The relationship of the urea clearance to the renal blood flow, Am. Jr. Physiol., 1934, cx, 387.
16. Rogers, L.: Further work on the reduction of the alkalinity of the blood in Asiatic cholera, and sodium bicarbonate injection in the prevention of uremia, Ann. Trop. Med. and Parasit., 1916–17, x, 129. Bowel diseases in the tropics, 1921, London.
17. Marshall, E. K., and Crane, M. M.: The influence of temporary closure of the renal artery on the amount and composition of the urine, Am. Jr. Physiol., 1923, lxiv, 387.
18. Scarff, R. W., and Keele, L. A.: The effects of temporary occlusion on the renal circulation of the rabbit, Brit. Jr. Exper. Path., 1943, xxiv, 147.
19. Phillips, R. A., and Hamilton, P. B.: Effects of renal ischemia in dogs. II. Effects of 20, 60 and 120 minutes of renal cachemia on glomerular and tubular function, Am. Jr. Physiol., 1948, in press.
20. Hamilton, P. B., Phillips, R. A., and Hiller, A.: Effects of renal ischemia. I. Duration of renal ischemia required to produce death in uremia, Am. Jr. Physiol., 1948, in press.

21. Van Slyke, D. D., Hiller, A., and Miller, B. F.: The clearance, extraction percentage and estimated filtration of sodium ferricyanide in the mammalian kidney. Comparison with inulin, creatinine, and urea, Am. Jr. Physiol., 1935, cxiii, 611.

22. Warren, J. V., and Brannon, E. S.: A method of obtaining renal venous blood in unanesthetized persons, with observations on the extraction of oxygen and sodium para-amino hippurate, Science, 1944, c, 108.

Bradley, S. E., and Curry, J., Cited by W. Goldring and H. Chasis *in* Hypertension and hypertensive disease, 1944, Publication of The Commonwealth Fund, New York.

23. Dole, V. P., Emerson, J., Jr., Phillips, R. A., Hamilton, P., and Van Slyke, D. D.: The renal extraction of oxygen in experimental shock, Am. Jr. Physiol., 1946, cxlv, 337.

24. Hamilton, A. S., and Collins, D. A.: The homeostatic rôle of a renal humoral mechanism in hemorrhage and shock, Am. Jr. Physiol., 1942, cxxxvi, 275.

25. Bahnson, H. T.: Rôle of the kidneys in the resistance of rats to hemorrhage, Am. Jr. Physiol., 1943, cxl, 416.

26. Page, I. H.: The occurrence of a vasoconstrictor substance in blood during shock induced by trauma, hemorrhage and burns, Am. Jr. Physiol., 1943, cxxxix, 386.

27. Dexter, L., Frank, H. A., Haynes, F. W., and Altschule, M. D.: Traumatic shock. VI. The effect of hemorrhagic shock on the concentration of renin and hypertensinogen in the plasma in unanesthetized dogs, Jr. Clin. Invest., 1943, xxii, 847.

28. Corcoran, A. C., Taylor, R. D., and Page, I. H.: Immediate effects on renal function of the onset of shock due to partially occluding limb tourniquets, Ann. Surg., 1944, cxviii, 871.

29. Shorr, E., Zweifach, B. W., and Furchgott, R. F.: On the occurrence, sites and modes of origin and destruction, of principles affecting the compensatory vascular mechanisms in experimental shock, Science, 1945, cii, 489.

30. Baez, S., Zweifach, B. W., and Shorr, E.: Hepato-renal factors in circulatory homeostasis. II. Disappearance of hepatic vaso-depressor material following intravenous administration, Proc. Soc. Exper. Biol. and Med., 1947, lxiv, 154.

31. Chambers, R., and Zweifach, B. W.: Blood-borne vasotrophic substances in experimental shock, Am. Jr. Physiol., 1947, cl, 239.

32. Van Slyke, K. K., and Evans, E. I.: The paradox of aciduria in the presence of alkalosis caused by hypochloremia, Ann. Surg., 1947, cxxvi, 545.

33. Van Slyke, K. K., and Evans, E. I.: The regulation of parenteral water and salt administration, Ann. Surg., 1948, in press.

34. Reimann, H. A., Chang, G. C. T., Chu, L. W., Liu, P. Y., and Ou, Y.: Asiatic cholera. Clinical study and experimental therapy with streptomycin, Am. Jr. Trop. Med., 1946, xxvi, 631.

35. Phillips, R. A., Van Slyke, D. D., Dole, V. P., Emerson, K., Jr., Hamilton, P. B., and Archibald, R. M.: Copper sulfate method for measuring specific gravities of whole blood and plasma, Bumed News Letter, 1943, 1, No. 9; Bull. U. S. Army Med. Dept., 1943, lxxi, 66. Publications of the Josiah Macy Jr. Foundation, 1945.

36. Sellards, A. W.: The relationship of renal lesions of Asiatic cholera to those of ordinary nephritis, Am. Jr. Trop. Dis., 1914–15, ii, 104.

37. Wiggers, J. C., and Ingraham, R. C.: Continuous intravenous infusion of alkalinizing agents during impending hemorrhagic shock conditions, Fed. Proc., 1946, Part II, v, 113.

38. Palmer, W. W., and Van Slyke, D. D.: Studies of acidosis. IX. Relationship between alkali retention and alkali reserve in normal and pathological individuals, Jr. Biol. Chem., 1917, xxxii, 499.

39. Martin, H. E., and Werkman, M.: Serum potassium, magnesium, and calcium levels in diabetic acidosis, Jr. Clin. Invest., 1947, xxvi, 217.

40. Hartmann, A. F.: Theory and practice of parenteral fluid administration, Jr. Am. Med. Assoc., 1934, ciii, 1349.

41. Kolff, W. J.: Personal communication.
42. Kolff, W. J.: The artificial kidney, Press of J. J. Kok N. V. Kampen (Holland), 1946.
43. Kolff, W. J., and Berk, H. R. J.: The artificial kidney: a dialyzer with great area, Acta med. Scandin., 1944, cxvii, 121.
44. Abel, J. J., Rowntree, L. G., and Turner, B. B.: On the removal of diffusible substances from the circulating blood of living animals by dialysis, Jr. Pharm. and Exper. Therap., 1913, v, 275.
45. Fine, J., Frank, H. A., and Seligman, A. M.: The treatment of acute renal failure by peritoneal irrigation, Ann. Surg., 1946, cxxiv, 857.

THE NEPHROTIC SYNDROME IN ADULTS: A COMMON DISORDER WITH MANY CAUSES *

By ROBERT M. KARK, F.A.C.P., F.R.C.P. (Lond.), CONRAD L. PIRANI, M.D., VICTOR E. POLLAK, M.B., M.R.C.P.E., ROBERT C. MUEHRCKE, M.D., and JOHN D. BLAINEY, M.D., M.R.C.P., *Chicago, Illinois*

THE metabolic, nutritional and clinical consequences of continued massive albuminuria constitute the nephrotic syndrome. Florid cases are readily recognized from infancy [1, 2] to extreme old age,[3] and the diagnosis can be confirmed rapidly in the laboratory by urinalysis and simple biochemical studies of the blood. The nephrotic syndrome was first described by Richard Bright,[4] who noted the association of proteinuria, hypoproteinemia and lipemia with edema of renal origin, and it has long been recognized as one manifestation of glomerulonephritis. From our experience with 98 adult patients studied by renal biopsy it is apparent that the syndrome may be due to a variety of causes and different pathologic changes in the kidney (table 4). Nevertheless, it is still considered by some to be a single disease entity.[5] The confusion which still exists about the different etiologies of the nephrotic syndrome has been caused by semantic difficulties, by the lack of correlation between pathologic findings and clinical data, by the disharmonious views of pediatricians and internists about the natural history of the syndrome, and by our imperfect knowledge of the mechanisms which produce its metabolic and clinical manifestations.

METABOLIC AND NUTRITIONAL CONSEQUENCES OF CONTINUED MASSIVE PROTEINURIA

The well known metabolic hallmarks of the nephrotic syndrome are proteinuria, hypoalbuminemia and hypercholesterolemia. But the full-blown picture presents many more biochemical aberrations than this. Albumin is the major protein lost in the urine, accounting for approximately 70% of the total. As can be seen from table 1, other plasma proteins, such as ceruloplasmin, also run to waste in the urine. The continued drain of nitrogen in the urine also compromises the tissue and cellular stores of protein, and

* Presented in part as a Morning Lecture at the Thirty-eighth Annual Session of The American College of Physicians, Boston, Massachusetts, April 12, 1957.

From the Departments of Medicine, Presbyterian, Cook County and Research and Educational Hospitals, and the Departments of Pathology and Medicine of the University of Illinois College of Medicine, Chicago, Illinois.

Supported in part by contract No. DA-49-007-MD637, Surgeon General's Office, Department of the Army, and grants from the U. S. Public Health Service (H-1029) and the Illinois Chapter of the American Rheumatism Foundation.

Requests for reprints should be addressed to Robert M. Kark, M.D., Presbyterian-St. Luke's Hospital, 1753 West Congress Street, Chicago 12, Illinois.

the clinical consequences of this impoverishment are tissue wastage, malnutrition, fatty metamorphosis of the liver, sodium retention, hydremia and edema. Depletion of complement makes the nephrotic patient particularly susceptible to infection, and loss of specialized proteins, such as those which bind thyroid hormone and iron, explains satisfactorily the apparent hypo-

TABLE 1

Some Biochemical Changes in the Urine of Patients with the Nephrotic Syndrome

Increased	Decreased	Variable
Albumin (6, 7)	Sodium chloride	Glucose (6)
Alpha$_1$ globulin (6, 7)		Potassium
Alpha$_2$ globulin (6, 7)		Amino acids (6)
Beta globulin (6, 7)		Nitrogen
Gamma globulin (6, 7)		
Protein-bound iodine (8, 9)		
Ceruloplasmin (10)		
Siderophilin (10, 11)		
Antidiuretic substance (12)		
Complement (13)		
Prothrombin (14)		
Antithrombin (14)		
Proconvertin (14)		

thyroidism and tendency to anemia. More difficult to explain is the marked increase in circulating serum lipids and relatively large plasma proteins, such as cholinesterase and fibrinogen (table 2).

These changes may develop as a result of disturbances in the transport of fats,[18] or they may be the result of some as yet unidentified mechanism. We have speculated elsewhere [19] that the metabolic changes seen in the nephrotic syndrome are the result of increased hepatic synthesis of proteins

TABLE 2

Some Biochemical Changes in the Blood of Patients with the Nephrotic Syndrome

Increased	Decreased	Variable
Total lipid (4)	Albumin	Alpha$_1$ globulin (6)
Triglycerides	Protein-bound iodine (9)	Gamma globulin (6)
Phospholipids	Siderophilin (10, 11)	Alpha lipoprotein (6)
Free cholesterol	Ceruloplasmin (10)	Sodium
Cholesterol esters	Complement (16)	Chloride
Beta lipoprotein (6)	Osmotic pressure (17)	Calcium
Alpha$_2$ globulin (6)	Plasma volume (6)	
Beta globulin (6)		
Fibrinogen (6)		
Cholinesterase (15)		

and fats, called forth by depletion of hepatic albumin and made evident by the retention of large molecular protein molecules in the blood stream and the loss of the small ones in the urine. Be this as it may, studies on nephrotic rats [20] and man [19, 21] have clearly demonstrated that infusion of large amounts of serum albumin can restore both the protein and the lipid abnormalities in the plasma to normal.

Massive loss of albumin in the urine is not invariably accompanied by

TABLE 3

Causes of the Nephrotic Syndrome

	Reference Number
1. *Heredofamilial*	(1)
2. *Infective*	
Syphilis	(22)
Malaria	(25, 26)
Subacute bacterial endocarditis	(27)
Tuberculosis*	(23)
Diphtheria*	(24)
3. *Toxins*	
Organic mercurials*	(33, 34)
Inorganic mercurials (teething powders)	(35)
Tridione, Paradione*	(40, 41, 42)
Bismuth*	(36)
Gold*	(37, 38, 39)
Trichlorethylene*	(52)
4. *Allergic*	
Poison oak*	(29)
Bee sting*	(31, 32)
Pollens and dust	(28)
Serum sickness	(30)
5. *Mechanical*	
Renal vein thrombosis	(43, 44, 45)
Constrictive pericarditis	(45)
Congestive cardiac failure	(46)
Tricuspid valve disease	(47)
Thrombosis or obstruction of inferior vena cava	(48)
6. *Generalized Disease Processes*	
Amyloidosis—primary	(51)
Amyloidosis—secondary	(4)
Myelomatosis	(46)
Systemic lupus erythematosus	(53)
Diabetic glomerulosclerosis	(55, 56)
Schönlein-Henoch purpura	(50)
Arteriolar nephrosclerosis	(62)
Progressive systemic sclerosis*	(52)
Polyarteritis nodosa*	(52)
Sickle cell anemia*	(52)
7. *Intrinsic Renal Disease*	
Membranous glomerulonephritis	(3)
Proliferative glomerulonephritis	(67)
Mixed membranous and proliferative glomerulonephritis	(61)
Tubular degeneration; no glomerular lesions (lipoid nephrosis)	(66)
Tubular degeneration; minimal glomerular lesions	(66)

* These causes have not been thoroughly validated.

all of the clinical or biochemical stigmata of the nephrotic syndrome. The loss of protein may not be sufficient to overwhelm the body's homeostatic mechanisms, and clinical edema may never appear. These patients with subclinical forms feel well, and rarely appear in the clinic unless proteinuria is detected on routine examination. In other *formes frustes* the serum lipid levels are normal or decreased in amount. The reasons for this are not clear. In our experience low or normal levels of serum cholesterol may accompany the nephrotic syndrome in generalized disease processes, e.g., systemic lupus erythematosus, and may well indicate a poor prognosis.

The Causes of the Nephrotic Syndrome

The many conditions reported to have been associated with the nephrotic syndrome are summarized in table 3. It is immediately evident that the nephrotic syndrome is not a single disease entity, but the metabolic expression of a wide variety of underlying disease states. It may be the

Table 4

Histologic Diagnoses in 98 Patients Ill with the Nephrotic Syndrome and Studied by Renal Biopsy

				No. of Cases
I.	Glomerulonephritis			46
	1. Membranous Type		28	
	Associated with superimposed pyelonephritis	3		
	Associated with severe vascular changes	2		
	Associated with margination of leukocytes (both patients were in heart failure)	2		
	Associated with sarcoidosis	1		
	Associated with subacute bacterial endocarditis	1		
	2. Mixed Type—membranous and proliferative		12	
	Associated with sarcoidosis	1		
	Associated with severe vascular changes	1		
	3. Proliferative Type		6	
	Edema appeared during organic mercurial therapy	1		
II.	"Lipoid Nephrosis"			11
	Associated with arteriosclerosis	3		
III.	Systemic Lupus Erythematosus (Lupus Nephritis)			18
IV.	Amyloidosis			3
	1. Primary		1	
	2. Secondary		2	
V.	Diabetes Mellitus			15
	1. Diffuse diabetic glomerulosclerosis		1	
	2. Diffuse and nodular diabetic glomerulosclerosis		14	
VI.	Severe Arterial and Arteriolar Nephrosclerosis			1
VII.	Increased Pressure in Renal Veins			4
	1. Renal vein thrombosis		2	
	2. Constrictive Pericarditis		1	
	3. Tricuspid stenosis		1	

result of: (a) primary renal disease, such as lipoid nephrosis or glomerulonephritis; (b) renal disease associated with systemic illnesses, such as diabetes mellitus, systemic lupus erythematosus, or amyloidosis; or (c) pressure effects on the venous system draining the kidney, e.g., renal vein thrombosis or constrictive pericarditis.

Rare causes today, but more common in the past, were infectious diseases such as secondary syphilis,[22] tuberculosis [23] and diphtheria.[24] In tropical climates the nephrotic syndrome has been reported occasionally in patients suffering from quartan malaria.[25, 26] More recently, the nephrotic syndrome has been observed in cases of subacute bacterial endocarditis.[27] In one such case observed by us, membranous glomerulonephritis was found by renal biopsy. *Staphylococcus aureus* was grown from both the kidney tissue and the blood, and the diagnoses of subacute bacterial endocarditis and membranous glomerulonephritis were confirmed post mortem.

The nephrotic syndrome has been reported as a manifestation of an allergic process.[28] Rytand observed its occurrence in seven patients who were sensitive to poison oak.[29] The nephrotic syndrome occurred three days to two months after the appearance of the poison oak dermatitis, but it did not recur subsequently when the patients were again exposed to poison oak, and when they again developed dermatitis. Rytand emphasized that there was no evidence of a direct nephrotoxic effect of poison oak, and suggested that the nephrotic syndrome might result from sensitization. If this is true, it is difficult to understand why the nephrotic syndrome did not recur with recurrent attacks of dermatitis. The development of the nephrotic syndrome has been reported during an attack of serum sickness,[30] and it has occurred in sensitive individuals following bee stings.[31, 32] Squire studied a patient in whom an allergic pathogenesis appeared to be the probable mechanism of development of the nephrotic syndrome.[28] This patient had seven separate episodes of the nephrotic syndrome, and each responded well to cortisone. He was found to be extremely sensitive to the pollens of trees and grass, and had an eosinophilia of over 1,000/mm.[3] The initial episode occurred while haymaking on a farm during his vacation, and all subsequent relapses occurred during the pollen season.

The nephrotic syndrome has also been reported in patients receiving drugs and chemicals, such as organic and inorganic mercury,[33, 34, 35] bismuth,[36] gold,[37, 38, 39] Tridione[40, 41] and Paradione.[42] When one considers the widespread use of all these agents, the occurrence of the nephrotic syndrome is extremely rare, and the evidence for a direct etiologic relationship is presumptive. In a single case, however, Barnett has demonstrated convincingly that the recurrent episodes and remissions of the nephrotic syndrome in his patient were directly associated with the administration and withdrawal of Tridione.[40] Several authors have reported the occurrence of the nephrotic syndrome in patients receiving prolonged treatment with mercurial diuretics,[33, 34] but the pathogenetic role of the mercurial diuretic agents has not been demonstrated satisfactorily, particularly as it appears likely that chronic heart failure may produce the nephrotic syndrome. In the renal biopsy of one such patient studied by us the tubules were dilated and lined by flattened epithelium in which regenerating tubular cells were seen. In addition, however, there was evidence of a proliferative glomerulitis. When the mercurial diuretic was withdrawn the patient's condition improved, and there was no recurrence of edema when he was treated with ammonium chloride.

Although the association of renal vein thrombosis and the nephrotic

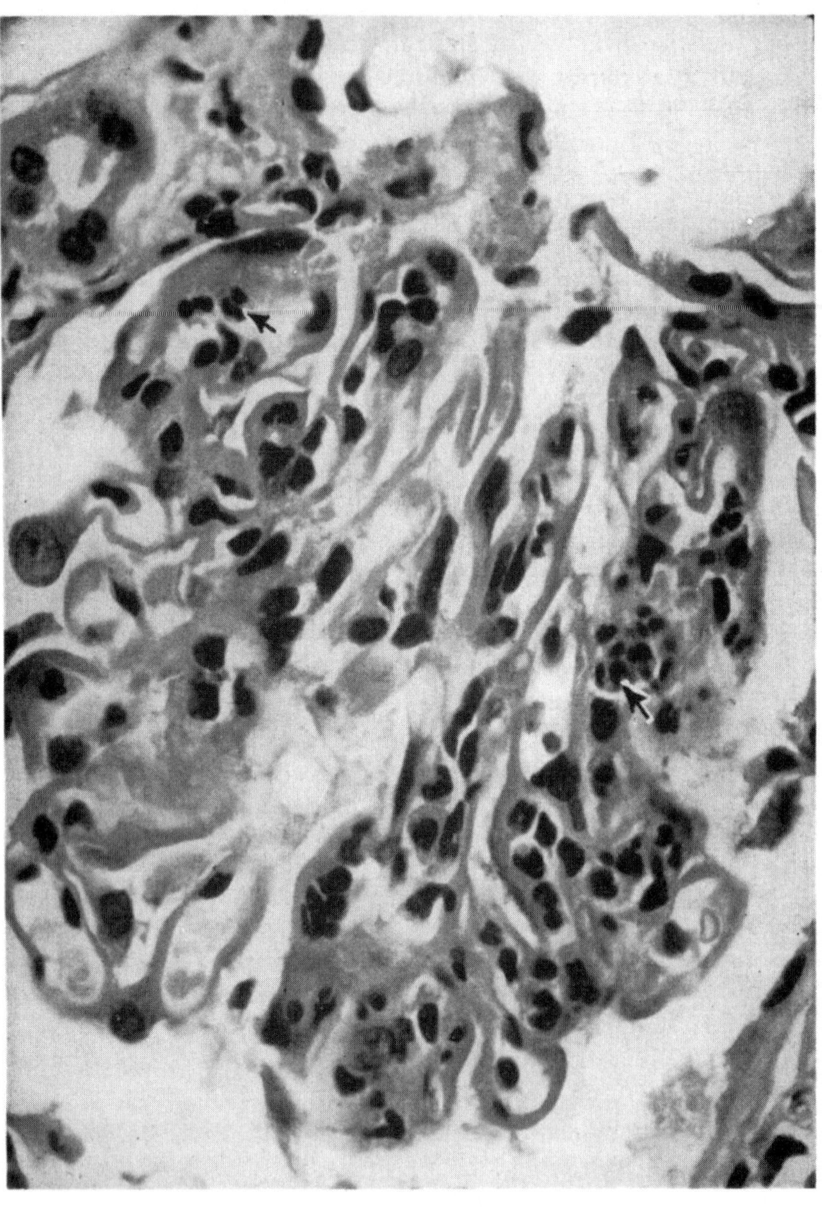

FIG. 1 (Legend on opposite page).

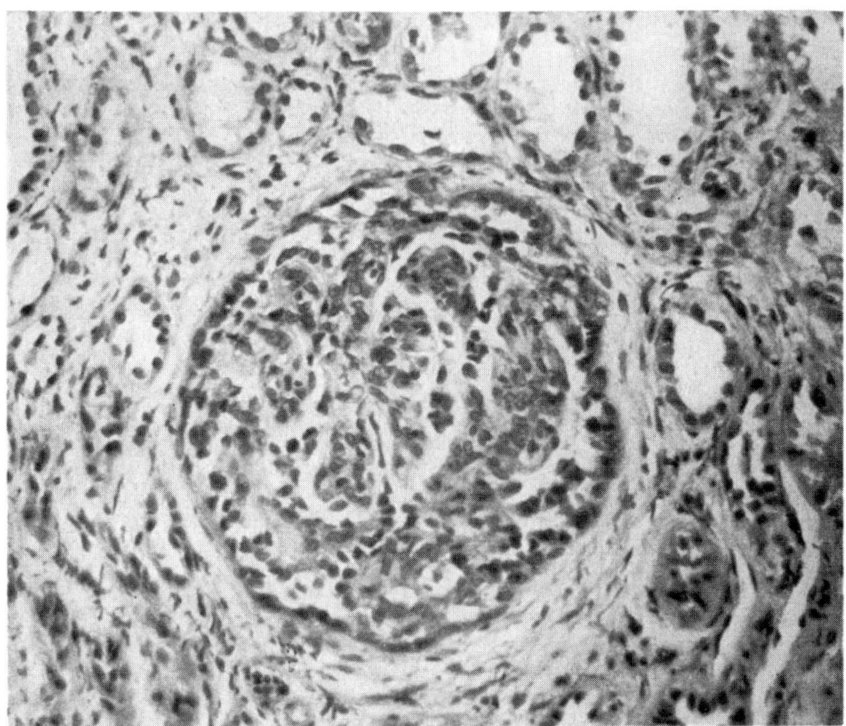

Fig. 2. *Systemic lupus erythematosus.* Renal biopsy from a 21 year old student who had been ill with systemic lupus erythematosus for 30 months. He developed generalized edema four months before the biopsy was taken. (Blood pressure, 140/108 mm. Hg; proteinuria, 3 to 10 gm./day; serum albumin, 2.4 gm./100 ml.; serum cholesterol, 460 mg./100 ml.) Advanced stage of lupus nephritis with proliferative and membranous glomerular lesions. Note the marked edema and some fibrosis in the interstitial tissue. In other glomeruli, fibrinoid changes and occasional hematoxylin bodies were seen (H & E × 300).

syndrome was first described by Rayer almost 120 years ago,[43] it is only recently that this condition has regained the attention of clinicians.[44] The main abnormality is extrarenal, and results primarily in interstitial renal edema and tubular degeneration. Diffuse thickening of the glomerular basement membrane develops, similar to that seen in cases of membranous glomerulonephritis. An unusual histologic feature seen in a number of these cases is margination of leukocytes in the glomerular capillaries.*[44] If the obstruction to the renal vein is sudden and complete no collateral cir-

* In two patients classified in table 4 as membranous glomerulonephritis, margination of leukocytes was noted in the glomerular capillaries. It is of interest that both patients were in congestive cardiac failure when the biopsies were made.

Fig. 1. *Constrictive pericarditis.* Renal biopsy from a 73 year old man with constrictive pericarditis and the nephrotic syndrome (edema, 3 plus; proteinuria, 5.4 gm./day; serum albumin, 1.2 gm./100 ml.; serum cholesterol, 327 mg./100 ml.). In this representative glomerulus there is a mild diffuse thickening of the capillary basement membrane. Note particularly the margination of polymorphonuclear leukocytes within the capillary lumina. This unusual feature was not seen in the usual type of membranous glomerulonephritis, but has been observed in the glomeruli of patients with the nephrotic syndrome due to renal vein thrombosis and congestive cardiac failure (H & E × 875).

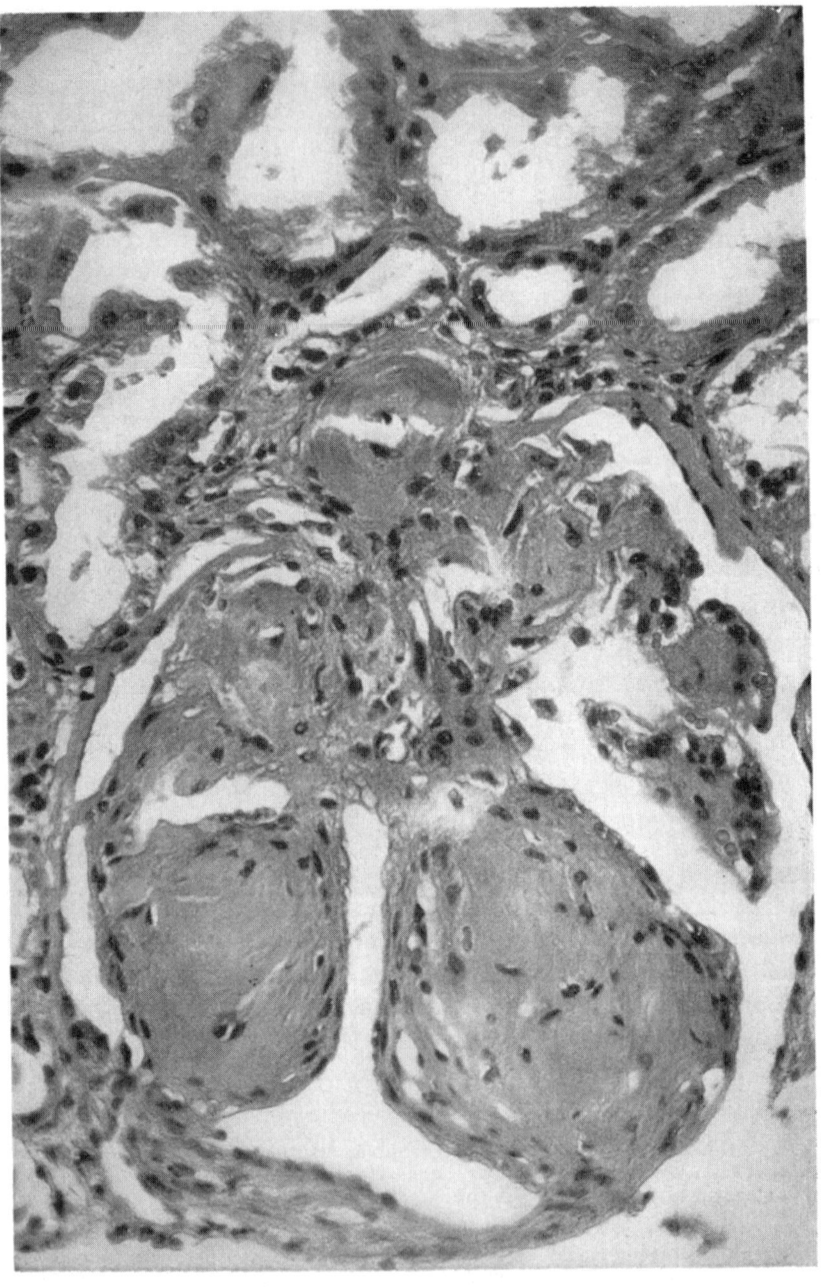

FIG. 3 (Legend on opposite page).

culation develops. The affected kidney is functionless, and the nephrotic syndrome does not appear. However, if adequate collateral venous drainage does develop the nephrotic syndrome occurs. Partial obstruction to the renal venous return may result not only from organic obstruction to the renal veins, but also from a functional obstruction due to considerable elevations of the pressure in the inferior vena cava. This may also result in the nephrotic syndrome. We have observed this in constrictive pericarditis,[45] severe congestive cardiac failure,[46] tricuspid valve disease,[47] and in thrombosis of, and pressure on, the inferior vena cava.[48] In these conditions the histology of the kidney (figure 1) is indistinguishable from that found in cases of renal vein thrombosis [49]; the conditions are of particular interest because they indicate that a simple mechanical disturbance of blood flow may initiate a complex metabolic derangement. Blainey, Hardwicke and Whitfield reported the occurrence of the nephrotic syndrome in a patient with constrictive pericarditis, in whom a pericardiectomy was done.[45] Two months after the operation the patient had no edema, the urine contained no protein, and the biochemical abnormalities had disappeared. Thus far this is the only case where it has been possible to lower the elevated inferior vena caval pressure, and to produce thereby a cure of the nephrotic syndrome.

The nephrotic syndrome occurs frequently in generalized disease processes which affect the kidney, such as systemic lupus erythematosus, diabetic glomerulosclerosis, Schönlein-Henoch purpura,[50] primary [51] and secondary amyloidosis,[4] and myelomatosis with or without amyloidosis.[46]

It is noteworthy that most of these are diseases which affect small blood vessels throughout the body. In the kidney they affect particularly the afferent arterioles and glomerular capillaries. It has also been reported to occur in polyarteritis nodosa, progressive systemic sclerosis [52] and sickle cell anemia.[52] It is not possible at the present time to be certain of the causal relationship of these three diseases to the nephrotic syndrome, as full case reports have not been presented in the literature.

The incidence of systemic lupus erythematosus appears to vary considerably from one country to another. In those areas where it has been recognized it is a common cause of the nephrotic syndrome. In our series of 98 patients with the nephrotic syndrome, lupus nephritis was the underlying cause in 18 (table 4 and figure 2). The course of the renal disease was usually rapid, and death occurred within a few months to three years in most patients so afflicted. In the more severely and acutely progressive cases the blood cholesterol levels were lower than those usually found in the

FIG. 3. *Diabetes mellitus.* Renal biopsy from a 35 year old man who had had diabetes mellitus for 13 years and edema for a few months (advanced diabetic retinopathy; blood pressure, 150/105 mm. Hg; urinary protein excretion, 6 to 18 gm./day; serum albumin, 2.4 gm./100 ml.; serum cholesterol, 522 mg./100 ml.). Representative glomerulus showing nodular and diffuse diabetic glomerulosclerosis. Note the characteristic lamination of the nodules and the sclerosis of the afferent arteriole. In the nephrotic syndrome associated with diabetes mellitus, nodular lesions are usually less prominent than in this case (H & E × 370).

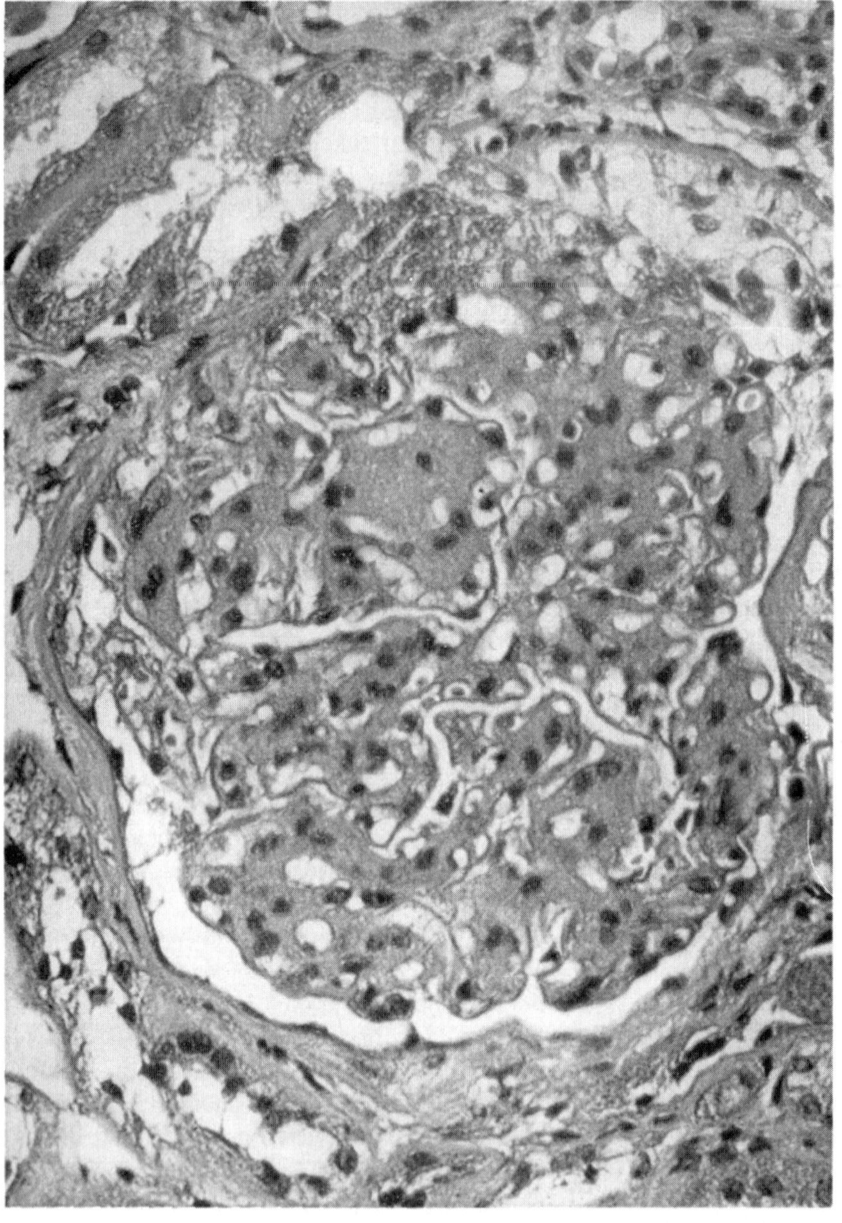

FIG. 4 (Legend on opposite page).

nephrotic syndrome, and these patients died within a few weeks or months of the onset of edema. The natural history and pathology of the nephrotic syndrome in systemic lupus erythematosus have been discussed fully elsewhere.[53]

Diabetes mellitus was the cause of the nephrotic syndrome in 15 patients (table 4). In our patients the occurrence of the nephrotic syndrome could not be related to the severity, duration or control of the diabetic state, nor was it related to the type of treatment given. In the past, attention has been focused particularly on the nodular glomerular lesion described by Kimmelstiel and Wilson.[54] In the present series these lesions (figure 3) were found in only 14 of the 15 diabetics with nephrotic syndrome. That the Kimmelstiel-Wilson lesions are not universally present in diabetics with nephrotic syndrome accords with the experience of others.[55, 56, 57, 58] It seems unlikely that the massive proteinuria characteristic of the nephrotic syndrome could be due to the nodular lesions in the glomeruli, which are often sparsely distributed. It is far more likely that the proteinuria was associated with diffuse diabetic glomerulosclerosis. Our observations [59] and those of Adams [56] support this concept, for we found the diffuse type of diabetic glomerulosclerosis described by Laipply, Eitzen and Dutra [60] and emphasized by Bell [61] in all 15 cases (figure 4). In addition, we have shown that the amount of protein in the urine is much more closely related to the severity of the diffuse lesions than to that of the nodular lesions.[59]

The nephrotic syndrome was also observed in one middle aged man who had had severe hypertension for from three to five years. When he was first seen the urine contained no protein; later, increasing amounts of protein appeared in the urine, and he ultimately developed the nephrotic syndrome. In addition to the severe tubular degeneration and interstitial edema seen in the renal biopsy sections, there were well marked sclerosis of afferent arterioles and hyaline arteriosclerotic changes in the glomeruli. These changes predominated in the hilar region of the tuft. The edematous phase was transitory, and he had a spontaneous diuresis. To our knowledge only one other case of the nephrotic syndrome associated only with arteriolar nephrosclerosis has been described.[62] Moreover when Bloom and Seegal reviewed 120 autopsies on patients who died with renal failure they found no history of the nephrotic syndrome in 50 patients who had had arteriolar nephrosclerosis.[63]

Diseases intrinsic to the kidney are the most common causes of the nephrotic syndrome. Glomerulonephritis was found in 46 of 98 patients

---

FIG. 4. *Diabetes mellitus.* Renal biopsy from a 31 year old woman who had had diabetes mellitus for 19 years and who had developed edema six months before the biopsy was taken (advanced diabetic retinopathy; blood pressure, 170/110 mm. Hg; proteinuria, 6 gm./day; serum albumin, 2.9 gm./100 ml.; serum cholesterol, 566 mg./100 ml.) Representative glomerulus showing moderately severe diffuse diabetic glomerulosclerosis. This type of glomerular lesion is always present when the nephrotic syndrome develops in diabetes mellitus; it is characterized by deposition of "hyaline" material within and between the capillary walls (H & E × 500).

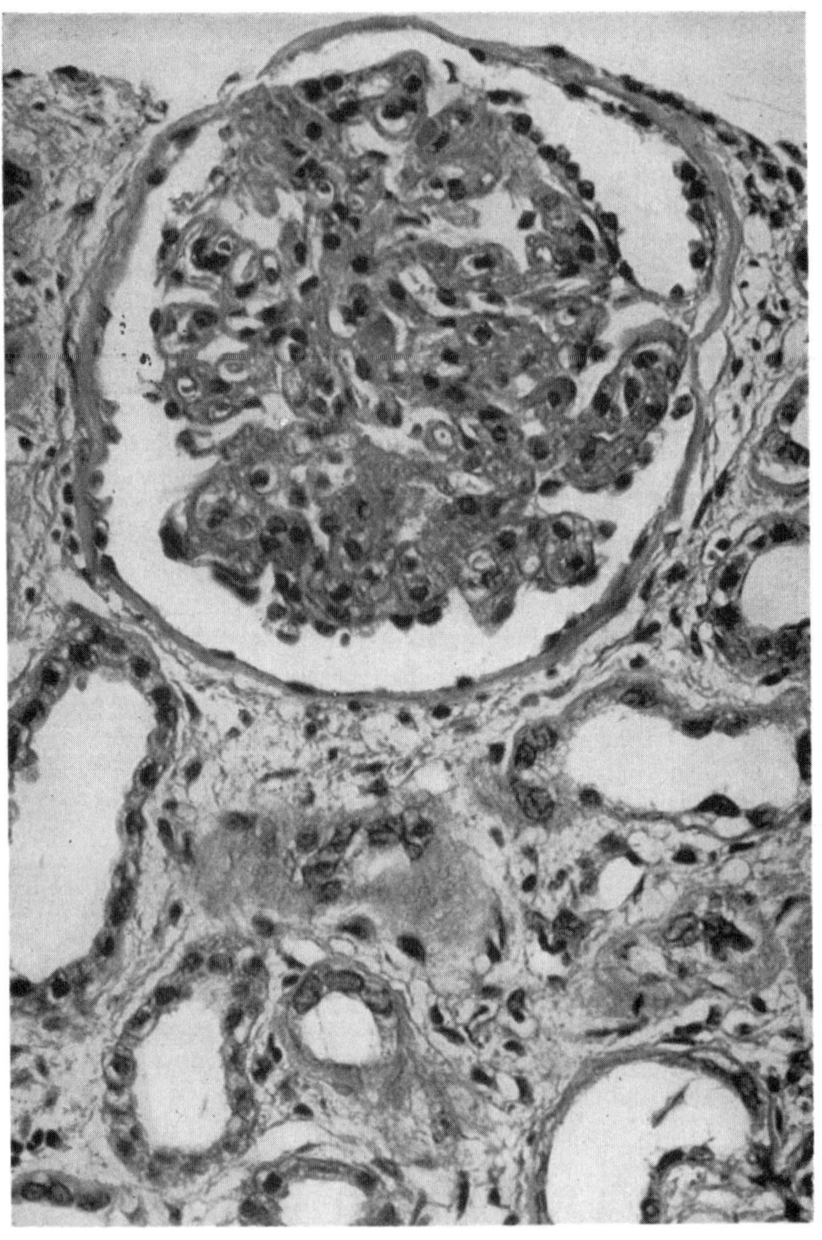

Fig. 5 (Legend on opposite page).

with the nephrotic syndrome (table 4). Although there are many histologic classifications of glomerulonephritis, we have preferred to limit our terminology to three types:

1. Membranous glomerulonephritis (figures 5 and 6), in which the pathologic change is seen predominantly or exclusively in the glomerular basement membrane (28 cases).
2. Proliferative glomerulonephritis, in which proliferation of endothelial and/or epithelial cells is the most prominent feature and in which epithelial or fibroepithelial crescents usually develop (six cases).
3. Mixed membranous and proliferative glomerulonephritis (figure 7), in which both membranous and proliferative changes were equally prominent (12 cases).

The histologic features of the first two groups correspond to Ellis' types II and I, respectively,[3] and to Longcope's types B and A.[64] It will be noted that membranous glomerulonephritis was considerably more frequent than was either of the other histologic types.

Lipoid nephrosis was originally recognized by Müller,[65] and described in detail by Munk[66] and by Volhard and Fahr.[67] The existence and nature of this entity have been the subject of controversy for many years. In essence, we understand by lipoid nephrosis a condition of unknown etiology characterized clinically by the nephrotic syndrome and having a good prognosis. The patient ultimately recovers completely unless, as was common in the past, he dies of intercurrent infection. There is no evidence of changes in the glomerular architecture by light microscopy, i.e., there is no glomerulonephritis (figure 8). However, the tubules are degenerated and filled with fat, while the interstitial tissue is edematous. Before the technic of renal biopsy was in use, it was usually impossible to make a definitive evaluation of the underlying renal pathology in many patients with the nephrotic syndrome. As a result, the diagnosis of lipoid nephrosis could be made only retrospectively many years after the edema and proteinuria had disappeared, or at the postmortem examination if the patient died of an intercurrent illness. From table 4 it can be seen that no definitive structural changes were observed in the glomeruli of 11 patients with the nephrotic syndrome when renal biopsies were made during or immediately after the edematous phase. In all there was degeneration of the tubules, the lining epithelium of which contained fat, and there was edema of the interstitial tissue. No significant abnormality could be demonstrated in the glomeruli in sections stained with hematoxylin and eosin, periodic

---

FIG. 5. *Membranous glomerulonephritis.* Renal biopsy from a 21 year old housewife who had had the nephrotic syndrome for four months (generalized edema; blood pressure, 130/75 mm. Hg; urinary protein excretion, 13 to 25 gm./day; serum albumin, 0.6 gm./100 ml.; serum cholesterol, 1,000 mg./100 ml.) In all glomeruli there was a diffuse, fairly regular thickening of the capillary basement membrane. Note the absence of significant glomerular hypercellularity. There is well marked edema of the interstitial tissue (H & E × 500).

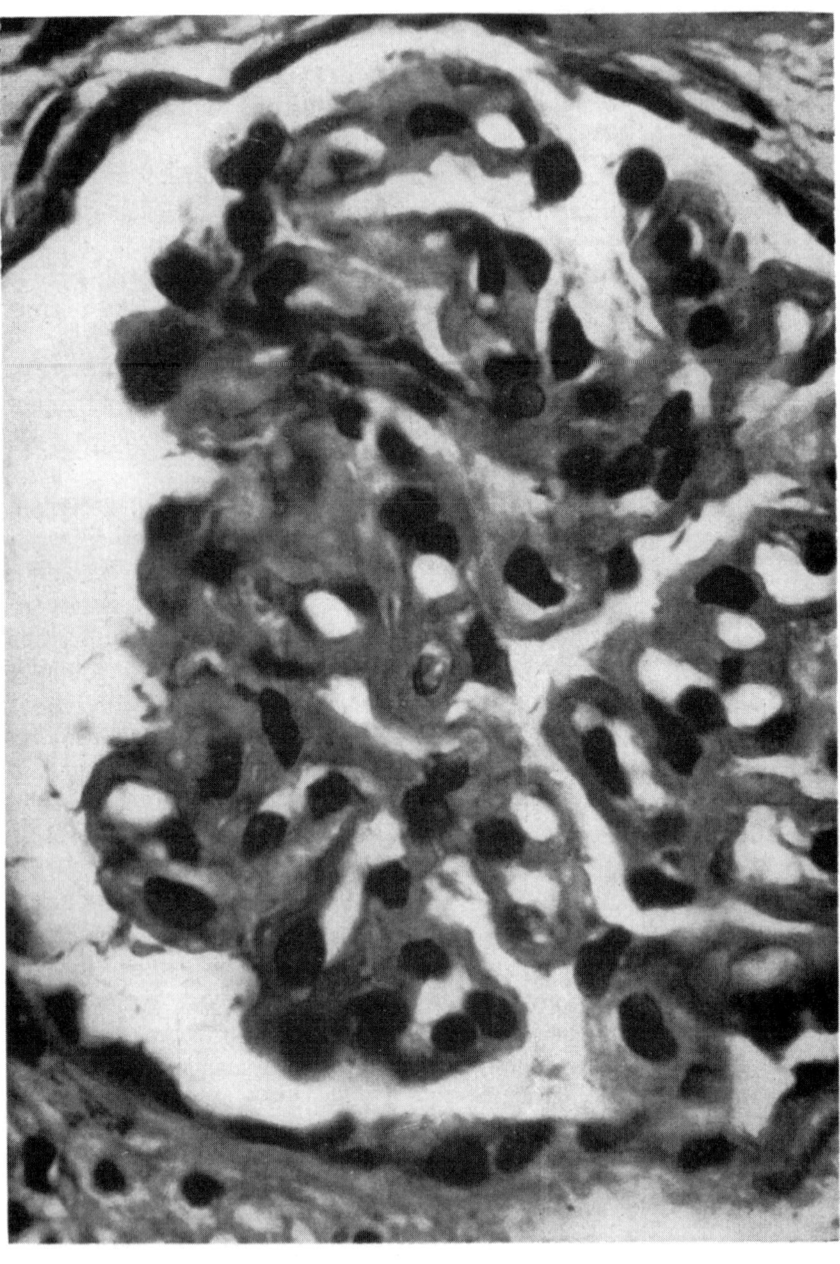

FIG. 6 (Legend on opposite page).

acid-Schiff and Mallory-azan. Clinically these patients have done well. All those treated with ACTH or adrenal corticosteroids had an excellent diuresis. No patient has developed permanent hypertension or evidence of renal failure. Proteinuria persists in some, but has disappeared completely in others.

It is at present impossible to classify these patients, either clinically or histologically. If they continue in excellent health without evidence of renal disease for many years, and if the renal histology remains normal, then we may consider that their original episode of nephrotic syndrome was truly associated with lipoid nephrosis. If, on the other hand, the glomerular basement membrane of these patients does eventually become thickened, we must consider that the nephrotic syndrome was due to early membranous glomerulonephritis. The earliest changes in the glomerular capillaries in these patients are detectable only by electron microscopy.[68, 69] From the clinician's point of view, however, the finding of normal or minimal glomerular changes in a patient with the nephrotic syndrome implies that the prognosis is considerably better than in those patients in whom the nephrotic syndrome is associated with definitive changes in the glomerular architecture.

Treatment

Treatment in the nephrotic syndrome should be directed toward the patient's principal complaint of edema, to the underlying renal condition, and to specific etiologic factors when these can be determined. At present much treatment is necessarily of a nonspecific nature, although with increasing accuracy in diagnosis this situation will change. Salt restriction is one of the most important of the measures designed to prevent edema and to initiate diuresis, and while low salt diets are widely prescribed, little attention is paid by many clinicians to ensuring that these are sufficiently low in sodium. An intake of less than 10 mEq./day (580 mg. sodium chloride) almost always prevents the accumulation of edema and will often start a diuresis, even without other forms of therapy. Limitation of salt intake to this level is now relatively easy with low sodium milk powders (Lonalac), as the diet can be given mainly in the form of drinks or, in severely edematous subjects with poor appetite, by intranasal drip feeding.

The level of protein intake required by these patients has been the cause of much argument. High protein diets of 150 gm. per day or more were originally advocated by Epstein,[70] and employed with considerable success. Later writers, however, observed a rise in the urinary protein loss on such diets,[71] and interpreted this as deterioration in the renal condition. On the

FIG. 6. *Membranous glomerulonephritis.* Renal biopsy from a 47 year old taxi driver who had been ill with the nephrotic syndrome for eight months (blood pressure, 140/70 mm. Hg; edema, 2 plus; urinary protein excretion, 12 gm./day; serum albumin, 2.7 to 4.3 gm./100 ml.; serum cholesterol, 300 to 600 mg./100 ml.). In this representative glomerulus, note the severe, diffuse thickening of the capillary basement membrane, characteristic of membranous glomerulonephritis (H & E × 1500).

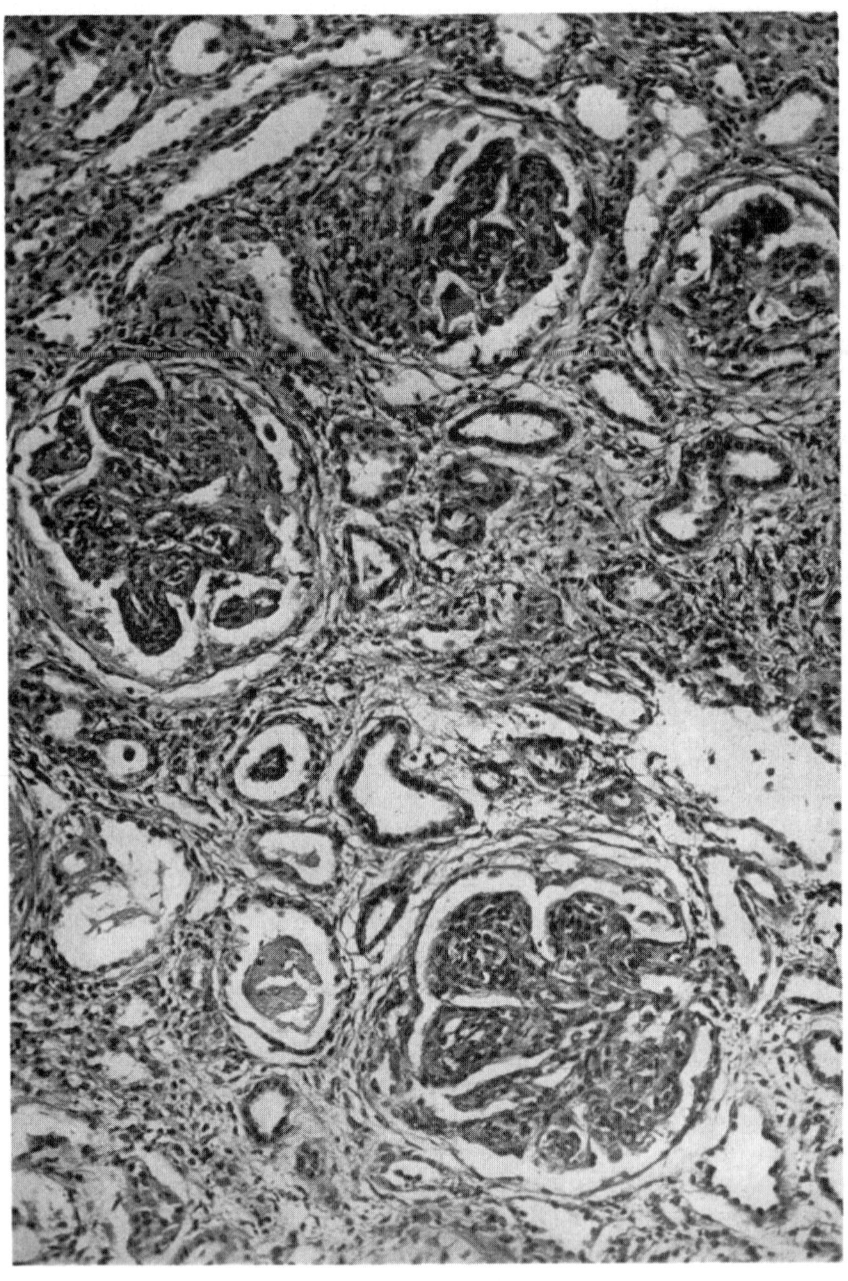

FIG. 7 (Legend on opposite page).

basis of animal studies it was also argued that high protein diets were undesirable, as the prognosis in nephrotoxic serum nephritis was worse when high protein diets were given, and the kidney was said to be required to do more "work" in excreting the additional urea load. Neither of these hypotheses is tenable, as it has been shown that increased proteinuria is to be expected with small rises of serum proteins,[72] and the work load caused by the excretion of urea is a very small fraction of that required by other tubular secretory processes in the kidney that occur normally in the nephrotic syndrome. The demonstration on high protein diets of prolonged positive nitrogen balances, at times amounting to 500 gm. nitrogen in some patients with proteinuria of many months' duration, suggests the presence of a severe body deficit of protein, of which the reduced serum proteins are only one manifestation. In adult patients no maximal level of protein intake could be observed other than that set by the patient's appetite,[73] and positive nitrogen balances were recorded with protein intakes ranging from 65 gm. to 200 gm., higher intakes leading to higher positive balance (figure 9). Since this body nitrogen deficit seems of fundamental importance in the patient with prolonged proteinuria, it would appear advisable to replace protein as rapidly as possible; in practice, it has been found that intakes of 120 gm. per day for the average adult, with high caloric intakes (50 to 60 cals./Kg.), have provided satisfactory repletion without unpalatable diets. Higher levels may be obtained on occasion with continuous tube feeding, and there seems to be no contraindication to their use. It is of course essential to ensure that patients actually take such diets; too often, high protein diets are advised but not consumed. The poor appetite of the edematous patient requires constant supervision and coaxing to ensure that adequate intakes are obtained.

In some patients with severe and prolonged proteinuria, deficiencies of both calcium and potassium may occur, with resulting bone rarefaction and hypokalemia. Both these defects are corrected by high protein diets, with the use of low sodium milk powder described, although additional potassium may be required in the early stages of treatment.

The precise value of steroid therapy in the nephrotic syndrome is still to be determined, since there has been considerable confusion in the rationale for the use of steroids, and great differences in dosage and in the type of steroid used in different reports. Many have used ACTH or cortisone in short courses for from 10 to 15 days, with large doses simply as a "diuretic," and there is little doubt that many patients will show loss of weight and edema with this treatment.[74, 75] The relapse rate, however, is

Fig. 7. *Proliferative and membranous glomerulonephritis.* Renal biopsy from a 14 year old schoolboy who gave a history of acute glomerulonephritis three months earlier, and who had had edema for two months (blood pressure, 140/70 mm. Hg; urinary protein excretion, 5 gm./day; serum albumin, 1.9 gm./100 ml.; serum cholesterol, 465 mg./100 ml.). Subacute glomerulonephritis with proliferative and membranous features. Note the fibroepithelial crescent around the glomerular tuft on the right, the marked interstitial edema, and the atrophy and dilatation of the convoluted tubules (H & E × 200).

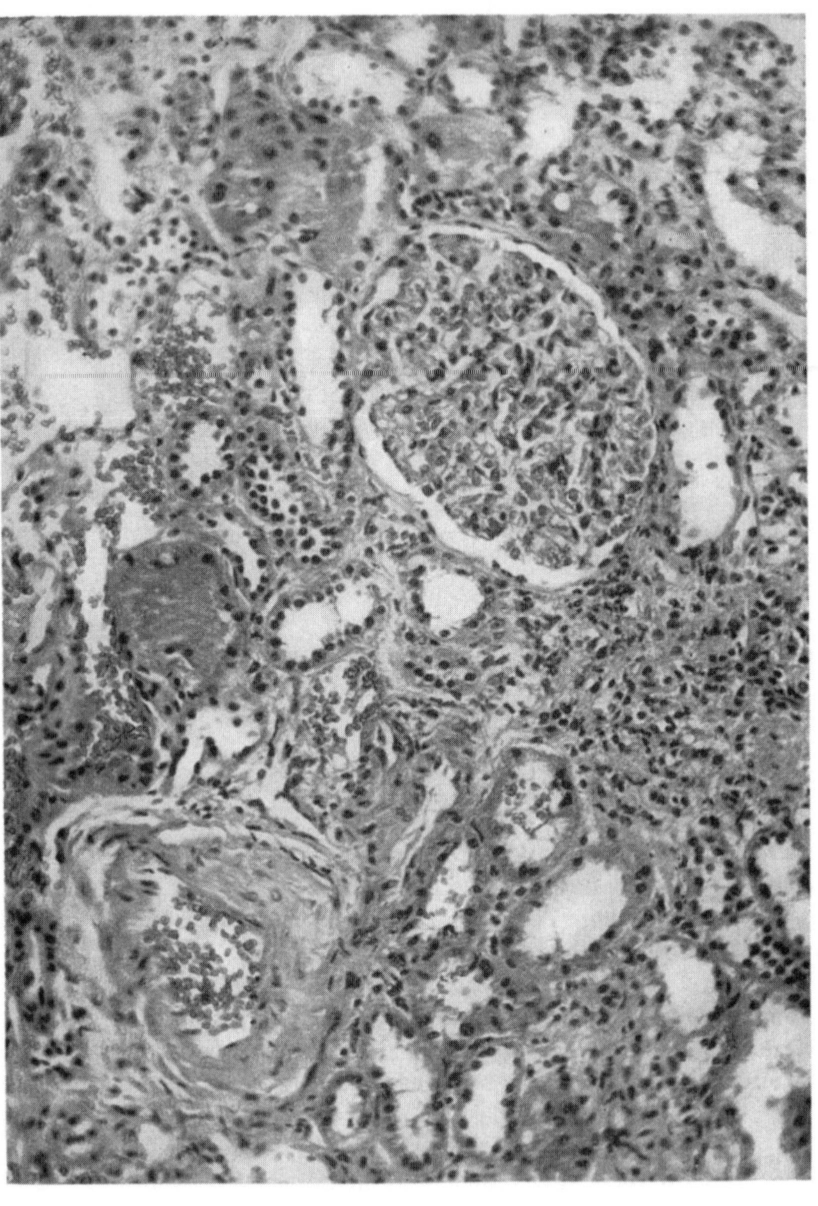

FIG. 8 (Legend on opposite page).

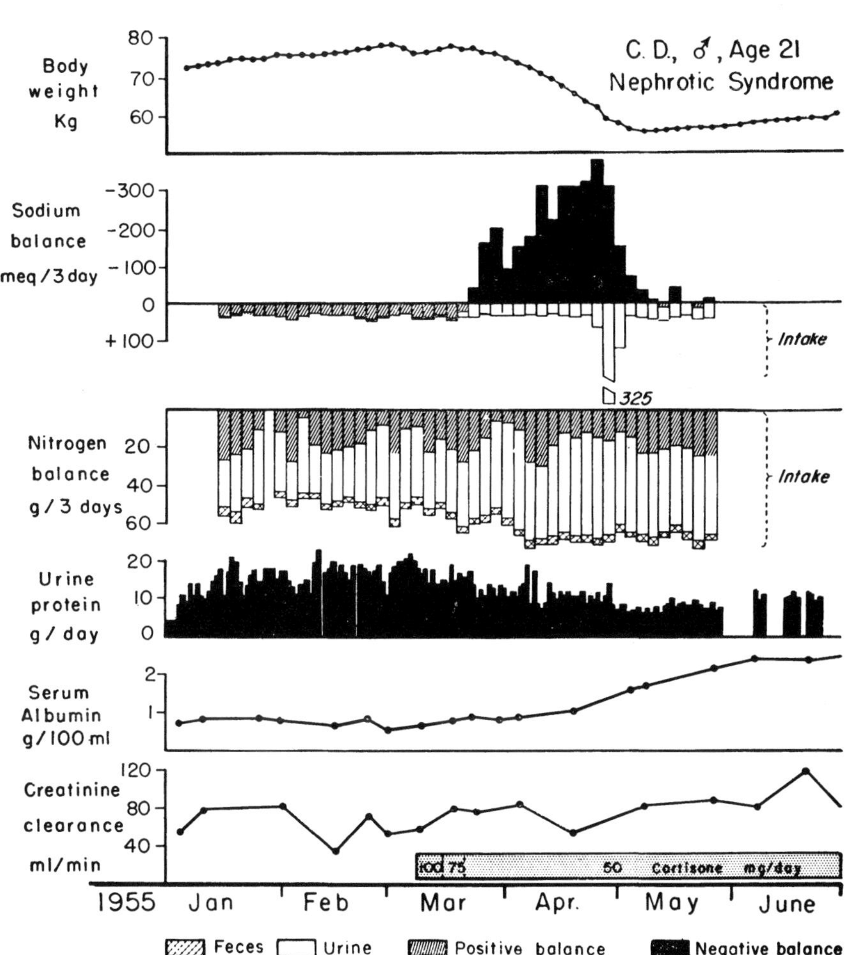

FIG. 9. Metabolic study in a 21 year old patient with the nephrotic syndrome. Note that this patient was in profound positive nitrogen balance throughout the five-month period during which he was studied—the result of an excellent intake of protein and calories.

high, and in many of the reported cases there has been little alteration in the proteinuria shortly after the cessation of a course of steroid. More prolonged treatment, either with cortisone in continuous dosage for many months,[46] or with intermittent courses three days per week for periods of from eight to 10 weeks,[75] has caused reduction in the proteinuria and decrease in the relapse rate in a number of patients; however, little reduction in the frequency of relapse was observed by Roscoe [5] in adults on intermittent dosage. While relief from edema is clearly important, alteration of

FIG. 8. *Lipoid nephrosis.* Renal biopsy from a 66 year old woman who had been ill with the nephrotic syndrome for four months (blood pressure, 160/88 mm. Hg; anasarca; urinary protein, 4 plus; serum albumin, 1.9 gm./100 ml.; serum cholesterol, 755 mg./100 ml.). The glomeruli were congested but were normal in other respects. Note the moderate arteriosclerosis and the interstitial edema (H & E × 225).

the renal abnormality that leads to proteinuria represents a more positive approach to therapy, and the present evidence suggests that continuous cortisone or ACTH does diminish proteinuria in a significant number of cases. Recent reports indicate further that the prognosis in cases of the nephrotic syndrome has been improved by continuous steroid therapy.[76, 77] Few complications have been observed in many cases treated in this way for prolonged periods,[46] provided adequate caloric protein and mineral intakes are ensured.

Considerable evidence suggests that the damage to the kidney in the nephrotic syndrome due to primary renal disease may be intermittent, relapses being associated with recurrent and often mild upper respiratory tract infections. In those cases where hemolytic streptococcal infection can be proved by throat swab or ASO titer levels, the prophylactic use of continuous penicillin seems worth further, prolonged trial. Unfortunately, there are many patients in whom no definite evidence for an association with streptococcal infection can be demonstrated, and it is possible that other agents which are known to cause upper respiratory infection may be involved. Until the relationship of specific infections to the renal lesion can be defined, it would certainly seem advisable to treat promptly any infection of this type with antibiotics in an attempt to prevent deterioration of renal function in patients with known renal disease.

Unfortunately, there are still few patients for whom specific treatment can be given for the nephrotic syndrome, but it is to be hoped that better methods of diagnosis will result in better treatment. Constrictive pericarditis,[45] congestive cardiac failure and possibly lupus nephritis are among the conditions in which treatment may be directed toward a specific cause with satisfactory improvement in the nephrotic syndrome.

Conclusion

The adult who is ill with the nephrotic syndrome comes to the doctor because he has edema. In most instances, physical examination and laboratory investigations, including tests of renal function, do not help in making a differential diagnosis. If azotemia is severe, and if renal function is markedly impaired, then one can usually predict that there is severe structural damage to the kidney. The converse does not hold: there can be marked structural changes to the glomeruli with little alteration in renal function; and with comparatively normal glomeruli, mild or moderate degrees of azotemia may be found. It is true that meticulous history taking is the best clue to the underlying disease. Nevertheless, in many patients with nephrotic syndrome the only complaint is edema. It is these circumstances that make renal biopsy so valuable a tool in the exact diagnosis of the disease—and, as has been indicated in the body of the paper, there may be a wide variety of pathologic patterns associated with the nephrotic syndrome.

As long as the physician considers that the nephrotic syndrome is a single entity with a poor prognosis, he will tend to adopt a pessimistic approach to its treatment. Discovering exactly what is wrong with the patient is useful, because it provides a rational approach to therapy, and stimulates the physician to continue to seek the latest therapeutic advances in the treatment of that particular disease.

Acknowledgment

We wish to thank Dr. George Babcock, Jr., and Dr. C. J. Szmal, Division of Clinical Research, Schering Corporation, Bloomfield, New Jersey, for the supplies of Meticorten used to treat some of the patients reported in this paper.

Summario in Interlingua

In adultos le syndrome nephrotic es le expression clinic de multe differente statos pathologic. Illo pote resultar ab damnification de glomerulos o de tubulos o ab augmento del pression in le venas renal. Nostre studios de biopsia renal in 98 adultos nephrotic ha reflectite un extense spectro de pathologia e de etiologia.

Glomerulonephritis subacute o chronic (membranose o proliferative o ambes) esseva trovate 46 vices. In 15 diabeticos, lesiones esseva trovate que esseva diffuse o diffuse e nodular o diffuse e nodular e exsudative. Dece-octo del patientes habeva systemic lupus erythematose.

In 11 patientes, le apparentia histologic esseva typic pro "nephrosis lipoide." Multo numerose erythrocytos esseva vidite in le glomerulos in que le membrana basal e le cellulas endothelial e epithelial esseva normal. Grados sever de degeneration tubular e de edema interstitial esseva observate. Le administration de hormones esseva sequite per un excellente diurese. Al tempore presente iste 11 patientes es vivente. Tres ha un sanitate excellente, e nulle has disveloppate signos de progressive morbo renal.

Esseva etiam observate casos de amyloidosis renal primari e secundari, de thrombosis de vena renal, de pericarditis constrictive, de insufficientia tricuspidal e stenosis, de nephrosclerosis arteriolar, e de myelomatosis sin amyloidosis. Un numero del casos esseva le resultato de diureticos mercurial. Con plus extense experientias il deveniva possibile establir exacte diagnoses histologic in plus que 90% del casos e, similemente, predicer le responsa a ACTH o corticosteroides e facer le prognose super le base del grado e del typo del compromissos glomerular.

BIBLIOGRAPHY

1. Darmady, E. M., and Stranack, F.: Discussion on the renal tubules. Microdissection of renal tubules, Proc. Roy. Soc. Med. **48**: 781, 1955.
2. Gruskay, F. L., and Turano, A.: Nephrosis in the newborn infant. A syndrome difficult to explain by existing theories of etiology, Arch. Dis. Childhood **94**: 117, 1957.
3. Ellis, A.: Natural history of Bright's disease. Clinical, histological and experimental observations. I. Nephritis, Lancet **1**: 1, 34, 72, 1942.
4. Osman, A. A.: Original papers of Richard Bright on renal disease, 1937, Oxford University Press, London.
5. Roscoe, M. H.: The nephrotic syndrome, Quart. J. Med **25**: 353, 1956.
6. Squire, J. R.: The nephrotic syndrome, *in* Advances in internal medicine, Vol. 7, edited by Dock, W., and Snapper, I., 1955, Year Book Publishers, Inc., Chicago, page 201.

7. Hardwicke, J., and Squire, J. R.: Relationship between plasma albumin concentration and protein excretion in patients with proteinuria, Clin. Sc. **14**: 509, 1955.
8. Kalant, N., MacIntyre, W. C., and Wilansky, D. L.: Thyroid function in experimental nephrosis, Clin. Res. **6**: 39, 1958.
9. Recant, L., and Riggs, D. S.: Thyroid function in nephrosis, J. Clin. Investigation **31**: 789, 1952.
10. Cartwright, G. E., Gubler, C. J., and Wintrobe, M. M.: Studies on copper metabolism. XI. Copper and iron metabolism in the nephrotic syndrome, J. Clin. Investigation **33**: 685, 1954.
11. Gitlin, D., Janeway, C. A., and Farr, L. E.: Studies on metabolism of plasma proteins in nephrotic syndrome. I. Albumin, gamma globulin and iron-binding globulin, J. Clin. Investigation **35**: 44, 1956.
12. Luetscher, J. A., Jr., Piel, C. F., and Curtis, R. H.: The nephrotic syndrome, J. Chron. Dis. **1**: 442, 1955.
13. Seifter, S., and Ecker, E. E.: Complement and isohemagglutinins in urinary proteins, J. Clin. Investigation **25**: 809, 1946.
14. Yatzidis, H., and Richet, G.: Activité de certaines protéines de la coagulation dans le plasma et les urines au cours du syndrome néphrotique, Rev. franc. d'études clin. et biol. **2**: 717, 1957.
15. Vorhaus, L. J., and Kark, R. M.: Serum cholinesterase in health and disease, Am. J. Med. **14**: 707, 1953.
16. Lange, K., Craig, F., Oberman, J., Slobody, L., Ogur, G., and LoCasto, F.: Changes during the course and treatment of glomerulonephritis, Arch. Int. Med. **88**: 433, 1951.
17. Armstrong, S. H., Jr., Kark, R. M., Schoenberger, J. A., Shatkin, J., and Sights, R.: Colloid osmotic pressures of serum proteins in nephrosis and cirrhosis. Relation to electrophoretic distribution and average molecular weights, J. Clin. Investigation **33**: 297, 1954.
18. Rosenman, R. H., Byers, S. O., and Friedman, M.: Plasma lipid interrelationships in experimental nephrosis, J. Clin. Investigation **36**: 1558, 1957.
19. Soothill, J. F., and Kark, R. M.: The effects of infusion of salt-poor human serum albumin on serum cholesterol, cholinesterase and albumin levels in healthy subjects and in patients ill with the nephrotic syndrome, Clin. Res. Proc. **4**: 140, 1956.
20. Rosenman, R. H., and Friedman, M.: In vivo studies of the role of albumin in endogenous and heparin-activated lipemia-clearing in nephrotic rats, J. Clin. Investigation **36**: 700, 1957.
21. Pollak, V. E., Dubin, A., and Kark, R. M.: Unpublished observations.
22. Moore, J. E.: Modern treatment of syphilis, 1933, Charles C Thomas, Springfield, Ill., p. 213.
23. Landouzy, L., and Bernard, L.: La néphrite parenchymateuse chronique des tuberculeux, Presse méd. **9**: 121, 1901.
24. Rosenberg, M.: Die Klinik der Nierenkrankheiten, 1927, S. Karger, Berlin, p. 58.
25. Giglioli, G.: Clinical notes, autopsy and histopathological findings from five fatal cases of quartan malarial nephritis from British Guiana, Tr. Roy. Soc. Trop. Med. and Hyg. **26**: 177, 1932.
26. Surbek, K. E.: A striking case of quartana nephrosis, Tr. Roy. Soc. Trop. Med. and Hyg. **25**: 201, 1931.
27. Eales, L.: Personal communication, 1957.
28. Squire, J. R.: Personal communication, 1957.
29. Rytand, D. A.: Fatal anuria, nephrotic syndrome and glomerular nephritis as sequels of dermatitis of poison oak, Am. J. Med. **5**: 548, 1948.
30. Fanconi, G., Kousmine, C., and Frischknecht, W.: Die konstitutionelle Bereitschaft zum Nephrosesyndrom, Helvet. paediat. acta **6**: 199, 1951.

31. Rytand, D. A.: Onset of the nephrotic syndrome during reaction to bee sting, Stanford M. Bull. **13**: 224, 1955.
32. Burch, G. E.: Personal communication, 1956.
33. Derow, H. A., and Wolff, L.: Oral administration of Mercupurin tablets in ambulatory patients with chronic congestive heart failure, Am. J. Med. **3**: 693, 1947.
34. Munck, O., and Nissen, N. I.: Development of nephrotic syndrome during treatment with mercurial diuretics, Acta med. Scandinav. **153**: 307, 1956.
35. Wilson, V. K., Thomson, M. L., and Holzel, A.: Mercury nephrosis in young children with special reference to teething powders containing mercury, Br. M. J. **1**: 358, 1952.
36. Beattie, J. W.: Nephrotic syndrome following sodium bismuth tartrate therapy in rheumatoid arthritis, Ann. Rheumat. Dis. **12**: 144, 1953.
37. Vallery-Radot, P., Mauric, G., Wolfromm, R., and Guiot, G.: Néphrose lipoïdique secondaire à un traitement aurique, Bull. et mém. Soc. méd. d. hôp. de Paris **58**: 96, 1942.
38. Weissenbach, R. J., Martineau, J., Brocard, J., and Malinsky, A.: Néphrose lipoïdique après chrysothérapie, Bull. et mém. Soc. méd. d. hôp. de Paris **52**: 1076, 1936.
39. Rathery, F., and Hurez, A.: Néphrose aurique ou néphrose lipoïdique, Bull. et mém. Soc. méd. de hôp. de Paris **52**: 1203, 1936.
40. Barnett, H. L., Simons, D. J., and Wells, R. E.: Nephrotic syndrome occurring during Tridione therapy, Am. J. Med. **4**: 760, 1948.
41. White, J. C.: Nephrosis occurring during trimethadione therapy, J. A. M. A. **139**: 376, 1949.
42. Wren, J. C., and Nutt, R. L.: Nephrotic syndrome occurring during paramethadione therapy, J. A. M. A. **153**: 918, 1953.
43. Rayer, P.: Traité des maladies des reins, 1840, Baillière, Paris.
44. Pollak, V. E., Kark, R. M., Pirani, C. L., Shafter, H. A., and Muehrcke, R. C.: Renal vein thrombosis and the nephrotic syndrome, Am. J. Med. **21**: 496, 1956.
45. Blainey, J. D., Hardwicke, J., and Whitfield, A. G. W.: The nephrotic syndrome associated with thrombosis of the renal veins, Lancet **2**: 1208, 1954.
46. Squire, J. R., Blainey, J. D., and Hardwicke, J.: The nephrotic syndrome, Brit. M. Bull. **13**: 43, 1957.
47. Goodwin, J. F.: Personal communication, 1956.
48. Shattock, S. G.: Occlusion of inferior vena cava as a result of internal trauma (dissecting varix?), Proc. Roy. Soc. Med. **6** (Path. Sect.): 126–132, 1913.
49. Pollak, V. E., Pirani, C. L., Muehrcke, R. C., Kark, R. M., and Folli, G.: Unpublished observations.
50. Derham, R. J., and Rogerson, M. M.: The Schönlein-Henoch syndrome with particular reference to renal sequelae, Arch. Dis. Childhood **31**: 364, 1956.
51. Muehrcke, R. C., Pirani, C. L., Pollak, V. E., and Kark, R. M.: Primary renal amyloidosis with the nephrotic syndrome studied by serial biopsies of the kidney, Guy's Hosp. Rep. **104**: 312, 1955.
52. Schreiner, G. E.: The differential diagnosis of acute and chronic glomerulonephritis, J. Chron. Dis. **5**: 45, 1957.
53. Muehrcke, R. C., Kark, R. M., Pirani, C. L., and Pollak, V. E.: Lupus nephritis: a clinical and pathologic study based on renal biopsies, Medicine **36**: 1, 1957.
54. Kimmelstiel, P., and Wilson, C.: Intercapillary lesions in glomeruli of kidney, Am. J. Path. **12**: 83, 1936.
55. Lambie, A. T., and Macfarlane, A.: A clinico-pathological study of diabetic glomerulosclerosis, Quart. J. Med. **24**: 125, 1954.
56. Adams, L. J.: Renal complications in young diabetics, Canad. M. A. J. **57**: 540, 1947.
57. Henderson, L. L., Sprague, R. G., and Wagener, H. P.: Intercapillary glomerulosclerosis, Am. J. Med. **3**: 131, 1947.

58. Reid, R. T. W.: Nodular glomerulosclerosis. A study of its incidence, morphology, and associated renal lesions in diabetes mellitus, Australasian Ann. Med. **4**: 44, 1955.
59. Gellman, D. D., Pirani, C. L., Soothill, J. F., Muehrcke, R. C., Maduros, W., and Kark, R. M.: Structure and function in diabetic nephropathy: the importance of diffuse glomerulosclerosis, Clin. Res. **6**: 293, 1958.
60. Laipply, T. C., Eitzen, O., and Dutra, F. R.: Intercapillary glomerulosclerosis, Arch. Int. Med. **74**: 354, 1944.
61. Bell, E. T.: Renal diseases, 2nd Ed., 1950, Lea and Febiger, Philadelphia.
62. Wilson, C.: Personal communication, 1956.
63. Bloom, W. L., and Seegal, D.: The nephrotic phase: its frequency of occurrence and its differential diagnostic value in determining the nature of the renal lesion in 120 patients who died of renal failure, Ann. Int. Med. **25**: 15, 1946.
64. Longcope, W. T.: Studies of the variations in the antistreptolysin titer of the blood serum from patients with hemorrhagic nephritis. II. Observations on patients suffering from streptococcal infections, rheumatic fever and acute and chronic hemorrhagic nephritis, J. Clin. Investigation **15**: 277, 1936.
65. Müller, F.: Morbus Brightii, Verhandl. d. deutsch. path. Gesellsch. **9**: 64, 1905.
66. Munk, F.: Pathologie und Klinik der Nephrosen, Nephritiden und Schrumpfnieren, 1918, Urban and Schwarzenberg, Berlin.
67. Volhard, F., and Fahr, T.: Die Brightsche Nierenkrankheit, 1914, Springer Verlag, Berlin.
68. Farquhar, M. G., Vernier, R. L., and Good, R. A.: Studies on familial nephrosis. II. Glomerular changes observed with the electron microscope, Am. J. Path. **33**: 791, 1957.
69. Folli, G., Pollak, V. E., Reid, R. T. W., Pirani, C. L., and Kark, R. M.: Electronmicroscopic studies of reversible glomerular lesions in adult nephrotic syndrome, Ann. Int. Med. **49**: 775, 1958.
70. Epstein, A. A.: The nature and treatment of chronic parenchymatous nephritis (nephrosis), J. A. M. A. **69**: 444, 1917.
71. Berglund, H., Scriver, W. deM., and Medes, G.: Proteinuria and plasma proteins, *in* Berglund, H., and Medes, G. (ed.): The kidney in health and disease, 1935, Henry Kimpton, London.
72. Hardwicke, J., and Squire, J. R.: Nephrotic syndrome, Brit. M. J. **1**: 875, 1954.
73. Blainey, J. D.: High protein diets in the treatment of the nephrotic syndrome, Clin. Sc. **13**: 567, 1954.
74. Rapoport, M., McCrory, W. W., Barbero, G., Barnett, H. L., Forman, C. W., and McNamara, H.: Effect of ACTH on children with the nephrotic syndrome, J. A. M. A. **147**: 1101, 1951.
75. Lange, K., Slobody, L., and Strang, R.: Prolonged intermittent ACTH and cortisone therapy in the nephrotic syndrome. Immunologic basis and results, Pediatrics **15**: 156, 1955.
76. Riley, C. M., Davis, R. A., Fertig, J. W., and Berger, A. P.: Nephrosis of childhood: statistical evaluation of the effect of adrenocortical-active therapy, J. Chron. Dis. **3**: 640, 1956.
77. Lange, K., Strang, R., Slobody, L. B., and Wenk, E. J.: The treatment of the nephrotic syndrome with steroids in children and adults, Arch. Int. Med. **99**: 760, 1957.

16 March 1999 Volume **130** Number **6**

Annals of Internal Medicine

A More Accurate Method To Estimate Glomerular Filtration Rate from Serum Creatinine: A New Prediction Equation

Andrew S. Levey, MD; Juan P. Bosch, MD; Julia Breyer Lewis, MD; Tom Greene, PhD; Nancy Rogers, MS; and David Roth, MD, for the Modification of Diet in Renal Disease Study Group*

Background: Serum creatinine concentration is widely used as an index of renal function, but this concentration is affected by factors other than glomerular filtration rate (GFR).

Objective: To develop an equation to predict GFR from serum creatinine concentration and other factors.

Design: Cross-sectional study of GFR, creatinine clearance, serum creatinine concentration, and demographic and clinical characteristics in patients with chronic renal disease.

Patients: 1628 patients enrolled in the baseline period of the Modification of Diet in Renal Disease (MDRD) Study, of whom 1070 were randomly selected as the training sample; the remaining 558 patients constituted the validation sample.

Methods: The prediction equation was developed by stepwise regression applied to the training sample. The equation was then tested and compared with other prediction equations in the validation sample.

Results: To simplify prediction of GFR, the equation included only demographic and serum variables. Independent factors associated with a lower GFR included a higher serum creatinine concentration, older age, female sex, nonblack ethnicity, higher serum urea nitrogen levels, and lower serum albumin levels ($P < 0.001$ for all factors). The multiple regression model explained 90.3% of the variance in the logarithm of GFR in the validation sample. Measured creatinine clearance overestimated GFR by 19%, and creatinine clearance predicted by the Cockcroft–Gault formula overestimated GFR by 16%. After adjustment for this overestimation, the percentage of variance of the logarithm of GFR predicted by measured creatinine clearance or the Cockcroft–Gault formula was 86.6% and 84.2%, respectively.

Conclusion: The equation developed from the MDRD Study provided a more accurate estimate of GFR in our study group than measured creatinine clearance or other commonly used equations.

This paper is also available at http://www.acponline.org.

Ann Intern Med. 1999;130:461-470.

* For members of the Modification of Diet in Renal Disease Study Group, see N Engl J Med. 1994;330:877-84.

The glomerular filtration rate (GFR) is traditionally considered the best overall index of renal function in health and disease (1). Because GFR is difficult to measure in clinical practice, most clinicians estimate the GFR from the serum creatinine concentration. However, the accuracy of this estimate is limited because the serum creatinine concentration is affected by factors other than creatinine filtration (2, 3). To circumvent these limitations, several formulas have been developed to estimate creatinine clearance from serum creatinine concentration, age, sex, and body size (4–12). Despite more recent studies that have related serum creatinine concentration to GFR (13–24), no formula is more widely used to predict creatinine clearance than that proposed by Cockcroft and Gault (4). This formula is used to detect the onset of renal insufficiency, to adjust the dose of drugs excreted by the kidney, and to evaluate the effectiveness of therapy for progressive renal disease. More recently, it has been used to document eligibility for reimbursement from the Medicare End Stage Renal Disease Program (25) and for accrual of points for patients on the waiting list for cadaveric renal transplantation (26). Major clinical decisions in general medicine, geriatrics, and oncology (as well as nephrology) are made by using the Cockcroft–Gault formula and other formulas to predict the level of renal function. Therefore, these formulas must predict GFR as accurately as possible.

The Modification of Diet in Renal Disease (MDRD) Study, a multicenter, controlled trial, evaluated the effect of dietary protein restriction and strict blood pressure control on the progression of renal disease (27–30). During the baseline period, GFR, serum creatinine, and several variables that affect the relation between them were measured in patients with chronic renal disease. The purpose of our study was to develop an equation from MDRD Study data that could improve the prediction of GFR from serum creatinine concentration.

Methods

Baseline Cohort and Measurement Methods in the Modification of Diet in Renal Disease Study

The overall study design and methods of recruitment for the MDRD Study have been described elsewhere (31, 32). A total of 1785 patients entered the baseline period. Of these patients, 1628 (91%) also underwent measurement of GFR and the other variables described below; these patients constitute the study group for these analyses.

Glomerular filtration rate was measured as the renal clearance of ^{125}I-iothalamate (33, 34). Creatinine clearance was computed from creatinine excretion in a 24-hour urine collection and a single measurement of serum creatinine. Serum and urine creatinine were measured by using a kinetic alkaline picrate assay with a normal range in serum of 62 to 124 μmol/L (0.7 to 1.4 mg/dL) (35). Glomerular filtration rate and creatinine clearance were expressed per 1.73 m^2 of body surface area by multiplying measured values by 1.73/body surface area (36). The serum and urine specimens were also used for other measurements, including serum albumin (bromcresol green method [35]), serum urea nitrogen (urease method [35]), and urine urea nitrogen (urease method [35]). Protein intake (g/d) was estimated as 6.25 [UUN (g/d) + 0.031 (g/kg per day) SBW (kg)], where UUN is urine urea nitrogen, SBW is standard body weight, and 0.031 g/kg per day is a constant reflecting the rate of excretion of nitrogen in compounds other than urine urea (37, 38). The diagnosis of diabetes and the cause of renal disease were assigned on the basis of chart review at the clinical center (39).

Statistical Analysis

Descriptive Statistics

The relation of renal function measurements to other baseline characteristics was assessed by using contingency tables, *t*-tests, analysis of variance, and linear regression, as appropriate. Nonparametric tests (Wilcoxon rank-sum tests and Kruskal–Wallis tests) gave consistent results. A *P* value less than 0.01 was considered statistically significant.

Multivariable Analysis of Glomerular Filtration Rate

We used stepwise multiple regression to determine a set of variables that jointly predicted GFR. The stepwise regression models were developed by using a training sample consisting of a random sample of 1070 of the 1628 patients. We found that the variability of the difference between the observed and predicted GFR values was greater for higher GFR values. This increase was eliminated by performing multiple regressions on log-transformed data. To facilitate clinical interpretation, the results were re-expressed in terms of the original units. Consequently, the prediction equation is a multiplicative model; regression coefficients refer to the change in geometric mean GFR associated with unit changes in the independent variable. Predicted GFR is expressed in mL/min per 1.73 m^2.

The following variables were considered for possible inclusion in the regression model: weight, height, sex, ethnicity, age, diagnosis of diabetes, serum creatinine concentration, serum urea nitrogen level, serum albumin level, serum phosphorus level, serum calcium level, mean arterial pressure, urine creatinine level, urine urea nitrogen level, urine protein level, and urine phosphorus level. The cause of renal disease was not included because in clinical practice, the cause may be unknown or clinicians may not use the same classification method as the investigators in the MDRD Study. A *P* value less than 0.001 was used as the criterion for entry of a variable into the model. Because of the difficulty in collecting complete 24-hour urine samples in clinical practice, an additional stepwise regression was performed to develop a prediction model that did not include urine biochemistry variables. Finally, because of the interest in developing a prediction equation to assess eligibility for Medicare reimbursement and listing for cadaveric renal transplantation, we repeated the analysis restricting the population to the subgroup of patients with higher serum creatinine concentrations (>221 μmol/L [2.5 mg/dL]; $n = 509$ in the training sample).

Methods for Comparing Equations To Predict Glomerular Filtration Rate

We first developed coefficients for each prediction equation (including the selection of the predictor variables for the stepwise regressions) using the data from the training sample to predict log GFR. Each prediction equation also included a multiplicative constant to account for any consistent bias in the application of that equation in the MDRD Study Group. This was particularly important for equations that are intended to estimate creatinine clearance, which is known to be higher than GFR. The regression coefficients determined in the training sample were then applied to obtain predicted GFRs in a separate validation sample consisting of the remaining 558 patients (172 patients with serum creatinine concentration > 221 μmol/L [2.5 mg/dL]). These predicted GFR values were compared with the actual GFRs in the validation sample to evaluate the performance of each prediction equation. In this way, separate data sets were used to construct the equations and assess their accuracy after removal of systematic bias. For each equation, we computed overall R^2 (percentage of variability in

Table 1. Association of Renal Function with Demographic and Clinical Characteristics, Protein Intake, and Blood Pressure in the Modification of Diet in Renal Disease Study Baseline Cohort*

Characteristic	Glomerular Filtration Rate	Creatinine Clearance	Serum Creatinine Concentration
	$mL \cdot s^{-2} \cdot m^{-2}$ (mL/min per 1.73 m^2)		µmol/L (mg/dL)
Overall (n = 1628)	0.38 ± 0.20 (39.8 ± 21.2)	0.47 ± 0.24 (48.6 ± 24.5)	203 ± 106 (2.3 ± 1.2)
Sex			
Male (n = 983)	0.39 ± 0.2 (40.2 ± 20.4)	0.48 ± 0.24 (49.6 ± 24.8)	212 ± 106 (2.4 ± 1.2)†
Female (n = 645)	0.38 ± 0.21 (39.1 ± 22.3)	0.45 ± 0.23 (47.0 ± 23.9)	177 ± 97 (2.0 ± 1.1)
Ethnicity			
Black (n = 197)	0.42 ± 0.21 (43.6 ± 21.4)†	0.48 ± 0.25 (49.8 ± 25.4)	212 ± 115 (2.4 ± 1.3)
White (n = 1304)	0.38 ± 0.2 (39.2 ± 20.8)	0.47 ± 0.23 (48.3 ± 23.8)	195 ± 97 (2.2 ± 1.1)
Age			
≤55 y (n = 947)	0.4 ± 0.22 (41.5 ± 22.7)†	0.49 ± 0.25 (50.4 ± 26.1)†	203 ± 106 (2.3 ± 1.2)
>55 y (n = 681)	0.36 ± 0.18 (37.4 ± 18.7)	0.44 ± 0.21 (46.0 ± 21.8)	194 ± 97 (2.2 ± 1.1)
Diabetes status			
Diabetic (n = 99)	0.38 ± 0.22 (39.3 ± 23.1)	0.46 ± 0.25 (47.6 ± 25.5)	186 ± 88 (2.1 ± 1.0)
Nondiabetic (n = 1529)	0.38 ± 0.2 (39.8 ± 21.1)	0.47 ± 0.24 (48.7 ± 24.4)	203 ± 106 (2.3 ± 1.2)
Cause of renal disease			
Polycystic kidney disease (n = 364)	0.38 ± 0.22 (39.9 ± 22.5)	0.46 ± 0.24 (47.3 ± 24.6)	203 ± 115 (2.3 ± 1.3)
Glomerular (n = 525)	0.37 ± 0.2 (38.6 ± 21.2)	0.47 ± 0.25 (48.9 ± 25.4)	203 ± 106 (2.3 ± 1.2)
Tubulointerstitial (n = 121)	0.36 ± 0.19 (37.5 ± 19.2)	0.44 ± 0.23 (45.8 ± 24.2)	186 ± 80 (2.1 ± 0.9)
Other or unknown (n = 618)	0.4 ± 0.2 (41.1 ± 20.7)	0.48 ± 0.23 (49.6 ± 23.6)	194 ± 97 (2.2 ± 1.1)
Protein intake‡			
<0.85 g/kg per day (n = 480)	0.32 ± 0.2 (32.9 ± 19.6)	0.35 ± 0.19 (36.6 ± 19.8)	230 ± 124 (2.6 ± 1.4)
0.85–1.05 g/kg per day (n = 585)	0.37 ± 0.18 (38.6 ± 19.1)	0.45 ± 0.2 (47.0 ± 21.2)	203 ± 106 (2.3 ± 1.2)
>1.05 g/kg per day (n = 562)	0.45 ± 0.22 (46.8 ± 22.3)	0.58 ± 0.25 (60.5 ± 25.8)	168 ± 80 (1.9 ± 0.9)
Mean arterial pressure§			
<98 mm Hg (n = 758)	0.4 ± 0.22 (41.0 ± 22.4)	0.48 ± 0.24 (49.7 ± 25.1)	194 ± 97 (2.2 ± 1.1)
98–107 mm Hg (n = 466)	0.38 ± 0.19 (39.3 ± 19.9)	0.47 ± 0.24 (49.2 ± 25.3)	203 ± 106 (2.3 ± 1.2)
>107 mm Hg (n = 404)	0.37 ± 0.19 (38.0 ± 20.1)	0.44 ± 0.21 (45.8 ± 22.1)	212 ± 106 (2.4 ± 1.2)

* Data are given as the mean ± SD and are moderately positively skewed so that mean is slightly higher than the median in each subgroup.
† Subgroup means differ from each other ($P \le 0.01$).
‡ Protein intake was significantly correlated with glomerular filtration rate, creatinine clearance, and serum creatinine concentration ($P < 0.01$).
§ Mean arterial pressure was significantly correlated with serum creatinine concentration ($P < 0.01$).

log GFR explained by the regression model) and the 50th, 75th, and 90th percentiles of the distribution of the percentage absolute difference between measured and predicted GFRs in the validation sample. The 50th percentiles indicate the typical size of the errors in prediction of GFR, and the 75th and 90th percentiles assess the sizes of the larger errors that occurred for each model.

Development of Final Prediction Equations

To improve the accuracy of the final MDRD Study prediction equations, the regression coefficients derived from the training sample were updated on the basis of data from all 1628 patients. As a result, the standard errors of the regression coefficients in the final MDRD Study prediction equations are slightly smaller than those derived from the training sample; thus, the accuracy of the final prediction equations may be slightly better (by about 0.1% to 0.2%) than their accuracy as assessed in the validation sample.

Results

Demographic and Clinical Characteristics

The mean age (± SD) of the cohort was 50.6 ± 12.7 years. Sixty percent of patients were male, 88% were white, and 6% were diabetic. Causes of renal disease were glomerular disease (32%), polycystic kidney disease (22%), tubulointerstitial disease (7%), and other or unknown renal diseases (40%). Mean protein intake was 0.99 ± 0.24 g/kg of body weight per day and mean arterial pressure was 99.4 ± 12.2 mm Hg. Mean weight was 79.6 ± 16.8 kg, body surface area was 1.91 ± 0.23 m^2, serum urea nitrogen concentration was 11.4 ± 5.7 mmol/L [32 ± 16 mg/dL], and serum albumin concentration was 40.0 ± 4.0 g/L [4.0 ± 0.4 g/dL], respectively.

Glomerular Filtration Rate, Creatinine Clearance, and Serum Creatinine Concentration

Renal function measurements for the study group and for various subgroups are shown in **Table 1**. Mean GFR for the population was 0.38 $mL \cdot s^{-2} \cdot m^{-2}$ (39.8 mL/min per 1.73 m^2), with lower values in patients with lower protein intake, white patients compared with black patients, and older patients (≥55 years) compared with younger patients ($P <$ 0.01). The mean value of creatinine clearance was 0.81 $mL \cdot s^{-2} \cdot m^{-2}$ (48.6 mL/min per 1.73 m^2) and was lower in older patients and patients with lower protein intake ($P \le 0.01$). The mean serum creatinine concentration was 203 µmol/L (2.3 mg/dL) and was higher in men, patients with lower protein intake, and patients with higher mean arterial pressure ($P \le 0.01$). **Figure 1** shows the well-known reciprocal relation of serum creatinine concentra-

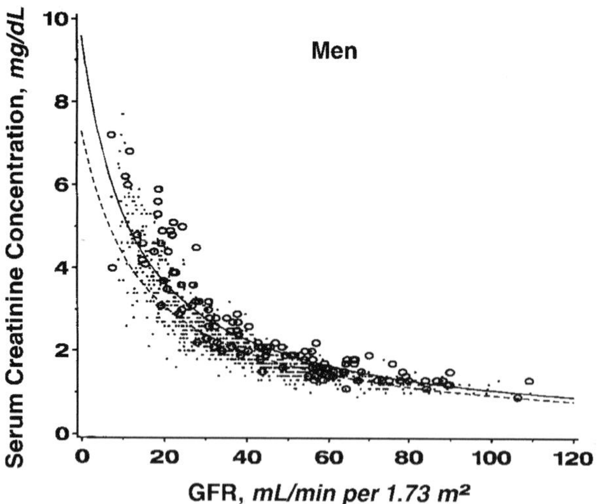

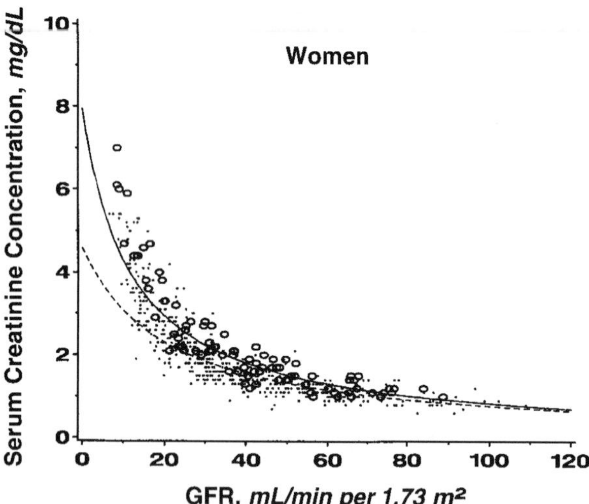

Figure 1. Relation of serum creatinine concentration to measured glomerular filtration rate (*GFR*). Each point represents the baseline measurement for one patient during the MDRD Study. Glomerular filtration rate was measured as the renal clearance of ^{125}I-iothalamate. Serum creatinine concentration (P_{cr}) was measured by using a kinetic alkaline picrate assay. Values are shown separately for men (n = 915) and women (n = 586) by ethnicity (white persons [*dashed lines and dots*] and black persons [*solid lines and circles*]). Regression lines were computed from the relation $1/P_{cr}$ compared with GFR. Black men (n = 113) have higher serum creatinine values than white men (n = 802) ($P < 0.001$); black women (n = 84) have higher serum creatinine values than white women (n = 502) ($P < 0.001$). To convert mL/min per 1.73 m² to $mL \cdot s^{-2} \cdot m^{-2}$, multiply by 0.00963. To convert mg/dL to μmol/L, multiply by 88.4.

tion to GFR for subgroups based on sex and ethnicity. At any given GFR, the serum creatinine concentration is significantly higher in men than in women and in black persons than in white persons ($P < 0.001$).

Relation among Clearance Measurements and Prediction of Glomerular Filtration Rate from Transformations of Serum Creatinine Concentration

The relations of GFR to creatinine and urea clearances are shown in **Figure 2**. Creatinine clearance usually exceeds GFR because of tubular secretion, whereas urea clearance is usually lower than GFR because of tubular reabsorption. The mean of creatinine and urea clearances provides a more accurate estimate of GFR. The relations of GFR to the reciprocal of serum creatinine (P_{cr}) × 100 ($100/P_{cr}$) and creatinine clearance predicted by the Cockcroft–Gault equation are also shown in **Figure 2**. As did measured creatinine clearance, the Cockcroft–Gault equation yielded values that were higher than the actual values for GFR.

Prediction of Glomerular Filtration Rate from Multiple Regression Models Derived from the Modification of Diet in Renal Disease Study

We developed equations to predict log GFR using stepwise regression applied to a randomly selected training sample of 1070 patients. We then validated the equations in the remaining 558 patients. Only variables with a P value less than 0.001 were included in the final models. In this section, we describe the final models on the basis of data from all 1628 patients. **Table 2** shows the variables in the final models. The prediction equations (equations 6 and 7) are shown in **Table 3**. As expected, predicted GFR does not systematically deviate from measured GFR (**Figure 3**), although a few values for measured GFR are below predicted values when GFR is normal or high.

As in the Cockcroft–Gault equation, the reciprocal of serum creatinine concentration is included in both models. The reciprocal of serum urea nitrogen concentration was also an independent predictor of GFR; this probably reflects the relation between GFR and urea clearance. Both urea and creatinine undergo glomerular filtration but are handled differently by the renal tubules; thus, it is not surprising that the serum levels of urea nitrogen and creatinine, although both are related to the level of GFR, would vary independently.

Older age and female sex were independent predictors of lower GFR, presumably reflecting the well-known relations of age and sex to muscle mass (40). Lower muscle mass, as observed in older persons and in women, causes lower urine creatinine excretion and, therefore, lower serum creatinine concentration at any GFR. Body size is also associated with urine creatinine excretion. However, because equations from the MDRD Study predict GFR adjusted for body surface area, neither height nor weight was an independent predictor of adjusted GFR. Black ethnicity was an independent predictor of higher GFR. Previous studies have shown that on average, black persons have greater muscle mass than white persons (41–43). In other analyses, we found that black ethnicity was an independent predictor of higher urine creatinine excretion (data not shown).

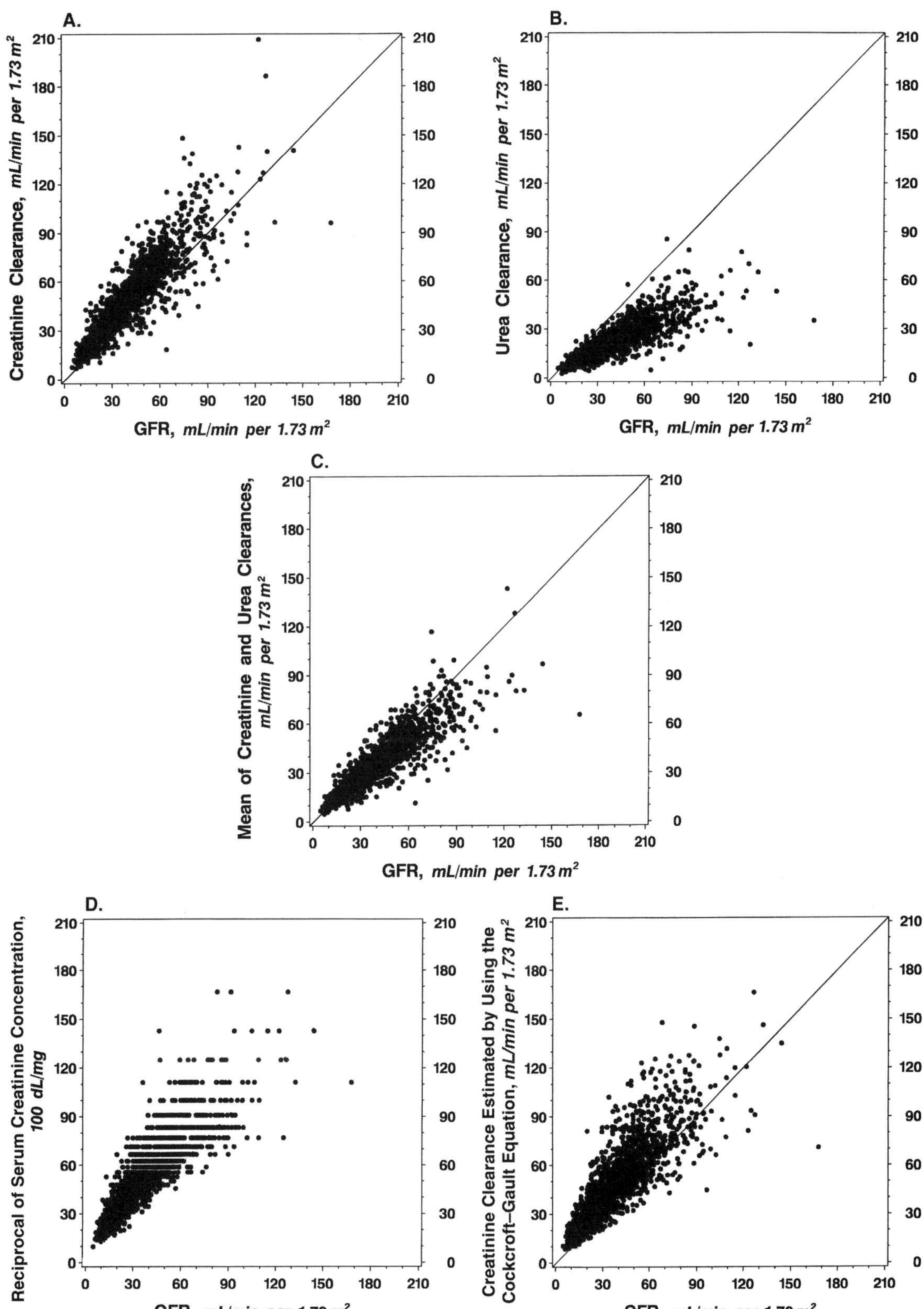

Figure 2. Relation of measured creatinine and urea clearances and transformations of serum creatinine concentration (P_{cr}) to measured glomerular filtration rate (*GFR*). Each point represents the baseline measurement during the Modification of Diet in Renal Disease Study (n = 1628). Correlations are shown for GFR, measured as the renal clearance of ^{125}I-iothalamate. Solid lines are lines of identity. **A.** Creatinine clearance. **B.** Urea clearance. **C.** The mean of creatinine and urea clearances. **D.** Reciprocal of serum creatinine, ×100. **E.** Creatinine clearance estimated by the Cockcroft–Gault formula: $C_{cr} = [(140 - \text{age}) \times \text{weight}]/(P_{cr} \times 72)$ for men or $C_{cr} = [(140 - \text{age}) - \text{weight}]/(P_{cr} \times 85)$ for women, where C_{cr} is creatinine clearance and is given in mL/min, P_{cr} is serum creatinine concentration and is given in mg/dL, age is given in years, and weight is given in kg. Estimated creatinine clearance was then adjusted for body surface area and expressed per 1.73 m^2. To convert mL/min to mL/s, multiply by 0.01667; to convert mL/min per 1.73 m^2 to mL · s^{-2} · m^{-2}, multiply by 0.00963; to convert mg/dL to μmol/L, multiply by 88.4.

Table 2. Multiple Regression Models To Predict Glomerular Filtration Rate (mL/min per 1.73 m²) from Serum Creatinine Concentration*

Variable	Change in GFR per 10% Change in Variable (95% CI)		Multiplication Factor for GFR (95% CI)	
	Model Based on Demographic, Serum, and Urine Variables (Equation 6)	Model Based on Demographic and Serum Variables Only (Equation 7)	Model Based on Demographic, Serum, and Urine Variables (Equation 6)	Model Based on Demographic and Serum Variables Only (Equation 7)
	%			
Continuous				
Serum creatinine concentration	−7.8 (−8.2 to −7.5)	−9.1 (−9.4 to −8.8)	–	–
Age	−1.6 (−1.9 to −1.3)	−1.7 (−2.0 to −1.4)	–	–
Serum urea nitrogen concentration	−2.7 (−3.1 to −2.4)	−1.6 (−1.9 to −1.3)	–	–
Urine urea nitrogen concentration	2.4 (2.1 to 2.7)	–	–	–
Serum albumin concentration	–	3.1 (2.1 to 4.0)	–	–
Dichotomous				
Sex (female)	–	–	0.82 (0.80 to 0.84)	0.76 (0.75 to 0.78)
Ethnicity (black)	–	–	1.18 (1.15 to 1.21)	1.18 (1.15 to 1.21)

* GFR = glomerular filtration rate; $P < 0.001$ for all variables.

In equation 6 (the model including urine biochemistry variables), lower urine urea nitrogen excretion was also an independent predictor of lower GFR, which could reflect the association of lower protein intake with lower GFR. In the randomized cohort of the MDRD Study, we previously showed that lower protein intake causes a reduction in GFR (44, 45). Alternatively, the relation between GFR and urine urea nitrogen that we saw in the baseline cohort may reflect a spontaneous reduction in protein intake that occurs as renal function declines in chronic renal disease. In equation 7 (the model excluding urine biochemistry values), serum albumin concentration seems to substitute for urine urea nitrogen concentration with little loss of accuracy; this may also reflect protein intake.

A diagnosis of diabetes was not an independent predictor of GFR. Some authors have suggested that the relation between serum creatinine concentration and GFR differs between diabetic and nondiabetic patients. In other analyses (data not shown), a term for diabetes forced into the multivariable model (equation 7) was nonsignificant ($P = 0.19$).

Table 3. Comparison of Equations To Predict Glomerular Filtration Rate (mL/min per 1.73 m²) from Serum Creatinine Concentration*

Equation 1: Serum creatinine
GFR = $0.69 \times [100/P_{cr}]$
Equation 2: Cockcroft–Gault formula
GFR = $0.84 \times$ [Cockcroft–Gault formula]
Equation 3: Creatinine clearance
GFR = $0.81 \times [C_{cr}]$
Equation 4: Average of creatinine and urea clearance
GFR = $1.11 \times [(C_{cr} + C_{urea})/2]$
Equation 5: Creatinine clearance, urea clearance, and demographic variables
GFR = $1.04 \times [C_{cr}]^{+0.751} \times [C_{urea}]^{+0.226} \times$ [1.109 if patient is black]
Equation 6: Demographic, serum, and urine variables
GFR = $198 \times [P_{cr}]^{-0.858} \times [\text{Age}]^{-0.167} \times$ [0.822 if patient is female] $\times$ [1.178 if patient is black] $\times [\text{SUN}]^{-0.293} \times [\text{UUN}]^{+0.249}$
Equation 7: Demographic and serum variables only
GFR = $170 \times [P_{cr}]^{-0.999} \times [\text{Age}]^{-0.176} \times$ [0.762 if patient is female] $\times$ [1.180 if patient is black] $\times [\text{SUN}]^{-0.170} \times [\text{Alb}]^{+0.318}$

* Cockcroft–Gault formula and creatinine clearance are adjusted for body surface area. Age, sex, and weight each had a P value > 0.75; none of them entered equation 5. Alb = serum albumin concentration (g/dL); C_{cr} = creatinine clearance (mL/min per 1.73 m²); C_{urea} = urea clearance (mL/min per 1.73 m²); P_{cr} = serum creatinine concentration (mg/dL); SUN = serum urea nitrogen concentration (mg/dL); UUN = urine urea nitrogen concentration (g/d).

For both multiple regression models, serum creatinine concentration was the most important predictor variable. Variability in serum creatinine concentration accounted for 80.4% of the variability in GFR (R^2, data not shown). **Table 2** shows the expected changes in mean GFR for 10% changes in continuous variables (serum creatinine level, age, serum urea nitrogen level, urine urea nitrogen level, and serum albumin level). For example, a 10% increase in serum creatinine was associated with a 7.8% and 9.1% decrease in mean GFR, respectively, in both multiple regression models (equations 6 and 7), assuming no change in the remaining variables. **Table 2** lists multiplication factors for dichotomous variables (sex and ethnicity). For example, in both models, black ethnicity was associated with a multiplication factor of 1.18, indicating that the expected mean GFR is 18% higher for black persons than for white persons when the same values are assumed for the other predictor variables.

Comparison of Prediction Equations

We compared the seven equations (**Table 3**) for their performance in predicting log GFR in the validation sample (**Figure 4**). The maximal R^2 value (91.2%) was associated with the multiple regression model that included urine biochemistry variables (equation 6). The multiple regression model derived from only demographic and serum biochemistry values (equation 7) was only slightly less precise ($R^2 = 90.3\%$). The differences in R^2 among the equations may seem small, but the accuracy of equations 6 and 7 compared with equation 1 reflects a reduction in unexplained variance ($1 - R^2$) by more than half (from 19.6% to a range of 8.8% to 9.7%).

The improvement in performance can also be shown by comparing the percentage absolute differences between the predicted and measured GFR values for each equation (**Figure 4**). A lower percentage absolute difference indicates a more narrow distribution of predicted GFR values, which reflects a more accurate estimate of measured GFR. The multiple regression models (equations 6 and 7) were the most accurate, especially for the 75th and 90th percentiles of the percentage absolute differences. Of note, equation 7, which does not require urine collection, provided a more precise estimate of GFR than the measured creatinine clearance (equation 3) or the equations based on measured creatinine and urea clearances (equations 5 and 6).

Each of the alternative prediction equations in **Table 3** included a multiplication factor derived from the training sample to correct for bias before comparisons with the MDRD Study prediction equations. For example, creatinine clearance predicted by the Cockcroft–Gault equation overestimated measured GFR by 16%. In clinical practice, such bias adjustments are not usually made. Thus, in clinical settings, the difference in performance among the equations from the MDRD Study and the alternative methods can be expected to be greater than that suggested by **Figure 4**. Without adjustments for bias, the median absolute errors (and the median percentage absolute errors) for the Cockcroft–Gault equation and equation 7 (from the MDRD Study) were 6.8 mL/min per 1.73 m^2 (19.8%) and 3.8 mL/min per 1.73 m^2 (11.5%), respectively. The 75th percentile of the percentage absolute errors was 12.2 mL/min per 1.73 m^2 (33.5%) for the Cockcroft–Gault equation and 6.9 mL/min per 1.73 m^2 (19.8%) for equation 7. The 90th percentile of the percentage absolute errors was 19.1 mL/min per 1.73 m^2 (47.5%) for the Cockcroft–Gault equation and 12.9 mL/min per 1.73 m^2 (28.4%) for equation 7.

Comparison of Prediction Equations in Patients with Higher Serum Creatinine Concentrations

In the subgroup of patients with serum creatinine concentrations greater than 221 μmol/L (2.5 mg/dL), the median percentage absolute differences in the validation sample between measured GFR and GFR predicted from equations 6 and 7 were similar to results obtained with data from the full study group (**Figure 4**). Values for R^2 were not computed for the subgroup because of the smaller range of GFR. We also compared the MDRD Study prediction equations to the three prediction equations reported by Walser and coworkers (22), which were derived from patients with higher concentrations of

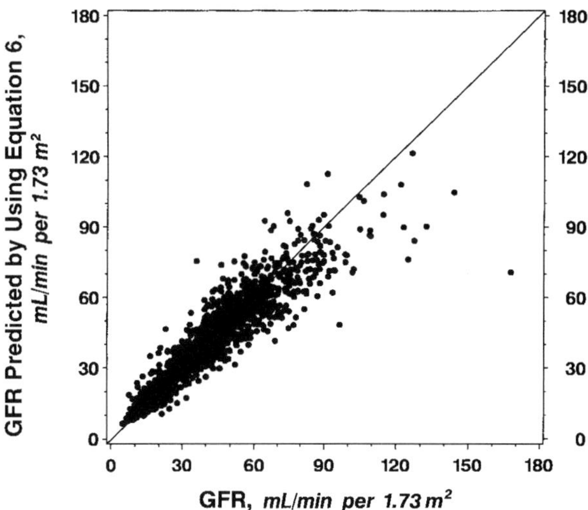

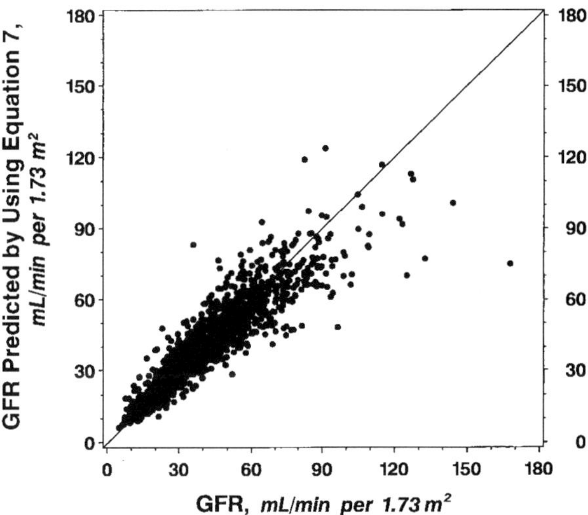

Figure 3. Relation of predicted glomerular filtration rate (*GFR*) to measured GFR. Each point represents the baseline measurement during the Modification of Diet in Renal Disease (MDRD) Study ($n = 1628$). **Top.** Glomerular filtration rate predicted by using MDRD Study equation 6. **Bottom.** Glomerular filtration rate predicted by using MDRD Study equation 7. Solid lines are lines of identity. To convert mL/min per 1.73 m^2 to $mL \cdot s^{-2} \cdot m^{-2}$, multiply by 0.00963.

serum creatinine ($\geq$177 μmol/L [2.0 mg/dL]) who underwent repeated measurement of GFR by renal clearance of ^{99m}Tc-diethylenetriamine pentaacetic acid. The absolute differences between predicted and measured GFR were consistently higher for the Walser equations than for the MDRD Study equations (14.2% to 16.7% for the median percentage absolute error, 25.7% to 25.9% for the 75th percentile of the absolute error, and 35.5% to 41.3% for the 90th percentile of the absolute error).

Discussion

The systematic evaluation of many patients with chronic renal disease during the baseline period of the MDRD Study allowed us to evaluate the relation of serum creatinine concentration to GFR. Using this large database and multiple regression analy-

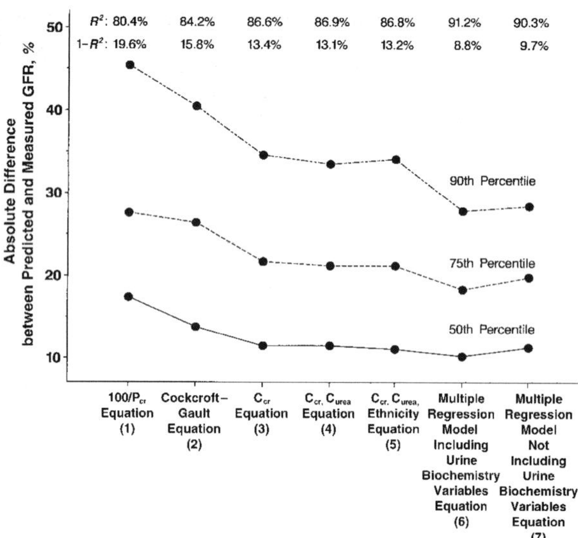

Figure 4. Comparison of equations to predict glomerular filtration rate (*GFR*). The values of R^2 indicate the percentage of variance of log GFR accounted for in the validation sample (n = 558) by equations derived from the training sample (n = 1070). The values of $1 - R^2$ indicate the percentage of variance in log GFR that is unexplained by each equation. C_{cr} = creatinine clearance; C_{urea} = urea clearance; P_{cr} = serum creatinine concentration.

ses, we developed equations for predicting GFR from the serum creatinine concentration and compared them with other equations. The equations based on measured or estimated creatinine clearance systematically overestimated GFR. Even after adjustment to correct for these systematic errors, variability in predicted GFR compared with measured GFR was lowest in the regression equations developed from the MDRD Study database (R^2 = 91.2% for equations 6 and 90.3% for equation 7) (**Table 3**). Furthermore, accuracy was maintained even when the validation sample was restricted to patients with higher concentrations of serum creatinine (≥221 μmol/L [2.5 mg/dL]). Therefore, the MDRD Study prediction equations seem to be more accurate (they demonstrate less bias and greater precision) in predicting GFR than measured creatinine clearance or other commonly used equations.

Factors associated with creatinine excretion, such as age, sex, and ethnicity, are included in the equations from the MDRD Study and contribute to their accuracy. However, equations 6 and 7 do not include urine creatinine excretion and both equations provide a more accurate estimate of GFR than does measured creatinine clearance. Eliminating 24-hour urine collections for the clinical estimation of renal function (equation 7) would simplify the procedures used in most general medicine, geriatric, oncology, and nephrology practices.

Inaccurate estimation of the level of renal function can lead to failure to identify the onset of renal insufficiency and end-stage renal disease and to errors in the prescribed dosage of drugs for patients with chronic renal disease. **Table 4** gives examples of creatinine clearance predicted from the Cockcroft–Gault equation and GFR predicted from the MDRD Study equation (equation 7) for hypothetical patients with varying serum creatinine concentrations and other characteristics. These examples demonstrate the wide range of values of renal function predicted in patients with the same value for serum creatinine (124 or 354 μmol/L [1.4 or 4.0 mg/dL]). Most important, these examples show that the predicted level of renal function is lower, especially in older persons and in women, than might have been anticipated from inspection of the serum creatinine alone, as is usually done in clinical practice. Patients with a serum creatinine concentration of 124 μmol/L (1.4 mg/dL), a value within the normal range in many clinical laboratories, would have renal insufficiency, as defined by serum creatinine concentration, creatinine clearance, or GFR less than two standard deviations below the normal range. Patients with a serum creatinine concentration of 354 μmol/L (4.0 mg/dL) would be approaching end-stage renal disease, as defined by a GFR less than 0.0963 $mL \cdot s^{-2} \cdot m^{-2}$ (10 mL/min per 1.73 m^2). These examples emphasize the importance of routinely using an equation to estimate the level of renal function.

The MDRD Study prediction equation (equation 7), which could be easily implemented in clinical practice, has several advantages over other equations. Equation 7 predicts GFR rather than creatinine clearance; uses a validated method for measuring GFR (renal clearance of ^{125}I-iothalamate) (33, 34); uses the method for measuring serum creatinine (the kinetic alkaline picrate reaction) that has been most widely accepted in U.S. clinical laboratories (46); has been validated in a cohort of patients (the validation sample) that differed from the cohort used to derive it (the training sample); predicts GFR over a wide range of values and can therefore be used for various purposes (including adjusting the doses of medications excreted by glomerular filtration, identifying renal insufficiency, assessing the progression of renal disease, and detecting the onset of end-stage renal disease); seems to be more accurate than the other equations tested; does not require collection of a timed urine sample or measurement of height and weight; includes a term for ethnicity (which is important because chronic renal disease is more prevalent among black persons); and does not require knowledge of the cause of renal disease. In addition, the required demographic data are readily available, and the measurements of urea nitrogen and albumin can be obtained from the same serum sample used for measurement of creatinine. The predicted GFR could be computed and reported by the clinical laboratory that receives the blood sample and patient demographic data.

However, there are disadvantages to using the MDRD Study prediction equation. First, the validation sample was drawn from the same population as the training sample. Thus, the performance of the MDRD Study equation in populations with different distributions of patient characteristics may not be the same as the performance seen in the MDRD Study validation sample. However, the MDRD Study prediction equation performed consistently well in each of the patient subgroups indicated in **Table 1** (data not shown), suggesting that it may perform relatively well in populations with different proportions of patients in these particular subgroups.

Second, the prediction equation has not been tested in all subgroups. For example, persons without renal disease, persons with type 1 diabetes, and persons with type 2 diabetes who receive insulin, children (persons < 18 years of age), elderly persons (persons > 70 years of age), pregnant women, patients with serious comorbid conditions, and renal transplant recipients were not eligible for entry into the MDRD Study during the baseline period. In addition, the prediction equation has been tested in relatively few black persons ($n = 197$; 12%) and persons with type 2 diabetes who are not receiving insulin ($n = 99$ [6%]). It has not been tested in patients with extreme values for serum albumin concentration. Reduction in serum albumin concentration may be caused by factors other than reduction in dietary protein intake, such as major surgery, liver disease, systemic inflammatory disease, malignant conditions, or severe cases of the nephrotic syndrome. However, to our knowledge, no other prediction equation has been tested in such a large number of patients with diverse characteristics and diverse causes of chronic renal disease. Studies in different populations would help establish further usefulness of the MDRD Study prediction equation.

Third, determination of the correct drug dosage may require computation of GFR that is not adjusted for body surface area (mL/min). Unadjusted GFR can be computed by multiplying the value of predicted GFR by the term body surface area/1.73 m^2 without loss of accuracy. Fourth, as with all prediction equations based on serum creatinine concentration, the MDRD Study prediction equation is inaccurate for patients not in a steady state of creatinine balance (such as patients with acute renal failure). The equation is also inaccurate for patients in whom drugs or medical conditions interfere with creatinine secretion (for example, cimetidine or trimethoprim therapy) or creatinine assay (for example, diabetic ketoacidosis or administration of certain cephalosporins). In these circumstances, accurate assessment of GFR requires clearance measurements.

In principle, the MDRD Study prediction equation could also be used to assess the level of renal function in clinical research studies. In particular, we and others (44) have shown that the serum creatinine concentration can be misleading when used to judge the efficacy of therapies designed to slow the progression of chronic renal disease, especially dietary protein restriction. Whether assessment of changes in predicted GFR would be more useful than measurements of changes in serum creatinine concentration has not been evaluated.

In summary, we have developed a new equation (**Table 3**, equation 7) to predict GFR that uses serum creatinine concentration, demographic characteristics (age, sex, and ethnicity), and other serum measurements (urea nitrogen and albumin concentrations) and is more accurate than other widely used prediction equations. The process of computing and reporting GFR that is predicted from serum creatinine concentrations could be implemented in clinical laboratories by routinely requesting patient demographic data and by measuring serum urea nitrogen and serum albumin levels in addition to serum creatinine levels. We recommend routinely using the MDRD Study prediction equation to predict GFR from serum creatinine concentration.

Note Added in Proof: Since submission of the manuscript, additional studies have been performed that

Table 4. Examples of Estimating Renal Function from Serum Creatinine by Using the Cockcroft–Gault Equation and Modification of Diet in Renal Disease Study Prediction Equation*

P_{cr}	Age	Sex	Ethnicity	Predicted C_{cr}†	Predicted GFR‡
mg/dL	*y*			*mL/min*	*mL/min per 1.73 m^2*
1.4	45	Male	White	71	58
1.4	45	Male	Black	71	68
1.4	45	Female	White	52	44
1.4	45	Female	Black	52	52
1.4	70	Male	White	52	54
1.4	70	Male	Black	52	63
1.4	70	Female	White	38	41
1.4	70	Female	Black	38	48
4.0	45	Male	White	25	17
4.0	45	Male	Black	25	20
4.0	45	Female	White	18	13
4.0	45	Female	Black	18	15
4.0	70	Male	White	18	15
4.0	70	Male	Black	18	18
4.0	70	Female	White	13	12
4.0	70	Female	Black	13	14

* C_{cr} = creatinine clearance; GFR = glomerular filtration rate; P_{cr} = serum creatinine concentration.

† Determined by using the Cockcroft–Gault formula, assuming body weight of 75 kg in men and 65 kg in women. Predicted C_{cr} is multiplied by 0.85 in women. The normal mean value for C_{cr} is 140 and 125 mL/min per 1.73 m^2 in young men and young women, respectively. The normal standard deviation is approximately 20 mL/min per 1.73 m^2. To convert mL/min to mL/s, multiply by 0.01667.

‡ Determined by using Modification of Diet in Renal Disease Study equation 7, assuming 1) serum urea nitrogen concentration of 20 mg/dL and serum albumin concentration of 4.0 mg/dL when serum creatinine concentration is 1.4 mg/dL and 2) serum urea concentration of 50 mg/dL and serum albumin concentration of 3.5 mg/dL when serum creatinine concentration is 4.0 mg/dL. The normal mean value for GFR (insulin clearance) is 130 and 120 mL/min per 1.73 m^2 in young men and young women, respectively. The normal standard deviation is approximately 20 mL/min per 1.73 m^2. To convert mL/min per 1.73 m^2 to $mL \cdot s^{-2} \cdot m^{-2}$, multiply by 0.00963.

validate the MDRD Study prediction equation in other groups of patients with chronic renal disease, including MDRD Study randomly assigned patients at the onset of end-stage renal disease (47), black persons with hypertensive renal disease (48), and renal transplant recipients (with a high proportion of diabetic patients) (49). The equation has not been validated in persons without renal disease.

Presented in part at the Seventh International Congress on Nutrition and Metabolism in Renal Disease, Stockholm, Sweden, 29 May–1 June 1994, and the 30th Annual Meeting of the American Society of Nephrology, San Antonio, Texas, 2–6 November 1997.

Grant Support: By the National Institute of Diabetes and Digestive and Kidney Diseases and the Health Care Financing Administration.

Requests for Reprints: Andrew S. Levey, MD, New England Medical Center, 750 Washington Street, Box 391, Boston, MA 02111.

Current Author Addresses: Dr. Levey: New England Medical Center, 750 Washington Street, Box 391, Boston, MA 02111; e-mail, Andrew.Levey@es.nemc.org.
Dr. Bosch: George Washington University, 901 23rd Street SW, Washington, DC 20037.
Dr. Lewis and Ms. Rogers: Vanderbilt University Medical Center, 1211 22nd Avenue S, Nashville, TN 37232.
Dr. Greene: Cleveland Clinic Foundation, 9500 Euclid Avenue, Cleveland, OH 44195.
Dr. Roth: University of Miami Medical Center, 1475 NW 12th Avenue, Miami, FL 33136.

References

1. **Smith HW.** Diseases of the kidney and urinary tract. In: The Kidney: Structure and Function in Health and Disease. New York: Oxford Univ Pr; 1951:836-87.
2. **Levey AS.** Measurement of renal function in chronic renal disease. Kidney Int. 1990;38:167-84.
3. **Perrone RD, Madias NE, Levey AS.** Serum creatinine as an index of renal function: new insights into old concepts. Clinical Chem. 1992;38:1933-53.
4. **Cockcroft DW, Gault MH.** Prediction of creatinine clearance from serum creatinine. Nephron. 1976;16:31-41.
5. **Parker RA, Bennett WM, Porter GA.** Clinical estimation of creatinine clearance without urine collection. Dialysis and Transplantation. 1980;9:251-2.
6. **Sawyer WT, Canaday BR, Poe TE, Webb CE, Gal P, Joyner PU, et al.** Variables affecting creatinine clearance prediction. Am J Hosp Pharm. 1983; 40:2175-80.
7. **Bjornsson TD, Cocchetto DM, McGowan FX, Verghese CP, Sedor F.** Nomogram for estimating creatinine clearance. Clin Pharmacokinet. 1983;8:365-9.
8. **Taylor GO, Bamgboye EA, Oyediran AB, Longe O.** Serum creatinine and prediction formulae for creatinine clearance. Afr J Med Med Sci. 1982;11:175-81.
9. **Gates GF.** Creatinine clearance estimation from serum creatinine values: an analysis of three mathematical models of glomerular function. Am J Kidney Dis. 1985;5:199-205.
10. **Jelliffe RW.** Creatinine clearance: bedside estimate [Letter]. Ann Intern Med. 1973;79:604-5.
11. **Hallynck T, Soep HH, Thomis J, Boelaert J, Daneels R, Fillastre JP, et al.** Prediction of creatinine clearance from serum creatinine concentration based on lean body mass. Clin Pharm Ther. 1981;30:414-21.
12. **Kampmann J, Siersbaek-Nielsen K, Kristensen M, Hansen JM.** Rapid evaluation of creatinine clearance. Acta Med Scand. 1974;196:517-20.
13. **Bröchner-Mortensen J, Rödbro P.** Selection of routine method for determination of glomerular filtration rate in adult patients. Scand J Clin Lab Invest. 1976;36:35-43.
14. **Tessitore N, Lo Schiavo C, Corgnati A, Previato G, Valvo E, Lupo A, et al.** 125I-iothalamate and creatinine clearances in patients with chronic renal diseases. Nephron. 1979;24:41-5.
15. **Bauer JH, Brooks CS, Burch RN.** Renal function studies in man with advanced renal insufficiency. Am J Kidney Dis. 1982;2:30-5.
16. **Van Lente F, Suit P.** Assessment of renal function by serum creatinine and creatinine clearance: glomerular filtration rate estimated by four procedures. Clin Chem. 1989;35:2326-30.
17. **Trollfors B, Alestig K, Jagenburg R.** Prediction of glomerular filtration rate from serum creatinine, age, sex and body weight. Acta Med Scand. 1987; 221:495-8.
18. **Groth S, Aasted M, Vestergaard B.** Screening of kidney function by plasma creatinine and single-sample 51Cr-EDTA clearance determination—a comparison. Scand J Clin Lab Invest. 1989;49:707-10.
19. **Lemann J, Bidani AK, Bain RP, Lewis EJ, Ronde RD.** Use of the serum creatinine to estimate glomerular filtration rate in health and early diabetic nephropathy. Collaborative Study Group of Angiotensin Converting Enzyme Inhibition in Diabetic Nephropathy. Am J Kidney Dis. 1990;16:236-43.
20. **DeSanto NG, Coppola S, Anastasio P, Coscarella G, Capasso G, Bellini L, et al.** Predicted creatinine clearance to assess glomerular filtration rate in chronic renal disease in humans. Am J Nephrol. 1991;11:181-5.
21. **Sampson MJ, Drury PL.** Accurate estimation of glomerular filtration rate in diabetic nephropathy from age, body weight, and serum creatinine. Diabetes Care. 1992;15:609-12.
22. **Walser M, Drew HH, Guldan JL.** Prediction of glomerular filtration rate from serum creatinine concentration in advanced chronic renal failure. Kidney Int. 1993;44:1145-8.
23. **Cochran M, St John A.** A comparison between estimates of GFR using [99mTc]DTPA clearance and the approximation of Cockroft and Gault. Aust N Z J Med. 1993;23:494-7.
24. **Pollock C, Gyory AZ, Hawkins T, Ross M, Ibels L.** Comparison of simultaneous renal clearances of true endogenous creatinine and subcutaneously administered iothalamate in man. Am J Nephrol. 1995;15:277-82.
25. **U.S. Department of Health and Human Services.** HCFA-2728-U4 (4-95). Form Approved: OMB No. 0938-0046, Health Care Financing Administration.
26. **American Society of Transplant Physicians.** Scientific Symposium on Listing Criteria: Kidney. Bethesda, MD; 30 January 1997.
27. **Klahr S, Levey AS, Beck GJ, Caggiula AW, Hunsicker L, Kusek JW, Striker G.** The effects of dietary protein restriction and blood-pressure control on the progression of renal disease. Modification of Diet in Renal Disease Study Group. N Engl J Med. 1994;330:877-84.
28. **Peterson JC, Adler S, Burkhart JM, Greene T, Hebert LA, King AJ, et al.** Blood pressure control, proteinuria, and the progression of renal disease. The Modification of Diet in Renal Disease Study. Ann Intern Med. 1995;123:754-62.
29. **Levey AS, Adler S, Caggiula AW, England BK, Greene T, Hunsicker LG, et al.** Effects of dietary protein restriction on the progression of advanced renal disease in the Modification of Diet in Renal Disease Study. Am J Kidney Dis. 1996;27:652-63.
30. Effects of dietary protein restriction on the progression of moderate renal disease in the Modification of Diet in Renal Disease Study. J Am Soc Nephrol. 1996;7:2616-25.
31. **Beck GJ, Berg RL, Coggins CH, Gassman JJ, Hunsicker LG, Williams GW.** Design and statistical issues of the Modification of Diet in Renal Disease Trial. The Modification of Diet in Renal Disease Study Group. Control Clin Trials. 1991;12:566-86.
32. **Kusek JW, Coyne T, de Velasco A, Drabik MJ, Finlay RA, Gassman JJ, et al.** Recruitment experience in the full-scale phase of the Modification of Diet in Renal Disease Study. Control Clin Trials. 1993;14:538-57.
33. **Perrone R, Steinman TI, Beck GJ, Skibinski CI, Royal H, Lawlor M, et al.** Utility of radioisotopic filtration markers in chronic renal insufficiency: simultaneous comparison of ^{125}I-iothalamate, ^{169}Yb-DTPA, ^{99m}Tc-DTPA, and inulin. The Modification of Diet in Renal Disease Study Group. Am J Kidney Dis. 1990;16:224-35.
34. **Levey AS, Greene T, Schluchter MD, Cleary PA, Teschan PE, Lorenz RA, et al.** Glomerular filtration rate measurements in clinical trials. Modification of Diet in Renal Disease Study Group and the Diabetes Control and Complications Trial Research Group. J Am Soc Nephrol. 1993;4:1159-71.
35. Astra-8 Operations Manual. Fullerton, CA: Beckman.
36. **DuBois D, DuBois EF.** A formula to estimate the approximate surface area if height and weight be known. Arch Intern Med. 1916;17:863-71.
37. **Frisancho AR.** Anthropometric Standards for the Assessment of Growth and Nutritional Status. Ann Arbor, MI: Univ of Michigan Pr; 1990.
38. **Maroni BJ, Steinman TI, Mitch WE.** A method for estimating nitrogen intake of patients with chronic renal failure. Kidney Int. 1985;27:58-65.
39. **Buckalew VM Jr, Berg RL, Wang SR, Porush JG, Rauch S, Schulman G.** Prevalence of hypertension in 1,795 subjects with chronic renal disease: the modification of diet in renal disease study baseline cohort. Modification of Diet in Renal Disease Study Group. Am J Kidney Dis. 1996;28:811-21.
40. **Heymsfield SB, Arteaga C, McManus C, Smith J, Moffitt S.** Measurement of muscle mass in humans: validity of the 24-hour urinary creatinine method. Am J Clin Nutr. 1983;37:478-94.
41. **Cohn SH, Abesemis C, Zanzi I, Aloia JF, Yasumura S, Ellis KJ.** Body elemental composition: comparison between black and white adults. Am J Physiol. 1977;232:E419-22.
42. **Harsha DW, Frerichs RR, Berenson GS.** Densitometry and anthropometry of black and white children. Hum Biol. 1978;50:261-80.
43. **Worrall JG, Phongsathorn V, Hooper RJ.** Racial variation in serum creatine kinase unrelated to lean body mass. Br J Rheumatol. 1990;29:371-3.
44. Effects of diet and antihypertensive therapy on creatinine clearance and serum creatinine concentration in the Modification of Diet in Renal Disease Study. J Am Soc Nephrol. 1996;7:556-65.
45. Short-term effects of protein intake, blood pressure, and antihypertensive therapy on glomerular filtration rate in the Modification of Diet in Renal Disease Study. J Am Soc Nephrol. 1996;7:2097-109.
46. **Hartmann AE.** Accuracy of creatinine results reported by participants in the CAP Chemistry Survey Program. Arch Pathol Lab Med. 1985;109:1068-71.
47. **Levey AS, Greene P, Burkart J.** Comprehensive assessment of the level of renal function at the initiation of dialysis in the MDRD study [Abstract]. MDRD Study Group. J Am Soc Nephrol. 1998;9:153A.
48. **Breyer-Lewis J, Agodoa L, Cheek D, Greene P, Middleton J, O'Connor D, et al.** Estimation of GFR from serum creatinine in the African-American Study of Kidney Disease [Abstract]. AASK Study Group. J Am Soc Nephrol. 1998;9:153A.
49. **Bedros FV, Kasiske BL.** Estimating glomerular filtration rate from serum creatinine in renal transplant recipients [Abstract]. J Am Soc Nephrol. 1998;9:666A.

SECTION IX

ONCOLOGY

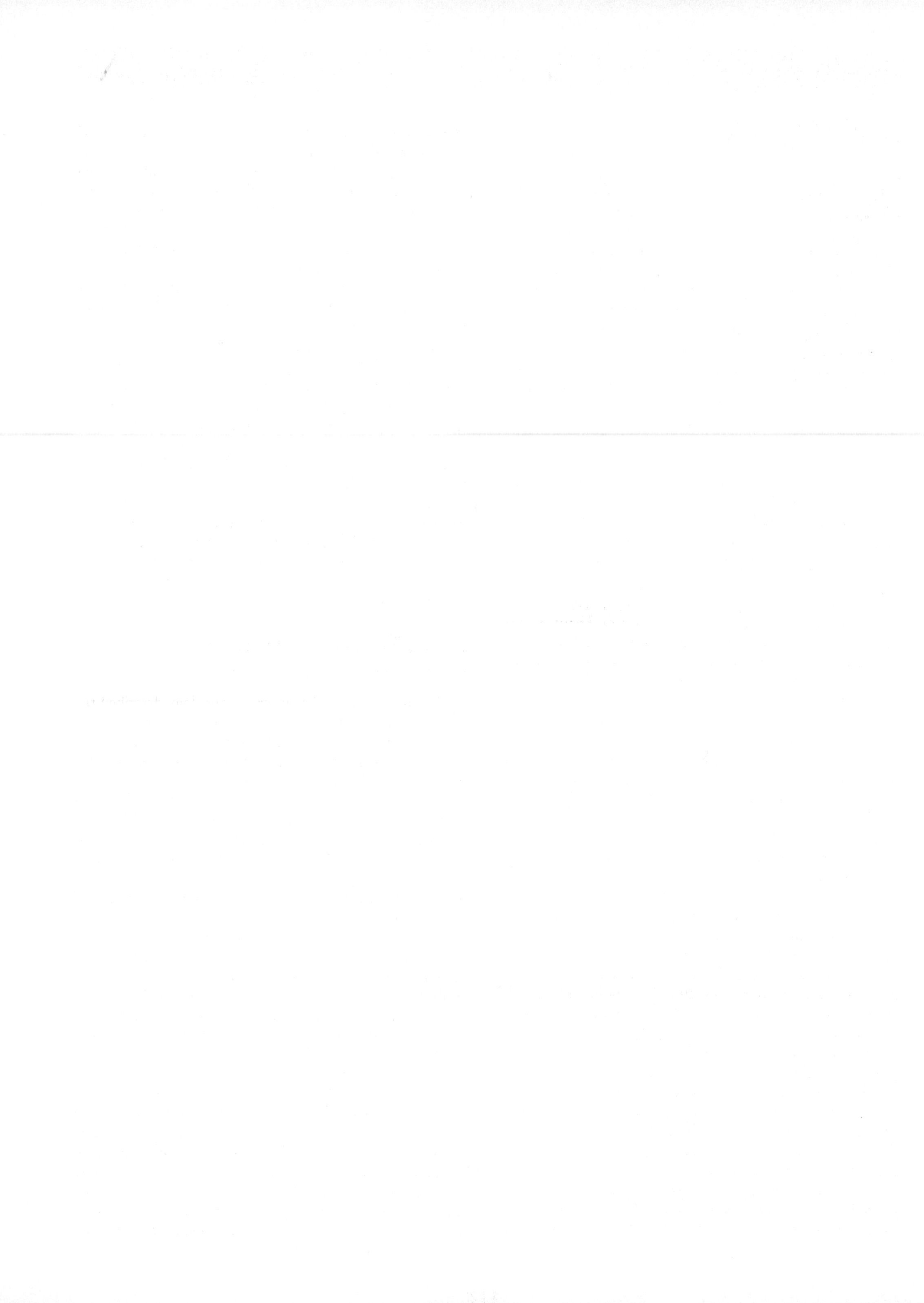

Cancer and heredity.

Slye M. Ann Intern Med. 1928;1:951-976.

Maud Slye (1879-1954) was a remarkable pathologist whose work in mice foresaw many aspects of the problem of hereditary susceptibility (and resistance) to human cancer. Her prescient *Annals* article foresaw a time when "the relation of heredity to predisposition to cancer and exemption from cancer" would "revolutionize preventive medicine". Dr Slye based this prediction on a body of fetchingly anthropomorphic work—she speaks of murine sons and daughters—focused on spontaneously arising malignancies among tens of thousands of mice that she maintained for their lifespans and necropsied at their natural deaths.

She interpreted her data to show that "protection" from neoplasia reflected a mendelian dominant effect and "susceptibility" a recessive one. She postulated a gene-environment interaction, viewing cancer as the result of "irritation of the appropriate kind and the appropriate degree applied to the cancer-susceptible tissue". She speculated that "if an individual susceptible to cancer will protect himself against irritation of locally susceptible tissues, he might avoid cancer even though he is a member of a family with much cancer". She wanted to empower society and individuals with genetic knowledge, calling for careful family histories and pedigree studies, prospective follow-up of cancer-prone families, and archiving tissues from biopsies and autopsies "so that man need not be blind as to what characters he is transmitting to his posterity".

Which of Dr. Slye's findings have we verified in our patients and their families?

She correctly predicted that occasional families would have multiple and multi-generational cases of common cancers, often of early onset. Some would have an organ-specific phenotype (breast cancer in families with germ line *BRCA1* and *BRCA2* mutations; colorectal cancer in those with *APC* mutations). Others would have a variety of cancer types (e,g,, in the Li-Fraumeni syndrome cause by mutations in *TP53*, "the guardian of the genome"). She was unable to specify the usual mechanism of such inheritance: that a person inherited "susceptibility" from a parent in the form of one mutated and inactivated copy of the causal tumor suppressor gene in all somatic cells and then began to develop a cancer when something, including the usual, error-prone processes of genetic housekeeping, inactivated the other copy in one somatic cell, freeing it and its daughters to start along a tumor progression pathway, initially by proliferating clonally.

She was right that identifying the albeit rare cancer-prone families would lead to a partnership of empowered patients, family members, and physicians that would try—through personal care and political processes—to ameliorate the burden of hereditary cancer. She could not have foreseen the remarkable complexity of decision making in cancer-prone families, the implications of variable gene penetrance, the problems of access to insurance, and the privacy issues. She might have been surprised how difficult it has proven to fix mutated genes.

Dr Slye was correct that genes and environments interact, that sun makes for more melanoma and smoking for more lung cancer in those rendered genetically susceptible to these cancers by inheriting a high penetrance, mutated gene. Her implication that all should avoid known carcinogenic exposures is a truism.

She overestimated the public health implications of hereditary cancer. Although a Darwinian, she did not recognize that high penetrance susceptibility genes would be rare in the population (because homozygous individuals would tend to die before bearing children). But her work is a reminder that in future genome-wide association studies of low-risk alleles ("polymorphisms" of genes individually having a small effect on susceptibility) may well allow identification of persons at sufficiently high risk (because of inheriting a group of low-risk alleles in complementary pathways to neoplasia) to warrant surveillance or intervention. Such individuals will likely be identified by risk models that integrate exposures, phenotype, family history and genotype. This approach to risk prediction and linked prevention will require the kind of collaborative and complex laboratory, clinical and population-based research that Dr Slye called for and that is still in evolution.

Lymphosarcoma cell leukemia.

Isaacs R. Ann Intern Med. 1937;11:657-662.

This article from a distant era in oncology described the evolution of a leukemic phase in 15 of 43 patients with what was then (~70 years ago) called *lymphosarcoma* (lymphosarcoma is now an obsolete term; it encompassed a number of lymphoid malignancies ranging from chronic lymphocytic leukemia (CLL) to the common, B-cell non-Hodgkin lymphomas, diffuse large B-cell lymphoma (DLBCL) and follicular lymphoma (FL)). The author believed that he was describing a single disease—many of his cases were likely FLs—whose natural history could include a terminal leukemic phase rather than the transformation of the original disease into another disease, "lymphatic leukemia". He described the change in the clinical course—weight loss and fever anemia, thrombocytopenia and hemorrhage—that accompanied the appearance of malignant cells in the blood. In the blood, these cells looked like the cells initially infiltrating the nodes. He noted a transient response to external beam radiation ("roentgen ray") therapy in 8 patients. The onset of the leukemic phase heralded a quick death (in an average of 26 days).

This paper has been widely cited as an early report of the phenomenon of tumor progression that describes a malignancy going from "good" to bad to worse. It described an uncommon event in FL, the evolution of a leukemic phase (more common is the evolution of DLBCL at a rate of about 3% per year). It is also a nice reminder of the immense progress in diagnosing, characterizing, understanding and treating the lymphoid malignancies, particularly DLBCL and FL. Isaacs was probably right in speculating that his cases did not have an entirely new disease. But neither did they simply have more of the same malignancy. We now understand that the abrupt change in disease course ("transformation") that he described commonly results from an array of genetic changes in subclones of the original malignancy (transformation may sometimes represent a new disease arising from a progenitor common to it and the original malignancy). The genetic changes that drive transformation are under active exploration and are likely numerous (ranging from activating chromosome translocations, e.g., of *c-MYC*; to mutation and inactivation of tumor suppressor genes, e.g., *TP53*; to amplification of oncogenes, e.g., *c-REL;* to other mechanisms and genes). Genotype-phenotype relationships reflect this complexity and are under study to relate a particular pattern of genetic alterations to alterations in a range of clinically important cellular behaviors—for example, in proliferation, in trafficking (e.g., into the blood in high numbers), and in therapy resistance.

Isaacs' report also reminds us that cell morphology no longer has the central role in classifying lymphoid malignancies (note his attention to the appearance of the nucleolus). It has given way to a widely validated system—promulgated by the World Health Organization (WHO)—that uses morphology, immunophenotyping, molecular genetic findings, and cytogenetic alterations to classify the hematologic malignancies, including the lymphomas. The WHO classification system is today's standard. It is highly reproducible, guides therapy, and drives clinical and translational studies. It is informed by a deep understanding of normal and neoplastic lymphoid cells. We now recognize that the diseases caused by malignant B-cell, T-cell, and natural killer (NK)-cells tend to reflect the phenotypes of their normal counterparts. This system is evolving. Ongoing research suggests that the WHO classification will eventually incorporate lessons from gene-expression profiling of the lymphoid malignancies.

Isaacs speculated about the role of radiation therapy in his patients. Combination chemotherapy together with the use of therapeutic monoclonal antibodies ("chemoimmunotherapy") has replaced radiation therapy (except in the rare cases of very low stage disease or for palliation) and revolutionized treatment of the common B cell non-Hodgkin lymphomas. In DLBCL, chemoimmunotherapy—for example, with R-CHOP (rituximab, cyclophosphamide, adriamycin, vincristine, prednisone)—produces complete response rates of ~75% and a failure-free survival rate of 50% at 3 years—a good surrogate for cure—in the young and the elderly. Comparable therapy prolongs survival in those with FL, although cure remains elusive.

Read Dr Isaacs' article as an early chapter in a history that is still unfolding.

Cis-diamminedichloroplatinum, vinblastine, and bleomycin combination chemotherapy in disseminated testicular cancer.

Einhorn LH, Donohue J. Ann Intern Med. 1977;87:293-298.

Chemotherapy of testicular cancer is one of the big success stories in treatment of metastatic cancer, and this article played an important role. The authors followed up on earlier work showing that multi-agent chemotherapy was modestly effective in patients with disseminated testicular nonseminomatous germ cell tumors. In this report of a case series of 50 patients with metastatic testicular cancer (4 with seminoma), the complete response rate was surprisingly high on a three-drug, platinum-based (cisplatin) chemotherapy regimen. The authors followed the paradigm of MOPP for Hodgkin lymphoma by using the combination of cisplatin/bleomycin/vinblastine, drugs with different mechanisms of action and relatively non-overlapping toxicities. 35 of 47 evaluable patients (74%) achieved a complete remission (the rate was 85% after including patients who required resection of residual disease); 29 were disease-free at 6-30+ months. Subsequent studies confirmed that the cure rate with this combination was 60%, which compares very favorably with the historical rate of 5%.

The article set the stage for what is now established as standard management of metastatic testicular cancer:

- Modification of the regimen to increase efficacy and decrease toxicity by using BEP (Bleomycin/Etoposide/cisPlatin)
- Risk-stratified therapy (by the International Germ Cell Cancer Collaborative Group [IGCCCG] staging system) with BEP that leads to an overall 80% cure rate and rates of 90%, 75%, and 40% in patients respectively with favorable, intermediate, and poor risk features. A feature of risk-stratified therapy is that patients with low risk disease are treated with lesser chemotherapy (three rather than four cycles of PEB) to blunt toxicity while maintaining the same high cure rate as for those treated with the more chemotherapy.
- Post-chemotherapy resection of residual masses 1 cm diameter
- New, more effective anti-emesis regimens for chemotherapy with high emetic risk in combination with dexamethasone and aprepitant
- Awareness of chemotherapy-induced long-term toxicities: secondary leukemia, therapy-related solid tumors, infertility, nephrotoxicity, neurotoxicity, and pulmonary and vascular toxicities.

Cancer and Heredity*

Maud Slye, *Chicago, Illinois*
From the Otho S. A. Sprague Memorial Institute and the University of Chicago.

THERE are two aspects of this work that I wish especially to stress at this time. First I wish to show with what complete accuracy problems in the relation of heredity to disease can be worked out; second, to emphasize how great a need there is that this relation of heredity to disease should be thoroughly worked out for man, and to suggest the almost incalculable value such studies would have for the future of preventive medicine. Indeed, as I see it, they would revolutionize preventive medicine.

Almost nowhere in the field of scientific research have the findings been so entirely ignored as have been the findings regarding the relation of heredity to disease. During the past thirty years, there have appeared from various research laboratories, suggestions more or less definite that there was a relation between heredity and the occurrence of cancer in experimental animals, the tests being made for the most part with experimentally induced cancer, mainly grafted cancer.

For the past nineteen years I have been making an exhaustive study of this problem of the relation of heredity to predisposition to cancer and exemption from cancer, with all its related problems dealing with the nature and the minutiae of behavior of malignant diseases. Mice were selected for the work for the following reasons: they are mammals and the disease problems they present closely approximate human disease problems. They are small and a sufficient number of them to furnish conclusive evidence can be maintained without an excessive budget. Also very many generations can be studied in the lifetime of one worker. Most important of all their cancers are almost identical with those of man in type, in the organs involved, and in clinical course and behavior.

The malignant growths which this stock has furnished have included practically every type and location known in human pathology and the stock has also yielded many cases of leukemia, both myelogenous and lymphatic; of pseudoleukemia and lymphosarcoma.

All conclusions have been based upon numbers so large as to be beyond all possibility of coincidence and to allow a very wide margin for possible error. The numbers involved are to date over 67,000 necropsies, including between 5,000 and 6,000 primary spontaneous neoplasms.

*Presented before the American College of Physicians, March 5, 1928, New Orleans, La.

These cancers are not caused by any experimental procedure, as are the tar cancers, the grafted cancers, the cancers arising after infesting the animals with large numbers of parasite larvae, or any other experimental method. They are spontaneous cancers, arising in the natural life of the animals, exactly as man's spontaneous cancers arise. Thus there is no chance in the study of spontaneous tumors of involving any unconsidered quantities not present in human cancer, as may possibly be done in all experimentally induced tumors. The relation which heredity has seemed to bear to the occurrence of all of these spontaneous tumors has been consistently identical.

Searching tests have been carried out which conclusively show that cancer is not contagious in my stocks of mice. Every mouse is allowed to live out his full span of life, and to die a natural death. The clinical course of cancer is closely studied throughout the life of the animal in every case where the tumor can be diagnosed during life. Necropsy is performed as quickly as possible after death, and all suspicious tissues are microscopically examined.

The Inheritability of the Cancer Tendency.—The methods of studying the relation of heredity to the occurrence of spontaneous cancer in the laboratory have been the same as those which would be followed in studying intensively the inheritability of any character whatever, and the criterion of the inheritance behavior of cancer has been identical with the most rigid criterion that could be applied in any study of heredity.

In 1865 Mendel worked out with garden peas a study of the method of heredity. Later Cuenot and others working with mice, found that the mendelian method applied also in the inheritance of the animal characters tested. Throughout these studies hereditary predisposition has been shown to bear a definite relation both to the tendency to be exempt from cancer and the tendency to be susceptible to it. In thousands of mice bred in the laboratory, the tendency to be exempt from spontaneous cancer was transmitted as a simple dominant character along mendelian lines.

Results of cross breeding.—When a cancer-free mouse was mated with a cancerous mouse, none of the first generation offspring had cancer. The tendency to be exempt from cancer thus behaved like a simple mendelian dominant. If however, two of these first generation hybrids were mated, one-fourth of their offspring were susceptible to cancer, while three-fourths were exempt from it. Thus the tendency to be susceptible to cancer behaved like a simple mendelian recessive. If, instead of mating two first generation hybrids, each first generation hybrid was mated with a cancer-free mouse, no cancer appeared in the second generation. In this manner, that is by mating all first-generation hybrids with cancer-free mice, all cancer susceptibility has been ruled out of the entire family for many generations.

The tendency to be susceptible to cancer is also inheritable, but it is inheritable as a recessive character. This means, that even though there has been a great deal of cancer in one side of the family, even 100%, if there is no cancer in the other side of the family, all of the immediate progeny have been cancer free. If they in their turn have been mated with cancer resistant individuals, cancer has been eliminated from their immediate families also.

By the successive mating of dominant non-cancerous mice with hybrid non-cancerous mice, cancer has been held off indefinitely but has still been present potentially, transmitted by the hybrid carrier through generation after generation, but never frankly shown as long as dominant non-cancer is mated with hybrid carriers. But when, in any generation, the 2nd, the 3rd, the nth, two hybrid non-cancerous mice have been mated, cancer has appeared in the next generation in almost mendelian ratio where the mice have lived well into cancer age. In the studies in this laboratory cancer has been held off for twenty-five generations by persistently mating analyzed dominant non-cancer with hybrid carriers through successive generations. But when eventually two of these hybrid carriers were mated, cancer has appeared in the next generation.

It is this possibility of transmitting cancer through successive generations by the right selective mating, without its frank appearance which would explain in human statistics the seemingly erratic occurrence of cancer sometimes in a family where no previous case has been known. Our human statistics however usually cover only two ancestral generations and the diagnoses in these were rarely based upon necropsy.

Out of the many hundreds of tests made in this laboratory a few typical ones have been selected and charted here to show both the method of procedure and the kind of results obtained. Note how exactly these results follow the mendelian expectation in heredity from the given type of cross made, and how rigid is the method of analysis by which the mice are classified in regard to their cancer tendency.

In this strain the parent female was 168. She was the daughter of parents neither of which had cancer. Her mother, female 499, died in old age of chronic nephritis; and her father, male 250, died of pulmonary infection. Female 168 herself died of uncertain causes but had no tumor. She had therefore been selected for this cross as she apparently was an extracted non-tumorous mouse.

The parent male 274 died of carcinoma of the lung. He came of a family which showed at necropsy 100% of cancer (strain 139). His mother 158, died of carcinoma of the mammary gland with metastases in the lungs; his father 193, with primary carcinoma of the lung. He was therefore used in this cross because he was an analyzed extracted cancerous individual.

We have here then a typical mendelian cross between the presence and the absence of a character: that is female 168 with the cancer-resistant tendency present and male 274 with the cancer-resistant tendency absent. The first hybrid generation showed no cancer whatever, which is the typical behavior in hybridization for a mendelian recessive. *The non-cancer tendency then was dominant over the cancer tendency in this cross,* just as pigmentation was dominant over the absence of

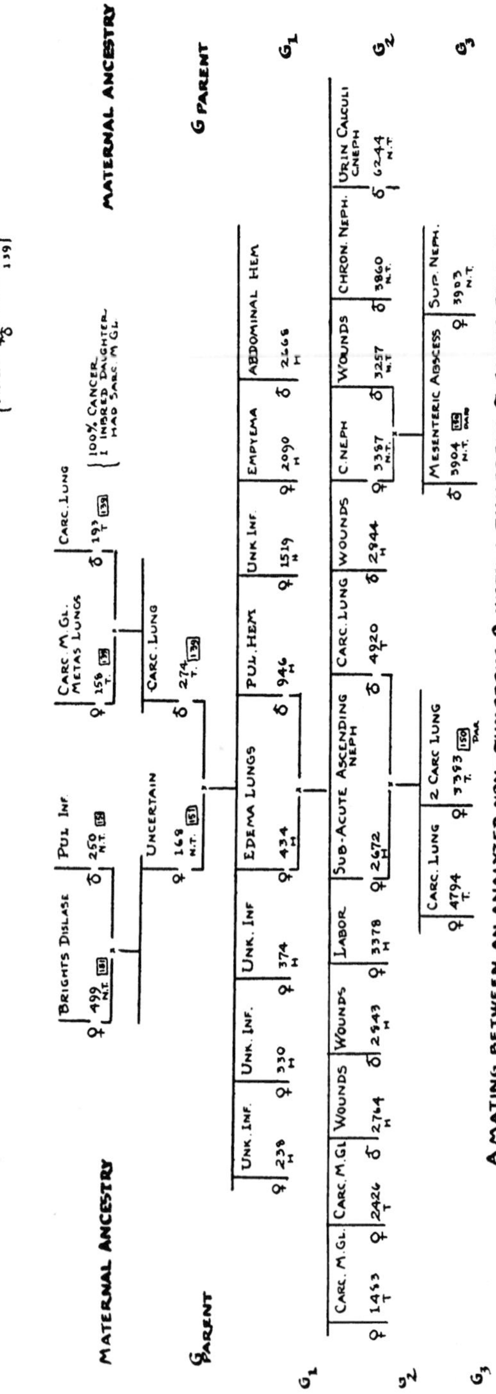

A MATING BETWEEN AN ANALYZED NON-TUMOROUS ♀ WITH A TUMOROUS ♂ GIVING PERFECT MENDELIAN RESULTS, SHOWING CANCER BEHAVING AS A SIMPLE MENDELIAN RECESSIVE.

CHART I

pigmentation in the standard mendelian diagram. When two of these first generation hybrid non-cancerous mice were mated, (female 434 who died with edema of the lungs without cancer, and male 946 who died of pulmonary hemorrhage without cancer) the resulting offspring showed the nearly perfect mendelian ratio of four dominant non-cancer, to six hybrid non-cancer to three recessive cancer mice. The cancer representatives were females 1483 and 2426 with carcinoma of the mammary gland, and male 4920 with a carcinoma of the lung.

Female 2672, in the second generation, who died of subacute ascending nephritis, was analyzed to determine whether she was dominant non-cancer or hybrid non-cancer, by being mated with male 4920 with cancer of the lung. Cancer appeared in her immediate offspring; female 4794 with carcinoma of the lung, and female 3383 with two primary carcinomas of the mammary gland. Female 2672 was thus shown to be a hybrid non-cancerous mouse capable of transmitting the disease though not herself frankly showing it. This mating also demonstrated the fact that when hybrid non-cancer is mated with recessive cancer, cancer appears in the immediate offspring, just as recessive albinism appears in the immediate offspring in the similar classic cross.

In the effort to derive an analyzed extracted dominant non-cancerous mouse, two others of the offspring of the same first generation hybrid carriers were selected, namely female 3387 who died of chronic nephritis without cancer, and male 3257 who died of wounds without cancer. Their son, male 3904, shown in this chart, who died of a mesenteric abscess without tumor, and their daughter, female 3903, dying of suppurative nephritis without cancer, appeared to be extracted dominant non-cancerous mice.

As all these mice were autopsied as are all others dying in this laboratory, and as every suspicious tissue is examined microscopically, it is absolutely known which mice have and which have not any form of neoplasm.

By this cross then there was obtained an analyzed cancerous female 3383 and an analyzed extracted non-cancerous male 3904 for further testing. Note that the types of tumors which appeared in this strain 145, and the organs in which they were located, were identical with those bred in, namely carcinoma of the mammary gland from ancestral female 158, and carcinoma of the lung from ancestral male 193 and parent male 274. Moreover no other types or locations of neoplasms occurred in this family.

Ancestral male 193 had one daughter in strain 139 (from which he was derived) with sarcoma of the mammary gland. Sarcoma of the mammary gland came out later in strain 145 as shown in chart 4, thus proving male 193 a hybrid carrier of sarcoma of the mammary gland as well as carcinoma of the mammary gland, though not himself frankly showing either, as he died with carcinoma of the lung.

The inheritance behavior then of the cancer-resistant tendency and the cancer-susceptible tendency are here identical with the pigmentation tendency and the non-pigmentation tendency. The cancer resistant tendency like the pigmentation tendency behaved like a mendelian dominant, and the cancer-susceptible tendency, like the non-pigmentation tendency, behaved like a recessive. Also, just as the type of color bred in is the one which appears in the offspring, so the types and locations of neoplasms bred in, were the ones which occurred in the offspring.

Chart 2 shows the inbred test which was given male 3904 to prove whether he was certainly an extracted pure bred cancer-resistant mouse. He was mated with his sister female 3903 (also shown in chart 1). She died of suppurative nephritis without tumor and appeared also to be an extracted pure-bred cancer-resistant mouse as did all other mice in this branch. No fraternity of this branch of strain 145 has ever shown a neoplasm either malignant or benign, although the strain still persists in the laboratory and has been in existence for over seventeen years, the original cross having been made in October, 1910. We have here then analyzed pure-bred cancer-resistant mice for hybridization testing.

To further test male 3904 as an extracted dominant non-cancerous mouse, he was hybridized with absolutely unrelated female 711 who was an analyzed non-cancerous member of strain 71 and who died in old age of an aortic rupture without tumor. No fraternity of this strain 224 ever showed a neoplasm malignant or benign, although it persisted in the laboratory for five years.

This is the method by which are analyzed all mice appearing in these studies. They are not chance mice picked up in the market or in the laboratory and mated by chance. They are analyzed individuals whose ancestry and inheritance potentialities are known facts and they can therefore be manipulated with a certain outcome.

Chart 4 shows a part of strain 150 which resulted from the cross of analyzed cancerous female 3383 and analyzed cancer-resistant male 3904. The first hybrid generation from this cross was all non-cancerous, that is, again the non-cancer tendency was dominant over the cancer tendency; but cancer appeared in the second generation in female 9778 with a carcinoma of the mammary gland, and male 5696 with a sarcoma of the mammary gland. Again when cancerous male 5695 was mated with non-cancerous female 5786, no cancer appeared in the next generation. In both tests then shown in this chart the non-cancer tendency was dominant over the cancer tendency.

This chart shows also the origins of Branches I, II, III, and IV of this strain. Branch I is made by the crossing of two *first generation* hybrids, female 6488 and male 5426. Branch II is derived from mating two other *first generation* hybrids, female 10852 and male 8035. Branch III is made by mating two hybrid non-cancerous mice, of the *second generation* female 12148 and male 11246. Branch IV is derived by mating two *second generation* extracted dominant non-cancerous mice, female 10911 and male 11346. Note how in every case the inheritance behavior is in exact accord with the standard mendelian expectation. That is, (1) the mating of a cancerous and a dominant non-cancerous mouse gives hybrid non-cancerous mice, with cancer appearing in the second generation. (2) The mating of two hybrid non-cancerous mice gives the standard three

PART OF STRAIN 145

INBRED ANALYSIS OF ♂ 3904 PROVING HIM NON-TUMOROUS

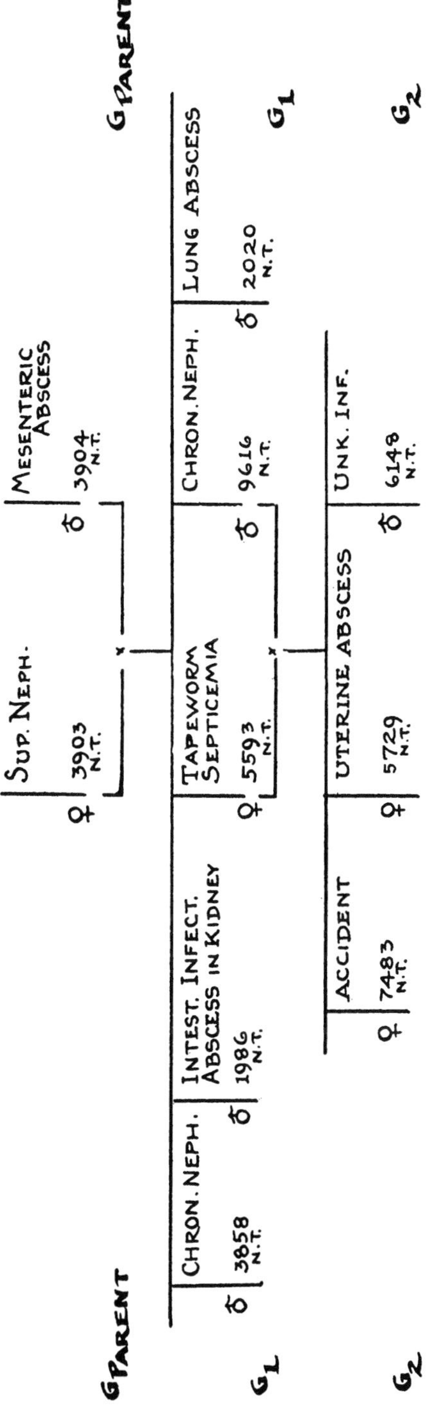

NO FRATERNITY IN THIS BRANCH OF THE FAMILY EVER PRODUCED A NEOPLASM EITHER MALIGNANT OR BENIGN.

CHART 2

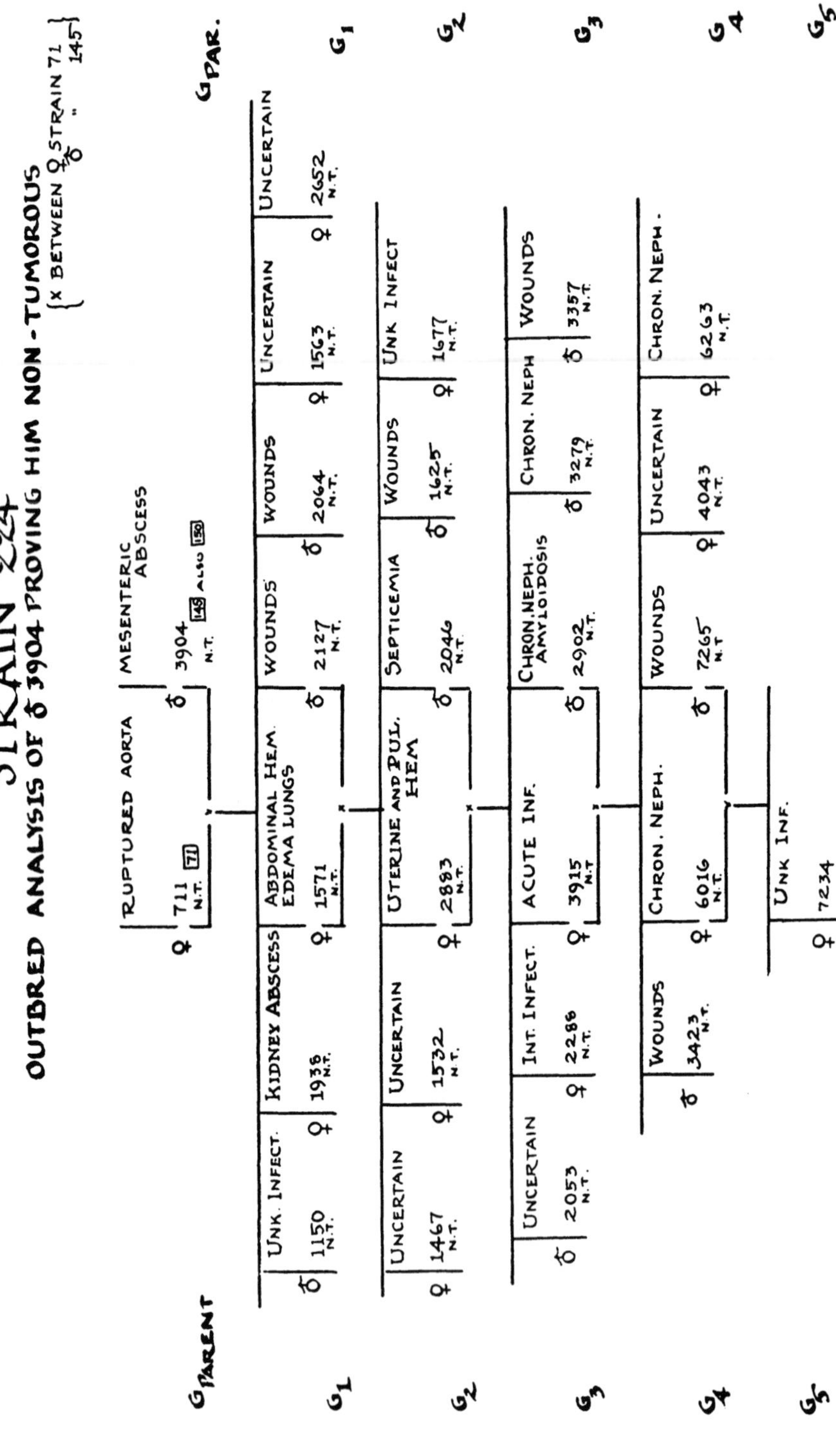
STRAIN 224
OUTBRED ANALYSIS OF ♂ 3904 PROVING HIM NON-TUMOROUS
{X BETWEEN ♀ STRAIN 71 ♂ " 145}
G PARENT
♀ 711 N.T. 71 RUPTURED AORTA
♂ 3904 N.T. 145 ALSO 150 MESENTERIC ABSCESS
G1
♂ 1150 N.T. UNK. INFECT.
♀ 1938 N.T. KIDNEY ABSCESS
♀ 1571 N.T. ABDOMINAL HEM. EDEMA LUNGS
♂ 2127 N.T. WOUNDS
♂ 2064 N.T. WOUNDS
♀ 1563 N.T. UNCERTAIN
♀ 2652 N.T. UNCERTAIN
G2
♀ 1467 N.T. UNCERTAIN
♀ 1532 N.T. UNCERTAIN
♀ 2883 N.T. UTERINE AND PUL. HEM
♂ 2046 N.T. SEPTICEMIA
♂ 1625 N.T. WOUNDS
♀ 1677 N.T. UNK INFECT
G3
♂ 2053 N.T. UNCERTAIN
♀ 2286 N.T. INT. INFECT.
♀ 3915 N.T. ACUTE INF.
♂ 2902 N.T. CHRON. NEPH. AMYLOIDOSIS
♂ 3279 N.T. CHRON. NEPH
♂ 3357 N.T. WOUNDS
G4
♂ 3423 N.T. WOUNDS
♀ 6016 N.T. CHRON. NEPH.
♂ 7265 N.T. WOUNDS
♀ 4043 N.T. UNCERTAIN
♀ 6263 N.T. CHRON. NEPH.
G5
♀ 7234 UNK INF.
NO FRATERNITY IN THIS FAMILY EVER PRODUCED A TUMOR MALIGNANT OR BENIGN.

CHART 3

PART OF STRAIN 150

SHOWING MATING OF ANALYZED NON-TUMOROUS ♂ 3904 WITH CARCIN-OMATOUS ♀ 3383

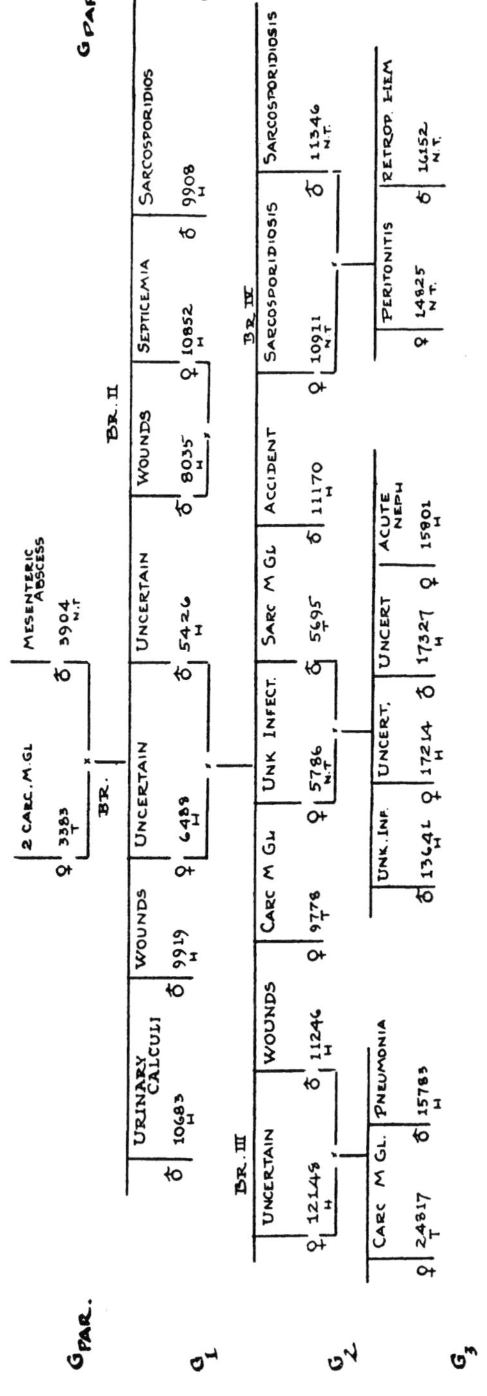

Chart 4

types, dominant non-cancer, hybrid non-cancer and recessive cancer. (3) The mating of two dominant non-cancerous mice gives extracted non-cancer only, no cancer ever appearing again in such branches.

Chart 5 gives the continuation of Branch I and shows the result of mating analyzed dominant non-tumorous female 5786 with her cancerous brother 5695 both of the second generation shown in chart 4. None of their immediate offspring ever showed tumor of any nature. Cancer thus again behaved like a recessive. Note that four branches of this family were made by mating four pairs of these hybrid non-cancerous mice, and in every case some cancer appeared in the next generation (generation 4 in the chart).

Note that throughout these charts the only tumors, both primary and secondary, which occurred, were tumors of the mammary gland and of the lung, like the ancestral tumors of the strain shown in chart I.

Chart 6 shows part of an extracted 100% cancerous strain (strain 338 Br. V) derived from double cancerous parentage, female 8619 with two carcinomas of the mammary gland and male 8751 with an adenoma of the liver. The ancestry behind this strain has been published previously. (1) It is here omitted in order to get the chart within the necessary size limits. The ancestry while in my hands, carried sarcomas, carcinomas and adenomas in most of the organs here represented.

Note the large number of liver tumors, sarcomas and adenomas, there being eleven cases of liver tumor, primary and secondary, out of twenty-four individuals, or nearly 50%. This is very noteworthy, because outside of this laboratory there have been only two spontaneous liver tumors in mice reported in all the literature, one by the Imperial Cancer Research Laboratory of England, (2) and one from the cancer laboratory of Harvard University in Boston, Mass (3).

The liver tumors in this strain 338 were deliberately bred for, in the effort to show that the uncommon internal tumors, as well as the more common mammary gland tumors, unquestionably were determined by heredity.

In line A note female 8865 with an osteosarcoma of the mammary gland metastasizing in the liver, succeeded by her grandson male 16370 with an osteosarcoma of the subcutaneous tissues of the leg, metastasizing in the liver.

Note the very frequent occurrence in this strain of multiple tumors, particularly females 9741, 12261, 22263, 30469 and 30501. The latter two mice had more neoplastic than normal tissues at the time of their death.

In this strain there is one case of pseudoleukemia, a disease which also occurred in the ancestry of this strain. In this laboratory chronic leukemia, pseudoleukemia, lymphosarcoma and kindred diseases have uniformly occurred in cancer strains only, and have followed the laws of heredity as surely as have neoplastic diseases. Their behavior in this laboratory would indi-

(1) Slye: Jour. Can. Res. Vol. I. No. 4, 1916.

(2) Murray: Third Scientific Report of the Imperial Cancer Research Fund, 1908, 69.

(3) Tyzzer: Jour. Med. Res. 1909, XXI, 479.

PART OF STRAIN 150 BR.I
CONTINUED ANALYSIS OF MATING OF CANCEROUS WITH NON-CANCEROUS MICE

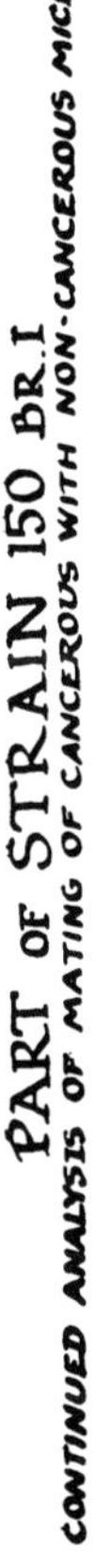

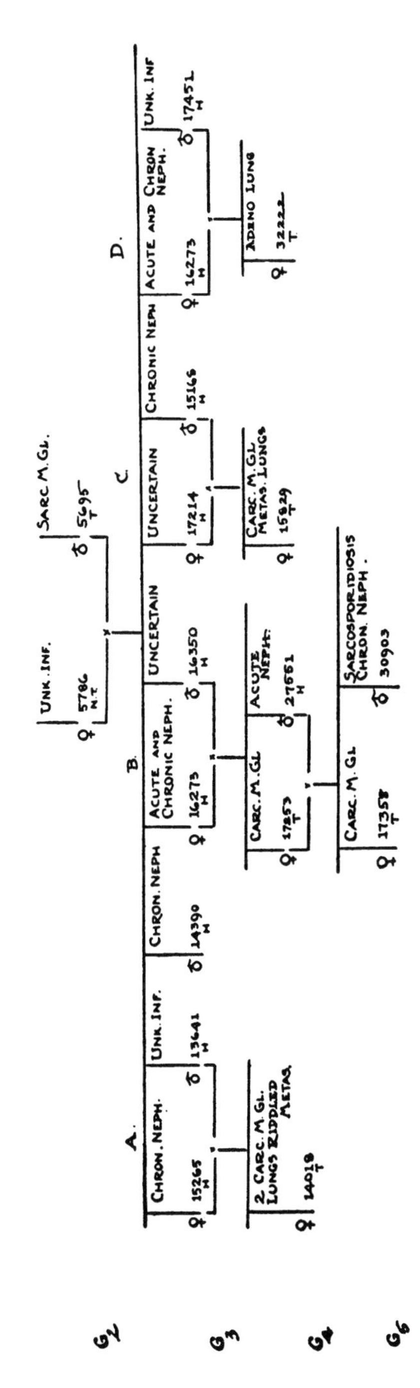

A CROSS BETWEEN A NON-TUMOROUS FEMALE AND A TUMOROUS MALE SHOWING HOW CANCER APPEARED IN THE SECOND HYBRID GENERATION FROM EVERY TESTING OF FIRST GENERATION HYBRID-CARRIERS IN LINES A·B·C·D~

CHART 5

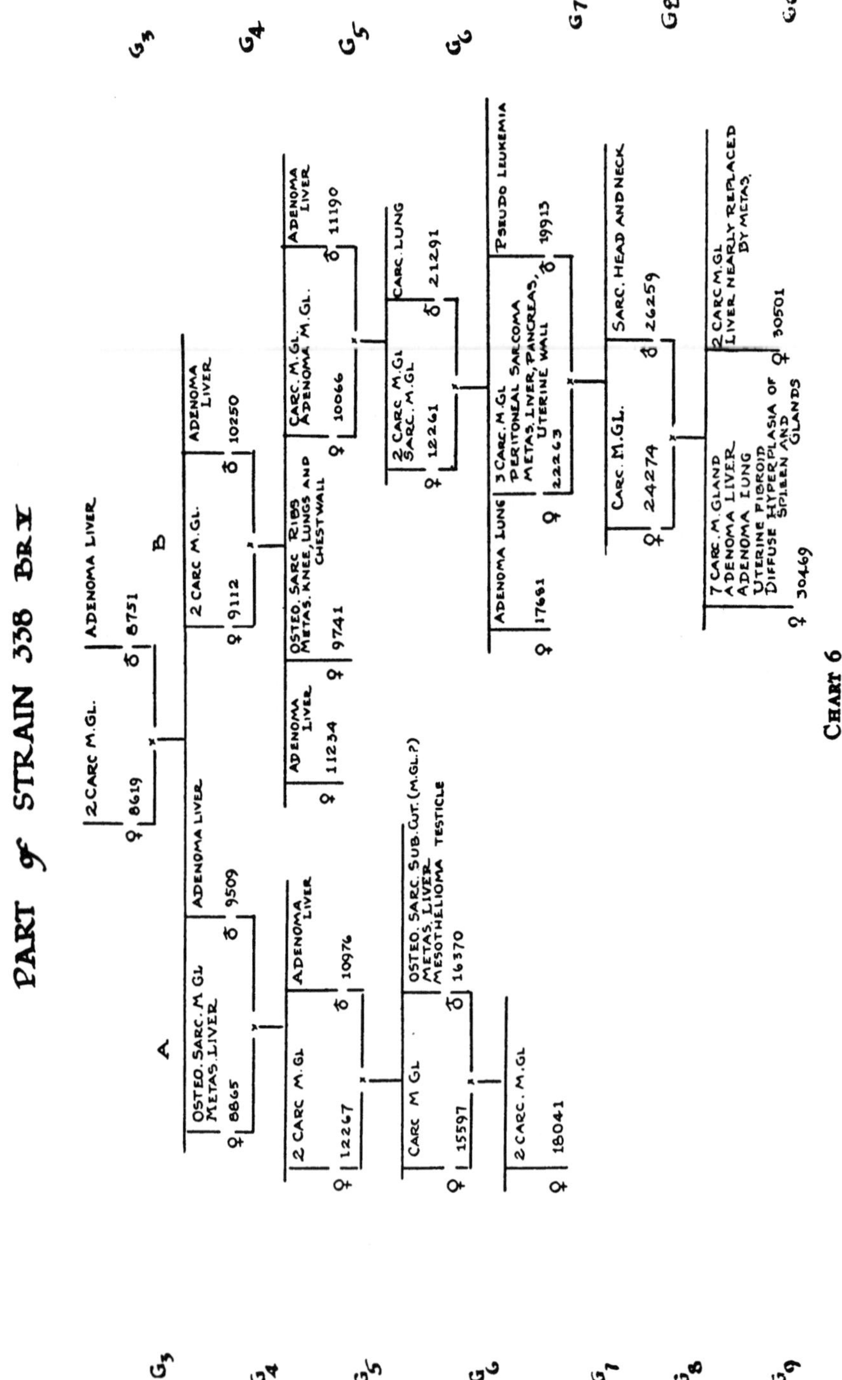
PART of STRAIN 338
2 CARC M.GL.
♀ 8619
ADENOMA LIVER
♂ 8751
A
B
G3
G4
G5
G6
G7
G8
G9
OSTEO. SARC. M GL METAS. LIVER
♀ 8865
ADENOMA LIVER
♂ 9509
2 CARC M.GL.
♀ 9112
ADENOMA LIVER
♂ 10250
2 CARC M.GL
♀ 12267
ADENOMA LIVER
♂ 10976
ADENOMA LIVER
♀ 11234
OSTEO. SARC RIBS METAS. KNEE, LUNGS AND CHESTWALL
♀ 9741
CARC. M.GL. ADENOMA M.GL.
♀ 10066
ADENOMA LIVER
♂ 11190
CARC M GL
♀ 15597
OSTEO. SARC. SUB.CUT. (M.GL.?) METAS. LIVER MESOTHELIOMA TESTICLE
♂ 16370
2 CARC M.GL SARC. M.GL
♀ 12261
CARC. LUNG
♂ 21291
2 CARC. M.GL
♀ 18041
ADENOMA LUNG
♀ 17681
3 CARC. M.GL PERITONEAL SARCOMA METAS. LIVER, PANCREAS, UTERINE WALL
♀ 22263
PSEUDO LEUKEMIA
♂ 19913
CARC. M.GL.
♀ 24274
SARC. HEAD AND NECK
♂ 26259
7 CARC. M.GLAND ADENOMA LIVER ADENOMA LUNG UTERINE FIBROID DIFFUSE HYPERPLASIA OF SPLEEN AND GLANDS
♀ 30469
2 CARC M.GL LIVER NEARLY REPLACED BY METAS.
♀ 30501
CHART 6

cate that they certainly are neoplastic diseases.

These charts are typical. Whenever in this laboratory two analyzed cancer-free mice have been mated, it has always been possible to secure 100% cancer-free families. In such crosses no instance of cancer in the succeeding strain has ever to date occurred. Also when two cancerous mice have been mated it has been possible to secure 100% cancer susceptible strains except for those mice that have died in infancy or that have been swept off by infections earlier in life than the normal age for the type of cancer to which they are predisposed. Occasionally a mouse in one of these 100% cancer strains derived from double cancerous parentage has developed a cancer when only two weeks old, although six months is an early cancer age in mice and is approximately the equivalent of about 32 years, an early cancer age in man.

In the hybridization test also susceptibility to cancer and exemption from cancer have uniformly proved to be inheritable. They have followed almost with exactness the standard expectation for a typical mendelian recessive and dominant respectively. Thus the tendency to exemption from cancer is unquestionably inheritable. Many hundreds of strains and branch strains have been carried in this laboratory, which have never shown a tumor growth of any kind. This means that in many families carried for fifty or more generations and comprising many thousands of members, there has been complete exemption from cancer. These cancer-free mice when bred into other families, carry with them exemption from cancer as a dominant character. Compare this with the record of man who pays no attention to heredity in his matings, and where one in eight over a given age is dying of cancer, and note how tremendously hopeful is this fact of the inheritability of the tendency to be exempt from cancer.

Even when a recessive cancer-susceptible mouse is mated with a hybrid carrier of the cancer tendency it is possible in the third generation to derive dominant pure breeding cancer-resistant individuals. This possibility of extracting wholly cancer-free families even where one parent was cancerous and the other is a cancer carrier is a most encouraging fact and it should be strongly emphasized. From every mating of a cancer-susceptible individual with a cancer-resistant individual, either dominant or hybrid, it has been possible by the right selective mating to produce families wholly resistant to cancer.

It is this hybridization test which proves beyond dispute the inheritability of any character, for nothing but heredity could explain the segregating out and the transmission unchanged of characters in which the two parents are unlike, and the perfect mendelian pattern which they follow: as for example, albinism and pigmentation, or cancer susceptibility and cancer resistance.

Where both parents die of the same disease and all the later members of the family die of the same cause, as in a 100% inbred test, we have no absolute demonstration that it might not be a case of epidemic contagion, either extra- or intra-uterine. But we cannot explain by contagion, the perfect mendelian pattern shown in a hybridization test. This pattern by every test that can be made, the cancer-susceptible and the cancer-resistant tendencies in mice of my stocks have uniformly followed.

The Influence of Heredity in Determining Secondary Neoplasms.

Not only has heredity definitely controlled the occurrence of primary tumors, but it has also controlled the occurrence of secondary tumors. (4) The tests made in this laboratory have shown that the only secondary tumors which occur in any strain, correspond with the primary tumors within that strain, both in type and in the organs in which they occur; thus showing that only those organs susceptible by heredity to primary tumors in any individual or strain, are susceptible to secondary growths.

These tests have demonstrated also that secondary tumors are as potent as primary tumors in heredity, in determining the type and the location of primary neoplasms in mice. That is, for example, the tendency to primary sarcoma of the kidney has followed from an ancestor with secondary sarcoma of the kidney, and vice versa. Note chart 7.

Strains 48 and 292. The parents in these strains are female 3 and male 360. Female 3 had a sarcoma-carcinoma of the mammary gland, a malignant adenoma of the liver, and sarcoma metastases in the kidney. She came of a family (strain 90) which carried also tumors of the mesenteric glands, ovary, spleen, adrenal and lungs, as well as leukemia and pesudoleukemia. She proved to be a hybrid carrier of the tendency of these organs to be susceptible to cancer, as well as of the tendency to leukemia and pseudoleukemia, and she transmitted the tendency to tumors in all of these organs to some of her posterity in hybrid crosses with analyzed dominant non-tumorous mice. She also frankly showed mammary gland, liver and kidney neoplasms of both carcinoma and sarcoma types.

Parent male 360 was the son of male 436 who died of carcinoma of the lung. This strain also carried mediastinal tumors primary and secondary. Male 360 then, was a 1st generation hybrid carrier of tumors of the lung and mediastinum, although not frankly showing tumor.

We have here then the mating of a tumorous female with a hybrid-carrier male. The first hybrid generation from this cross showed some tumorous individuals and some hybrid carriers in about equal numbers.

Note that both the primary tumors and the secondary tumors are of the same types and occur in the same organs as those bred in.

These strains were selected because they show locations of neoplasms in mice which have not been reported at all or else rarely reported from other laboratories. This chart shows that these internal tumors, difficult to diagnose clinically, follow exactly the same laws of heredity as do the easily noted mammary gland and skin tumors.

It is very difficult and laborious to secure these strains yielding high percentages of internal tumors, because it is so difficult to diagnose them before the death of the mouse and in time to secure offspring from such a selected

(4) Slye: Jour. Can. Res. Vol. VI, No. 3, 1921.

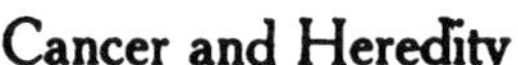

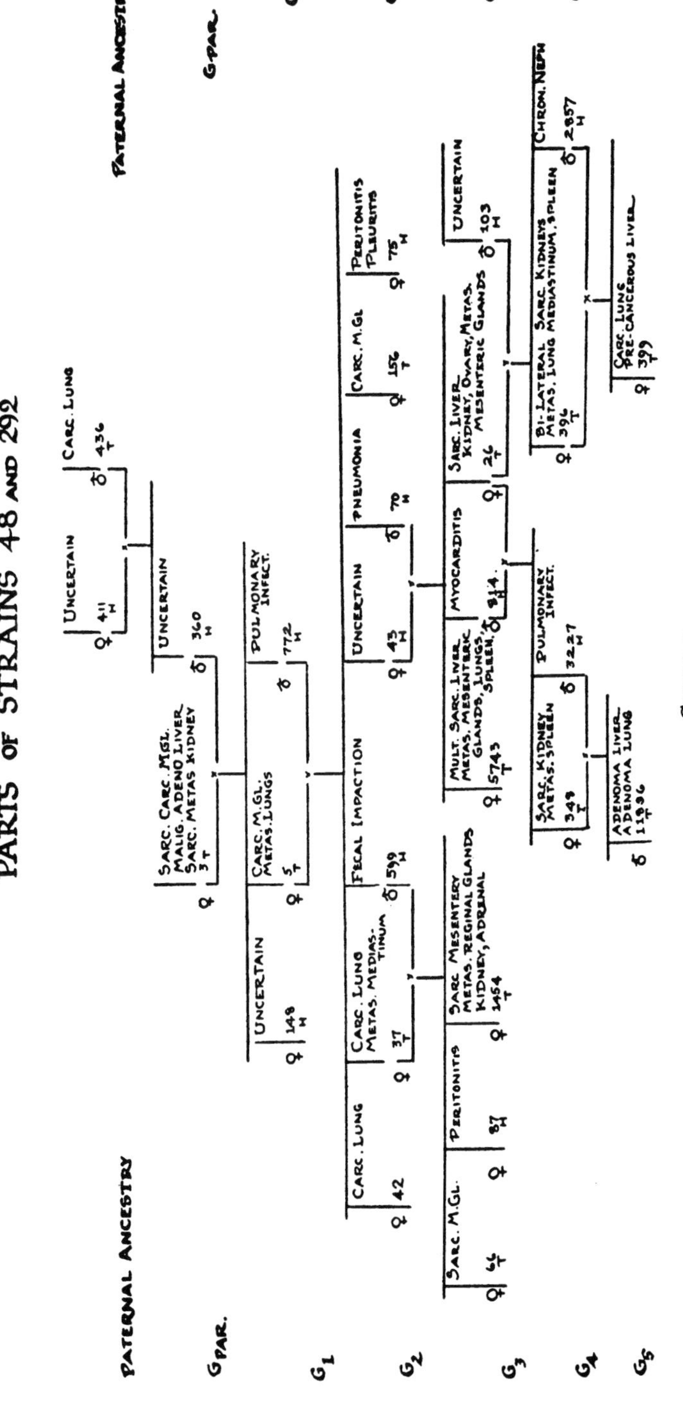

PARTS OF STRAINS 48 AND 292

CHART 7

cancerous parentage. Only by long continued and painstaking effort is it possible to obtain them, but when we find 5 sarcomas of the kidney, 4 sarcomas of the liver, 3 sarcomas of the mesentery, 1 sarcoma of the adrenal, 3 sarcomas of the spleen, and 1 sarcoma of the ovary, in addition to numerous carcinomas of the mammary gland and lung, in a little family of sixteen members, whose ancestry was known to carry all these types of tumors, the certainty of heredity control is evident.

It has been suggested that mammary gland cancer being the most commonly reported tumor in mice, might occur by chance in these large numbers, but it is not possible to think that such rarely reported internal tumors as those shown in this typical chart, could have occurred in such numbers by chance.

Many strains in this laboratory (4) have been so manipulated in selective breeding as to exclude primary tumors of the lung, which are common tumors in mice. The lung is also one of the most frequently reported seats of secondary growths in mice. In such strains in my stocks where primary lung tumors never occur, no tumor metastases grow in the lungs even where tumor emboli are very numerous in the lung blood vessels.

Chart 8 shows a 100% lung tumor strain, strain 139. Every member of this family that lived to be six months of age or over, showed lung carcinoma either primary or secondary.

Chart 9 shows another lung tumor strain. Every member of this family except male 2501 had lung carcinoma either primary or secondary. Male 2501 had a testicular tumor only.

Chart 10 shows a part of strain 392. Note female 12058 of the fourth generation shown in the chart. If her statistics had been taken for three generations only no tumor would have been shown in the family. But if we examine one generation farther back we find almost the duplicate of the new growths shown in female 12058. This indicates how deceptive may be the results of an examination of the death causes in the ancestry for even three generations. It also indicates how the tendency to cancer persists in hybrid carriers through generation after generation, until the right mating is made; when the cancer tendency appears in the next generation.

Charts 11 and 12 show the almost perfect inheritance behavior of thyroid malignancy as a simple mendelian recessive, occurring in strain J. D. 30-62-68. The mating is between female 24843 with thyroid carcinoma, and non-cancerous male 24383. The first hybrid generation (gen. 15 in the chart) showed no tumor. No tumor appeared in the second hybrid generation, where it might have been expected; but all of these mice died rather early for the occurrence of thyroid malignancy. When two of the 16th generation mice were mated however, thyroid malignancy occurred in the next generation. Again in generation 18, from the mating of cancerous female 31909 with non-cancerous male 32556, no cancer occurred in the next generation. But when two of these hybrid carriers were mated, thyroid carcinoma occurred in the next generation, female

(4) Slye: Jour. Can. Res. Vol. VI, No. 2, 1921.

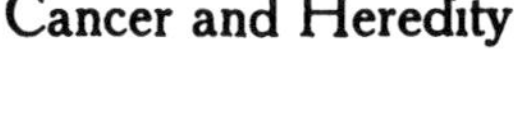

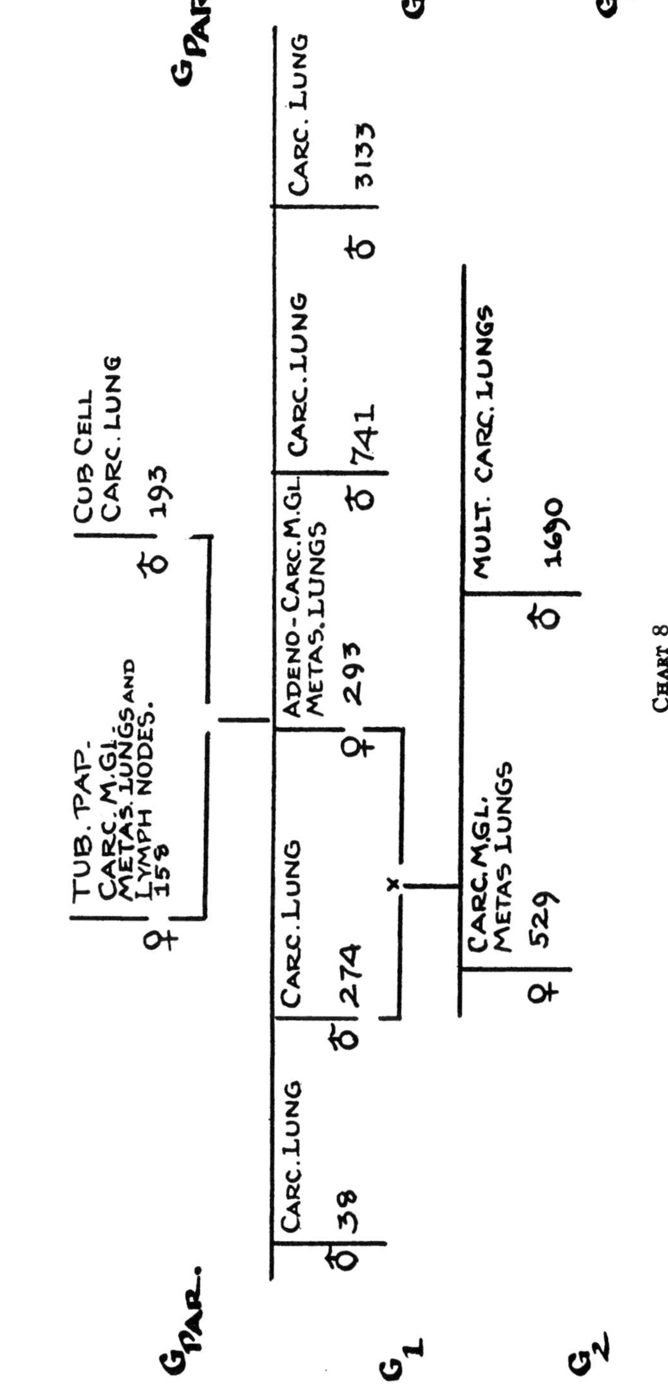
STRAIN I39
G PAR.
G1
G2
TUB. PAP.
CARC. M.GL.
METAS. LUNGS AND
LYMPH NODES.
158
CUB CELL
CARC. LUNG
193
CARC. LUNG
38
CARC. LUNG
274
ADENO-CARC. M.GL
METAS. LUNGS
293
CARC. LUNG
741
CARC. LUNG
3133
CARC. M.GL.
METAS LUNGS
529
MULT. CARC. LUNGS
1690

Chart 8

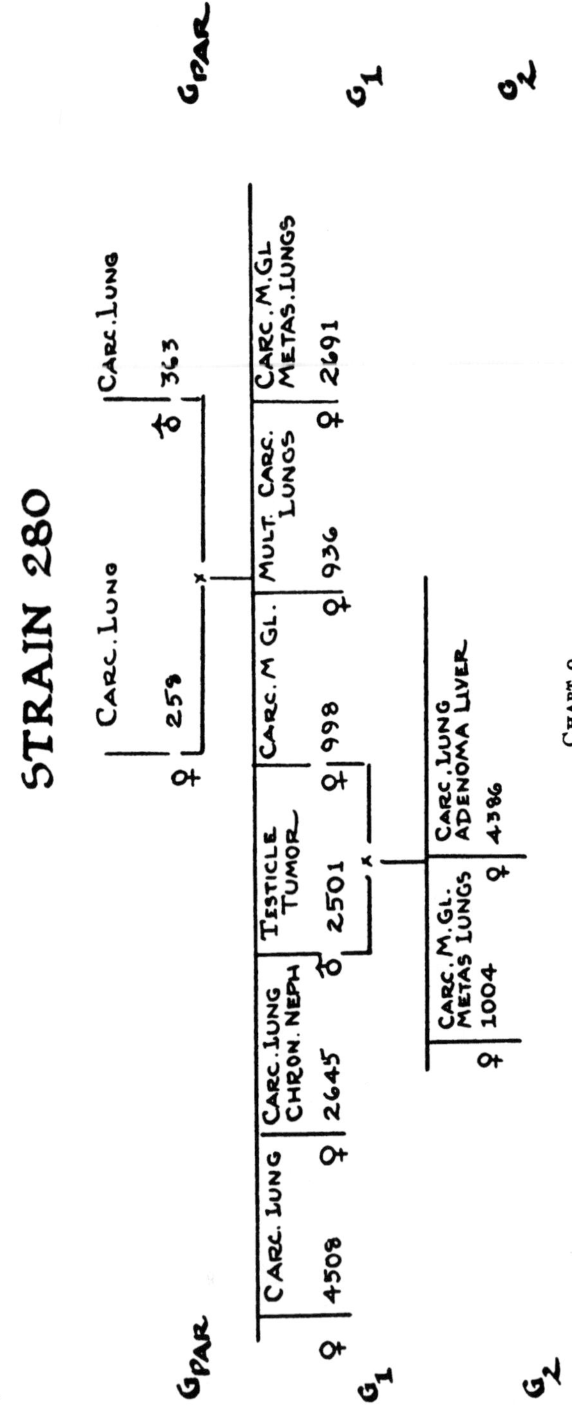
STRAIN 280
G PAR
G 1
G 2
Carc. Lung
♀ 259
Carc. Lung
♂ 363
Carc. Lung
♀ 4508
Carc. Lung
Chron. Neph
♀ 2645
Testicle
Tumor
♂ 2501
Carc. M Gl.
♀ 998
Mult. Carc.
Lungs
♀ 936
Carc. M. Gl
Metas. Lungs
♀ 2691
Carc. M. Gl.
Metas Lungs
♀ 1004
Carc. Lung
Adenoma Liver
♀ 4386

Chart 9

37841. When this female 37841 was mated with hybrid carrier male 35938, thyroid malignancy occurred in the next generation. This chart shows the almost perfect inheritance behavior of a given type and location of malignancy, (that is sarcoma-carcinoma of the thyroid) as a simple mendelian recessive character. This is very striking, because thyroid malignancy in mice has nowhere else been reported. This classic occurrence of this type of tumor deliberately bred for in one family of mice, is noteworthy.

Chart 12 shows how by the continuous mating of a non-cancerous individual with a hybrid carrier in each successive generation of this same family after the 22nd generation, all malignancy was held off for five generations. The tendency however was still present in the family, transmitted by the hybrid carriers through generation after generation. When in the 27th generation two of these hybrid carriers were mated, sarcoma-carcinoma of the thyroid occurred again in the 28th generation. This is the most stringent

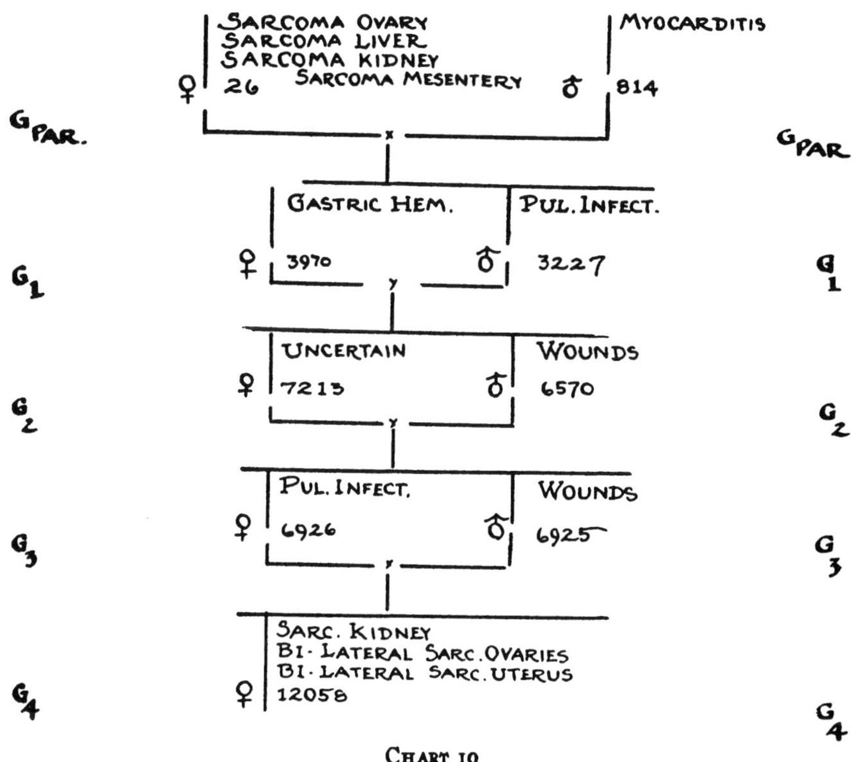

Chart 10

test that can be made to show whether or not any character has a hereditary basis. The occurrence of thyroid malignancy in the 28th generation of this family showed the perfect mendelian ratio of one-fourth cancer free, to two-fourths hybrid carrier, to one-fourth cations. This branch of the family was chosen to show this particular type of proliferation. Other branches of the family showed malignancy in other locations, according to the matings made. In my experience, these pre-cancerous proliferations of muzzle skin and eye-

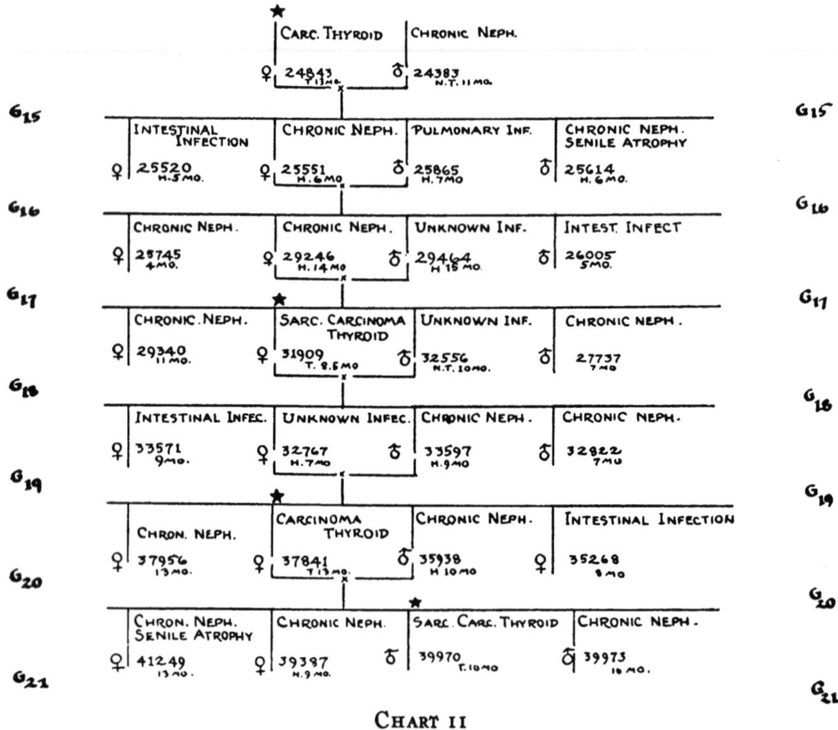

CHART 11

thyroid malignancy. Some of the non-tumorous members of the family are omitted, in order to get the chart within the necessary limits.

Chart 13 shows a family of strain 150 derived from the mating of two cancerous parents. Note the high percentage of basal-cell carcinoma of the eyelids and muzzle skin and pre-cancerous proliferation in these same lo-lids have gone on to malignancy in every case where the mouse has lived long enough for this to occur.

Chart 14 shows two branches of strain 215. Note the high percentage of carcinoma and adenoma of the lung in branch A and the high percentage of liver adenomas in branch B (each according to the matings made). The frequency of liver tumors in branch B

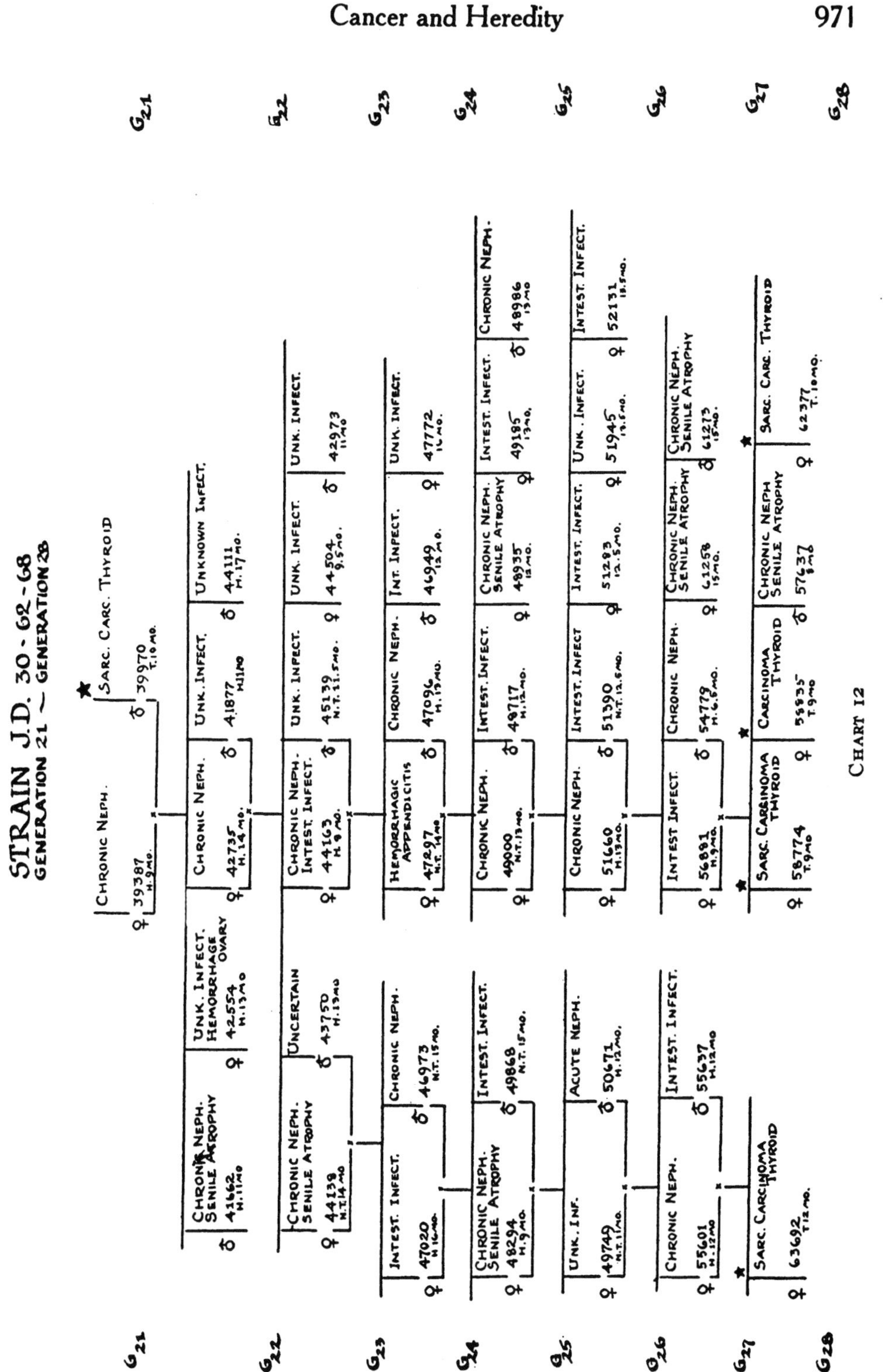

CHART 12

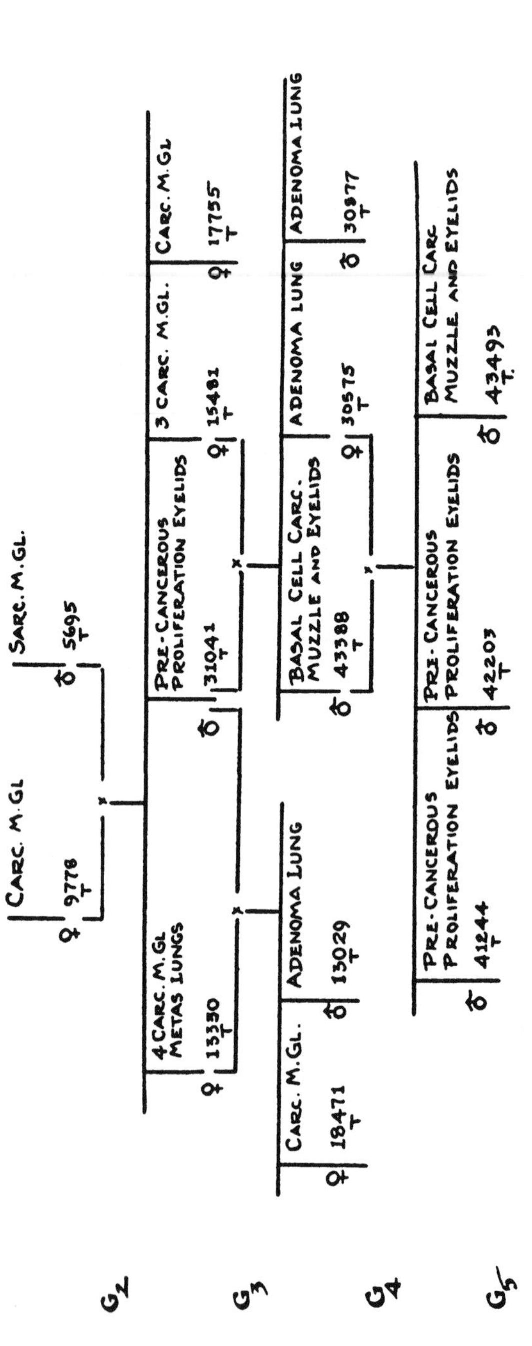

A 100% Tumerous Strain from the Mating of Two Tumorous Parents

Chart 13

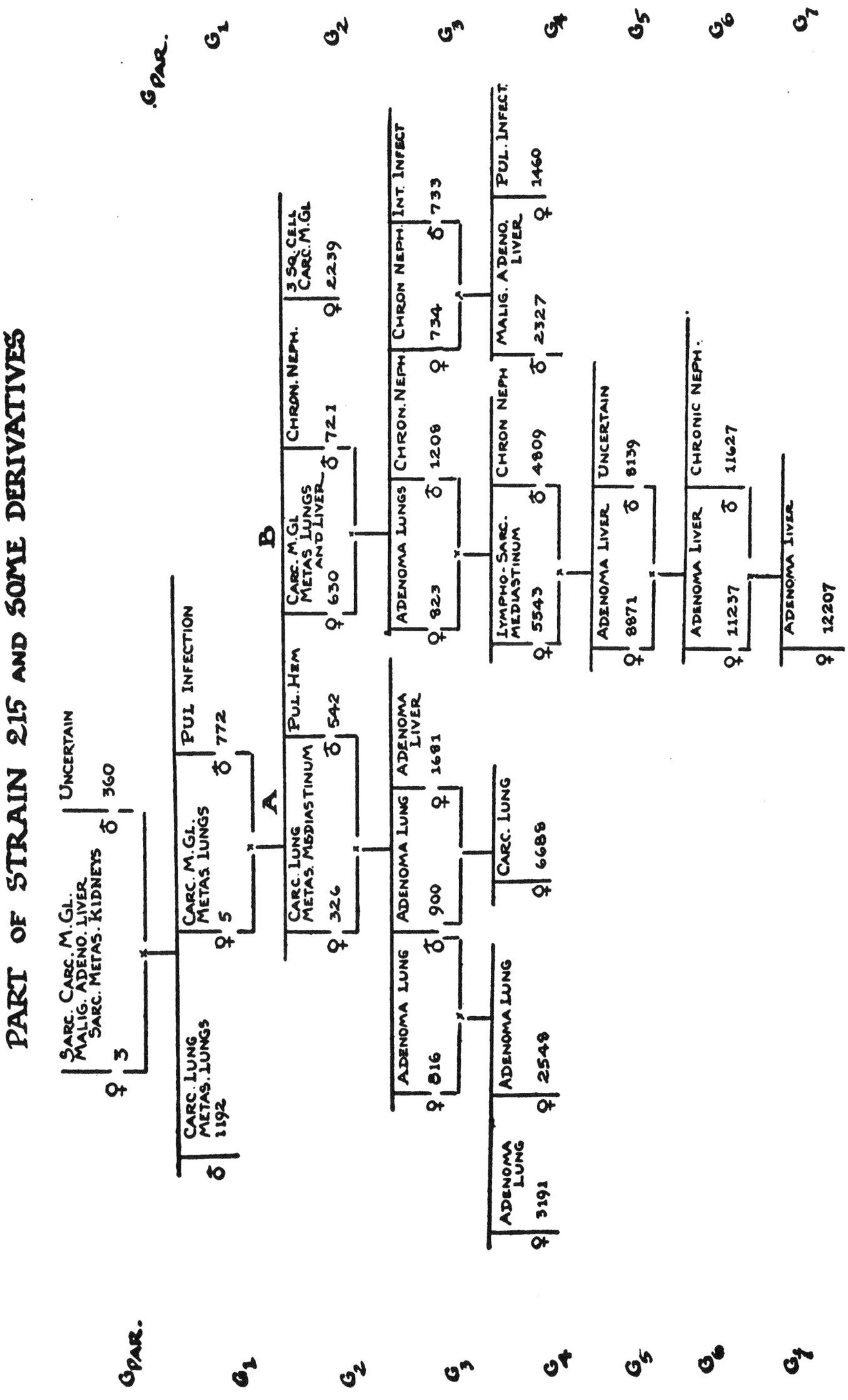

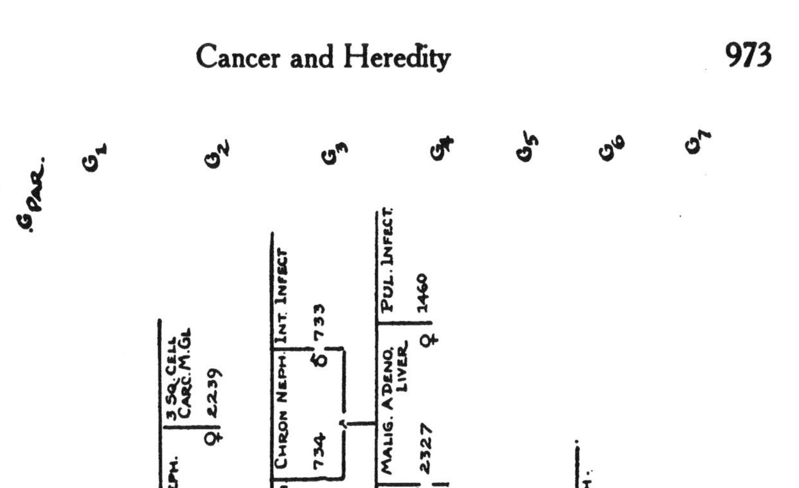
PART OF STRAIN 215 AND SOME DERIVATIVES
G PAR.
G1
G2
G3
G4
G5
G6
G7
SARC. CARC. M. GL. MALIG. ADENO. LIVER SARC. METAS. KIDNEYS
♀ 3
UNCERTAIN
♂ 360
CARC. LUNG METAS. LUNGS
♂ 1192
CARC. M. GL. METAS. LUNGS
♀ 5
PUL INFECTION
♂ 772
A
B
CARC. LUNG METAS. MEDIASTINUM
♀ 326
PUL. HEM
♂ 542
CARC. M. GL. METAS LUNGS AND LIVER
♀ 630
CHRON. NEPH.
♂ 721
3 SQ. CELL CARC. M. GL.
♀ 2239
ADENOMA LUNG
♀ 816
ADENOMA LUNG
♂ 900
ADENOMA LIVER
♀ 1681
ADENOMA LUNGS
♀ 823
CHRON. NEPH.
♂ 1208
CHRON NEPH.
♀ 734
INT. INFECT
♂ 733
ADENOMA LUNG
♀ 3191
ADENOMA LUNG
♀ 2548
CARC. LUNG
♀ 6688
LYMPHO-SARC. MEDIASTINUM
♀ 5543
CHRON NEPH
♂ 4809
MALIG. ADENO. LIVER
♂ 2327
PUL. INFECT.
♀ 1460
ADENOMA LIVER
♀ 8871
UNCERTAIN
♂ 8139
ADENOMA LIVER
♀ 11237
CHRONIC NEPH.
♂ 11627
ADENOMA LIVER
♀ 12207

CHART 14

is very striking as this is a tumor very rarely reported. These were malignant adenomas.

In strains which do not carry liver tumors, no secondary growths have appeared in the liver, even when multiple emboli have been present throughout the liver vessels, whereas in those strains where primary liver tumors occur, the liver is a frequent site for secondary growths, as shown in strain 338 Br. C, in strains 48 and 292.

There are apparently two factors necessary to induce cancer. If either of them could be wholly avoided, it might be possible to prevent cancer. These factors are (1) an inherited local susceptibility to the disease, and (2) irritation of the appropriate kind and the appropriate degree applied to the cancer-susceptible tissues. Experiments eliminating one or the other of these two factors, in order to see whether cancer can be avoided in this way, are being carried on in this laboratory with a promise of some success. In these experiments by avoiding either the cancer susceptible factor or the irritation factor, cancer has in some cases been avoided. The experiments thus suggest that both inherited susceptibility and local irritation are necessary in inducing cancer. They suggest that cancer susceptibility is local and not systemic. In mice susceptible to only one location of cancer, no amount of irritation or stimulation applied to other parts of the body has ever to date induced a cancer. Avoidance of irritation to the locally susceptible tissues has prevented cancer in some cases, even in susceptible individuals. This would suggest that if an individual susceptible to cancer will protect himself against irritation of locally susceptible tissues, he might avoid cancer even though he is a member of a family with much cancer.

The fact of the inheritability of exemption from cancer is one of the few hopeful observations ever made concerning the disease, because it means that instead of every one being susceptible, large numbers are wholly exempt. It also means that it is possible wholly to eliminate cancer from any family by the right genetic procedure, as I have eliminated it from hundreds of families involving thousands of individuals.

What I have said regarding the certainty of the relation of heredity to exemption from spontaneous cancer and to the tendency to be susceptible to cancer has to do with the mice of my stocks. Its application to man and to most other animals remains to be tried. But mice are mammals like man, organ for organ their anatomy and functions are markedly similar in all fundamentals which we can test.

We find marked similarity in such types of tissue behavior, both normal and abnormal, as we are able to study in man and the lower mammals. Tissue reactions in reproduction, regeneration and all the fundamental vital processes are markedly similar. The differences in refinements and complexities attach themselves only to the less basic entities.

The spontaneous cancers in mice are also similar to those of man in every essential of structure and of behavior of which we are informed. Heredity is the most fundamental of all basic biologic facts next to the fact of the existence of life itself, and it plays the leading rôle in evolution, keeping species and even varieties pure. Heredity applies in man and it applies in mice. Man has neoplasms and mice have similar neoplasms. The suggestion that the relation between heredity and cancer must be similar in both, surely offers itself, unless we discard evolution as the explanation of organic life as it exists today. For if evolution means anything, it must mean that down the full line from the single cell to man, similar tissues derived from ancestral tissues have responded in the same way as the ancestral tissues to the same types of stimulation. Only so could an unbroken series of organisms evolve each from the preceding. The methods and facts of heredity in man would therefore seem to be similar to the methods and facts of heredity in mice, unless there is a break in the evolutionary series between man and all other forms of life, thus isolating him from every other form of life.

Therefore since it is possible wholly to eliminate spontaneous cancer from families of mice by the appropriate genetic procedure, it might prove to be possible so to eliminate cancer from families of man. This does not mean that we can relax our vigilance against any forms of chronic irritations in any case, since we have not as yet even begun to apply the facts of heredity to the human species, and we have few adequate statistics of human heredity in relation to disease. But it does mean that we should begin to get correct scientific human statistics regarding diseases in man, based upon operation, biopsy, or necropsy in every case, and not upon opinion, so that we could make such an application because in this procedure lies much hope.

Moreover since there is in man the beginning of a genetic sense, (that is a sense for the fitness of matings) it should be possible to educate this genetic sense. This is the great hope for humanity. The way to educate it is to make generally known the facts and operation of heredity, so that man need not be blind as to what characters he is transmitting to his posterity. If, moreover, we would uniformly permit necropsy as is the invariable rule in this laboratory, the exact facts concerning diseases in man could be obtained. If these facts were then kept in permanent record in the laboratory, in two generations by the right selective matings it might prove to be possible to begin to eliminate cancer, as I have consistently and completely eliminated it from hundreds of families of mice in the laboratory.

I am aware that the problem of founding permanent correct human cancer archives is a difficult one as every great work is difficult, but it is largely for the purpose of presenting the necessity of such a foundation and to urge this society to begin it, that I am here.

Two generations of medical men will handle at least four generations of cancer patients. If we had a sufficient number of cases on record and available for study, four generations of accurate records would almost certainly give us the necessary data in each possible type of mating, to demonstrate the relation of heredity to cancer susceptibility and cancer exemption in man, or to prove that there is no such relation.

With all the experimental evidence which is now at hand on this subject of heredity, the time obviously has come when permanently available human records are the immediate requirement. The great mass of valuable human records which exists today, is, with a few notable exceptions like those of Warthin, Broca and some others, so buried in widely scattered masses of local data as to be unavailable.

If we would begin, each in his own location, to make duplicate permanent heredity records of every suspected cancer case, with duplicate permanent slides from operation, biopsy or necropsy in every case, the solution of the problem would be at hand. These duplicates, records and slides from every location should in every case be deposited in a central permanent bureau, where they can be studied together. That central bureau I greatly desire to see located in Chicago which is a central city, so that it would be possible for me to organize the data, and to begin to analyze it, thus starting the permanent foundation. Indeed I would receive it in the beginning in my own laboratory and carry on the necessary work of organization, until the permanent location should be established.

I have brought this matter before this body, because most cancer cases in their beginnings come to you. How you handle them largely determines the outcome. It lies within your possibility to keep track of them from the beginning to the end. It is easily within your power to begin such a foundation if it appeals to you as a necessary thing to be done, and I have therefore brought the matter first to you.

There is open to you now, in my opinion, the greatest opportunity for a tremendous advance in medical science that anywhere presents itself today, that is, the practical incorporation of the immeasurable benefits of the facts of heredity into future preventive medicine. Such an incorporation will revolutionize preventive medicine. If the time were at my disposal I would show you how.

I am here therefore to beg that a committee of your organization be appointed to consider ways and means by which permanent scientific human cancer archives can be founded. I promise you every co-operation of ideas and of service that lies within my power now and in the future. I also beg the local co-operation of every member of this great society toward this end.

For if the findings in regard to the relation of heredity to malignant diseases in mice should prove to hold for man, and every biologic fact at our disposal indicates that they would thus hold, and if we make our data available, for the first time in the history of the study of this disease, the way of the complete elimination of cancer is open.

AN ARTICLE CONTRIBUTED TO AN ANNIVERSARY VOLUME IN HONOR OF DOCTOR JOSEPH HERSEY PRATT

LYMPHOSARCOMA CELL LEUKEMIA *

By Raphael Isaacs, *Ann Arbor, Michigan*

It has been observed frequently that the blood of patients with lymphosarcoma may become leukemic. This syndrome has been characterized as leukosarcoma by Sternberg [1] or as lymphosarcoma terminating in lymphatic leukemia.[2, 3, 4] Flashman and Leopold [5] noted 107 cases of this type in the literature and described an additional case. On the basis of a lymphosarcoma presumably terminating in lymphatic leukemia, numerous speculations have been published concerning the relationship of these two conditions. A careful cytological study of the cell types in this form of leukemia has shown, however, that the cells are not lymphocytes, but lymphosarcoma cells, so that the condition is a true lymphosarcoma cell leukemia.

Material and Methods

Of 43 patients with known lymphosarcoma, 15 developed a leukocytosis during the course of the disease. This group comprised 10 males and five females. There were eight positive biopsies and six autopsies. The ages of the patients ranged from six to 70 years, with a fairly even distribution in the intervening decades, except that between 21 and 30 years, which included one third of the patients. Warthin [6] noted leukemic transformation in nine cases of lymphosarcoma, out of a group of 134 biopsies.

To note how a lymphosarcoma cell would appear if it was in the blood stream, pieces of fresh lymphosarcoma glands were stirred in blood serum, and films were made of this suspension. These were stained with Wright's stain alone or preceded by brilliant cresyl blue while the cells were in the moist state.

The Lymphosarcoma Cell

The lymphosarcoma cell in the blood stream is usually mistaken for a lymphocyte. There are certain differentiating features, however, the most marked being the peculiar characteristics of the nucleolus. This is usually eccentrically placed, single, very rarely multiple. In the films made on brilliant cresyl blue containing cover glasses, later stained with Wright's stain, the nucleolus stands out as a sky blue, round area, surrounded by a deep, blue black rim of chromatin which is piled up around it. (Figure 1.) In the true immature lymphocyte or lymphoblast, under these conditions, the

* Presented to the Michigan Academy of Science, Arts and Letters, March 8, 1935, and, in abstract, to the American Society of Experimental Pathology, Washington, March 25, 1936. (Arch. Path., 1936, xxii, 287.)

From the Thomas Henry Simpson Memorial Institute for Medical Research, University of Michigan, Ann Arbor, Michigan.

nucleolus appears as a light blue " hole " or area in the chromatin structure, without the heavily staining rim. The nucleoli are more likely to be multiple in the immature lymphocytes or lymphoblasts than in the lymphosarcoma cell.

The lymphosarcoma cell, in films, varies in size from 7.5 by 9 microns to 12 by 13.5 microns. The nucleus is usually oval or oblong, occasionally being egg shaped (thicker at one end) in films. Kidney shaped or notched forms are common in some specimens. The stained chromatin is coarsely reticular and somewhat spongy in structure and the chromatin around the edge is thickened into a fairly definite nuclear wall, differing in this respect from the monocyte. The cytoplasm of the cell is sparse, deeply basophilic, and with the brilliant cresyl blue, Wright's stain, appears as a fine, blue lacework.

In sections of fixed tissue, the lymphosarcoma cell is large and round, resembling the lymphoblast in size and proportion of practically non-granular cytoplasm. The nucleus may be irregular in size and shape, many showing indentations on lobulation.

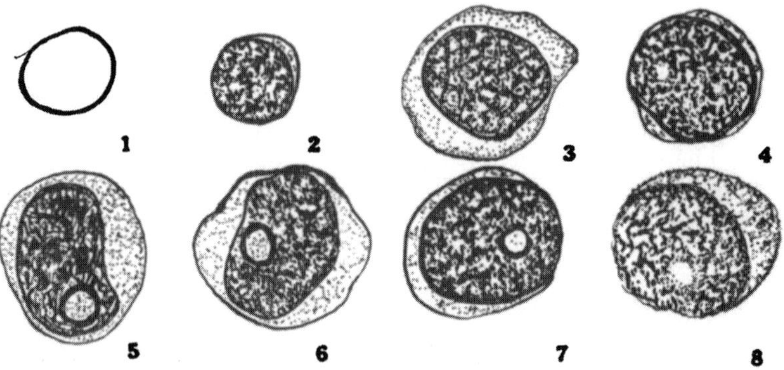

FIG. 1. Cells from peripheral circulation. Stained supravitally with brilliant cresyl blue and counterstained with Wright's stain. (Camera lucida drawings) 1–4 normal blood. 1. Normal red blood cell, for size comparison. 2. Small lymphocyte. 3. Large lymphocyte. 4. Large immature lymphocyte, with several small nucleoli. 5, 6, 7. Cells from lymphosarcoma cell leukemia. 8. Lymphocyte from lymphatic leukemia.

These cells were studied supravitally by Wiseman[7] who found that unlike mature lymphocytes, they did not show motility, although both types did not show evidence of phagocytosis. The mitochondria were described as dust-like, as compared to the large rods and spheres of the mature lymphocyte and the small spheres of the lymphatic leukemia cell. Deep scarlet neutral-red vacuoles, 1 to 10, were present at the periphery of the nucleus in the " sarcoma cell " although they were absent in the leukemic cell and, when present in the mature lymphocyte, they stained rose red.

The Blood

There appear to be two phases of the blood in patients with lymphosarcoma—an aleukemic and a leukemic phase. In the aleukemic phase, the leukocyte count varies from 6,000 to 10,000 per cubic millimeter with 30 to 40 per cent "lymphocytes." Many of these cells are not lymphocytes, but lymphosarcoma cells. The percentage varies from 3 or 4 to 25 or 30 in this group. In the leukemic phase, the count rapidly increases to an average of 70,000 $\pm$ 43,200 per cubic millimeter, the highest count in this series being 156,000 per cubic millimeter. As the count increases, the bulk of the cells are lymphosarcoma cells, which in some cases form 98 per cent of the total.

As the leukemic process progresses, anemia becomes more marked, the average red blood cell count being around 2.5 million per cu. mm. In some patients it reached a much lower level (0.8 to 1.0 million). The color index was most frequently around 1 or slightly below. The blood platelets were increased in number in the early stages, but decreased in the late stages.

Clinical Course

In most of the patients, enlargement of lymph nodes was the first sign noted. Visible tumors in the neck region were the first evidence in three patients; inguinal nodes in two; mediastinal (cough, dyspnea, pleural effusion) in three; abdominal symptoms in two; sore throat in four; weakness in two and submaxillary enlargement in one. Symptoms, in order of their frequency, were weight loss (average 15 pounds); fever; bleeding (petechiae, hemoptysis, hematuria, epistaxis, hematemesis, gross bleeding from mucous membranes, retinal hemorrhages); joint pains; pulmonary and hilar lesions (roentgen-ray changes, pleural effusion, dyspnea, chest pain, cough); allergic symptoms; herpes; skin lesions (toxic erythema, erythema multiforme); bone lesions; facial palsy; diplopia; local edema. Albuminuria (trace), during some stage of the disease was common. The spleen size varied from 15 to 23 centimeters (average 16.5 cm.); and at autopsy the weights varied from 490 to 700 grams. The spleen was palpable in seven patients.

With the onset of the leukemic phase, fever was common (100 to 105° F.). Terminally, 104° to 107° F. were noted. Lung involvement was not always definitely indicated on the roentgen-ray plates, although autopsy in some of these patients showed infiltration of the alveolar walls and of the perivascular and peribronchial tissue with lymphosarcoma cells. This type of lesion was most common in patients dying in the leukemic state, whereas in two who were aleukemic on the day of death, the lungs were not involved. The degree of leukemia was more parallel to the lung involvement than to the degree of peripheral lymph node enlargement.

The duration of the disease varied from 2.5 to 36 + months. The duration of the leukemic phase varied from two days to 60 days in eleven patients in whom approximate data were available. One patient, however, gave a history of a leukemic blood picture (94,000 per cu. mm.), diagnosed as lymphatic leukemia, for over seven years. This patient had a white blood cell count of 37,000 when first observed at this clinic, with 84 per cent lymphosarcoma cells. He died 27 days later. The maximum count was 73,000. The average duration of the leukemic phase in all of the other patients was 26 days.

Nine patients gave a history of one or more of the common childhood diseases. Of the others, three gave a history of a symptom complex which they were told was influenza.

Lymphosarcoma and Pregnancy

One patient with lymphosarcoma showed a remission during a period of pregnancy. The patient, a 31-year-old woman, was first studied after she had had cervical and axillary glandular enlargement for 18 months. Her blood count at that time was as follows: Red blood cell count 3,500,000 per cu. mm.; white blood cell count 47,800; hemoglobin 67 per cent (Sahli), 9.38 grams per cent; atypical "lymphocytes" 65 per cent; blasts 0.5 per cent. She became pregnant six months later, and during the third month she returned to the clinic for examination. At that time her red blood cell count was 4 million per cu. mm., white blood cells 7,100 per cu. mm., hemoglobin, 12.93 grams per cent, polymorphonuclear neutrophiles 71 per cent, large lymphocytes 15 per cent, small lymphocytes 9 per cent, monocytes 5 per cent. The adenopathy had practically disappeared. A perfectly normal child was born in due course of time, and eight months after this the blood count was still normal, but lymphosarcoma cells were noted on the blood films. About nine months after this, the patient returned in complete relapse, with a red blood cell count of 800,000 per cu. mm., white blood cells 4,200, hemoglobin 2.88 grams per cent. Lymphosarcoma cells, 27 per cent, and one blast were noted. She received two blood transfusions and had another remission. An examination four months later showed her red blood cells at a level of 3,600,000 per cu. mm., white blood cells 6,100 and hemoglobin 75 per cent (Sahli) (10.5 grams per cent), "lymphocytes" 59 per cent.

Effect of Roentgen-Ray Irradiation

In 11 of the patients the leukemic phase started after roentgen-ray therapy, in two no roentgen therapy was given, and in two it is uncertain whether the patients had received roentgen therapy before they reported to the hospital or not. A decrease in the number of leukocytes followed roentgen-ray therapy during the leukemic phase, in 8 patients, with severe leukopenia (3,500, 1,800 and 350 per cu. mm.) developing in three patients. In five patients there was a subsequent increase in number after the initial decrease. There appeared to be two stages in the effect of roentgen-ray therapy, an initial decrease in the number of leukocytes, followed by a marked and rapid increase. Thus in one man with a leukocyte count of 50,000 per cu. mm. (96 per cent lymphosarcoma cells), 2800 r were given over 12 positions from May 20 to June 4. On the last day the count was

33,000 per cu. mm. Two days later the count was 156,000 per cu. mm. and the patient died. In another patient the initial count was 10,500 leukocytes per cu. mm. On five successive days, 150 r were given. The leukocyte count fell to 5,500 per cu. mm. It then rose gradually to 15,200 with 66 per cent lymphosarcoma cells 43 days later. Three days before death, which followed in two weeks, the count was 92,000, with 85 per cent lymphosarcoma cells. A third example is that of a patient with 7,800 leukocytes per cu. mm., who received 1,200 r over a five day period. At the close of the treatments the leukocyte count was 6,800 per cu. mm. An observation 41 days later showed that the count had increased to 50,000 per cu. mm. and three days later to 70,800 per cu. mm. The patient died within four weeks.

Pathological Changes in the Organs

Autopsy studies of the organs of patients dying during the leukemic phase showed transformation, in varying degrees, of all lymphoid tissue in the body, into the lymphosarcoma type. The lymphoid follicles of the intestine and colon, as well as the tonsil showed this change. There was marked invasion of the bone marrow and subperiosteal extension, which also involved the surrounding tissues. All of the organs showed invasion with lymphosarcoma cells. Among those showing perivascular or tissue infiltration were the brain, capsule of the pituitary, the fatty envelope of all the organs (heart, kidneys, aorta), the myocardium, beneath the epicardium, bronchi, pulmonary alveolar walls, thyroid, esophagus, thymus, spleen, diaphragm, stomach, liver, gall-bladder, adrenal, kidney, ureter, skin, testes, epididymis, seminal vesicles and vas deferens. The skull, when involved, showed osteolytic lymphosarcomatous infiltration.

Discussion

The frequent occurrence of the leukemic state of lymphosarcoma after roentgen-ray therapy is of interest in connection with the observations of Krebs, Rask-Nielsen and Wagner [8] on the production of a " leukosarcomatosis " (aleukemic and leukemic) in white mice after irradiation. They found that the leukemic phase developed late in the course of the disease, and that, as in the cases cited here, the prognosis was bad.

In view of the tendency of the lymphosarcoma cell to invade the tissues, it is not surprising that some of the cells enter the blood stream. However, it appears that the number does not reach leukemic proportions until there is extensive growth in moving organs, as the lungs. This phenomenon is similar to that found in other types of leukemia (Isaacs [9]).

Summary and Conclusions

1. The characteristics of 15 cases of lymphosarcoma cell leukemia are given.

2. The lymphosarcoma cell has characteristic cytologic features which facilitate its recognition in the blood stream. This cell type may constitute 4 to 98 per cent of the leukocytes in the peripheral circulation.

3. The leukemic phase is usually ushered in with exacerbation of symptoms and fever.

4. The leukocyte count may reach a maximum of from 23,000 to 156,000, and there is progressive anemia and thrombocytopenia.

5. The duration of the leukemic phase varies from two to 60 days (average 26 days) although one patient had a history of leukemia for over seven years.

6. There may be relapses and remissions, but the prognosis is poor. A temporary remission may be induced by roentgen-ray therapy, but this is followed by a relapse and death.

7. The disease appears to be a true lymphosarcoma cell leukemia, rather than lymphosarcoma turning into lymphatic leukemia.

REFERENCES

1. Sternberg, C.: Ueber Leukosarcomatose, Wien. klin. Wchnschr., 1908, xxi, 475.
2. Webster, L. T.: Lymphosarcoma, lymphatic leukemia, leukosarcoma, Hodgkin's disease, Johns Hopkins Hosp. Bull., 1920, xxi, 458–461.
3. Evans, W. A., and Leucutia, T.: The neoplastic nature of lymphatic leukemia and its relation to lymphosarcoma, Am. Jr. Roentgenol., 1926, xv, 497–513.
4. Doub, H. P., and Hartman, F. W.: Lymphocytic, myelocytic and monocytic neoplasms; roentgen diagnosis and treatment, Jr. Am. Med. Assoc., 1935, cv, 942–948.
5. Flashman, D. H., and Leopold, S. S.: Leukosarcoma; with report of a case beginning with a primary retroperitoneal lymphosarcoma and terminating with leukemia, Am. Jr. Med. Sci., 1929, clxxvii, 651–663.
6. Warthin, A. S.: The genetic neoplastic relationships of Hodgkin's disease, aleukaemic and leukaemic lymphoblastoma, and mycosis fungoides, Ann. Surg., 1931, xciii, 153–161.
7. Wiseman, B. K.: Lymphopoiesis, lymphatic hyperplasia, and lymphemia: Fundamental observations concerning the pathologic physiology and interrelationships of lymphatic leukemia, leukosarcoma and lymphosarcoma, Ann. Int. Med., 1936, ix, 1303–1329.
8. Krebs, C., Rask-Nielsen, H. C., and Wagner, A.: The origin of lymphosarcomatosis and its relation to other forms of leucosis in white mice. Lymphomatosis infiltrans leucemica et aleucemica, Acta Radiologica, 1930, supp. X, Stockholm.
9. Isaacs, R.: The physiologic histology of bone marrow. The mechanism of the development of blood cells and their liberation into the peripheral circulation, Folia haemat., 1930, xl, 395–405.

Cis-Diamminedichloroplatinum, Vinblastine, and Bleomycin Combination Chemotherapy in Disseminated Testicular Cancer

LAWRENCE H. EINHORN, M.D., F.A.C.P.; and JOHN DONOHUE, M.D.; Indianapolis, Indiana

Fifty patients with disseminated testicular cancer were treated with a three-drug combination consisting of *cis*-diamminedichloroplatinum, vinblastine, and bleomycin. Three patients were considered inevaluable due to early death. This chemotherapy regimen produced 74% complete and 26% partial remissions. Furthermore, five patients with partial remission became disease-free after surgical removal of residual disease, producing an overall 85% disease-free status. Toxicity, although significant during remission induction with *cis*-platinum, vinblastine, and bleomycin, was usually manageable, although there were two drug-related deaths during this period. Thirty-eight of these patients remain alive and 32 remain alive and disease-free at 6+ to 30+ months. We believe this regimen represents a major advance in the management of patients with disseminated testicular cancer.

ALTHOUGH TESTICULAR CANCER accounts for only 1% of all malignant tumors in men, it ranks first in incidence of cancer deaths in the 25 to 34 age group (1). Thus cancer of the testis has a significant impact on the social, economic, and emotional status of this young population.

Radiotherapy is the treatment of choice for pure seminoma, as this tumor is very radiosensitive, producing a 90% to 95% cure rate, and retroperitoneal node dissection is rarely indicated (2). Indeed, radiotherapy for metastatic lesions produces an excellent 55% 5-year survival (3). However, the treatment for nonseminomatous germinal neoplasms has produced much less satisfactory results with considerably more controversy as to the preferred treatment for all stages of disease.

In 1960, Li and associates (4) introduced the first major thrust of chemotherapy in advanced testicular cancer with the combination of dactinomycin (actinomycin-D), chlorambucil, and methotrexate. Subsequent studies confirmed a 50% to 70% response rate, which included 10% to 20% complete remissions (5, 6). The past 15 years have also seen the development of many new agents with substantial activity, notably vinblastine (7), bleomycin (8), and mithramycin (9). One of the major significant achievements of these single-agent studies was not only the demonstration that a complete remission could be obtained in disseminated testicular cancer, but that approximately half of these complete remissions were permanent cures (5-7, 9). Most relapses occurred within 2 years of initiation of chemotherapy.

Combination chemotherapy has produced excellent long-term complete remissions in other chemosensitive tumors such as Hodgkin's disease (10). Likewise, most recent attempts at improved chemotherapy in testicular cancer have been with combination chemotherapy. One of the most widely used combinations has been vinblastine plus bleomycin (11).

Cis-diamminedichloroplatinum is one of a group of coordination compounds of platinum identified by Rosenberg, VanCamp, and Krigas (12) that strongly inhibits bacterial replication. This agent has significant activity in refractory advanced testicular cancer, and, furthermore, it is ideal for combination chemotherapy because of its relative lack of myelosuppression (13).

In 1974, we began a study using vinblastine, bleomycin, and *cis*-diamminedichloroplatinum in disseminated testicular cancer. The primary goal was to increase the complete remission rate and potential cure rate. The results of treatment of the first 50 patients are the subject of this paper.

Materials and Methods

Fifty patients with germ-cell tumors of the testis were the subjects of this study. The median age was 26 years with a range of 15 to 63. All patients with metastatic measurable disease not refractory to any of the study agents were eligible for this study. Three patients died within 2 weeks of initiation of chemotherapy and were considered inevaluable.

Platinum was given in a dosage of 20 mg/m^2 body surface area as a 15-min intravenous infusion for 5 consecutive days (Days 1 to 5) every 3 weeks for three courses. Eight patients were given additional courses of platinum because they had no significant nephrotoxicity and had persistent evidence of residual disease after the first three courses. Vinblastine was given on Days 1 and 2 in a total dosage of 0.4 mg/kg body weight (0.2 mg/kg body weight each day) for a total of five courses every 3 weeks, and then given as a single injection in a dosage of 0.3 mg/kg body weight every 4 weeks for a total of 2 years of therapy. The vinblastine dosage was lowered 25% if the patient received previous radiotherapy. Bleomycin was given on Days 2, 9, and 16 of each platinum course, and was given with the platinum 6 h after vinblastine and then given weekly for a total of 12 weeks in a dosage of 30 U per week by intravenous push injection. Vinblastine and bleomycin were used in sequential

▶ From the Indiana University Medical Center; Indianapolis, Indiana.

combination in an attempt to make bleomycin more effective. Thusly vinblastine was given 6 h before bleomycin to take advantage of potential synergism between these two drugs (14). Bleomycin was shown to be most effective in killing Chinese hamster ovary cells in mitosis (15), and because vinblastine, like vincristine, also produces an arrest in the mitotic phase of the cell cycle, vinblastine and bleomycin were used in sequential combination for potential maximal tumor destruction by bleomycin. The bleomycin was stopped at a total dosage of 360 U because this drug can cause cumulative pulmonary fibrosis. Tice bacillus Calmette-Guérin (BCG) immunotherapy was started after completion of the 12 weeks of bleomycin in those patients who achieved complete remission, and was given by scarification 1, 2, and 3 weeks after each vinblastine injection for a total of 4 months and thereafter was given 1 and 3 weeks after each vinblastine injection. The dosage was 6×10^8 organisms with each scarification. This immunotherapy was used in an attempt to augment host cell-mediated immunity and prolong the duration of remission, and improve the prospects for total cell kill and eventual cure as has been shown in other diseases (16, 17).

The criterion for a partial response was a decrease of 50% or more in the sum of the products of diameters of all measurable lesions. A complete response was defined as a complete disappearance of all clinical, radiographic, and biochemical evidence of disease, including normal whole-lung tomograms, serum beta subunit of human chorionic gonadotrophin, and serum alpha-fetoprotein.

Blood cell counts, platelet counts, and differentials were determined weekly for all patients, and liver and renal function tests were done every 3 weeks. Arterial blood gas and pulmonary function studies were done every 3 weeks while patients were on bleomycin. Tumor measurements were recorded at least every 3 weeks, and appropriate radiologic and biochemical studies, including radioimmunoassay alpha-fetoprotein and beta subunit of human chorionic gonadotrophin, were repeated at least every 6 to 8 weeks.

Results

Fifty patients with disseminated testicular cancer were the subject of this study. Two patients died within 1 week of institution of chemotherapy, and a third patient died 2 weeks after initiation of chemotherapy, all presumably due to massive tumor, leaving 47 evaluable patients. All three of these patients had significant respiratory symptomatology due to massive pulmonary metastases.

Thirty-five of 47 patients (74%) achieved complete remission and 29 of these complete remissions remain alive and disease-free at from 6+ to 30+ months. Four patients died in complete remission. All four of these deaths were during the first 6 months of this study; there have been no drug-related deaths or deaths of patients in complete remission during the past 2 years. Two of these deaths were due to Gram-negative sepsis, one from bleomycin-induced pulmonary fibrosis, and one from multiple small-bowel fistulae and obstruction secondary to previous surgery. One of the above two deaths from Gram-negative sepsis was from klebsiella pneumonia in a chronic alcoholic who had no evidence of leukopenia during this episode.

Only three of these 35 complete remissions have relapsed. One patient relapsed on maintenance therapy with recurrent pulmonary disease and died shortly thereafter; a second patient refused any form of maintenance therapy and developed rapidly progressive pulmonary metastases and died within 24 h of readmission; a third patient developed headaches and right hemiparesis due to bilateral central nervous system metastases and is presently grossly free of disease and asymptomatic after whole-brain radiotherapy. All three relapses occurred within 9 months of initiation of chemotherapy.

In addition, five of the 12 patients in partial remission were rendered disease-free following surgical removal of residual disease after significant reduction of tumor volume with chemotherapy. Three of these five patients had complete removal of a teratoma, one via thoracotomy and two via laparotomy, and all three of these patients remain alive and disease-free on maintenance vinblastine plus BCG for 9+ to 24+ months after their surgery. The other two patients had residual embryonal and choriocarcinoma removed completely at laparotomy, but both eventually died with progressive tumor. Thus, the chemotherapy regimen of *cis*-diamminedichloroplatinum, vinblastine, and bleomycin produced 74% complete and 26% partial remissions in 47 evaluable patients. With the addition of surgical removal of residual disease in five of the patients in partial remission, an 85% overall disease-free status was obtained. Thirty-eight of these 47 patients remain alive and 32 remain alive and disease-free from 6+ to 30+ months later.

The relation of histology to response to chemotherapy is shown in Table 1. Excellent complete remission rates were seen in all cell types, although there was a suggestion of a lower complete remission rate in teratocarcinoma and choriocarcinoma. Obviously, these numbers are too small to make any valid conclusions concerning histology and complete remission; however, it was our impression that the lower complete remission rates in these histologies were primarily due to more extensive disease. Samuels, Johnson, and Holoye (11) have devised a classification for extent of disease, and the relation of extent of disease to complete remission is shown in Table 2. Twenty of 22 patients with minimal disease (Groups A, C, and E) achieved complete remission with this chemotherapy, and 18 of these patients are at present alive and disease-free.

The relation of previous therapy to complete remission is shown in Table 3. Patients with previous radiotherapy had considerably more prolonged and severe hematologic and gastrointestinal toxicity.

Radioimmunoassay alpha-fetoprotein was elevated in 50% of the patients and beta subunit of human chorionic gonadotrophin was elevated in 80% of these patients. Only three patients failed to have one of these two markers elevated. Generally speaking, we tended to see a one-log reduction in these tumor markers with each course of *cis*-platinum therapy. Eight patients received more than three courses of platinum. Each of these patients had extensive pulmonary (with or without abdominal) disease and achieved significant cytoreduction clinically, radiographically, and biochemically with each preceding course, but still had not yet achieved a complete remission. Five of these patients received a fourth course of platinum; three of these five patients achieved a complete remission with this course and have all remained in complete remission for longer than 12 months. The other two patients did not achieve complete remission, but the fourth course did normalize their tumor markers and they both have remained in partial remission for more than a year. The three patients who had more than four courses of *cis*-platinum achieved further cytoreduction, but never achieved complete remission.

Toxicity

Toxicity could be best described by separating this three-drug combination into its individual components:

Cis-platinum caused moderate-to-severe nausea and vomiting in all patients during each 5-day course. During the first year of this study, intravenous hydration was only used for very severe nausea and vomiting. Although only three of these earlier patients had significant azotemia (blood urea nitrogen greater than 50 mg/dl, or serum creatinine greater than 3.0 mg/dl, or both), many of these earlier patients now have a 25% to 50% reduction from their baseline creatinine clearance and have serum creatinine of 1.5 to 2.0 mg/dl. None of these patients show progressive nephrotoxicity or azotemic symptomatology, and the long-term effects of *cis*-platinum on renal function are still being studied. One patient required hemodialysis for acute renal failure and is the subject of a separate case report (18). In the past 18 months, we have been using vigorous intravenous hydration on all patients during each course of *cis*-platinum, using 100 ml/h of normal saline for 12 h before administration of chemotherapy (prehydration) and then continuous saline hydration during all 5 days of *cis*-platinum administration. Since we have been using this form of intravenous hydration, we have only rarely encountered any of the above biochemical manifestations of platinum nephrotoxicity, and none of these patients have had serum creatinines above 1.5 mg/dl. We have not used mannitol diuresis in any of our patients. Although occasional patients had a decrease in high-frequency hearing, there were no observed clinical audiologic abnormalities. Mild hyperuricemia and hypokalemia were occasionally seen, but were not a clinical problem.

Bleomycin produced fever, chills, and cutaneous striae in all patients, but these were not a clinical problem and did not require alteration of the bleomycin dosages. All patients had significant alopecia and most had weight loss

Table 1. Classification of Primary Tumor

Dixon-Moore	Histology	Patients	Complete Remissions*
		no.	*%*
I	Pure seminoma	4	75
II	Embryonal, with or without seminoma	25	84
III	Teratoma	2	50
IV	Teratocarcinoma with embryonal or choriocarcinoma	9	55
V	Choriocarcinoma with embryonal carcinoma	5	60
	Yolk sac	2	100

* Complete disappearance of all clinical, radiographic, and biochemical evidence of disease, including normal whole lung tomograms and serum alpha-fetoprotein and beta subunit human chorionic gonadotrophin.

Table 2. Extent of Disease

	Patients	Complete Remissions*
	no.	*%*
A. Minimal pulmonary disease	10	90
B. Advanced Pulmonary disease	9	67
C. Minimal abdominal and pulmonary disease	9	88
D. Advanced abdominal disease	16	56
E. Elevated human chorionic gonadotropin	3	100

* Complete disappearance of all clinical, radiographic, and biochemical evidence of disease, including normal whole lung tomograms and serum alpha-fetoprotein and beta subunit human chorionic gonadotrophin.

(from *cis*-platinum and bleomycin) during the 12 weeks of bleomycin. No patient required intravenous hyperalimentation, and all patients completely regained their weight after the completion of bleomycin therapy. There was one death from bleomycin pulmonary fibrosis in a patient who inadvertently received a total of 420 U of bleomycin. There were no other cases of clinically significant pulmonary fibrosis.

Vinblastine produced myalgia in half of the patients. Although this was occasionally severe enough to require narcotic analgesics during the first 12 weeks of therapy, it was not a clinical problem during maintenance therapy with the lower dosage (0.3 mg/kg body weight) of vinblastine. Anemia and thrombocytopenia were observed in several patients but no patient had thrombocytopenic bleeding or required platelet transfusions. Only four patients experienced thrombocytopenia below 100 000 mm^3 and these were all in patients who had had previous radiotherapy. Anemia was more of a problem, especially in patients who had had previous radiotherapy. Packed erythrocyte transfusions were required periodically on four patients during the first several months of therapy, and all four of these patients had received previous radiotherapy. Leukopenia also was more severe and prolonged in patients with previous irradiation, and they were started on a lowered dosage of vinblastine (0.15 mg/kg body weight for 2 consecutive days). The most serious side-effect, which was seen in all patients, was severe leukopenia. The nadir of the leukocyte usually was 1000 mm^3 between Days 7 and 14. Eighteen patients required hospitalization for presumed sepsis with granulocytopenic fever and were cultured and started on antibiotic coverage with broad-spectrum antibiotics. Seven of these patients had documented Gram-negative sepsis and one of these patients died of sepsis.

The BCG immunotherapy caused local erythema, pruritus, fever, and myalgia but was generally well tolerated by all patients except one who had severe local reactivity and an ulcerated regional lymph node requiring cessation of the BCG.

Despite the aforementioned significant toxicity, this occurred primarily during the 12 weeks of remission induction therapy. Maintenance therapy with vinblastine and BCG was well tolerated and all patients regained their hair growth and weight during this period. No patient

Table 3. Previous Therapy

	Patients	Complete Remissions*
	no.	%
Surgery alone	21	76
Surgery and chemoprophylaxis	9	88
Surgery and chemotherapy (for metastatic disease)	10	70
Surgery and radiotherapy	3	67
Surgery, chemotherapy, and radiotherapy	4	50

* Complete disappearance of all clinical, radiographic, and biochemical evidence of disease, including normal whole lung tomograms and serum alpha-fetoprotein and beta subunit human chorionic gonadotrophin.

required hospitalization for complications of therapy during vinblastine and BCG maintenance and were all able to continue school or work full-time.

The value of maintenance therapy vinblastine and BCG was impossible to ascertain especially with the clear definitions of complete remission that were used.

Discussion

Since the original report by Li and associates (4) in 1960 showing activity of chemotherapy in disseminated testicular cancer, there have been numerous clinical trials evaluating a variety of drugs in these diseases (Table 4). Although it is not possible to extract present survival data on all patients reported in Table 4, there does appear to be a general trend showing that more than 50% of all complete remissions in disseminated testicular cancer have prolonged survival and potential cure. Indeed, in testicular cancer in general, most relapses occur within 2 years of initiation of chemotherapy or surgery (23, 24). It seems quite reasonable to expect that many of the patients in this study who are currently alive and disease-free will be cured of their malignancy.

Generally speaking, the only meaningful response for the patient has been complete remission, as partial remissions were usually of brief duration. However, it is noteworthy that of our 12 patients who achieved partial remission, five of these patients had significant enough reduction of tumor volume to make an attempt at surgical removal of residual disease feasible, and three of these five patients remain alive and disease-free 9+ to 24+ months after their surgery. Five of the other seven patients in partial remission have remained in their original partial remission for 7+ to 23+ months. Aggressive chemotherapy appears capable of changing the histology to a more mature and benign form, as has been previously reported (25, 26), and this may be partly responsible for the prolonged duration of partial remissions seen in some of these patients.

The rationale behind combination chemotherapy is to combine antineoplastic drugs that are all individually active against the specific tumor, exhibit different toxicities, have different mechanisms of action, and have shown clinical synergism. Vinblastine, bleomycin, and *cis*-platinum all have activity against testicular cancer as single agents (7, 8, 13). These three agents have individual and separate side-effects, with the dose-limiting toxicity of vinblastine, bleomycin, and *cis*-platinum being leukopenia, pulmonary fibrosis, and nephrotoxicity respectively. Vinblastine, a vinca alkaloid, produces a mitotic arrest (27). Bleomycin combines with DNA in the presence of a sulfhydryl compound or hydrogen peroxide, resulting in a decrease of the DNA melting point and scission of the DNA strands (28). *Cis*-platinum produces inhibition of DNA synthesis, possibly through template inactivation (29). The combination of vinblastine and bleomycin appears to represent a truly synergistic combination as the complete remission rate for this two-drug combination is higher than would be predicted from the single-agent data of these two drugs (7, 8).

Although the treatment of choice for seminoma is orchiectomy plus radiotherapy, a word of caution needs to be interjected. Patients who have a "pure seminoma" diagnosed by orchiectomy should not have an elevated beta subunit of human chorionic gonadotrophin or alpha-fetoprotein level, as such patients have nonseminomatous elements present elsewhere and should be managed as a nonseminomatous testicular cancer (30).

It is attractive to consider adjuvant aggressive chemotherapy with regimens such as *cis*-platinum, vinblastine, and bleomycin in stage B nonseminomatous testicu-

Table 4. Results with Chemotherapy in Disseminated Testicular Cancer

Authors	Treatment	Total Patients	Complete Remissions*		Prolonged Survivors†
			no.	(%)	
Wyatt, McAninch (19)	Methotrexate	10	4	(40)	4
MacKenzie (6)	Dactinomycin (alone or in double or triple therapy)	154	24	(16)	13
Mendelson, Serpick (20)	Cyclophosphamide, vincristine, methotrexate, and flourouracil (COMF)	17	5	(29)	1
Jacobs (21)	Vincristine, dactinomycin and cyclophosphamide (VAC)	58	7	(12)	4
Kennedy (9)	Mithramycin	23	5	(22)	5
Samuels, Howe (7)	Vinblastine	21	4	(19)	2
Samuels, Johnson, Holoye (11)	Vinblastine and bleomycin	23	9	(39)	. . .
Cvitkovic, Hayes, Golbey (22)	Vinblastine, bleomycin, cyclophosphamide, dactinomycin and *cis*-platinum (VAB III)	26	18	(69)	. . .

* Complete disappearance of all clinical, radiographic, and biochemical evidence of disease, including normal whole lung tomograms and serum alpha-fetoprotein and beta subunit human chorionic gonadotrophin.

† Those patients remaining alive and disease-free at the time of publication.

lar cancer (tumor metastatic to retroperitoneal nodes but not beyond) as about 40% of these patients are going to relapse postoperatively (31). Clearly this three-drug regimen has significant activity in advanced disease. The use of adjuvant aggressive combination chemotherapy would certainly lower the recurrence rate, but only a randomized prospective study could ascertain whether it would improve the survival in stage B nonseminomatous testicular cancer. There is a certain morbidity and mortality associated with such chemotherapy, and it is our feeling that we can avoid such aggressive chemotherapy in most patients with stage B disease without lowering the survival probability by following such patients postoperatively once a month for the first year with chest roentgenogram, beta subunit human chorionic gonadotrophin, and alphafetoprotein determinations. This allows us to find relapses at a relatively early time when they have minimal recurrent disease, and institute chemotherapy with *cis*-platinum, vinblastine, and bleomycin at that time with a very high probability of complete remission. Twenty of 22 patients with "minimal" disease (Table 2) achieved complete remission, and the only two patients failing to achieve complete remission included a patient who had been heavily treated with previous chemotherapy and another patient who had complete disappearance of bilateral pulmonary metastases except for a solitary nodule, which was removed at thoracotomy and found to have changed histologically from an embryonal carcinoma to a teratoma. Thus, only two of 22 patients with "minimal" disease failed to achieve a disease-free status. At this institution, we have been using dactinomycin chemoprophylaxis postoperatively for stage B disease and have had eight of 24 such patients relapse and develop pulmonary metastases. However, all eight of these patients achieved complete remission and are presently alive and disease-free after institution of *cis*-platinum, vinblastine, and bleomycin chemotherapy. One patient had the rare clinical situation of developing recurrent advanced pulmonary metastases 7 years after completion of a course of adjuvant dactinomycin, and this patient failed to achieve complete remission.

Recommendations for Platinum-Vinblastine-Bleomycin

Our experience with this regimen of combination chemotherapy in 50 patients with advanced testicular cancer allows us to suggest the following guidelines.

[1] The goal of therapy in all patients should be complete remission and if a clinical complete remission is not achieved after three courses of *cis*-platinum in a responding patient with no significant nephrotoxicity, a fourth course should be given. We have not found any value in exceeding four courses. Most patients achieved a clinical complete remission by the end of two courses of *cis*-platinum.

[2] If a clinical complete remission has not been achieved with chemotherapy, surgical excision of residual disease should be considered if feasible. The two clinical situations where this occurs are:

(a) Complete disappearance of pulmonary metastases except for a solitary residual nodule or nodules confined to a single lobe of the lung; wedge resection is the preferred surgical approach.

(b) Complete disappearance of all supradiaphragmatic disease in a patient who initially presented with a large palpable abdominal mass. It has been our policy to do an exploratory laparotomy with removal of any residual tumor in all such patients who initially presented with pulmonary disease and a large palpable abdominal mass after the 12 weeks of bleomycin therapy. We have done seven such surgical explorations; four patients had complete excision of residual tumor and three others had no evidence of remaining abdominal tumor. Interestingly, one of these patients had a persistent palpable abdominal mass that was removed at surgery and proved to be fibrous tissue only. Thus, as has been previously reported (32), the presence of a persistent retroperitoneal mass in this circumstance does not invariably mean the presence of persistent malignant tissue. We have not felt it necessary to do laparotomies or retroperitoneal node dissection in any of the other patients in this series, despite the fact that many of them had evidence of abdominal disease initially.

[3] The major toxicity with this therapeutic regimen has been the significant leukopenia and potential granulocytopenic sepsis secondary to vinblastine. It is quite possible that we could achieve the same therapeutic results without such significant leukopenia and potential sepsis by starting with a 25% reduction in the vinblastine dosage. This question is currently being evaluated at this institution in a randomized prospective study, and although the numbers are small, thus far, we have achieved the same complete remission rate with the lowered dosage of vinblastine. Any patient who has had previous irradiation should have a 25% to 50% dosage reduction of vinblastine.

[4] It has been our practice to hospitalize any patient with a temperature above 38.3 °C and less than 1000 granulocytes/mm^3, obtain appropriate cultures, and institute broad-spectrum antibiotic coverage with cephalothin and carbenicillin. We try to avoid gentamicin in this situation because of the possible synergistic renal tubular damage between *cis*-platinum and aminoglycoside antibiotics. Some of our more significant transient nephrotoxicity in our earlier patients was seen in this clinical situation where gentamicin was used.

[5] Vigorous attention is paid to saline hydration, regardless of the patient's oral intake. All patients receive 100 ml/h normal saline intravenous hydration for 12 h before institution of the chemotherapy and for the entire 5-day course of *cis*-platinum.

This present regimen has produced the highest complete remission rate in testicular cancer reported thus far. Furthermore, chemotherapy can significantly alter the course of the disease, even without complete remission. Present aggressive chemotherapy regimens appear to be capable of changing the histology to a more benign form and transferring previously inoperable patients (who fail to achieve a chemotherapy complete remission) to potentially operable and, it is hoped, curable patients.

The results of recent regimens and this regimen clearly indicate that disseminated testicular cancer is a very responsive disease to chemotherapy, and many patients are probably curative, even with far-advanced disease. The complete remission rate of 74% and overall disease-free status of 85% is as high as has been seen in any adult malignancy treated with chemotherapy.

ACKNOWLEDGMENTS: Received 26 January 1977; revision accepted 18 May 1977.

► Requests for reprints should be addressed to Lawrence H. Einhorn, M.D., F.A.C.P.; Indiana University School of Medicine; 110 West Michigan Street; Indianapolis, IN 46202.

References

1. MacKay EN, Sellers AH: A statistical review of malignant testicular tumors based on the experience of the Ontario Cancer Foundation Clinics, 1938-1961. *Can Med Assoc J* 94:889-899, 1966
2. Maier JG, Mittemeyer BT, Sulak MH: Treatment and prognosis in seminoma of the testis. *J Urol* 99:72-78, 1968
3. Freedman M, Purkayastha MC: Recurrent seminoma: management of late metastases, recurrence of a second primary tumor. *Am J Roentgenol Radium Ther Nucl Med* 83:25-42, 1960
4. Li MC, Whitmore WF, Golbey R, Grabstald H: Effects of combined drug therapy on metastatic cancer of the testis. *JAMA* 174:145-153, 1960
5. Ansfield FJ, Korbitz BD, Davis HL Jr, Ramirez G: Triple therapy in testicular tumors. *Cancer* 24:442-446, 1969
6. MacKenzie AR: Chemotherapy of metastatic testis cancer—results in 154 patients. *Cancer* 19:1369-1376, 1966
7. Samuels ML, Howe CD: Vinblastine in the management of testicular cancer. *Cancer* 25:1009-1017, 1970
8. Blum RH, Carter S, Agre K: A clinical review of bleomycin—a new antineoplastic agent. *Cancer* 31:903-914, 1973
9. Kennedy BJ: Mithramycin therapy in advanced testicular neoplasms. *Cancer* 26:755-766, 1970
10. DeVita VT, Serpick AA, Carbone PP: Combination chemotherapy in the treatment of advanced Hodgkin's disease. *Ann Intern Med* 73:881-895, 1970
11. Samuels ML, Johnson EE, Holoye PY: Continuous intravenous bleomycin therapy with vinblastine in stage III testicular neoplasia. *Cancer Chemother Rep* 59:563-570, 1975
12. Rosenberg B, VanCamp L, Krigas T: Inhibition of cell division in *E. Coli* by electrolysis products from a platinum electrode. *Nature* 205:678-699, 1965
13. Higby DJ, Wallace HJ, Albert DJ, Holland JF: Diaminodichloroplatinum: a phase I study showing responses in testicular and other tumors. *Cancer* 33:1219-1225, 1974
14. Livingston RB, Bodey GP, Gottlieb JA, et al: Kinetic scheduling of vincristine (NSC-67574) and bleomycin (NSC-125066) in patients with lung cancer and other malignant tumors. *Cancer Chemother Rep* 57:219-224, 1973
15. Barranco SC, Humphrey RM: The effects of bleomycin on survival and cell progression in Chinese hamster cells in vitro. *Cancer Res* 31:1218-1223, 1971
16. Gutterman JU, Rodriguez V, Mavligit G, et al: Chemoimmunotherapy of adult acute leukemia. Prolongation or remission in myeloblastic leukemia with BCG. *Lancet* 2:1405-1409, 1974
17. Gutterman JU, Mavligit G, Gottlieb JA, et al: Chemoimmunotherapy of disseminated malignant melanoma with dimethyl triazeno imidazole carboxamide and bacillus Calmette-Guerín. *N Engl J Med* 291:592-597, 1974
18. Crooke ST, Luft F, Broughton A, et al: Bleomycin serum pharmacokinetics as determined by a radioimmunoassay and a microbiologic assay in a patient with compromised renal function. *Cancer,* in press for 1977
19. Wyatt JK, McAninch LH: A chemotherapeutic approach to advanced testicular carcinoma. *Can J Surg* 10:421-426, 1967
20. Mendelson D, Serpick AA: Combination chemotherapy of testicular tumors. *J Urol* 103:619-623, 1970
21. Jacobs E: Combination chemotherapy of metastatic testicular germinal cell tumors and soft part sarcomas. *Cancer* 25:324-332, 1970
22. Cvitkovic E, Hayes D, Golbey R: Primary combination chemotherapy (VAB III) for metastatic or unresectable germ cell tumors. *Proc Am Soc Clin Oncol* 17:296, 1976
23. Nefzger MD, Mostofi FK: Survival after surgery for germinal malignancies of the testis. *Cancer* 30:1225-1232, 1972
24. Lefevre RE, Levin HE, Banowsky LH, et al: Testis tumors: review of 125 cases at the Cleveland Clinic. *Urology* 6:588-593, 1975
25. Willis GW, Hajdu SI: Histologically benign teratoid metastasis of testicular embryonal carcinoma: report of five cases. *Am J Clin Pathol* 59:338-343, 1973
26. Merrin C, Takita H, Weber R, et al: Combination radical surgery and multiple sequential chemotherapy for the treatment of advanced carcinoma of the testis (stage III). *Cancer* 37:20-29, 1976
27. Creasey W: Effect of the vinca alkaloids on RNA synthesis in relation to mitotic arrest. *Fed Proc* 27:760, 1968
28. Nagai K, Suzuk H, Tanaka N, et al: Decrease of melting temperature and single strand scission of DNA by bleomycin in the presence of hydrogen peroxide. *J Antibiot* 22:624-628, 1969
29. Harder HC, Smith RG, LeRoy A: Template inactivation: the mechanism of action of *cis*-dichlorodiammineplatinum. *Proc Am Assoc Cancer Res* 17:80, 1976
30. Lange PH, McIntire R, Waldmann TA, et al: Serum alpha-fetoprotein and human chorionic gonadotropin in the diagnosis and management of non-seminomatous germ-cell testicular cancer. *N Engl J Med* 295:1237-1240, 1976
31. Skinner DG, Leadbetter WF: The surgical management of testis tumors. *J Urol* 106:84-93, 1971
32. Comisarow RH, Grabstald H: Re-exploration for retroperitoneal lymph node metastases from testis tumor. *J Urol* 115:569-571, 1976

Section X

Pulmonary Medicine

Continuous or nocturnal oxygen therapy in hypoxemic chronic obstructive lung disease: a clinical trial.

Nocturnal Oxygen Therapy Trial Group. Ann Intern Med. 1980;93: 391-398.

Through the 1960s, treatment of chronic obstructive pulmonary disease (COPD) was limited to potassium iodide as a mucolytic, antibiotics for pneumonia, and combinations of theophylline and ephedrine. Phlebotomy was commonly performed for erythrocytosis caused by hypoxemia. Oxygen use and exercise were contraindicated. Reports of oxygen therapy surfaced, however, including an influential 1967 paper by Levine and colleagues in *Annals* describing impressive results in hypoxemic patients with COPD patients treated with ambulatory oxygen. Pulmonary pressures and erythrocytosis were ameliorated, while exercise tolerance increased (1).

Because the prognosis of COPD was so terrible, prescriptions for continuous oxygen grew despite the lack of firm data, as did the associated costs. Thus, in 1976, the National Heart, Lung, and Blood Institute organized a trial to assess whether nocturnal oxygen alone might be sufficient. It was postulated that 12 hours of oxygen each night might achieve equivalent reductions in pulmonary vascular resistance and hematocrit, but without the inconvenience and cost associated with the ambulatory delivery systems required for continuous daytime therapy (2). The Nocturnal Oxygen Therapy Trial (NOTT), published in *Annals* in 1980, provided a clear-cut answer: Continuous oxygen therapy was indicated for hypoxemic patients with COPD.

Twenty-one percent of the patients in the nocturnal oxygen group died within 12 months as compared with 12% of those receiving continuous oxygen; mortality at 24 months was 41% and 22%, respectively. Of note, survival was improved in patients without erythrocytosis or pulmonary hypertension, as well as those with poor baseline exercise tolerance. These findings, complemented by the results of the British Medical Research Council trial published in 1981 demonstrating improved survival with 15 hours of oxygen daily compared with room air (3), firmly established the scientific basis and insurance requirements that persist today for oxygen therapy.

Long-term oxygen for hypoxemic patients with COPD, or those with cor pulmonale, is the standard of care and the only intervention and to date it is the proven to increase survival. The NOTT findings remain paramount in our management of COPD. Indeed, when was the last time you ordered therapeutic phlebotomy for your patient with COPD? Sounds as crazy today as prescribing a blood-letting!

References

1. **Levine BE, Bigelow DB, Hamstra RD, Beckwitt HJ, Mitchell RS, Nett LM, et al.** The role of long-term continuous oxygen administration in patients with chronic airway obstruction with hypoxemia. Ann Intern Med. 1967;66:639-50.

2. **Lenfant C.** Twelve- or 24-hour oxygen therapy: why a clinical trial? [Editorial]. JAMA. 1980;243:551-2.

3. Long term domiciliary oxygen therapy in chronic hypoxic cor pulmonale complicating chronic bronchitis and emphysema. Report of the Medical Research Council Working Party. Lancet. 1981;1:681-6.

Is embolic risk conditioned by location of deep venous thrombosis?

Moser KM, LeMoine JR. Ann Intern Med. 1981;94(Part 1):439-444.

In the late 1970s, Moser and LeMoine sought to establish whether emerging diagnostic modalities could reliably identify which patients with deep vein venous thrombosis (DVT) needed anticoagulation. Recent studies had shown non-invasive radiofibrinogen leg scans and impedance plethysmography (IPG) to be highly sensitive for DVT and potential substitutes for contrast venography (1,2). And while clot confined to the calf appeared not to pose a risk of pulmonary embolism (PE), the safety of withholding anticoagulation in this setting had not been shown. Indeed, as the availability of highly sensitive and non-invasive tests grew, so did the apparent over-diagnosis and inappropriate treatment of DVT. By the mid 1970s, an editorialist in *Annals* cautioned that heparin had become the most common cause of drug-related toxicity and iatrogenic death in U.S. hospitals (3).

Moser and LeMoine performed contrast venography, leg scanning, and IPGs in 68 hospitalized patients with clinical findings or risks for DVT and correlated these results with baseline ventilation-perfusion scans and clinical evaluations 3 months later. The combination of leg scanning and IPG successfully identified all patients with venographically evident clot and accurately determined its location as either proximal or confined to the calf. Uniquely useful to the practicing physician, however, was the demonstration that no patient with clot confined to the calf had PE on ventilation-perfusion scanning. Most importantly, this study showed for the first time that heparin could be safely withheld in these patients; none had clinical evidence of PE by 3 months, and none had received anticoagulation. Thus, not only could non-invasive testing be used to localize clot within the leg, but the results could be used to guide therapy and avoid needless exposure to the risk of anticoagulation.

Since then, our diagnostic approach has been refined several times (4). Today, we can identify certain low- risk patients by blood testing alone. Neither radiofibrinogen leg scanning nor IPG is routinely performed in U.S. hospitals. But the measures employed by Moser and LeMoine—correlating test results and treatments with clinical outcomes at 3 months—, remains the standard for judging the prudence of any diagnostic or management algorithm for venous thromboembolic disease.

References

1. **Moser KM, Brach BB, Dolan GF.** Clinically suspected deep venous thrombosis of the lower extremities. A comparison of venography, impedance plethysmography, and radiolabeled fibrinogen. JAMA. 1977;237: 2195-8.

2. **Hull R, Hirsh J, Sackett DL, Powers P, Turpie AG, Walker I.** Combined use of leg scanning and impedance plethysmography in suspected venous thrombosis. An alternative to venography. N Engl J Med. 1977;296:1497-500.

3. **Robin ED.** Overdiagnosis and overtreatment of pulmonary embolism: the emperor may have no clothes. Ann Intern Med. 1977;87:775-81.

4. **Goodacre S.** In the clinic. Deep venous thrombosis. Ann Intern Med. 2008;149:ITC3-1.

Antibiotic therapy in exacerbations of chronic obstructive pulmonary disease.

Anthonisen NR, Manfreda J, Warren CP, Hershfield ES, Harding GK, Nelson NA. Ann Intern Med. 1987;106:196-204.

In the early 1980s, Anthonisen and colleagues designed a double-blind randomized controlled trial to assess the effect of antibiotics on acute exacerbations of chronic obstructive pulmonary disease (COPD). Conventional wisdom since the mid-1970s was that bacterial infection was an epiphenomenon of worsened symptoms in COPD, rather than their cause (1). Yet, courses of antibiotics remained standard practice for such disease "flares." The findings of the landmark study published in *Annals*, therefore, have since affected (or at least justified) the care of millions of patients with COPD exacerbations. Ten days of an oral antibiotic decreased the duration of symptoms, increased the likelihood of their resolution, and reduced by nearly one half the number of patients who deteriorated further. Antibiotics were beneficial regardless of whether corticosteroids were also used, and few antibiotic-related side effects were noted. (There was no report of whether antibiotic resistance occurred, an interesting contrast to a major concern of in antimicrobial therapy studies performed today.)

Despite many subsequent studies, with at times conflicting data, Anthonisen and colleagues' trial remains one of the largest and most rigorously conducted, and its findings have been confirmed by recent systematic reviews (2,3). But the study contributed more than solid data; by establishing a standardized method to characterize an exacerbation's severity, it provided an essential tool to report and compare results. The presence of one, two, or three cardinal symptoms (increased dyspnea, sputum volume, or purulence) continues to define an exacerbation as mild, moderate, or severe, respectively. Anthonisen and colleagues' results and method of patient evaluation continue to be cited as the sentinel work supporting national and international practice guidelines (4,5).

Approximately half of the patients treated with placebo got better without antibiotics. We now believe that approximately half of exacerbations are triggered by bacterial infection (6). The problem of identifying which half, however, remains. Until we find better ways, Anthonisen and colleagues' conclusion about who should receive antibiotics remains valid—that is, patients with moderate or severe exacerbations.

References

1. **Tager I, Speizer FE.** Role of infection in chronic bronchitis. N Engl J Med. 1975;292:563-71.
2. **Bach PB, Brown C, Gelfand SE, McCrory DC.** American College of Physicians-American Society of Internal Medicine. Management of acute exacerbations of chronic obstructive pulmonary disease: a summary and appraisal of published evidence. Ann Intern Med. 2001;134:600-20.
3. **Ram FS, Rodriguez-Roisin R, Granados-Navarrete A, Garcia-Aymerich J, Barnes NC.** Antibiotics for exacerbations of chronic obstructive pulmonary disease. Cochrane Database Syst Rev. 2006:CD004403.
4. **Snow V, Lascher S, Mottur-Pilson C.** Joint Expert Panel on Chronic Obstructive Pulmonary Disease of the American College of Chest Physicians and the American College of Physicians-American Society of Internal Medicine. Evidence base for management of acute exacerbations of chronic obstructive pulmonary disease. Ann Intern Med. 2001;134: 595-9.
5. **The Global Initiative for Obstructive Lung Disease home page.** Accessed at www.goldcopd.com; 2 February 2009.
6. **Sethi S, Murphy TF.** Infection in the pathogenesis and course of chronic obstructive pulmonary disease. N Engl J Med. 2008;359:2355-65.

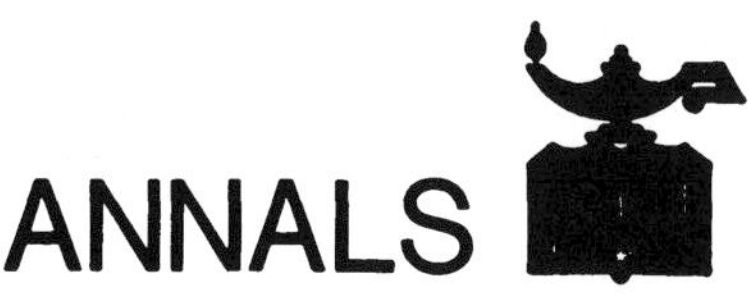

ANNALS of Internal Medicine

SEPTEMBER 1980 • VOLUME 93 • NUMBER 3

Published Monthly by the American College of Physicians

Continuous or Nocturnal Oxygen Therapy in Hypoxemic Chronic Obstructive Lung Disease

A Clinical Trial

NOCTURNAL OXYGEN THERAPY TRIAL GROUP*

At six centers, 203 patients with hypoxemic chronic obstructive lung disease were randomly allocated to either continuous oxygen (O_2) therapy or 12-hour nocturnal O_2 therapy and followed for at least 12 months (mean, 19.3 months). The two groups were initially well matched in terms of physiological and neuropsychological function. Compliance with each oxygen regimen was good. Overall mortality in the nocturnal O_2 therapy group was 1.94 times that in the continuous O_2 therapy group ($P = 0.01$). This trend was striking in patients with carbon dioxide retention and also present in patients with relatively poor lung function, low mean nocturnal oxygen saturation, more severe brain dysfunction, and prominent mood disturbances. Continuous O_2 therapy also appeared to benefit patients with low mean pulmonary artery pressure and pulmonary vascular resistance and those with relatively well-preserved exercise capacity. We conclude that in hypoxemic chronic obstructive lung disease, continuous O_2 therapy is associated with a lower mortality than is nocturnal O_2 therapy. The reason for this difference is not clear.

PATIENTS WITH chronic obstructive lung disease and hypoxemia have a poor prognosis in spite of treatment regimens aimed at improving the mechanical function of the lungs (1). Because of this, such patients are often treated with supplementary oxygen on an outpatient basis. Early studies of this treatment, which compared patients before and after oxygen therapy, indicated that chronic O_2 therapy resulted in improved exercise tolerance, decreased pulmonary hypertension and erythrocytosis, and improved neuropsychological function (2-6). A trial in which oxygen was given to one group of patients but withheld from a similar control group has not been done in North America, but such a trial is underway in the United Kingdom, and a preliminary report indicates that oxygen administration was associated with a reduced mortality (7).

Long-term oxygen administration is an expensive form of treatment, particularly when ambulatory patients are supplied with portable units. It is not clear whether continuous O_2 therapy is necessary; patients suffer their most severe hypoxemia while sleeping (8), and it is possible that hypoxemic sequelae such as erythrocytosis and pulmonary hypertension could be prevented by exclusively nocturnal oxygen administration. Indeed, there is some evidence that pulmonary hypertension can be reduced by as little as 15 hours of oxygen administration per day (9, 10).

On the basis of this rationale, the Division of Lung Diseases of the National Heart, Lung, and Blood Institute initiated a multicenter clinical trial comparing continuous O_2 therapy with nocturnal O_2 therapy in patients with hypoxemic chronic obstructive lung disease (11).

Methods

The protocol for the trial has been published elsewhere in detail (12) and therefore will be presented briefly here. Six treatment centers recruited 203 patients over 27 months and followed each surviving patient at least 1 year. The number of patients at each center varied from 26 to 44. Entry and exclusion criteria are shown in Table 1. The most important entry criterion was, of course, hypoxemia. The protocol required that this criterion be fulfilled on at least two occasions more than 1 week apart during a 3-week observation period while the subject was free of exacerbations and was managed without supplemental oxygen and with intensive bronchodilator therapy. In practice, patients were initially identified as fitting the entry but not the exclusion criteria, recruited in a preliminary way, and observed for 3 weeks to ensure stability. At the end of this time, if the patients still met these criteria, informed consent was obtained and the patient was hospitalized for a week of baseline studies. At the end of these studies, each patient was randomly allocated by the Data Center to either continuous O_2 or nocturnal O_2 therapy. Randomization schedules were developed sepa-

*For acknowledgment of contract support, a list of participants in the Nocturnal Oxygen Therapy Trial, and lists of other supporting personnel, see Acknowledgments at the end of this article.

Table 1. Entry and Exclusion Criteria

Entry criteria
- Clinical diagnosis of chronic obstructive lung disease
- Hypoxemia
  - $Pa_{O_2} \leqslant 55$ mm Hg
  - $Pa_{O_2} \leqslant 59$ plus one of the following:
    - Edema
    - Hematocrit $\geqslant 55\%$
    - P pulmonale on ECG: 3 mm in leads II, III, aVf
- Lung function*
  - $FEV_1/FVC < 70\%$ after inhaled bronchodilator
  - TLC $\geqslant 80\%$ predicted
  - Age > 35

Exclusion criteria
- Previous O_2 therapy: 12 h/d for 30 days during previous 2 months
- Other disease that might be expected to influence mortality, morbidity, compliance with therapy, or ability to give informed consent

* FEV_1 = forced expiratory volume in 1 second; FVC = forced vital capacity; TLC = total lung capacity.

rately for each investigative center. Treatment assignments were preset in blocks of four with an equal number of patients receiving nocturnal O_2 therapy and continuous O_2 therapy in each block. The order of treatment assignment was randomly computer-generated within each block of four.

Baseline studies included a complete history and physical examination, blood count, urinalysis, measurements of blood urea nitrogen and electrolytes, ECG, and chest radiograph. Lung function was assessed by measuring forced expiratory volume in 1 second (FEV_1) and forced vital capacity (FVC) spirometrically and functional residual capacity (FRC) with a plethysmograph. Arterial blood was obtained while the patient, breathing room air, rested semirecumbent and was analyzed for Po_2, Pco_2, and pH with appropriate electrodes. Exercise performance was studied with bicycle ergometry, using a progressive multi-stage technique. Right heart catheterization was done with measurements of pulmonary artery and wedge pressures and of cardiac output. Oxygen saturation during sleep was measured with an ear oximeter while the patient breathed air and O_2 on separate nights. Neuropsychological function was assessed by study of neuropsychological history and administration of a modified Halstead-Reitan battery (13) of tests. These tests were evaluated collectively, in terms of the Russell-Neuringer average impairment index (14), and a clinical rating scale of 1 to 6 with 6 representing maximal impairment (15). This rating was made by two neuropsychologists without knowledge of the treatment assignment of the patient. The patient's quality of life was assessed by the administration of the Minnesota Multiphasic Personality Inventory (16), the Sickness Impact Profile (17), and the Profile of Mood States (18).

After 6 months of nocturnal or continuous O_2 therapy, all baseline tests except sleep studies were repeated. Thereafter, at 6-month intervals, all baseline studies were again repeated except sleep studies, right heart catheterization, and neuropsychological testing.

After randomization, patients were instructed in the use of their oxygen equipment and discharged for follow-up as outpatients. Oxygen was administered by nasal prongs at a measured flow rate of 1 to 4 L/min. Each patient received the lowest flow in whole litres per minute that demonstrably increased resting, semirecumbent arterial Po_2 at least 6 mm Hg and maintained a resting arterial Po_2 of 60 to 80 mm Hg. This dose was increased by 1 L/min for periods of exercise and sleep. Oxygen delivery systems varied; oxygen concentrators, liquid oxygen systems, and compressed gas were all used. Compliance with therapy was checked in two ways. The patient and a family member were required to keep written records of oxygen use, and oxygen reservoirs or concentrators were fitted with timers that recorded the duration of gas flow. Because only stationary systems had such timers, oxygen use was recorded accurately in nocturnal O_2 therapy patients but underestimated in some continuous O_2 therapy patients who, in addition to a stationary system, used a portable system such as liquid oxygen walkers or small tanks of compressed gas.

Besides oxygen, all patients were treated with oral theophylline and inhaled beta-2 agonists. Diuretics and antibiotics were used as clinically indicated. Use of other drugs, such as steroids, cardiac glycosides, sedatives, tranquilizers, antidepressants and oral beta agonists, was discouraged. Therapeutic phlebotomies were not done.

All patients were followed closely to assure compliance and to assess changes in clinical state. For the first 6 months of the study, they were visited weekly in the home by a nurse practitioner, and were seen each month in outpatient clinic. After the first 6 months, they were visited at home at least once a month and were seen in the outpatient clinic at least every 3 months. At 1-month intervals during the first 6 months and at 3-month intervals thereafter, samples of arterial blood were obtained while the patient breathed his prescribed dose of oxygen and the dose adjusted if arterial Po_2 was not 60 to 80 mm Hg. Unscheduled clinic or emergency room visits were recorded. When a patient became ill enough to be hospitalized, the assigned treatment regimen was suspended but was resumed as soon as possible thereafter. Oxygen dose was reassessed after each hospitalization. If a patient died, an attempt was made to obtain a postmortem examination.

All observations were made under specified conditions at predetermined time intervals and recorded on standardized data forms to assure uniform collection of data by all participants. Immediately after each recorded event, copies of the completed data forms were mailed directly to a designated Data Center for editing, analysis, and storage. All the data on the study forms were subjected to an initial clerical review and were then keypunched and verified. All keypunched information was subjected to an extensive computer edit. Errors detected in this editing process were sent to the clinics for correction. Measurements based on analogue recordings, notably records of cardiac catheterization and sleep studies, were verified by the submission of a random sample amounting to 10% of the original records to single readers. All neuropsychologic data were reviewed by experts who checked them for accuracy and consistency. An Advisory Board including clinicians, epidemiologists, and other experts periodically reviewed confidential interim data on the progress of the trial. In particular, follow-up measurements and other outcome criteria were examined so that the trial could be terminated promptly if a clinically significant difference between treatments emerged. In fact, the scheduled end of the trial coincided with the development of a difference in mortality that would have necessitated termination of the trial.

Percentage of events in the nocturnal and the continuous O_2 therapy groups as well as life tables calculated according to Kaplan and Meier (19) are reported. Survivorship of all patients as of 26 May 1980, regardless of the extent of their participation, was ascertained by individual follow-up observation.

For comparison of survival in the nocturnal O_2 therapy and the continuous O_2 therapy groups, the Cox actuarial procedure (20) was applied. This statistical procedure, which is based on a proportional hazard model, takes into account the ranking of the times of follow-up and death in the two treatment groups.

Mortality data were monitored at regular intervals throughout the trial to detect treatment differences as soon as possible. Also, many other end points were evaluated in the final data analysis. Because of this, if nocturnal O_2 and continuous O_2 therapy regimens were alike in every respect, by chance alone 5% of the secondary outcome variables would show a difference significant at the 5% level (21). It is clear that, because multiple variables were evaluated and key variables analyzed during the trial, one should be cautious in assessments of statistical significance.

Results

The 203 patients who were recruited were selected

from 1043 patients who were screened for the study. Of these, 809 patients never entered the stabilization phase: 31% of them were found to have other major disease, 15% refused, 12% were discovered to have previously received chronic O_2 therapy, and in 21% the arterial Po_2 rose so that the patient was no longer eligible. The remainder of these 809 patients were ineligible for a variety of reasons, such as living too far from a study center. In all six centers, a total of only four patients fulfilled the entry criteria but were judged by the investigators to be "too sick" to undergo 3 weeks of observation off O_2. Thirty-one patients entered stabilization but did not complete it and were not randomized to the study. Failure of completion was chiefly due to an absence of informed consent or a rise in arterial Po_2 during stabilization such that the patient was ineligible.

Table 2 shows selected mean baseline characteristics of both nocturnal O_2 therapy and continuous O_2 therapy groups and indicates that they were comparable: The randomization process was successful. The average patient age was more than 65 years; most patients were male. They were hypoxemic with a slightly elevated hematocrit value and borderline CO_2 retention. Expiratory flow was severely compromised, and they were hyperinflated. Maximum exercise performance, as tested by bicycle ergometry, was sharply limited. The average patient showed resting tachycardia, modest pulmonary hypertension, and increased pulmonary vascular resistance. During sleep, patients were hypoxemic while breathing air but generally not while breathing their prescribed dose of O_2. Neuropsychological test results showed that the average patient had impaired brain function; patients on continuous O_2 therapy appeared to be slightly less impaired than those on nocturnal O_2, the difference approaching significance when the overall clinical rating and the Russell-Neuringer average impairment index were considered. Quality of life measures indicated relatively low level of patient self-satisfaction, reduced physical and social capabilities, and increased levels of depression, anxiety, and hostility. More detailed analyses of these baseline data will be presented in other reports.

Compliance was assessed both by timers and by examining patient logs. The former was objective but systematically underestimated O_2 use by continuous O_2 therapy patients with portable systems. In nocturnal O_2 therapy patients, timer and log data were in excellent agreement, both indicating that more than 82% of the nocturnal O_2 therapy patients used 13 hours or less of O_2 per day. According to timers, nocturnal O_2 therapy patients averaged 12.0 h/d (SD = 2.5 h/d) whereas continuous O_2 therapy patients averaged 17.7 h/d (SD = 4.8 h/d). Figure 1 shows data from patient logs and indicates that

Table 2. Baseline Characteristics of Nocturnal O_2 Therapy and Continuous O_2 Therapy Groups

Characteristics*	Nocturnal O_2 Therapy	Continuous O_2 Therapy	*P* Value
General and cardiopulmonary characteristics			
Patients, *no.*†	102	101	
Age, *yrs*	65.7	65.2	0.72
Male, %†	80.4	77.2	0.58
White, %†	78.4	77.2	0.84
Pa_{O_2}, *mm Hg*	51.5	50.8	0.32
Pa_{CO_2}, *mm Hg*	43.9	43.4	0.70
pH	7.41	7.40	0.19
Hematocrit, %	47.3	47.7	0.60
FEV_1, *% predicted*	29.9	29.5	0.82
FVC, *% predicted*	53.6	52.6	0.70
FRC, *% predicted*	177.6	175.7	0.78
Mean sleep Sa_{O_2}, air, %	83.5	83.0	0.66
Mean sleep Sa_{O_2}, O_2, %	94.0	94.1	0.83
Maximum workload, air, *W*	37.3	37.5	0.95
Heart rate, min^{-1}	92.6	93.1	0.83
Mean pulmonary artery pressure, *mm Hg*	29.0	30.0	0.58
Cardiac index, $L/min \cdot m^2$	2.91	2.95	0.69
Pulmonary vascular resistance, $dyne/s \cdot cm^5$	330	333	0.91
Neuropsychiatric characteristics‡			
Overall rating (3.5)	4.5	4.2	0.06
Halstead impairment index (0.63)	0.78	0.73	0.15
Russell-Neuringer average impairment index (1.8)	2.3	2.1	0.08
Brain age quotient (89)	75.4	80.4	0.11
Quality of life‡			
MMPI, average scales 0.9 (54.5)	60.9	61.4	0.68
SIP			
Physical scale (0.6)	20.5	19.8	0.78
Psychosocial scale (1.6)	23.9	20.5	0.22
POMS—mood disturbance (26.4)	48.4	49.7	0.76

* FEV_1 = forced expiratory volume in 1 second; FVC = forced vital capacity; FRC = functional residual capacity; MMPI = Minnesota Multiphasic Personality Inventory; SIP = Sickness Impact Profile; POMS = Profile of Mood States.

† All values reported for the two groups are mean values except numbers of subjects, sex, and race.

‡ Normal values are shown in parentheses.

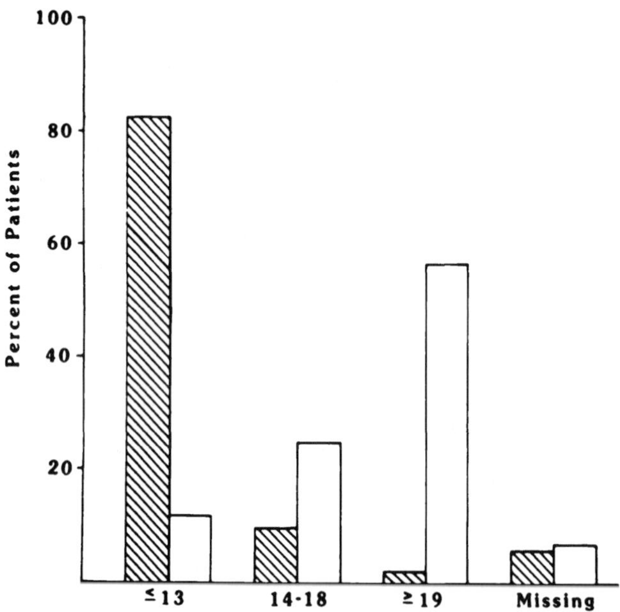

Figure 1. Compliance with treatment regimens as assessed by patient log, expressed as a frequency distribution of daily O_2 use. Hatched bars represent patients on nocturnal O_2 therapy, open bars, those on continuous O_2 therapy. "Missing" indicates patients in whom data are missing.

82% of nocturnal O_2 therapy patients used O_2 for 13 hours or less per day and that 56% of continuous O_2 therapy patients used O_2 for 19 or more hours per day.

The 203 patients were followed for an average of 19.3 months. Of the total group, 80 nocturnal O_2 and 87 continuous O_2 therapy patients were followed for 12 months and 29 nocturnal O_2 and 37 continuous O_2 therapy patients were followed for 24 months. Two continuous O_2 therapy patients were lost to follow-up 2 months before the trial was ended, one after 12 months of treatment and the other after 15 months. A total of 64 patients died, 41 in the nocturnal O_2 therapy group and 23 in the continuous O_2 therapy group. Life table cumulative survival rates, shown in Figure 2, indicate the pattern of mortality throughout the study period. Based on the Cox model, unadjusted for baseline characteristics, this difference in survival was significant ($P = 0.01$). The 12-month mortality was 20.6% (SE = 4.0%) in the nocturnal O_2 therapy group and 11.9% (SE = 3.2%) in the continuous O_2 therapy group, whereas the 24-month mortality was 40.8% (SE = 5.5%) and 22.4% (SE = 4.6%), respectively. Overall mortality was 31.5% for all patients and varied from 15.4% to 41.9% among centers. At all centers, mortality for the nocturnal O_2 therapy group exceeded that for the continuous O_2 therapy group. The relative risk of death for the nocturnal O_2 therapy group compared with the continuous O_2 therapy group was 1.94 with 95% confidence limits ranging from 1.17 to 3.24. The above analyses were done according to treatment assignment and did not consider compliance. However, compliance was very good, and compliance failure could not account for the difference between groups.

Mortality was examined in subgroups defined according to variables thought to be clinically important; the median overall baseline values of these variables were used to separate groups. Figure 3 shows mortality in patients with arterial P_{CO_2} equal to or greater than 43 mm Hg, the median value fór all patients at baseline; survival was better in the continuous O_2 therapy group, and this difference was highly significant ($P < 0.002$). This and other selected baseline values are related to mortality in Table 3. In two other subgroups, those with low pH and those who showed high levels of mood disturbance such as depression and anxiety (Profile of Mood States test), the continuous O_2 therapy group demonstrated very significantly greater survival than the nocturnal O_2 therapy group. Also, in a number of other subgroups mortality differed ($0.01 < P < 0.05$). Patients with low FVC, high FRC, more severe nocturnal hypoxemia, low hematocrit values, and more severe indexes of brain dysfunction all tended to have lower mortality on continuous than on nocturnal O_2 therapy. The same was true of patients with pulmonary artery pressure and pulmonary vascular resistance values that were below the median and for those whose work capacity on the cycle ergometer was above the median.

Although patients on continuous O_2 therapy tended to be hospitalized less often and to have fewer long hospitalizations than nocturnal O_2 therapy patients, differences were not statistically significant.

The effects of treatment on the physiological and psychological variables listed in Table 2 were examined by comparing baseline and follow-up data in individual patients. For some variables, such as those resulting from cardiac catheterization, only 6-month follow-up data were available. For other indexes, such as arterial P_{O_2} and P_{CO_2}, results at 6 months, 12 months, and 18 months could be compared with baseline values. With the exception of hematocrit and pulmonary vascular resistance, none of the variables listed in Table 2 showed statistically significant changes that were dependent on treatment regimen. Hematocrit values fell more in patients on con-

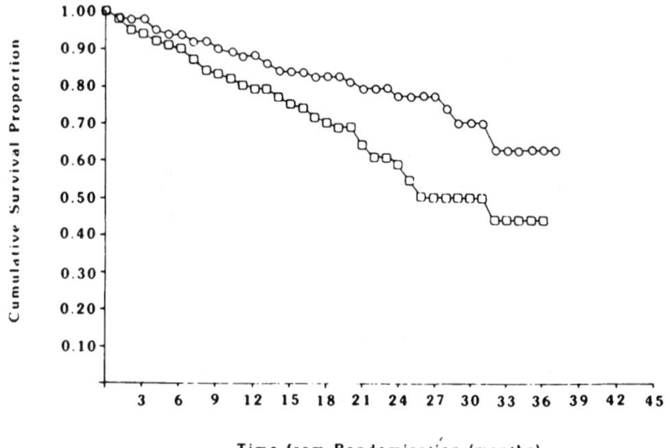

Figure 2. Overall mortality. Ordinate is fraction of patients surviving; abscissa is time from randomization or duration of treatment. Open circles represent continuous O_2 therapy group; squares represent nocturnal O_2 therapy group. Of the total group, 80 nocturnal O_2 and 87 continuous O_2 therapy patients were followed for 12 months, and 29 nocturnal O_2 and 37 continuous O_2 therapy patients were followed for 24 months.

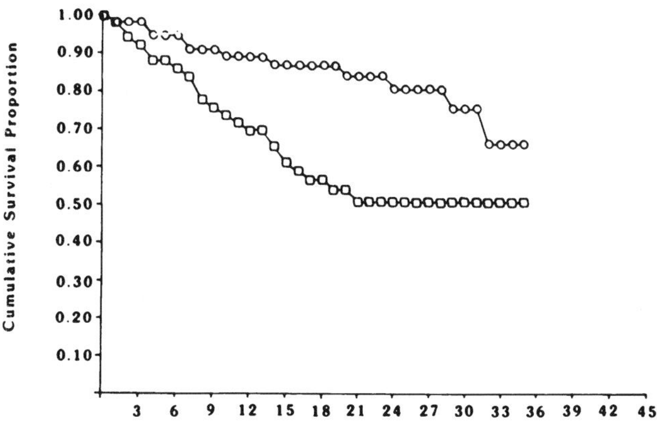

Figure 3. Survival of patients with arterial Pco_2 over 43 mm Hg. Ordinate is fraction of patients surviving; abscissa is time from randomization or duration of treatment. Open circles represent continuous O_2 therapy patients; squares represent nocturnal O_2 therapy patients. Of these patients, 35 nocturnal O_2 therapy patients and 50 continuous O_2 therapy patients were followed for 12 months, and 13 patients on nocturnal and 25 on continuous O_2 therapy were followed for 24 months.

tinuous O_2 therapy than in those on nocturnal O_2 therapy: This was not significant at 6 months ($P = 0.06$) but was significant at both 12 months ($P = 0.005$) and 18 months ($P = 0.008$). At 18 months hematocrit values showed, on the average, a fall of 2.0% from baseline in 36 nocturnal O_2 therapy patients and had decreased an average of 9.2% in 40 patients on continuous O_2 therapy. Pulmonary vascular resistance was measured in follow-up only at 6 months; at that time 49 nocturnal O_2 therapy patients showed a mean increase of 6.5% while 52 continuous O_2 therapy patients showed a mean decrease of 11.1% ($P = 0.04$).

When data for all patients were combined and baseline and follow-up data compared, significant changes in hematocrit and pulmonary vascular resistance were observed. Hematocrit values fell from a mean at baseline of 47.5% to a mean of 44.3% at 6 months. Pulmonary vascular resistance fell from a mean of 322 dyne/s • cm^5 at baseline to a mean of 281 dyne/s • cm^5 at 6 months. No significant change occurred in arterial blood gas levels, lung volumes or FEV_1, maximum work attained, mean pulmonary artery pressure, or cardiac index. With the exception of the Minnesota Multiphasic Personality Inventory, all the measures of neuropsychological function and quality of life listed in Table 2 improved significantly when all patients were considered.

Discussion

The patients studied were probably representative of patients in general with hypoxemic chronic obstructive lung disease. The study centers attempted to recruit every patient who fulfilled the entry criteria and presented no reason for exclusion (Table 1). Over 1000 patients were screened for the study; a large fraction of these were not eligible for the study chiefly because of other disease and failure to demonstrate persistent hypoxemia. Very few patients did not enter the study because they were thought "too sick" to endure 3 weeks' observation without oxygen. The only biases that operated in patient selection were that the patient live near a study center, that he or she have no serious extrapulmonary disease, and that he or she not previously have been treated with long-term oxygen therapy. Thus, except that they were largely urban dwellers and did not have major disease of other organ systems, these patients probably were representative of the type of person with obstructive disease currently thought to merit long-term low-flow oxygen therapy. As indicated in Table 2 the patients were randomized successfully. At baseline, there was no significant difference between nocturnal O_2 and continuous O_2 therapy groups in any of the variables listed, although in some neuropsychological test results there were trends favoring the continuous O_2 therapy group. The effectiveness of the prescribed dose of O_2 in relieving hypoxemia was established and repeatedly checked. Therapy other than that involving O_2 was the same in both groups and therefore could not have biased the results. Finally, as indicated in Figure 1, patients complied well with their prescribed treatment regimens; few continuous O_2 therapy patients used O_2 for 13 hours or less, and few nocturnal O_2 therapy patients used it for 19 hours or more. This record of compliance is unusually good (22) and probably occurred both because the patients were followed very closely and because they found it easy to believe that oxygen was beneficial to them. In any event, this clinical trial appeared to fulfill several important criteria: The patients were representative of the general clinical population addressed by the trial, the treatment groups were similar at the beginning of the trial, the treatment was shown to achieve its short-term goal, and each group generally followed its assigned treatment plan.

We believe that the trial gave a clear-cut answer in terms of the variable of ultimate clinical importance: mortality. Mortality in the nocturnal O_2 therapy group was nearly twice that in the continuous O_2 therapy group. The analysis of treatment-dependent differences in overall mortality was the first statistic derived from the trial data because it was considered the most important. Therefore it cannot be argued that the difference in overall mortality was a chance result of many tests being applied to the data. The probability was truly 1% that the difference in mortality between the nocturnal O_2 and the continuous O_2 therapy groups was due to chance. Had the trial been prolonged, an even more impressive statistic might have emerged; this would have reflected an even greater differential mortality that would have been ethically unacceptable. Had the trial been scheduled to last longer, the Advisory Board would have terminated it at the time that it did stop because of the mortality difference reported here.

In analyzing mortality, we analyzed all deaths. Nonrespiratory factors contributed to the deaths of some patients: Two committed suicide, one had leukemia, four had carcinoma of the lung, and one had a cerebrovascular accident. These deaths were randomly distributed between the nocturnal O_2 and the continuous O_2 therapy groups. When these patients were eliminated from consideration, survival in the continuous O_2 therapy group

Table 3. Mortality According to Baseline Characteristics*

Characteristic†	Number of Patients	Deaths			P Value
		Total	Nocturnal O_2 Therapy	Continuous O_2 Therapy	
	no.	←	%	→	
Pa_{O_2}, *mm Hg*					
<52	89	39.3	47.7	31.1	0.06
≥52	113	25.7	34.5	16.4	0.06
Pa_{CO_2}, *mm Hg*					
<43	96	31.2	34.6	27.3	0.78
≥43	106	32.1	46.0	19.6	0.002
pH					
<7.40	95	28.4	42.2	16.0	0.004
≥7.40	107	34.6	38.6	30.0	0.46
Hematocrit, %					
<47.4	99	32.3	41.5	21.7	0.03
≥47.4	102	31.4	38.8	24.5	0.20
FEV_1, *L*					
<0.69	97	35.0	43.4	25.0	0.07
≥0.69	101	29.7	39.1	21.8	0.08
FVC, *L*					
<1.89	99	31.3	43.5	20.8	0.01
≥1.89	99	33.3	39.6	26.1	0.20
FRC, *L*					
<6.06	81	30.9	40.0	22.0	0.10
≥6.06	82	32.9	42.9	22.5	0.05
Sleep, mean Sa_{O_2}, air breathing, %					
<85	89	37.1	50.0	24.4	0.02
≥85	92	23.9	31.1	17.0	0.14
Maximum work load, *W*					
<35	85	42.4	48.8	35.7	0.13
≥35	113	23.9	33.9	14.0	0.02
Resting heart rate, *beats/min*					
<92	101	28.7	38.8	19.2	0.08
≥92	102	34.3	41.5	26.5	0.06
Mean pulmonary artery pressure, *mm Hg*					
<27	86	27.9	37.0	17.5	0.03
≥27	98	31.6	39.6	24.0	0.14
Pulmonary vascular resistance, *dyne/s·cm*^{5}					
<279	84	23.8	33.3	12.8	0.03
≥279	84	36.9	45.2	38.6	0.11
Neuropsychological rating					
<4.5	92	25.0	31.7	19.6	0.24
≥4.5	94	39.4	48.0	29.5	0.04
Russell-Neuringer average impairment index					
<2.17	85	25.9	31.7	20.5	0.30
≥2.17	89	37.1	45.8	26.8	0.03
Halstead impairment index					
<0.75	87	26.4	34.1	19.6	0.19
≥0.75	87	36.8	43.8	28.8	0.05
Mood disturbance (POMS)					
<43	89	29.2	30.2	28.3	0.80
≥43	92	37.0	52.2	21.7	0.005

* Groups defined according to the median value for each characteristic. Data percentages for the continuous and nocturnal therapy groups are for deaths in each group divided according to the criteria for "Characteristic" and are not percentages of the totals in Column 2.

† FEV_1 = forced expiratory volume in 1 second; FVC = forced vital capacity; FRC = functional residual capacity; POMS = Profile of Mood States.

was still significantly ($P = 0.03$) greater than in the nocturnal O_2 therapy group. We have included all patients in our major analysis of mortality because we believe that even in the cases cited above, it is impossible to argue that the patient's severe respiratory disease did not contribute to their death. An example of this complexity is afforded by our experience with coronary artery disease. Three patients (two on nocturnal O_2, one on continuous O_2 therapy) died of arrhythmias after documented myocardial infarctions. On the other hand, nine other patients had sudden deaths—they were found dead in bed—some with a history of increasing respiratory difficulty but most without. Presumably these patients had fatal arrhythmias, but few would argue that their deaths were not primarily respiratory.

In an effort to discern if certain types of patients benefited from continuous O_2 therapy, we split nocturnal O_2 and continuous O_2 therapy patients into subgroups according to median values of baseline characteristics thought to be clinically important. Many subgroups showed significant survival benefit with continuous O_2 therapy (Table 3), reflecting the reduced overall mortality associated with this treatment. Generally patients with hypoventilation and relatively poor pulmonary function—high arterial P_{CO_2}, low pH, low nocturnal oxygen saturation, low FVC, and high FRC—showed increased survival with continuous O_2 therapy. The same was true of patients with more severe brain impairment of neuropsychological testing and of patients who demonstrated high levels of mood disturbance. These results could be synthesized to reach the conclusion that the effect of continuous O_2 therapy was most striking in the sickest patients. On the other hand, it was patients with the least disturbed pulmonary hemodynamics—relatively low mean pulmonary artery pressure and pulmonary vascular resistance—and relatively well preserved exercise capacity who showed benefit from continuous O_2 therapy. Thus the composite patient showing the most benefit from continuous O_2 therapy would have relatively severe derangements of life quality and brain and lung function but relatively mild disturbances of pulmonary hemodynamics and exercise capacity.

Although there was overlap between subgroups showing benefit from continuous O_2 therapy, this overlap was never total. For example, of the 95 patients with baseline pH under 7.40, 24 also had arterial P_{CO_2} less than 43 mm Hg, and of the 107 patients with baseline pH over 7.40, 35 had arterial P_{CO_2} greater than 43 mm Hg.

Most of the differences in mortality noted in Table 3 that we have cited as significant were significant at the 5% level. It might be argued that these differences are not impressive considering that we made many statistical comparisons and that some therefore might attain these levels of significance in the absence of a difference between nocturnal O_2 and continuous O_2 therapy groups. We do not believe that this explains the results shown. Subgroups with high arterial P_{CO_2}, low pH, and more serious mood disturbance showed differences in mortality that were an order of magnitude more significant than those likely to be achieved by chance alone. Groups of independent variables, such as those concerning hypoventilation and lung function, showed concordant differences in mortality that would have been unlikely had they been due to chance. Finally, too many of the variables shown in Table 3 showed $P < 0.05$ to be due to chance; the items shown were selected from analysis of the characteristics shown in Table 2, and probabilities of less than 5% occurred in many more than 5% of the subgroups tested.

The reason for the decreased mortality associated with continuous O_2 therapy is unclear. Of the numerous physiological and psychological variables measured during the study, only two showed a significant treatment-related change with time. Hematocrit value decreased in patients on continuous O_2 therapy but not in those on nocturnal O_2 therapy. Although this result is in accord with the results of animal studies (23), the decline in hematocrit values in the continuous O_2 therapy group was small, averaging 9.2% at 18 months, and assigning any clinical significance to a change of this magnitude is difficult. Overall mortality (Table 3) was very similar in patients with high and low hematocrit values at baseline; having a low hematocrit value at baseline was not associated with increased survival. Further, though continuous O_2 therapy lowered hematocrit values, it appeared to decrease mortality in patients who entered the study with low hematocrit values (Table 3). It appears therefore that although continuous O_2 therapy decreased hematocrit values and increased survival, there is no evidence that these results are related to one another.

Pulmonary vascular resistance also showed a differential effect of treatment, which is also consistent with animal studies showing that intermittent normoxia does not reverse anatomical evidence of hypoxia-induced pulmonary hypertension whereas continuous normoxia does (23). The treatment-related change in pulmonary vascular resistance was more substantial than the hematocrit change, and the 11% decline in resistance seen in the continuous O_2 therapy group may have been partially responsible for its longevity. This is not supported by examining mortality data in relation to pulmonary vascular resistance (Table 3). Although patients who entered the study with high pulmonary vascular resistances had relatively high overall mortality, patients with a low baseline pulmonary vascular resistance showed a mortality benefit from continuous O_2 therapy, whereas those with high resistance did not. The effect of change in pulmonary vascular resistance on mortality also suggested that changes in resistance were not the cause of the lower mortality in patients on continuous O_2 therapy. The median change of pulmonary vascular resistance for 101 patients was a decrease of 20 dyne/s • cm^5 at 6 months. Of patients with a greater decrease 14 subsequently died, nine in the nocturnal O_2 therapy group and five in the continuous O_2 therapy group. Of patients who demonstrated a smaller decrease in pulmonary vascular resistance, nine subsequently died, all from the nocturnal O_2 therapy group. Thus, when both groups were combined, patients with large decreases in pulmonary vascular resistance tended to have a greater mortality than patients with small decreases. Further, it appeared that continuous O_2 therapy had more striking beneficial effect in the patients with small decreases of pulmonary vascular resistance. These data strongly suggest that although continuous O_2 therapy reduced both mortality and pulmonary vascular resistance, the two phenomena were not related.

The present study may be compared with others in which the effects of oxygen therapy have been examined through testing of patients before and after some months of treatment (2-6, 9, 10). Qualitatively, our results are similar. When nocturnal O_2 and continuous O_2 therapy groups were combined, oxygen therapy apparently resulted in a fall in hematocrit value and pulmonary vascular resistance and improvements in neuropsychologic function and the patients' perceptions of their quality of life. However, changes were not large, averaging about 10% in all instances, and whether even these changes were in fact due to oxygen is uncertain. It is entirely possible that these improvements, especially those of quality of life, were due not to oxygen but to the more intensive medical and nursing care the patients received as study participants. Further, mean pulmonary artery pressure did not change significantly, falling from 28.0 mm Hg to 26.4 mm Hg in 6 months, and exercise tolerance as tested by maximum work achieved on a bicycle ergometer did not improve, findings that differ from those of others. The reasons are not clear for the relatively small impact of oxygen therapy on the physiological and neuropsychological functions that we measured. Our study had many more patients than did previous ones and may have contained subgroups that showed greater benefits, but the nature of our mean results indicates that were there such subgroups, there must have been others showing nearly equal deterioration. As has been discussed above, there is no reason to believe that our patient sample was biased so as to minimize the effects of oxygen therapy. A more likely cause for the relatively small oxygen effect observed is that our protocol required a 3-week observation period before baseline studies and entrance into the study. During this period, arterial blood gas levels in many patients improved to the point that the patient was no longer eligible for the study. Most previous studies have been less meticulous in assuring patient stability, raising the question that some of their subjects were unstable on entry and therefore likely to improve whether given oxygen or not.

In this trial, mortality was lower in continuous O_2 therapy patients than in nocturnal O_2 therapy patients, particularly in those with more severe derangements of lung and brain function and high levels of mood disturbance. We believe such patients should be treated with continuous O_2. This does not necessarily mean that there is no place for nocturnal O_2 therapy in the treatment of hypoxemic chronic obstructive lung disease. Indeed, the current British trial that compares supplemental O_2 with no supplemental O_2 involves 15 hours of O_2 administration a day. This regimen is closer to our nocturnal O_2 regimen than to continuous O_2 therapy and is reported to be associated with a lower mortality than that experienced by patients receiving no outpatient oxygen (7). Thus it appears that some oxygen is better than none and that continuous oxygen is better than nocturnal, at least in severely ill patients.

ACKNOWLEDGMENTS: Supported by contracts N01-HR-6-2942, 2943, 2944, 2945, 2946, and 2947 from the Division of Lung Diseases, National Heart, Lung, and Blood Institute, National Institutes of Health, U.S. Department of Health and Human Services.

Participants in the Nocturnal Oxygen Therapy Trial were the following.

Clinical Centers: Henry Ford Hospital, Detroit, Michigan: Paul A. Kvale, M.D.*; William A. Conway, M.D.; E.O. Coates, Jr., M.D.; George C. Bower, M.D.; Fareed U. Khaja, M.D.; Kenneth M. Adams, Ph.D.; Julia A. Lee, M.S.; Marcia Kopacz, R.N., M.S.N.; and Jennifer Reeves, R.N.

Northwestern University, Chicago, Illinois: David W. Cugell, M.D.*; Norman Solliday, M.D.; John Campbell, M.D.; William Kuczerpa, M.D.; Diane Judge, R.N.; and Carmen Zych, R.N.

University of Manitoba, Winnipeg, Manitoba: Nicholas R. Anthonisen, M.D.*; Morley M. Lertzman, M.D.; John A. Fleetham, M.D.; Janet Clarke, R.N.; and Ann McBurney, R.N.

University of California and Scripps Clinic Research Foundation, San Diego, California: Richard M. Timms, M.D.*; Patty Nordgren, R.N.; Richard Bordow, M.D.; Dale Kocienski, M.D.; and Connie Neveu, M.T.

University of Colorado, Denver, Colorado; Thomas L. Petty, M.D.*; Thomas A. Neff, M.D.; Enrique Fernandez, M.D.; Louise M. Nett, R.N., RRT; Robert Maulitz, M.D.; Ruth Harada, M.D.; and Michael D. Baird, B.S.

University of Southern California, Los Angeles, California: C. Thomas Boylen, M.D.*; John Mohler, M.D.; Hugo Chiodi, M.D.; Daniel Kanada, M.D.; Elaine Layne, R.N.; Sylviane Herzog, M.S.; and Peggy Pegg, R.N.

Data Center: University of Michigan, Ann Arbor, Michigan: George W. Williams, Ph.D.; and Sandy M. Snedecor, B.S.

Neuropsychology Centers: Veterans Administration Medical Center and University of California, San Diego: Igor Grant, M.D.; Robert Reed, M.S.

University of Colorado, Denver, Colorado: Robert H. Heaton, Ph.D.; and Susan Heaton, B.A.

Quality of Life Assessment: University of West Virginia, Morgantown, West Virginia: A. John McSweeny, Ph.D.

Pathology Center: University of Manitoba, Winnipeg, Manitoba: William M. Thurlbeck, M.D.

Advisory Board: Marvin A. Sackner, M.D. (Chairman); Stephen M. Ayres, M.D.; B. William Brown, Ph.D.; Millicent Higgins, M.D., Dr. P.H.; Philip Kimbel, M.D.; Jeanne K. Malchon; Harold Menkes, M.D.; William F. Miller, M.D.; and Louis Vachon, M.D.

National Heart, Lung, and Blood Institute: Lynn H. Blake, Ph.D.; David DeMets, Ph.D.; Claude Lenfant, M.D.; Hannah Peavy, M.D.; and Richard Sohn, Ph.D.

*Principal Investigators

References

1. BURROWS B, EARLE RH. Course and prognosis of chronic obstructive lung disease, a prospective study of 200 patients. *N Engl J Med.* 1969;**280**:397-404.
2. LEVINE BE, BIGELOW DB, HAMSTRA RD, et al. The role of long-term continuous oxygen administration in patients with chronic airway obstruction with hypoxemia. *Ann Intern Med.* 1967;**66**:639-50.
3. PETTY TL, FINIGAN MM. The clinical evaluation of prolonged ambulatory oxygen therapy in patients with chronic airway obstruction. *Am J Med.* 1968;**45**:242-52.
4. ABRAHAM AS, COLE RR, BISHOP JM. Reversal of pulmonary hypertension by prolonged oxygen administration to patients with chronic bronchitis. *Circ Res.* 1968;**23**:147-57.
5. KROP HD, BLOCK AJ, COHEN E. Neuropsychologic effects of continuous oxygen therapy in chronic obstructive pulmonary disease. *Chest* 1973;**64**:317-22.
6. STEWARD BN, HOOD CI, BLOCK AJ. Long term results of continuous oxygen therapy at sea level. *Chest.* 1975;**68**:486-92.
7. FLENLEY DC, DOUGLAS NJ, LAMB D. Nocturnal hypoxemia and long term domiciliary oxygen in blue and bloated bronchitics. *Chest.* 1980;**77**:305-7.
8. KOO KW, SAX DS, SNIDER GL. Arterial blood gases and pH during sleep in chronic obstructive lung disease. *Am J Med.* 1975;**58**:663-70.
9. STARK RD, FINNEGAN P, BISHOP JM. Daily requirement of oxygen to reverse pulmonary hypertension in patients with chronic bronchitis. *Br Med J.* 1972;**3**:724-8.
10. STARK RD, FINNEGAN P, BISHOP JM. Long-term domiciliary oxygen in chronic bronchitis with pulmonary hypertension. *Br Med J.* 1973;**3**:467-70.
11. LENFANT C. Twelve- or 24-hour oxygen therapy: why a clinical trial? *JAMA.* 1980;**243**:551-2. Editorial.
12. NATIONAL HEART, LUNG, AND BLOOD INSTITUTE, DIVISION OF LUNG DISEASE. *Protocol for Nocturnal Oxygen Therapy Collaborative Program.* Bethesda: National Institutes of Health; 1978. (Available from the National Heart, Lung, and Blood Institute.)
13. REITAN RM, DAVIDSON LA. *Clinical Neuropsychology: Current Status and Applications,* New York: John Wiley and Sons; 1974.
14. RUSSELL EW, NEURINGER C, GOLDSTEIN G. *Assessment of Brain Damage: a Neuropsychological Key Approach.* New York: John Wiley and Sons; 1970.
15. GRANT I, HEATON RK, MCSWEENEY AJ, ADAMS KM, TIMMS RM. Brain dysfunction in COPD. *Chest.* 1980;77 (suppl.):308-9.
16. DAHLSTROM WG, WELSH GS, DAHLSTROM LE. *An MMPI Handbook. Vol. I.* Minneapolis: University of Minnesota; 1972.
17. BERGNER M, BOBBIT RA, POLLARD WE, MARTIN DP, GILSON BS. The sickness impact profile: validation of health and status measure. *Med Care.* 1976;**14**:57-67.
18. WASKOW IE, PARLOFF MB. *Psychotherapy Change Measures.* Washington, D.C.: U.S. Government Printing Office; 1975.
19. KAPLAN EL, MEIER P. Non-parametric estimation from incomplete observation. *J Am Statist Assoc.* 1958;**53**:457-81.
20. COX DR. Regression models and life tables. *J R Stat Soc. [Series B].* 1972;**35**:187-220.
21. ARMITAGE P. *Sequential Medical Trials.* Springfield, Illinois: Charles C Thomas; 1970.
22. Report of the Committee for the Assessment of Biometric Aspects of Controlled Trials of Hypoglycemic Agents. *JAMA.* 1975;**231**:583-608.
23. KAY JM. Effect of continuous and intermittent normoxia on chronic hypoxic pulmonary hypertension, right ventricular hypertrophy, and polycythemia in rats. *Am Rev Respir Dis.* 1980; in press.

Is Embolic Risk Conditioned By Location of Deep Venous Thrombosis?

KENNETH M. MOSER, M.D.; and JOHN R. LeMOINE, M.D.; San Diego, California

Sixty-eight patients clinically suspected of having (33), or at high risk for (35), deep venous thrombosis were studied with contrast venography, radiofibrinogen leg scanning, and impedance plethysmography as well as ventilation and perfusion lung scans. Thrombosis limited to the veins in the calf of the leg (unilateral or bilateral) was shown by venography in 21 patients. None of these patients had clinical symptoms or scan results indicating embolism. Fifteen patients had thrombosis involving proximal (thigh) as well as distal (calf) veins by venography. Eight had scan evidence of embolism, although only one was symptomatic. The combination of radiofibrinogen and impedance tests allows accurate detection of both the presence and location of deep venous thrombosis. The availability of sensitive and specific, noninvasive methods for detecting and localizing venous thrombosis, as well as the apparently low embolic risk of calf-only thrombosis may condition future approaches to prophylaxis and treatment of patients with or at high risk for deep venous thrombosis.

IN THE past, the diagnosis of deep venous thrombosis of the lower extremities, identified as the source of most clinically significant pulmonary thromboemboli (1-3), has been a mandate for the institution of anticoagulant therapy. Pulmonary embolism is a frequent cause of death, particularly among patients hospitalized for other remediable, and often minor, problems. Therefore, immediate treatment of deep venous thrombosis is essential to prevent development of its potentially lethal complication, pulmonary embolism. Other reasons for therapy include: preventing extension and hastening resolution of deep venous thrombosis, thus shortening the hospital stay as well as the extent of residual venous obstruction. These secondary objectives, however, may not warrant the institution of anticoagulant treatment for all patients because of the risk associated with the therapy itself.

The treatment of all patients with deep venous thrombosis, in order to prevent embolism, is a simplistic translation of diagnosis into therapy, and may no longer be tenable. Despite the implicit assumption that all forms of deep venous thrombosis have the same natural history and potential to cause emboli, recent evidence indicates this assumption may not be valid.

The use of sensitive techniques for diagnosis, such as radiolabeled fibrinogen leg scans and impedance plethysmography, has emphasized the long evident fact that not all deep venous thrombi give rise to emboli (4-10). Furthermore, previous studies with these techniques have indicated that thrombi limited to the calf of the leg rarely result in emboli and often resolve spontaneously (4). More proximal thrombi pose greater risk in terms of both embolism and local residua (4-11).

Emergence from an era in which clinical judgment and contrast venography constituted the entire diagnostic armamentarium for deep venous thrombosis into this new age in which highly sensitive, noninvasive techniques have become available requires a reevaluation of the indications for anticoagulant therapy. Some forms of deep venous thrombosis of the lower extremities may have low embolic risk (for example, the distal deep venous thrombi, limited to the calf), while others are more dangerous (such as the proximal deep venous thrombi, above the knee). This distinction, if proved valid, could provide a framework for selecting patients who require therapy.

▶ From the Pulmonary Division, Department of Medicine, University of California, San Diego, California.

Table 1. Venogram Results by Patient Groups

Group*		Distal Thrombosis		
		No	Yes	Total
Group I				
Proximal	No	17	6	23
Thrombosis	Yes	0	10	10
Total		17	16	33
$\chi^2 = 15.24$				
$p < 0.0001$				
Group 2				
Proximal	No	14	7	21
Thrombosis	Yes	0	3	3
Total		14	10	24
$p = 0.059$ (Fisher's exact test)				
Group 3†				
Proximal	No	0	8	8
Thrombosis	Yes	0	2	2
Total		0	10	10
All groups				
Proximal	No	31	21	52
Thrombosis	Yes	0	15	15
Total		31	36	67
$\chi^2 = 16.6$				
$p < 0.0001$				

* χ^2 = chi-square test. Chi-square not computed for Group 2 because of small expected values in two cells. In Group 3, no test of independence is possible because only patients with distal thrombosis were observed.
† Excludes patient who declined venogram.

This framework, however, demands that reliable methods exist for locating the thrombosis.

This study was undertaken to determine whether a category of relatively safe deep venous thrombosis exists, and if so, whether current noninvasive diagnostic techniques can reliably differentiate between the types (5, 7-10).

Methods

Group 1 consisted of 33 medical service patients with clinically suspected lower-extremity thrombosis. All patients referred, who consented to the study, were accepted except those with coexisting chronic obstructive pulmonary disease. Each patient received radiofibrinogen leg scans and impedance and contrast venography to detect the presence and extent of deep venous thrombosis. Venography was performed within 24 hours of the impedance test and initiation of radiofibrinogen counting. Four of these patients had been receiving heparin before the injection of radiofibrinogen.

Group 2 consisted of 24 patients undergoing hip surgery, and group 3 comprised 11 patients with acute traumatic spinal cord paralysis. These patients were followed prospectively to assess the incidence of deep venous thrombosis and pulmonary embolism. Radiofibrinogen leg scans and impedance were done daily during the study period. Venography was done in all patients (except one in group 3 who refused): at the request of the attending physician, after the radiofibrinogen test had become positive, or 5 to 7 days after admission to the study. No patient in groups 2 or 3 received heparin during the study.

In all patients, ventilation and perfusion lung scans as well as a chest roentgenogram on the same day were done either at the request of the attending physician (one patient), when a positive venogram was obtained (36 patients), or 5 to 7 days after admission to the study (31 patients). Patients with abnormal scans were asked to return for follow-up scans 2 weeks later. Three months after hospital discharge, all patients were recalled or visited, and a history and physical examination were performed.

The radiolabeled fibrinogen leg scans and the impedance plethysmography were done by methods described elsewhere (7, 8). Criteria for a positive leg scan included a difference of 15% in count rates between adjacent or contralateral counting sites that persisted for 24 hours. Venography was done according to standard technique (12).

An Anger camera was used to record perfusion (Q) and ventilation (V) scans. Perfusion lung scans were done with ^{99}Tc-labeled macroaggregated albumin. Ventilation scans were done with ^{133}Xe radioisotope and included wash-in and wash-out studies. A ventilation/perfusion scan was considered positive for pulmonary embolism if, associated with a negative chest roentgenogram, the perfusion scan showed one or more zones of absent perfusion that were normally ventilated during wash-in and wash-out of ^{133}Xe. The scan was recorded as normal when no perfusion defects were present, as not diagnostic of embolism when perfusion defects were matched by ventilation defects (13). Pulmonary angiography was not an investigational component of this study, although the attending physicians, apprised of the results of the other studies, were encouraged to prescribe it. Only four pulmonary angiograms were done.

All patients gave their informed consent before participation. Venogram and ventilation-perfusion (V/Q) lung scans were assessed by different persons without knowledge of the results of any other tests.

Patients with thrombi limited to the calf veins were not treated with heparin, nor was any patient with a negative venogram. All patients with above-knee thrombi were treated with heparin within 48 hours of the positive venogram. Chi-square analyses and determination of confidence limits were done by standard technics (by Dr. C. Berry, University of California, San Diego).

Results

Deep venous thrombosis was detected by venography in 36 of the 67 patients (Table 1): in 21 of these 36 patients, thrombosis was confined to the distal (calf) veins; in 15 thrombosis involved the proximal (thigh) veins as well as the distal veins. No patient in this series had thrombosis only involving the thigh veins. Eight of the 36 patients with venous thrombosis had bilateral involvement. The association of distal and proximal thrombosis in the total patient group is statistically significant ($p < 0.0001$). This significance is also present, though weakly, in Group 2 ($p = 0.059$). In Group 3 the association cannot be examined as all patients had distal thrombosis.

Of the 134 legs studied (Table 2), 90 were negative by venography; 28 had calf involvement only; and 16 had proximal plus distal vein involvement. Chi-square analyses, applied to both patient and leg data, strongly rejects the hypothesis that proximal and distal thrombosis are independent phenomena in the patients studied.

The correlation of radiofibrinogen, impedance and ven-

Table 2. Venogram Results by Leg

Group	Total Number	Positive			Negative
		Distal Only	Proximal Only	Distal and Proximal	
1	66	8	0	11	47
2	48	10	0	3	35
3*	20	10	0	2	8
Total	134	28	0	16	90

* Excludes patient who declined venogram.

Table 3: Correlation, by Patient, Among Test Results

Venogram	Radiofibrinogen Scan		Impedance Plethysmography	
	Positive	Negative	Positive	Negative
Negative	3*	28	0	31
Distal only	21	0	6	15
Distal and proximal	9	6†	15	0

* Calf only.
† In four patients, radiofibrinogen scan was positive in calf only.

ography results was analyzed in terms of patients and legs. The patient data are shown in Table 3. Three of 31 patients with negative venograms had positive radiofibrinogen scans (calf only). Radiofibrinogen scanning detected all 21 patients with thrombosis limited to the distal veins. Of the 15 patients with proximal plus distal thrombosis, radiofibrinogen detected both locations in nine. Of the six patients recorded as negative by radiofibrinogen in Table 3, radiofibrinogen was positive in four, in the calf only. The other two patients had negative scans for the calf and thigh; both had received heparin for more than 24 hours before radiofibrinogen injection.

The impedance test detected six of 21 patients who had thrombosis limited to the distal veins, and was abnormal in all 15 patients with distal plus proximal thombosis. No false positives occurred in the 31 patients with negative venograms. Thus, in terms of patients, the two techniques detected all 36 patients with venographically proven deep venous thrombosis and correctly identified the 15 with proximal vein involvement. Although radiofibrinogen scanning detected three apparent false positive calf vein thromboses, these may represent small thrombi not seen on venogram.

In terms of legs studied (Table 4), the radiofibrinogen scan detected 26 of the 28 legs with thrombi limited to the distal veins. Of the 16 with distal plus proximal vein involvement, radiofibrinogen detected both locations in 10. Four of the six legs reported as negative by radiofibrinogen, were positive in the calf only. As noted previously, both legs that were reported as totally negative by radiofibrinogen scanning were of patients who had received heparin for 24 hours before radiofibrinogen injection. The impedance test detected seven of 28 thrombi limited to the calf veins and 15 of 16 that involved proximal plus distal veins. The one leg missed by impedance showed large collaterals by venography on that side (although not on the other side, which was positive by impedance). None of the 90 legs reported negative by venography was positive by impedance.

One patient from Group 3 refused venography. His radiofibrinogen study was positive in one calf; the impedance was normal bilaterally.

Perfusion and ventilation scans were done in all 68 patients (Table 5). Of the 15 patients with thrombosis detected proximally (above the knee), eight disclosed a V/Q pattern characteristic of embolism, that is, absence of perfusion and normal ventilation in the zone(s) involved. All showed this V/Q pattern in at least one lobe. One of these eight patients (with two lobes plus a segmental defect shown) had symptoms suggestive of embolism. In all eight patients, follow-up perfusion scans showed substantial-to-complete clearing of the perfusion defect(s) within 2 weeks.

The scans of the 31 patients with negative venograms were normal or not diagnostic in all. This was also the case in the 21 patients with thrombosis limited to the calf. Thus, by these scan criteria, embolism occurred in eight of 15 patients with proximal vein thrombosis, and in none of 21 with thrombosis limited to the calf veins. In those patients with distal thrombosis only, we may take upper 95% confidence limit as the upper bound on the embolic risk in patients like those in our study; in patients with distal thrombi only, as detected by venography, this upper bound is 13%; and in patients with only distal thrombi, as detected by radiofibrinogen, the upper bound is 11%.

The frequency of not diagnostic scans was similar in the different venographic groups: eight of 31 among those with negative venograms; six of 21 among those with distal-only deep venous thrombosis; and three of 15 among those with distal and proximal deep venous thrombosis. Furthermore, of the 15 patients with matched defects in whom no angiogram was done, 12 had follow-up scans 2 weeks later showing no significant change. In the very unlikely worst case possibility that all abnormal scans represented embolic disease, embolic incidence would have been 26% among patients with negative venograms and impedance, 28% among those with distal only deep venous thrombosis and 73% among those with distal and proximal deep venous thrombosis.

Only four patients, all in group 1, were tested by pulmonary angiography. Reluctance to do this procedure in Groups 2 and 3 patients is understandable. Angiography of the two Group 1 patients having distal and proximal deep venous thrombosis (including the one with symptoms) and V/Q scan mismatch showed emboli. The two with only distal thrombosis and minor matching V/Q scan abnormalities had normal angiograms. These negative angiograms would reduce the worst-case embolic incidence in the distal-only group to four of 21 bringing it below the worst case for patients with negative venograms.

Three of the 15 patients with proximal vein thrombosis

Table 4. Correlation, by Leg, Among Test Results

Venogram	Radiofibrinogen Scan		Impedance Plethysmography	
	Positive	Negative	Positive	Negative
Negative	3*	87	0	90
Distal only	26	2	7	21
Distal and proximal	10	6†	15	1
Not done	1	1	0	2

* Positive in calf only.
† In four legs, positive in calf only.

Table 5. Results of Ventilation and Perfusion Scans in 68 Patients

Venogram	V/Q Scan*	
	Normal or Not Diagnostic	Mismatch
Negative	31 (8)	0
Distal only	21 (6)	0
Distal and proximal	7 (3)	8
Not done	1 (0)	0
Total	60 (17)	8

* Figures in parentheses indicate patients with abnormal scans classified as not diagnostic of embolism. Of the eight patients with ventilation/perfusion (V/Q) mismatch: five were in group 1; two, group 2; and one, group 3. Only one patient (in group 1) had the V/Q study done because of symptoms suggesting embolism; and it was one of the eight showing mismatch.

were lost to follow-up, and one (with severe spinal cord injury) died of nonembolic causes. At the time of follow-up, 3 months after hospital discharge, none of the remaining patients reported interval events suggesting embolism, although two of these 11 had signs or symptoms suggestive of the postphlebitic syndrome.

All 21 patients with venographically demonstrated distal-only thrombosis were evaluated. None had been treated with heparin, had an interval history of venous thrombosis or embolism, or had physical findings or symptoms of the postphlebitic syndrome.

None of the 31 patients with negative venograms was treated with heparin. Two were lost to follow-up, but none of the other 29 had interval events or physical findings suggesting venous thrombosis or pulmonary embolism.

Discussion

Most of the recent attention received by venous thrombosis of the lower extremities has been directed towards its prevention (5-11). Coupled with this research are the development and increased usage of noninvasive techniques for detecting deep venous thrombosis (5-11). These investigations, enhancing its diagnosis and appreciation of its natural history, have also generated new questions. For example, the radiofibrinogen test is so sensitive that deep venous thrombosis is now discovered in many prospectively studied asymptomatic patients. Must all patients identified by such studies as being at high risk of deep venous thrombosis be provided with antithrombotic prophylaxis or, alternatively, must all with positive radiofibrinogen tests receive anticoagulant therapy, presumably with full-dose heparin?

Firm data are needed to demonstrate that: some forms of deep venous thrombosis are relatively safe, with very low embolic incidence and postphlebitic sequelae; and these forms of thrombosis can reliably be distinguished from those that pose greater hazard. Although our data do not provide complete answers, they do suggest the value of examining these important questions using larger patient samples.

In this study, distal thrombi were associated with very limited, if any, embolic risk. None of the 21 patients with venographic evidence of such thrombi developed symptoms or scan evidence of pulmonary embolism. Statistical analysis of those cases with distal thrombi only shows the upper 95% confidence limit for embolic risk is 13%. No heparin therapy was administered and all patients were asymptomatic after at least 3 months of follow-up. Further, radiofibrinogen detected four additional patients who were positive only in the calf (three with negative venograms; one refused venogram). In these patients also, V/Q scans were not indicative of embolism, heparin was not given, and they remained asymptomatic for at least 3 months. The upper 95% confidence limit for embolic risk in patients with distal only thrombi detected by radiofibrinogen is 11%. Thus, the hospital and follow-up outcome of 25 patients with untreated known or suspected calf-only thrombi was satisfactory. None has had postphlebitic symptoms thus far, although only further follow-up will show whether these salutary results persist.

Proximal thrombi, however, posed a major threat of pulmonary embolization. Over half the patients with thrombosis above the knee had scintiphotographic evidence compatible with pulmonary embolism. The earlier observations of McLaughlin and Paterson (3) as well as more recent studies by Havig (2), based on autopsy specimens, also suggest the relatively high embolic risk associated with proximal venous thrombi. In addition, postphlebitic signs or symptoms were present in two of these patients.

While the differential embolic hazard of below-knee versus above-knee thrombi has been suggested by these and other investigators (2, 4-10), precise information bearing on this point is difficult to find in the literature, either because the location of the venous thrombosis is not clearly stated (or identified), or the diagnosis of pulmonary embolism was based exclusively on clinical evidence. Only one of our eight patients with a positive ventilation/perfusion study for embolism had *symptoms* suggesting that diagnosis, and all had negative chest roentgenograms. Because all mismatches seen on ventilation/perfusion scanning involved at least one lobe and since all these patients (except perhaps the one with spinal cord injury) were capable of reporting symptoms, the absence of symptoms does not seem to be explained by embolic size or peculiarities of the subject population. Our data may indicate that asymptomatic emboli are rather common. Although the documentation of embolic occurrence by ventilation/perfusion scans can be debated (14), this will remain a moot point because it is difficult to endorse pulmonary angiography in asymptomatic patients as an investigative alternative to scanning. We believe that scanning is a sensitive and reliable tool in this context. No scans showed mismatch in those patients in whom all three diagnostic tests for deep venous thrombosis were negative, or in whom one or more tests indicated thrombosis limited to the calf. Furthermore, all eight patients with mismatch on ventilation/perfusion scans had negative chest roentgenograms and showed resolution of the perfusion defects in follow-up scans.

The 43 normal scans, plus the two with matched abnormalities in which angiogram was negative, certainly did not have emboli. How many of the 15 with matched abnormalities and no angiogram did have emboli remains unknown, as does the absolute incidence of embolism in the six patients with mismatch in whom angiography was not done. However, if we were to speculate, accepting the highly unlikely assumption that embolism was present in all mismatched scan defects plus all matched defects without angiography, the embolic incidence would have been eight of 31 of patients with negative venograms; four of 21 among those with distal-only venous thrombosis; and 11 of 15 among those with proximal vein involvement. The fact that, 2 weeks later, perfusion distribution was not altered in 12 of the 15 nonangiogramed patients with initial matched defects makes such assumptions of incidence even more unlikely.

The reason for the major difference in embolic potential that appears to exist between proximal and distal venous thrombi is not entirely clear. Speculations that calf thrombi are more securely attached or more susceptible to rapid spontaneous resolution may be valid. Kakkar and associates (4) have reported that thrombi confined to the calf often resolve in 72 hours without therapy. An alternative explanation may be that no difference in embolic incidence actually exists, but that the difference is based on the ability of emboli of differing size to produce symptoms or be detected by V/Q scanning (or standard angiography). Thrombi in proximal leg veins are larger. Certainly the size of vessels obstructed by emboli is a major determinant of both the extent of the signs and symptoms that alert the clinician and of the sensitivity of detection by scanning and angiography. Thus, whether calf-only venous thrombi fail to embolize or merely give rise to small, clinically inapparent emboli remains an unanswered question.

Even if these differences in embolic risk are fully validated, they would be of little benefit unless physicians were able to categorize patients reliably. Clearly, venography can distinguish between proximal and distal deep venous thrombosis, but this approach has definite drawbacks. Venography is time-consuming to the radiographer, frequently painful to the patient and associated with a definite incidence of untoward reactions (15), including thrombosis (16). Thus, initial, and particularly repetitive applications of this test are difficult to justify outside an investigative context.

We believe that our study indicates that the combination of radiofibrinogen leg scans and impedance can be used reliably to diagnose the *presence* of deep venous thrombosis, and categorize the detected thrombosis into proximal (dangerous) or distal-only (safer) classification. This approach has previously been proposed by Hull and colleagues (7, 9). In our study, impedance was positive in all 15 patients, as well as in 15 of the 16 limbs, with venogram-proven proximal deep venous thrombosis. Impedance was positive in only six of 21 patients with thrombosis limited to the calf shown by venogram. The insensitivity of impedance to calf thrombi is widely appreciated and, actually, confers a high degree of specificity in the diagnosis of proximal deep venous thrombosis (7-10).

The radiofibrinogen leg scan was positive in nine of 15 patients with proximal (plus distal) deep venous thrombosis. Of the six false negative studies, four were positive in the calf and the two completely negative results were associated with antecedent heparin therapy (8). In the detection of distal deep venous thrombosis, the radiofibrinogen test excelled. All 21 patients with calf-only disease by venogram had positive radiofibrinogen studies. The three false positive radiofibrinogen leg scans raise an unanswerable question as to which test, venogram or radiofibrinogen leg scan, is more sensitive, an issue others also have raised (4, 17, 18).

Three interesting features of our data warrant comment. Although it has been reported that 15% to 20% of initially calf-limited thrombi extend to the thigh veins under observation (4), none did so in our series. Further, even in patients with hip surgery, we encountered no instance of above-the-knee-only thrombosis. Finally, we encountered a relatively high incidence of thigh-vein thrombosis. We have no explanation for the first two features. However, the third is explained by the fact that all medical patients were referred because of clinical suspicion of venous thrombosis. In our experience and that of others (5), when this clinical suspicion is confirmed, above-knee involvement is frequent. Furthermore, the high overall prevalence of venous thrombosis among the medical patients (Group 1) is explained by the fact that they entered the study because venous thrombosis was clinically suspected, while groups 2 and 3 were studied only because of high risk. Interestingly, the Group 1 data confirm previous studies in which a clinical suspicion of venous thrombosis proved correct about 50% of the time (5-8).

Thus, our data are compatible with previous suggestions that distal (calf) deep venous thrombosis poses a low risk of embolization, contrary to proximal (thigh) thrombi; and that radiofibrinogen leg scans plus impedance can be used to identify both the presence and location of deep venous thrombosis. If these trends are confirmed by future investigations, such concepts may provide the clinician with increased flexibility in his therapeutic approach to patients with, or at high risk for, deep venous thrombosis. Proximal thrombosis, with its high embolic risk, would continue to require antithrombotic therapy, but thrombosis confined to the calf might allow continued patient observation by noninvasive techniques (radiofibrinogen, impedance), and treatment with smaller doses of heparin or no therapy. Considering the many patients who are now automatic candidates for heparin treatment, these provocative issues merit consideration and further investigation.

ACKNOWLEDGMENTS: Grant support: HL-18576, University of California Thrombosis Project.

▶ Requests for reprints should be addressed to Kenneth M. Moser, M.D.; University Hospital; 225 Dickinson Street; San Diego, CA 92103.

References

1. Sevitt S, Gallagher N. Venous thrombosis and pulmonary embolism: a clinico-pathological study in injured and burned patients. *Br J Surg.* 1961;**48**:475-89.
2. Havig GO: Source of pulmonary emboli. *Acta Chir Scand.* 1977;**478**(Suppl):42-7.

3. McLaughlin AD, Paterson J. Some basic observations on venous thrombosis and pulmonary embolism. *Surg Gynecol Obstet.* 1951;**93:**1-7.
4. Kakkar VV, Flanc C, Howe CT, Clark MB. Natural history of postoperative deep vein thrombosis. *Lancet.* 1969;**2:**230-2.
5. Hirsh J, Hull R. Comparative value of tests for the diagnosis of venous thrombosis. *World J Surg.* 1978;**2:**27-38.
6. Kakkar, VV. Deep vein thrombosis: detection and prevention. *Circulation.* 1975;**51:**8-19.
7. Hull R, Hirsh J, Sackett DL, Powers P, Turpie AGG, Walker I. Combined use of leg scanning and impedance plethysmography in suspected venous thrombosis: an alternative to venography. *N Engl J Med.* 1977;**296:**1497-500.
8. Moser KM, Brach BB, Dolan GF. Clinically suspected deep venous thrombosis of the lower extremities; a comparison of venography impedance plethysmography and radiolabeled fibrinogen. *JAMA.* 1977;**237:**2195-8.
9. Hull R, Van Aken WG, Hirsh J, et al. Impedance plethysmography using occlusive cuff technique in the diagnosis of venous thrombosis. *Circulation.* 1976;**53:**696-700.
10. Wheeler HB, O'Donnell JH, Anderson FA, Benedict K. Occlusive imedance plethysmography: a diagnostic procedure for venous thrombosis and pulmonary embolism. *Prog Cardiovasc Dis.* 1974;**17:**199-205.
11. Kakkar VV, Corrigan TP, Fossard DP. Prevention of fatal postoperative pulmonary embolism by low doses of heparin: an international multicenter trial. *Lancet.* 1975;**2:**45-51.
12. Rabinov K, Paulin S. Roentgen diagnosis of venous thrombosis in the leg. *Arch Surg.* 1972;**104:**134-44.
13. Moser KM. Clinical applications of ventilation/perfusion scintiphotography. In: Baum, GL, ed. *Textbook of Pulmonary Diseases.* Boston: Little, Brown and Company; 1974:103-27.
14. Robin ED. Overdiagnosis and overtreatment of pulmonary embolism: the emperor may have no clothes. *Ann Intern Med.* 1977;**87:**775-81.
15. Bettman MA, Paulin S. Leg phlebography: the incidence, nature and modification of undesirable side effects. *Radiology.* 1977;**122:**101-4.
16. Albrechtsson U, Olsson CG. Thrombotic side-effects of lower limb phlebography. *Lancet.* 1976;**1:**723-4.
17. O'Brien JR. Peripheral venous scanning with ^{125}I tagged fibrinogen. *Lancet.* 1972;**1:**909-10. Letter.
18. Mavor GE, Walker MG, Dhall DP. et al. Peripheral venous scanning with ^{125}I-tagged fibrinogen. *Lancet.* 1972;**1:**661-3.

Antibiotic Therapy in Exacerbations of Chronic Obstructive Pulmonary Disease

N. R. ANTHONISEN, M.D.; J. MANFREDA, M.D.; C. P. W. WARREN, M.D.; E. S. HERSHFIELD, M.D.; G. K. M. HARDING, M.D.; and N. A. NELSON, Ph.D.; Winnipeg, Manitoba, Canada

The effects of broad-spectrum antibiotic and placebo therapy in patients with chronic obstructive pulmonary disease in exacerbation were compared in a randomized, double-blinded, crossover trial. Exacerbations were defined in terms of increased dyspnea, sputum production, and sputum purulence. Exacerbations were followed at 3-day intervals by home visits, and those that resolved in 21 days were designated treatment successes. Treatment failures included exacerbations in which symptoms did not resolve but no intervention was necessary, and those in which the patient's condition deteriorated so that intervention was necessary. Over 3.5 years in 173 patients, 362 exacerbations were treated, 180 with placebo and 182 with antibiotic. The success rate with placebo was 55% and with antibiotic 68%. The rate of failure with deterioration was 19% with placebo and 10% with antibiotic. There was a significant benefit associated with antibiotic. Peak flow recovered more rapidly with antibiotic treatment than with placebo. Side effects were uncommon and did not differ between antibiotic and placebo.

EXACERBATIONS of chronic obstructive pulmonary disease are commonly characterized by increases in dyspnea, cough, and sputum production with increased purulence in sputum. It is recommended that these exacerbations be treated with a 7- to 10-day course of broad-spectrum antibiotics (1-4), though the role of bacterial infection in exacerbations is recognized as unclear. Surprisingly, the efficacy of the therapy is also not clear. Tager and Speizer (5) reviewed the problem in 1975 and concluded that no good evidence existed that antibiotic therapy was of either short-term or long-term benefit, and they suggested that this form of treatment be reassessed. Since 1975, the problem has been little investigated; one recent report has found antibiotic therapy to be of no benefit in patients hospitalized with exacerbations (6).

Because chronic obstructive pulmonary disease is a common disease, and patients are reported to have an average of one to four exacerbations per year, antibiotic therapy of these exacerbations is a frequently used unproven treatment. For this reason, we conducted a trial of antibiotic therapy for such exacerbations.

Materials and Methods

PATIENTS

We recruited patients with stable chronic obstructive pulmonary disease, characterized them in terms of symptoms and lung function, and followed them. When an exacerbation developed, the patient was given, in a double-blinded manner, a 10-day course of either placebo or antibiotic according to a prearranged random schedule, and the exacerbation was followed closely for 3 weeks. Subsequently, the patient continued to be followed, and further exacerbations were treated in a crossover manner alternating placebo and antibiotic. Patients were seen in the clinic at least every 3 months and fully reevaluated at yearly intervals.

Patients were eligible for the trial if they were at least 35 years old and had a clinical diagnosis of chronic obstructive disease, not asthma. In addition, they had to live close enough to the clinical center for home visits and to be reliable (that is, to keep two consecutive outpatient appointments). They were

▶ From the Sections of Respiratory and Infectious Diseases, Department of Internal Medicine, and the Department of Social and Preventive Medicine, University of Manitoba; Winnipeg, Manitoba, Canada.

required to have a forced expired volume in 1 second (FEV_1) that was less than 70% of the predicted value and less than 70% of the forced vital capacity. The total lung capacity was required to be greater than 80% of the predicted value. Patients were excluded if the FEV_1 increased to 80% of the predicted value with use of an inhaled bronchodilator product. Patients were also excluded if they had other disease serious enough to influence their quality of life or clinical course, such as cancer, left ventricular failure, or stroke, or if they had other disease likely to require antibiotic therapy, such as recurrent sinusitis or urinary tract infection.

STUDY PROTOCOL AND TESTING

When suitable patients were identified, they were placed on a standard regimen (*see* below) and followed for 2 weeks. At the end of that time, if they still fulfilled the entry criteria, they had baseline studies. These studies consisted of a symptom history in the form of a modified American Thoracic Society questionnaire (7), an examination of the heart and lungs, a chest radiograph and an electrocardiogram if one was not available from less than 1 year previously, and lung function tests. Forced vital capacity and FEV_1 were measured with a rolling seal spirometer. Of three efforts, the one with the largest sum of FEV_1 and forced vital capacity was recorded and compared with normal values (8). Measurements were repeated after the inhalation of 250 μg of isoproterenol. Peak flow was measured with a Wright peak flow meter (Clement Clark International, London, England), with the best of three efforts being recorded. Functional residual capacity was measured by plethysmography and compared with normal values (9). Inspiratory capacity and expiratory reserve volume were measured by spirometry, allowing computation of total lung capacity and residual volume that were also compared with normal values (9). Arterial blood samples were obtained while the patients were semirecumbent at rest and were analyzed for (Po_2) and (Pco_2) with appropriately calibrated electrodes.

When not having an exacerbation, patients were seen at the clinical center at 3-month intervals. At these visits, symptoms were evaluated, the heart and lungs reexamined, and FEV_1, forced vital capacity, and peak flow measured. At yearly intervals, all baseline studies were repeated. Patients were managed between exacerbations with a standard regimen. All patients received inhaled albuterol supplied by metered-dose inhalers or compressor nebulizers, or both. All patients received oral theophylline, usually in the long-acting form and usually in standard doses. Some patients who had serious symptoms and who were thought to be steroid responsive (10) were maintained on prednisone, 5 to 10 mg/d. Diuretics were used to manage edema, and patients who fulfilled standard criteria for home oxygen therapy received such therapy for at least 18 h/d (11). All patients received polyvalent anti-influenza vaccine each autumn. Patients thought to be steroid responsive received increased doses of these agents during exacerbations. The regimen employed usually consisted of 40 mg of prednisone for 3 days, with the dosage being tapered to the maintenance dose in 9 to 12 days. Although the dose schedule varied somewhat among patients, it was the same during all exacerbations in any given patient.

PROTOCOL DURING EXACERBATIONS

Exacerbations were defined in terms of symptoms. The occurrence of increased dyspnea, sputum volume, and sputum purulence was defined as a type-1 exacerbation. Type-2 exacerbations were defined as occurring when two of these three symptoms were present. Type-3 exacerbations were defined as occurring when one of the three symptoms was present in addition to at least one of the following findings: upper respiratory infection (sore throat, nasal discharge) within the past 5 days; fever without other cause; increased wheezing; increased cough; or increase in respiratory rate or heart rate by 20% as compared with baseline. If during the course of an exacerbation new symptoms appeared, reclassification was done; that is, an exacerbation that was initially type 3 could be reclassified as type 1 or 2, but not the reverse. It should be noted that the classification of exacerbations was done prospectively and for analytical purposes only, as management was the same for all exacerbations.

Patients who had an increase in symptoms notified the center and were seen on the same day by an experienced nurse-practitioner, who decided whether the symptoms fulfilled the criteria outlined earlier. If the patient was judged to be dangerously ill, the patient's physician was notified and participated in the decision as to whether the patient would begin the study protocol. If the patient was thought to have an exacerbation, the nurse-practitioner checked symptoms, measured peak flow, and prescribed a ten-day course of either antibiotic or placebo at the initial visit. All exacerbations were treated in the same way. During all exacerbations, repeat visits were made at 3-day intervals until day 15, and if symptoms had not resolved by then, another visit was made at day 21. On each occasion, symptoms and peak flow were checked, the patient questioned about symptoms associated with the medication, and the remaining antibiotic or placebo pills counted. Peak flow was measured three times at each visit, and the largest value recorded.

The antibiotics and regimens used were trimethoprim-sulfamethoxazole, one tablet (160 mg/800 mg) twice daily; amoxicillin, 0.25 g four times daily; or doxycycline, 200 mg initially followed by 0.1 g daily. The choice of antibiotic was made by the patient's physician, since these agents appear not to differ in effectiveness in this situation (12-15). We were supplied an appropriate placebo for each drug, so that neither the patient nor the medical staff knew which medication was active.

The outcome of the exacerbations was defined in terms of symptoms. A "treatment success" was defined as resolution within 21 days of all symptoms that accompanied the exacerbation. The date of resolution was noted. Treatment failures were of two types: "no resolution" included exacerbations in which all symptoms did not resolve in 21 days but no further intervention was deemed necessary; in "failure with deterioration," symptoms worsened during the exacerbation to the point that further intervention (hospitalization or treatment with antibiotic in unblinded fashion) was deemed necessary. These interventions could only be instituted after consultation with a physician, usually the patient's own, and only after more than 72 hours of antibiotic or placebo treatment had been given. If intervention was thought necessary less than 72 hours after treatment was begun, the treatment was not designated a success or failure because we believed that such rapid deterioration was unlikely to be related to antibiotic or placebo therapy.

After an exacerbation, patients were required to have a 2-week period with the same symptoms as those present before the exacerbation before another exacerbation was studied. If patients were hospitalized, new baseline measurements were made before another exacerbation was studied. At their quarterly clinic visits, patients were questioned closely about episodes of illness that were not studied; if these had the characteristics of an exacerbation, they were classified as a "missed" exacerbation.

ANALYSIS OF DATA

In 61 exacerbations, the symptom questionnaire administered by the nurse-practitioners was checked for accuracy and repeatability. This was done by the patient's physician, who telephoned the patient and administered the same questionnaire within 24 hours of the nurse-practitioner's visit. Calls were made after the first visit and again at the end of the observation period—days 15 or 21. The physicians were not informed of the patient's progress.

All data were recorded on special forms, checked for accuracy, and entered into a computer file. The SAS statistical package (SAS Institute Inc., Cary, North Carolina) was used in analysis. For discrete variables such as treatment success or failure, the chi-square test statistic was used when only the first exacerbation for each patient was analyzed. When exacerbation outcomes were analyzed in patients with multiple exacerbations, and when comparisons were made within patients, the

Table 1. Symptoms at Baseline in Patients with Chronic Obstructive Pulmonary Disease

	Patients
	%
Cough	
None	15.0
Morning only	60.1
Episodes during day	20.8
Nearly continuous	4.0
Sputum quantity	
None	16.2
Less than 30 mL	57.2
30-100 mL	22.5
More than 100 mL	4.0
Sputum quality	
Mucoid	62.4
Mucopurulent	18.5
Purulent	2.9
Dyspnea	
None	6.3
Only on unusual exertion	28.3
Present during normal activity	48.4
Present at rest	16.7
Wheezing	
None	30.0
Present only on unusual activity or exacerbations	52.6
Present on many daily activities	15.6
Present at rest	1.7

likelihood-ratio chi-square statistic was used. We used the *t*-test and repeated-measures analyses of variance to assess continuous variables such as duration of exacerbations.

In the analyses of success and failure rates, several approaches were used. The simplest and easiest to understand was the comparison of results in all antibiotic-treated and placebo-treated exacerbations. However, many patients had exacerbations treated in each way, and consequently exacerbation outcomes may not have been independent of each other because of differences among patients and similarities (between exacerbations) within patients.

We therefore analyzed only the first exacerbation for each patient, using independent treatment groups that were, however, relatively small. Also, in patients who had at least two exacerbations, we analyzed exacerbations as matched sets, because each of these patients had at least one exacerbation treated with antibiotic and another treated with placebo. The first two to four exacerbations in each patient were used for this analysis; the fifth and subsequent ones were excluded to prevent the result from being biased by the few patients who had more than four exacerbations. The likelihood chi-square test statistics were generated for this group. To describe our experience more completely, we pooled the results from these patients who had multiple exacerbation with those results from patients who had only one exacerbation. This pooling was permissible because the two data sets were independent, and the analysis consisted of calculating an average value for the two data sets after weighting each of them according to the variability of the estimates. Odds ratios and one-tailed confidence limits for these results were calculated in the usual way (16-18).

Sets with discordant outcomes—that is, sets containing exacerbations with both successful and unsuccessful outcomes—were examined by using outcome (success or failure) as the dependent variable. Independent variables were exacerbation order (first or second), exacerbation type (1, 2, or 3) and treatment (antibiotic or placebo).

The same matched-set model was used to examine the association between presenting symptoms (present or absent) at the onset of exacerbations and the treatment. In patients who had more than one exacerbation, duration was analyzed by examining the first two to four exacerbations. Again, a pair-type analysis was used, the general linear model for repeated observations (19).

Peak flow results were also analyzed by a paired-within-patient format. We examined peak flow data from 64 patients who had at least one antibiotic-treated and one placebo-treated exacerbation followed for 15 to 21 days (this excluded failures with deterioration). If a patient had more than one exacerbation with a 15- to 21-day follow-up and the same treatment, peak flow values were averaged. Effects of treatment on peak flow were examined with a repeated-measures analysis of variance using peak flow as the dependent variable and days of testing (0, 3, 6, 12, or 15) and treatment as the independent variables.

Agreement between nurse-practitioners and physicians with regard to symptoms was analyzed by the computation of kappa scores, which correct for concordance due to chance (19, 20).

Results

Between 1 November 1981 and September 1984, 173 patients were enrolled in the study. The group was 79.8% male, and the average age was 67.3 ± 9.0 (SD) years. Nearly all (93.6%) had a history of smoking, averaging 39.9 ± 28.9 pack-years, although only 21.4% were smoking at the time of enrollment. Other baseline characteristics are shown in Tables 1 and 2. At baseline, most patients had morning cough with scanty mucoid sputum, developed dyspnea with mild exertions, but wheezed only with severer exertion (Table 1). Lung function studies (Table 2) showed that the average patient had moderately severe airways obstruction with a poor bronchodilator response and hyperinflation but near-normal arterial blood gases. The standard deviations for these average values (Table 2) are relatively large, however, indicating that a wide range of lung function was represented. Seven patients were on home oxygen therapy for chronic respiratory failure.

More than 4000 patient-months were observed during the study; the average patient was followed for 23.7 ± 11.3 months. Of the 173 patients, 59 dropped out before the study was ended on 1 March 1985. Of these, 18 died, although only 1 death occurred during an exacerbation managed by our protocol and this was due to a ruptured aortic aneurysm. Fifteen patients were dropped because they did not cooperate with the study protocol, and another 17 patients were dropped because they developed other disease or because their physicians believed that the study was not in their best interest (usually because they were "too sick" for the study). The patients who dropped out did not differ significantly from the remainder of the

Table 2. Lung Function at Baseline in Patients with Chronic Obstructive Pulmonary Disease*

Forced expiratory volume in 1 second, *% predicted*	33.9 ± 13.7
Forced vital capacity, *% predicted*	59.5 ± 16.8
Functional residual capacity, *% predicted*	164.6 ± 34.4
Total lung capacity, *% predicted*	128.9 ± 19.7
Residual volume, *% predicted*	205.3 ± 51.5
Bronchodilator response, *% FEV_1*	111.8 ± 17.6
Peak flow, *L/min*	227.5 ± 96.1
Arterial Po_2, *mm Hg*	68.3 ± 9.9
Arterial Pco_2, *mm Hg*	36.6 ± 6.1
Arterial pH	7.42 ± 0.03

* Data given as mean ± SD. FEV_1 = forced expiratory volume in 1 second.

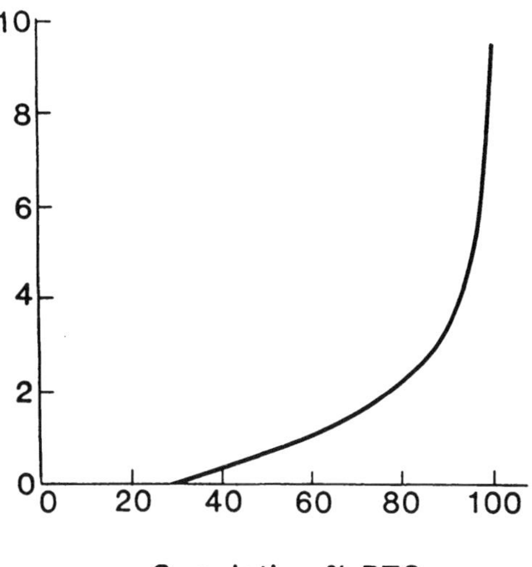

Figure 1. Cumulative distribution of exacerbations frequency in patients with chronic obstructive pulmonary disease followed at least 6 months. The ordinate shows the exacerbation frequency, and the abscissa, the percentage of patients (*PTS*).

patients in symptoms (Table 1) or lung function (Table 2).

The 173 patients had 448 exacerbations while under observation. Of these, 86 were "missed," that is, not treated according to protocol. In 35 cases the patient was judged by the study team to be "too sick" for the protocol; in 21 the patient or an outside physician began antibiotic therapy before notifying the study team; and in 16 the exacerbation occurred when the patient was out of town. The other 14 exacerbations were missed for various reasons. When all patients and all exacerbations were considered, the average patient had 1 exacerbation each 9.2 months. This statistic is somewhat misleading, however, because 10 patients were followed for less than 6 months. When these patients were excluded, the average was 1 exacerbation each 8.5 months, or an average frequency of 1.3 ± 1.5/yr. A cumulative distribution of exacerbation frequency in patients followed at least 6 months is shown in Figure 1. About 25% of the patients had no exacerbations; the median for the whole group was 0.8 exacerbations per year; and a small number of patients had many exacerbations (10% had more than 3.4/yr, and 1 averaged 9.6/yr).

Symptoms present at the onset of the 362 exacerbations treated according to protocol are shown in Table 3. Increased dyspnea, cough, sputum, sputum purulence, and wheeze were common, whereas fever and tachycardia were relatively uncommon. Approximately 40% of the exacerbations were type 1 at onset, and another 40% were type 2. The distribution of exacerbation types was essentially the same in antibiotic- and placebo-treated exacerbations. The frequency of individual symptoms was not significantly different between antibiotic- and placebo-treated exacerbations except for wheeze, which occurred more often ($p < 0.01$) at the onset of antibiotic-treated exacerbations. Systemic steroid thereapy was used in 42.8% of antibiotic-treated exacerbations and in 43.5% of placebo-treated ones.

The success and failure rates in 180 placebo-treated and 182 antibiotic-treated exacerbations are shown in the top of Table 4. A few episodes were not classified as treatment success or failure, because the patients' condition deteriorated less than 72 hours after treatment began or they developed another illness unrelated to the exacerbation. The success rate in antibiotic-treated exacerbations was about 1.24 times higher than the success rate in placebo-treated episodes. Failures with deterioration (those in which the patient's symptoms worsened so that further intervention was thought necessary) were nearly twice as common with placebo treatment.

When matched sets of exacerbations and single exacerbations were pooled, the relative odds favoring success with antibiotic treatment were 2.32 times the odds for placebo, with a lower 95% confidence limit of 1.38. In these data, the success rate with antibiotics was 18.9% greater than that with placebo, with a lower 95% confidence limit of 7.8%. Similarly, when odds ratios obtained from matched sets and single exacerbations were pooled, deterioration was 0.467 times as common in antibiotic-treated exacerbations as in placebo-treated ones, with an upper 95% confidence limit of 0.88. In these data there was a 9.1% difference in the frequency of deterioration, with a lower 95% confidence limit of 1.9%. By matched-set analysis, exacerbation outcome was not significantly related to order of treatment or exacerbation type.

We also analyzed the first exacerbation recorded in each patient, 59 of which were treated with placebo and 57 with antibiotic. The results (Table 4 Bottom) were similar to these when all exacerbations were analyzed together. The difference in success rates just missed being statistically significant ($p = 0.06$, chi square) in this relatively small series.

Because both wheeze (Table 3) and success (Table 4) were associated with antibiotic therapy, their relationship with each other was examined. Wheeze was not associat-

Table 3. Findings at Onset of Exacerbations of Chronic Obstructive Pulmonary Disease*

	Placebo Group ($n = 180$)	Antibiotic Group ($n = 182$)
Exacerbation type, %		
Type 1	39.7	38.5
Type 2	41.9	42.3
Type 3	18.4	19.2
Individual findings, %		
Recent upper respiratory tract infection	54.7	48.9
Increased dyspnea	87.2	92.3
Increased sputum production	71.7	67.6
Change in sputum color	60.6	58.8
Increased wheeze	67.2	79.1
Increased cough	82.2	82.4
Fever	29.4	29.1
Increased heart rate	21.6	21.7
Increased respiratory rate	44.1	40.7

* Increased wheeze was commoner ($p = 0.01$) at the onset of antibiotic-treated exacerbations when results from matched-set and single exacerbations were pooled. There was no significant difference ($p > 0.10$) for any other finding shown.

Table 4. Outcome of Exacerbations of Chronic Obstructive Pulmonary Disease

	Placebo Group	Antibiotic Group
	%(n)	%(n)
All exacerbations		
Success	55.0(99)	68.1(124)*
No resolution	23.3(42)	18.7 (34)
Deterioration	18.9(34)	9.9 (18)†
Other‡	2.9 (5)	3.2 (6)
First exacerbations		
Success	52.3(31)	66.8 (38)§
No resolution	27.1(16)	17.5 (10)
Deterioration	17.0(10)	12.3 (7)
Other‡	3.4 (2)	3.4 (2)

* $p < 0.01$ when results from matched-set and single exacerbations were pooled.

† $p < 0.05$ when matched-set and single exacerbation data were pooled.

‡ Includes exacerbations in which patients had deterioration in less than 72 hours or developed unrelated illnesses.

§ $p = 0.06$, chi-square test.

ed with a successful outcome. In placebo-treated exacerbations, the success rate was 57.6% in those episodes without increased wheezing at onset, and it was 53.7% in those episodes with increased wheezing. In antibiotic-treated exacerbations, the success rate was 76.3% in those episodes without increased wheezing at onset and 65.8% in those with wheezing. The presence of wheeze, though associated with antibiotic therapy (Table 3), was not associated with treatment success, as was antibiotic therapy. The same result was obtained when the effect of wheezing on outcome was examined with the matched-set model. The inclusion of wheeze in the model did not alter the relative odds favoring antibiotic treatment and did not significantly improve the fit of the model.

Table 5 presents success and failure rates for exacerbations classified as to type, both at onset and when the maximum number of symptoms was present (if additional symptoms occurred during an exacerbation, it was reclassified accordingly). By either method of classification, placebo treatment showed a graduation of success rates from type-1 to type-3 exacerbations, with the rate being highest in the type-3 exacerbations. Differences in success rate between antibiotic and placebo were greatest in exacerbations classified as type 1 at onset, and in these exacerbations deterioration was over twice as common with placebo as with antibiotic. In type-2 exacerbations, antibiotic success rates were somewhat greater and deterioration somewhat less common than with placebo, but differences between treatments were less striking than in type-1 exacerbations and deterioration was much less common whatever the treatment. By both classification systems, type-3 exacerbations showed essentially the same rates of success and deterioration for antibiotic and placebo treatment. Of exacerbations classified as type 3 at onset, 20 of 33 treated with placebo were reclassified due to an increase in symptoms, as compared with 14 of 35 treated with antibiotic. However, the outcomes of exacerbations that worsened were not different from those of exacerbations that did not worsen. Of the 20 placebo-treated exacerbations that were associated with an increase in symptoms, 8 were treatment failures, 3 with deterioration; of 14 similar antibiotic-treated exacerbations, 6 were failures, 4 with deterioration.

When all exacerbations without deterioration were considered, with treatment failures being assigned a duration of 22 days, antibiotic-treated exacerbations were shorter than those treated with placebo (14.1 ± 6.3 days compared with 15.5 ± 6.1 days). Duration was also analyzed by the general linear model technique, which examined data from the first two to four exacerbations in patients who had multiple exacerbations. When treatment failures were assigned a duration of 22 days, the duration of antibiotic-treated exacerbations averaged 2.2 days less than those treated with placebo ($p = 0.02$). When all treatment failures were eliminated, antibiotic-treated exacerbations averaged 11.9 ± 5.3 days in length and those treated with placebo were 12.8 ± 5.2 days in length, values that were not significantly different. Treatment order did not affect these differences.

Peak flow data were analyzed in patients with paired exacerbations that were followed for 15 to 21 days. Peak flow declined from a mean of 215 L/min during stable baseline conditions to 190 L/min at the onset of exacerbations ($p < 0.05$, paired t-test). Furthermore, peak flow increased during the exacerbation (Figure 2), and the rate of increase was faster in antibiotic-treated exacerbations than in placebo-treated ones ($p < 0.02$, repeated-measures analysis of variance).

Table 5. Exacerbation Result by Type*

	Placebo Group			Antibiotic Group		
	Type 1	Type 2	Type 3	Type 1	Type 2	Type 3
	←		%(n)			→
Exacerbation onset						
Success	43.0(31)	60.0(45)	69.7(23)	62.9(44)	70.1(54)	74.2(26)
No resolution	22.2(16)	26.7(20)	18.2 (6)	20.0(14)	20.8(16)	11.4 (4)
Deterioration	30.5(22)	10.7 (8)	12.1 (4)	14.3(10)	5.2 (4)	11.4 (4)
Maximum symptoms						
Success	46.0(52)	66.7(36)	84.6(11)	57.7(60)	80.7(46)	85.7(18)
No resolution	24.8(28)	24.1(13)	7.7 (1)	22.1(23)	15.8 (9)	9.5 (2)
Deterioration	26.6(30)	5.6 (3)	7.7 (1)	15.4(16)	3.5 (2)	0

* Sum of percents is less than 100% because of patients who had deterioration in less than 72 hours or who developed unrelated disease. For definition of types 1, 2, and 3, see Methods.

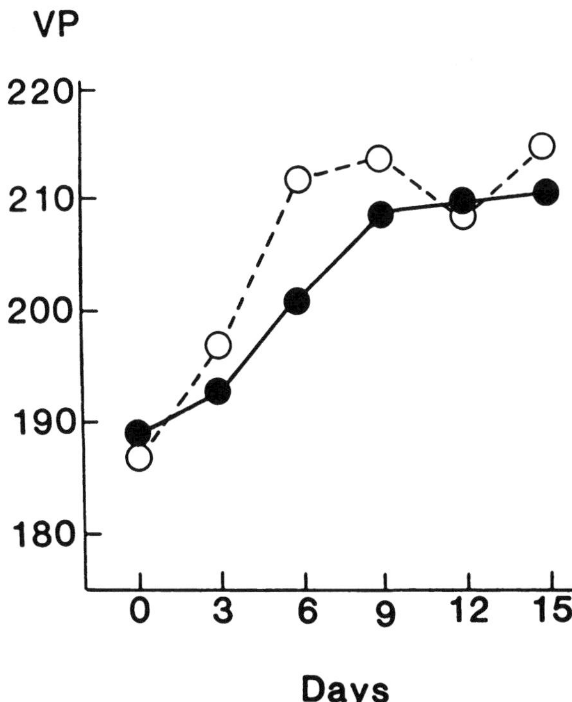

Figure 2. Recovery of peak flow ($\dot{V}P$) in 64 patients with paired exacerbations that were observed for 15 to 21 days. Open symbols show antibiotic-treated exacerbations; closed circles, those treated with placebo.

No significant differences were seen in success rates that depended on the individual antibiotic used. About 20% of the exacerbations were treated with doxycycline or its placebo, whereas the remainder were evenly divided between trimethoprim-sulfamethoxazole and amoxicillin or their placebos. The choice of antibiotic was not systematically related to baseline lung function or number of exacerbations. At the onset of exacerbations, the frequency of individual findings was similar for all three antibiotics; and with all of them the success rate was greater than that achieved with placebo, although differences were not statistically significant between placebo and individual agents considered separately. The use of systemic steroid treatment during exacerbations did not influence the results. In exacerbations treated with steroids, the success rate with antibiotic was higher (though not significantly so) than that with placebo, and these rates were similar and not significantly different from those in exacerbations not treated with steroids.

The incidence of side effects was low and not significantly different between antibiotic and placebo therapy (Table 6). (Table 6 lists individual symptoms during exacerbations, not patients, and many patients had more than one side effect during a given exacerbation.) Although gastrointestinal symptoms were slightly commoner in antibiotic-treated exacerbations, all other symptoms were commoner during placebo treatment. Symptoms regarded as serious enough to withdraw therapy occurred slightly more often during placebo-treated exacerbations.

Kappa scores for the comparison of nurse-practitioner and physician evaluations of symptoms are shown in Table 7. In general, agreement was fair to good (20, 21). In particular, agreement as to whether an exacerbation had ended or not was 78.4% (kappa = 0.57, Table 7).

Discussion

POTENTIAL BIASES

This study shows that, compared to placebo, antibiotic treatment of chronic obstructive pulmonary disease in exacerbation produced significantly earlier resolution of symptoms. Before this conclusion can be accepted, however, biases in the study must be examined. The most notable was that increased wheezing was commoner in antibiotic-treated exacerbations than in those treated with placebo (Table 3); this observation raises the question of whether treatment success was associated with the increased wheezing and not antibiotics. This was not the case. In both antibiotic- and placebo-treated episodes, exacerbations having increased wheezing at onset were associated with lower success rates than those without wheezing. The reason for the higher assignment of exacerbations with increased wheezing to antibiotic treatment is not clear, but because wheezing was not associated with successful resolution of symptoms, the increased success rate observed with antibiotics cannot be ascribed to wheeze.

A few other systemic biases existed in our study. The study was conducted in double-blinded fashion; placebo medications were not distinguishable from antibiotics, and neither the patients nor the study team knew which tablets were active medication. Aside from the use of antibiotic or placebo, treatment regimens during exacerbations did not differ, and our crossover design ensured that therapy between exacerbations was not different. Systemic steroid therapy was used in approximately 42% of both antibiotic- and placebo-treated exacerbations, and the success rate with antibiotics was greater in both steroid-treated and non-steroid-treated exacerbations. Some patients dropped out of the study because their physicians judged them "too sick" to participate (that is, too sick to have exacerbations treated with placebo half the time), and some exacerbations in study patients were not treated on the study protocol for similar reasons. Thus, our results may not apply to such patients or exacerbations. However, we believe it unlikely that antibiotics would be less successful than placebo in severely ill patients. The judgment of whether a patient was "too sick"

Table 6. Percentage of Exacerbations with Side Effects During the First 9 Days of Therapy*

Side Effect	Placebo Group	Antibiotic Group
	%	%
Nausea	8.0	10.1
Vomiting	1.9	2.8
Abdominal cramps	4.2	3.2
Diarrhea	2.9	5.0
Rash	1.0	1.2
Other	6.1	1.5
Treatment discontinued	2.5	1.5

* Incidence of each side effect recorded separately. Many patients had more than one.

Table 7. Kappa Scores for Agreement on Symptoms Between Physician and Nurse-Practitioner

	Onset of Exacerbation	End of Exacerbation
Upper respiratory infection	0.39	...
Increased dyspnea	0.70	0.53
Increased sputum production	0.51	0.25
Change in color	0.73	0.48
Increased wheezing	0.50	0.49
Increased cough	0.56	0.57
Number of symptoms (out of five)	0.49	0.47
None at end	...	0.57

was totally subjective, and there likely was considerable overlap between these patients and exacerbations and those treated on our protocol. Patients who dropped out did not differ significantly from the remainder in symptoms or lung function. Furthermore, failures with deterioration occurred nearly twice as often in placebo-treated exacerbations, which argues that antibiotic treatment was advantageous in severe exacerbations.

Some might argue that our criteria for the onset and resolution of exacerbations were "soft" and subjective, because they depended on patient reports of symptoms. We deliberately used symptoms to define the onset of exacerbations, because these are the criteria applied in medical practice, and once onset was defined in these terms, resolution had to be defined in similar ones. Agreement was fair to good between our nurse-practitioners and the patients' physicians as to whether increased symptoms were present or absent. The kappa scores in Table 7 are substantially higher—indicating better agreement—than those between radiologists reading xeromammograms (22). This agreement was achieved despite some differences in methods. The nurse-practitioners interviewed patients directly whereas the physicians did so by telephone, and the timing of the interviews could vary by as much as 24 hours. Thus, though our criteria may have been "soft," they were reproducible.

Symptomatic evidence favoring the efficacy of antibiotic therapy was supported by the peak flow results shown in Figure 2. In antibiotic-treated exacerbations, peak flow, an objective measurement, increased more rapidly than it did in exacerbations treated with placebo. It should be noted that our analysis of the peak flow results was, if anything, biased against an antibiotic advantage. We studied pairs of exacerbations from single patients that were observed for 15 to 21 days; exacerbations with deterioration were excluded from the analysis. Because such failures occurred more often in placebo-treated episodes and were probably associated with prolonged depressions of peak flow, their exclusion tended to increase apparent recovery of peak flow more in the placebo than in the antibiotic group.

Others might argue that our classifying treatment outcome as success or failure at 21 days was arbitrary and that a different result might have been observed had a different time period been used. Had we used a shorter time period for our criterion, failure rates would have been higher for both placebo- and antibiotic-treated exacerbations, and the difference between the two would have been greater because the duration of successfully treated exacerbations was shorter for antibiotic than for placebo. Had we used a longer time period, the final day of evaluation would have been at least 2 weeks after the end of the 10-day course of antibiotic therapy, and it would have become unclear whether we were dealing with single exacerbations. In any event, treatment failures with deterioration largely occurred within the first 15 days of exacerbations, and their definition was not dependent on an arbitrary decision about the acceptable duration of exacerbations. These failures were nearly twice as common with placebo.

In summary, we found that antibiotic-treated exacerbations were significantly more likely to resolve in 21 days than were placebo-treated ones, and they were significantly less likely to be associated with clinically alarming deterioration after the first 72 hours. This conclusion was supported by the more rapid recovery of peak flow in patients with antibiotic-treated exacerbations. We do not believe that these results were due to biases in the study or methods of analysis. Finally, the close similarity of rates in the two panels of Table 4 indicates that our result was not due to data from a few patients with many exacerbations; success and failure rates for all exacerbations were similar to those when only each patient's first exacerbation was considered. This conclusion was supported by the results of the matched-set analyses, which considered only the first four exacerbations in each patient.

COMPARISON WITH OTHER STUDIES

How did our findings differ from those of others who have studied this question? In 1975, Tager and Speizer (5) reviewed six adequately controlled studies of antibiotic therapy in chronic obstructive pulmonary disease in which the patient populations were reasonably well defined. Two studies were "positive," purporting to show an advantage for antibiotic, but one (13) used questionable statistical methods. The other (12) compared a group of 86 placebo-treated patients with two groups of approximately equal size, one of patients treated with tetracycline and the other of patients treated with chloramphenicol. The antibiotic-treated groups improved more rapidly in terms of "general assessment" and "sputum purulence," but early relapse was seen, particularly for sputum purulence, in all groups. Of four "negative" studies, three (23-25) showed a trend favoring antibiotic therapy; the largest examined results from 71 antibiotic-treated and 75 placebo-treated exacerbations (23). The last of the six studies reviewed had only 9 patients in the antibiotic treatment group (26).

More recently, Nicotra and coworkers (6) completed a careful study of 40 patients with chronic obstructive pulmonary disease hospitalized with acute exacerbations, comparing tetracycline treatment with placebo. Their assessment was based on lung function tests and blood gases, and at 7 days there was no difference between treatment groups. However, both arterial Po_2 and peak flow increased more in the tetracycline group. Indeed, the differences they observed in peak flow at 7 days were very similar to those we found at 6 days (Figure 2). Presumably, our differences were statistically significant because we had a larger patient group and because our paired, within-patient analysis reduced the variability of the result. Thus, our results were not qualitatively different from those in the literature, and the reason we found statistically significant advantages for antibiotic therapy is probably that we observed many more exacerbations than others did.

CLINICAL SIGNIFICANCE

If the statistical validity of our results is accepted, what is their clinical significance? The difference in success rate between antibiotic and placebo treatment approximated 13%, with more than half of the placebo treatments being successful. This percentage does not appear to be a great clinical advantage. The difference in failures with deterioration was probably of greater clinical significance; patients having such failures were thought to need additional treatment, which certainly resulted in increased cost and likely was associated with increased patient morbidity. Although these failures were relatively uncommon, they occurred nearly twice as often with placebo treatment and probably afford the best argument for antibiotic therapy.

Arguments against antibiotic therapy would be cost and side effects. The cost of broad-spectrum antibiotics like the ones we used is relatively small and should not deter their use. Side effects were not severe and occurred no more often than with placebo (Table 7). It should be noted that the incidence of side effects in our study was almost certainly less than that which would be noted if patients were randomly exposed to the antibiotics we used. Most, if not all, of our patients had had courses of broad-spectrum antibiotics before they entered this trial, and presumably their physicians specified a particular antibiotic in light of this past experience. A drug was avoided if a patient was thought to be sensitive to it, thereby decreasing the side effects seen in this study. It would appear, however, that side effects are likely to be very uncommon and of little significance in patients with established chronic obstructive pulmonary disease.

Antibiotic therapy would be more attractive if we were able to identify kinds of exacerbations that are associated with the greatest difference between antibiotic and placebo therapy. Furthermore, if these exacerbations could be identified at their onset, the expense of close follow-up in all patients could be avoided. Table 5 indicates that exacerbations classified as type 1 at onset showed a relatively large advantage for antibiotic therapy. There was nearly a 20% difference in success rates, and deterioration occurred in 30% of placebo-treated episodes, more than twice as often as with antibiotic. Clearly, exacerbations presenting with increased dyspnea, sputum, and sputum purulence should be treated with antibiotic. Antibiotics appeared to confer no benefit in type-3 exacerbations and apparently should not be used when only one symptom (dyspnea, sputum, or sputum purulence) is present. Type-2 exacerbations, in which two of the three symptoms were present at onset, had a 70% success rate with antibiotic and a 60% success rate without it; and although deterioration was relatively uncommon, it occurred more often in placebo-treated exacerbations (Table 5). Antibiotic therapy could probably be justified for such exacerbations in patients known to tolerate the proposed antibiotic.

We also analyzed individual symptoms (Table 3) to see if any were associated with a greater difference between antibiotic and placebo therapy than the group as a whole. We found that although some (notably increased dyspnea, cough, sputum, and sputum purulence) were associated with a difference between treatments similar to that of the study as a whole, none clearly exceeded it or approached the treatment-related differences noted for type-1 exacerbations.

ACKNOWLEDGMENTS: The authors thank the nurse-practitioners who did the study, L. A. Mendella, B. N. Nord, I. Warner, D. Gaborieau, A. Szabo, and M. A. Robinson; and thank Dr. V. A. Taraska, who contributed patients to the study.

Grant support: by a grant from Health and Welfare Canada. Drugs and placebos were supplied free of charge by the following manufacturers: Burroughs Wellcome Co. (trimethoprim-sulfamethoxazole, Septra DS, Ayerst Laboratories (amoxicillin, Amoxil), and Pfizer Canada, Inc. (doxycycline, Vibramycin).

▶ Requests for reprints should be addressed to N. R. Anthonisen, M.D.; F-2 General Centre, Health Sciences Centre, University of Manitoba, 700 William Avenue; Winnipeg, Manitoba, Canada R3E 0Z3.

References

1. INGRAM RH JR. Chronic bronchitis, emphysema, and airways obstruction. In: PETERSDORF RG, ADAMS RD, BRAUNWALD E, ISSELBACHER KJ, MARTIN JB, WILSON JD, eds. *Harrison's Principles of Internal Medicine.* 10th ed. New York: McGraw-Hill Book Co.; 1983:1550.
2. WELCH MH. Obstructive diseases. In: GUENTER CA, WELCH MH, eds. *Pulmonary Medicine.* 2nd ed. Philadelphia: J. B. Lippincott Company; 1982:697.
3. HOWELL JBL. Chronic lung disease with airflow obstruction—chronic bronchitis and emphysema. In: EMERSON P, ed. *Thoracic Medicine.* London: Butterworth; 1981:456.
4. STUART-HARRIS C. Acute respiratory infection in the patient with chronic bronchitis and emphysema. In: FISHMAN AP, ed. *Pulmonary Diseases and Disorders.* New York: McGraw-Hill Book Co.; 1980:455.
5. TAGER I, SPEIZER FE. Role of infection in chronic bronchitis. *N Engl J Med.* 1975;**292:**563-70.
6. NICOTRA MB, RIVERA M, AWE RJ. Antibiotic therapy in acute exacerbations of chronic bronchitis: a controlled study using tetracycline. *Ann Intern Med.* 1982;**97:**18-21.
7. NATIONAL HEART, LUNG AND BLOOD INSTITUTE, DIVISION OF LUNG DISEASES. *Protocol Intermittent Positive Pressure Breathing Collaborative Program.* Bethesda, Maryland: National Institutes of Health; 1978.
8. MORRIS JF, KOSKI A, JOHNSON LC. Spirometric standards for healthy nonsmoking adults. *Am Rev Respir Dis.* 1971;**103:**57-67.
9. GOLDMAN HI, BECKLACKE MR. Respiratory function tests: normal values at medium altitudes and the prediction of normal results. *Am Rev Tuberc.* 1959;**79:**457-67.
10. MENDELLA LA, MANFREDA J, WARREN CPW, ANTHONISEN NR. Steroid responses in stable chronic obstructive pulmonary disease. *Ann Intern Med.* 1982;**96:**17-21.
11. NOCTURNAL OXYGEN THERAPY TRIAL GROUP. Continuous or nocturnal oxygen therapy in hypoxemic chronic obstructive lung disease: a clinical trial. *Ann Intern Med.* 1980;**93:**391-8.
12. PINES A, RAAFAT H, GREENFIELD JSB, LINSELL WD, SOLARI ME. Antibiotic regimens in moderately ill patients with purulent exacerbations of chronic bronchitis. *Br J Dis Chest.* 1972;**66:**107-15.
13. PINES A, RAAFAT H, PLUCINSKI K, GREENFIELD JSB, SOLARI M. Antibiotic regimens in severe and acute purulent exacerbations of chronic bronchitis. *Br Med J.* 1968;**2:**735-8.
14. HUGHES DTD, DREW CD, JOHNSON TBW, JARVIS JD. Trimethoprim and sulphamethoxazole in the treatment of chronic chest infections. *Chemotherapy.* 1969;**14:**151-7.

SECTION XI

RHEUMATOLOGY

The spectrum of vasculitis: clinical, pathologic, immunologic and therapeutic considerations.

Fauci AS, Haynes BF, Katz P. Ann Intern Med. 1978;89(Part 1):660-676.

Fauci and associates' article, an edited transcription of a Combined Clinical Staff Conference at the Clinical Center of the National Institutes of Health (NIH) in Bethesda, Maryland, probably had more influence than any other in attracting medical students and residents in internal medicine to the rapidly evolving subspecialty of rheumatology. The attraction of the field, as highlighted by the authors, was the combination of a sophisticated base of knowledge in immunology, biochemistry, and pathology matched with the challenge of diagnosis by careful history and physical examination of multisystem diseases with protean manifestations and pathology that, if biopsy sites were chosen carefully, could be diagnostic. More significant for patients with vasculitic syndromes, a base of evidence for the efficacy of new therapies was evolving rapidly.

If you were a bright senior medical student in the late 1970s with a strong interest in learning to apply new information from basic science to clinical disease, this article might have been your epiphany. Fauci and associates collated the best of published studies. Many of the patients had been studied as inpatients and outpatients at the Clinical Center of the NIH. The initial paragraphs focus on the immunopathogenic mechanisms of systemic and localized vasculitis, including the 1976 publication of a study (1) that established hepatitis B as the cause polyarteritis in some cases. This section was followed by a careful classification of systemic vasculitis that emphasized its wide spectrum of presentations. In 1978, giant cell arteritis, which manifests clinically as polymyalgia rheumatica or temporal arteritis, was little known to U.S. physicians; it had been defined only a short time earlier in Great Britain. Fauci and associates provided a still-unrivaled presentation of the similarities and differences between temporal arteritis and Takayasu's arteritis. For many students, this article was their first introduction to the mucocutaneous lymph node syndrome, better known now as Kawasaki's disease, with changes of vasculitis along the main trunk and branches of the coronary arteries.

In addition to a superb review of immunopathology, classification, and clinical manifestatios of vasculitis, Fauci and colleagues presented a comprehensive analysis of therapy, with emphasis on the evidence that cyclophosphamide could, when given alone or in combination with glucocorticoids, induce remission in Wegener's granulomatosis and produce beneficial effects in polyarteritis. The observations of Fauci and Sheldon Wolff in 1977 on 21 patients treated with cyclophosphamide were holding true. These findings gave rheumatologists confidence and optimism.

Another major contribution of this article was documentation of the unique benefit of the Clinical Center at NIH, where patients with selected diseases are comprehensively studied over a long period, and new clinical protocols put to thorough testing.

References

1. **Sergent JS, Lockshin MD, Christian CL, Gocke DJ.** Vasculitis with hepatitis B antigenemia: long-term observation in nine patients. Medicine (Baltimore). 1976;55:1-18.

Glucocorticoid-induced osteoporosis: pathogenesis and management.

Lukert BP, Raisz LG. Ann Intern Med. 1990;112:352-364.

The danger of glucocorticoids to bone health has been known since the late 1950s; however, Lukert and Raisz's review served for at least a decade as the best source for evidence on the pathogenesis of glucocorticoid-associated osteoporosis. The senior author, Larry Raisz was a leading clinical investigator who contributed much to our understanding of bone physiology and calcium homeostasis.

The statement that "bone loss with resulting fractures is the most incapacitating sequela of steroid therapy" told the reader early in the article that what followed was of great importance. Table 1, which summarized results of 16 studies on the effect of glucocorticoids in humans, provided convicing evidence that 30% to 50% of patients receiving glucocorticoids for a disease process would become osteoporotic and that approximately 50% would experience fractures. The section on pathogenesis was more complete and current than information in any available textbook material and included summaries of the latest published data on glucocorticoid effects on secretion of sex hormones, intestinal calcium absorption, vitamin D metabolism, and renal excretion of calcium and phosphorus. This section remains current today. Table 3 outlined the major mechanisms in the pathogenesis of this form of osteoporosis: decreased gastrointestinal calcium absorption and increased renal excretion of calcium, leading to secondary hyperparathyroidism; decreased gonadal hormone secretion; inhibited insulin-like growth factor-1; inhibited osteoblast function and cytodevelopment (due to steroids) and prostaglandin E_2 production; increased sensitivity to parathyroid hormone; and probable stimulation of osteoclastic activity.

The section on prevention and treatment stated that any dose higher than the equivalent of 7.5 mg prednisone daily would be harmful to bone. Studies from the 1990s revealed that even 5 mg prednisone daily could lead to decreased bone density. The treatment section is relatively short because evidence on the use and availability of bisphosphonate therapy, now a mainstay of treatment as well as prevention, was just emerging. Instead, use of estrogens was encouraged, reflecting the beliefs of the era that preceded the discovery that estrogens increase the risk for cardiovascular adverse events.

Wegener granulomatosis: an analysis of 158 patients.

Hoffman GS, Kerr GS, Leavitt RY, et al. Ann Intern Med. 1992;116: 488-498.

Before 1970, the diagnosis of Wegener's granulomatosis was usually a death sentence: The disease killed 50% of its victims in 5 months and 80% in 1 year. That dramatically changed when Anthony Fauci and Sheldon Wolff and their colleagues conducted the first prospective protocol-driven studies of vasculitis in the late 1960s at the National Institutes of Health (NIH) (1). The legacy of these studies was profound. Treatment with corticosteroids and daily cyclophosphamide produced remission in over 90% of cases. Hoffman and colleagues enlarged the cohort from 21 to 158 patients, each of whom was studied with the same rigor characteristic of clinical studies from the NIH Clinical Center. Their study provided important guidance and sounded several warnings. First, corticosteroids alone almost never produced remissions in Wegener's granulomatosis. Second, 86% and 47% of patients, respectively, had permanent disease- and treatment-related morbidity. Third, serious infections and cancer, especially bladder cancer and lymphomas, were far more common than first recognized in earlier studies from the NIH. The latency period between cyclophosphamide exposure and cancer diagnoses was often years, which meant long-term surveillance of patients, including those who enjoyed prolonged remissions. Finally, antineutrophil cytoplasmic antibodies were commonly associated with Wegener's granulomatosis, but a change in antibody titer correlated only crudely with change in disease status.

These observations made it clear that safer and effective approaches to vasculitis care were sorely needed. Hoffman and associates included preliminary data on the efficacy of methotrexate for patients with less severe forms of disease in whom renal failure did not increase the risk of methotrexate-induced bone marrow suppression. They and others subsequently confirmed these results and set the stage for exploration of other interventions. Hoffman and colleagues also demonstrated that in desperate circumstances, cyclophosphamide is still a life-saving drug, but its use can be limited to the several months required to induce remission, whereas agents that pose far less risk often successfully maintain remission—-thereby avoiding many most of the toxicities of long-term cyclophosphamide exposure (2,3).

In addition to reviewing therapies, Hoffman and colleagues expanded the knowledge base on unusual manifestations of Wegener's granulomatosis that could help clinicians avoid misdiagnosis. Some of these included fever and weight loss masquerading as cancer; polyarticular arthritis and positive tests for rheumatoid factor appearing to be rheumatoid arthritis; and cardiac, optic and retro-orbital manifestations.

References

1. **Fauci AS, Haynes BF, Katz P, Wolff SM.** Wegener's granulomatosis: prospective clinical and therapeutic experience with 85 patients for 21 years. 1983;98:76-85.

2. **Jayne D, Rasmussen N, Andrassy K, et al., European Vasculitis Study Group.** A randomized trial of maintenance therapy for vasculitis associated with antineutrophil cytoplasmic autoantibodies. N Engl J Med. 2003; 349:36-44.

3. **Villa-Forte A, Clark TM, Gomes M, et al.** Substitution of methotrexate for cyclophosphamide in Wegener granulomatosis: a 12-year single-practice experience. Medicine (Baltimore). 2007;86:269-77.

The Spectrum of Vasculitis

Clinical, Pathologic, Immunologic, and Therapeutic Considerations

Moderator: ANTHONY S. FAUCI, M.D., F.A.C.P. *Discussants:* BARTON F. HAYNES, M.D.; and PAUL KATZ, M.D.; Bethesda, Maryland

Vasculitis is a clinicopathologic process characterized by inflammation and necrosis of blood vessels. Certain disorders have vasculitis as the predominant and most obvious manifestation, whereas others have various degrees of vasculitis in association with other primary disorders. Within the entire spectrum of vasculitis virtually any size or type of blood vessel in any organ system can be involved. Most of the vasculitides can be associated directly or indirectly with immunopathogenic mechanisms. In this regard, immune complex mediation is being increasingly recognized as the underlying mechanism in several of the vasculitides. With clinical, pathologic, and immunologic criteria, certain vasculitic disorders can be clearly recognized and categorized as distinct entities, whereas in others there is an overlap of different diseases within a broader category. in recent years, several of the more serious vasculitides, such as Wegener's granulomatosis and the systemic necrotizing vasculitides of the polyarteritis nodosa group, which formerly had extremely poor prognoses, have been shown to be extraordinarily responsive to chronic low-dose cytotoxic therapy, particularly cyclophosphamide.

DR. ANTHONY S. FAUCI (Head, Clinical Physiology Section, Laboratory of Clinical Investigation, Deputy Clinical Director, National Institute of Allergy and Infectious Diseases): Vasculitis is a clinicopathologic process characterized by an inflammation and necrosis of blood vessels. It can exist as the major and primary manifestation of a number of clinical syndromes, or it may represent a relatively minor component of other primary disease processes.

Necrotizing vasculitis was first described more than 100 years ago in a 27-year-old man by Kussmaul and Maier (1). That patient had what is now called classic polyarteritis nodosa. With this early description, all vasculitides were originally thought to be polyarteritis nodosa. However, it soon became clear that the disseminated vasculitides comprised a broad spectrum of disorders involving vessels of different types, sizes, and locations characterized by various clinical manifestations, with or without identifiable precipitating factors. In many cases, attempts at classification of the vasculitides into separate categories either resulted in an oversimplified grouping or a cumbersome series of categorizations with little appreciation of overlap. Such approaches were of little consequence at a time when identification of precipitating antigens was not feasible, and the few available therapeutic modalities were generally ineffective.

The following discussions will focus on recent advances in the appreciation of the pathogenesis, immunologic mechanisms, and clinical manifestations of several of these diseases, leading to a clearer understanding of the distinctions and overlaps among these disorders and, most importantly, to more rational and directed therapeutic approaches resulting in striking remissions and improved prognosis in several heretofore devastating diseases.

Pathophysiology and Immunologic Mechanisms

It has now become clear that a substantial proportion of the necrotizing vasculitides are either directly caused by, or closely associated with, immunopathogenic mechanisms. Also, as advanced technology becomes progressively more available, it is likely that offending antigens and immunologic phenomena will be directly associated with virtually all of the vasculitides. In this regard, it is reasonable to extrapolate an immunopathogenisis or association from certain diseases with well-established immunopathogenesis to that spectrum of vasculitides with suggestive, but less definitive, immunopathogenesis. For example, systemic vasculitis is an important clinicopathologic feature of several of the connective tissue or collagen vascular diseases, such as systemic lupus erythematosus and rheumatoid arthritis, in which immunopathogenic mechanisms are well established (2-6). Additionally, clear-cut immunopathogenesis has been established in several of the primary vasculitides, particularly in cases of hepatitis B antigen-associated necrotizing vasculitis

▶ An edited transcription of a Combined Clinical Staff Conference at the Clinical Center, Bethesda, Maryland, 2 February 1978, by the National Institute of Allergy and Infectious Diseases, National Institutes of Health, U.S. Department of Health, Education, and Welfare.

▶ Authors who wish to cite a section of this conference and specifically indicate its author can use this example for the form of reference:
HAYNES BF: Treatment of the granulomatous vasculitides, pp. 671-673 in FAUCI AS (moderator): The spectrum of vasculitis. Clinical, pathologic, immunologic, and therapeutic considerations. *Ann Intern Med* 89 (Part 1):660-676, 1978

(7). Similarities of immunologic aberrancies found in these diseases, to that substantial portion of patients with vasculitis of questionable or unknown origin, make the interrelation between the two groups obvious (3, 4, 8, 9). Such abnormalities include hypergammaglobulinemia, rheumatoid factor, cryoglobulinemia, circulating immune complexes, and hypocomplementemia. Furthermore, the temporal relation of various vasculitic syndromes to drug ingestion, antigen exposure, or certain infections (10) lends further support to the concept of hypersensitivity or disordered immunologic reactivity playing a role in the pathogenesis of these diseases.

The prevailing theory, for which there is now substantial evidence, is that most of the vasculitic syndromes are caused by, or closely associated with, deposition of immune complexes in blood vessel walls. Elegant studies in animal models (11) have enabled the construction of hypotheses for the stepwise series of events most likely operable in the immune complex mediated vascular damage of systemic vasculitis.

Figure 1 details the proposed mechanisms of immune complex vasculitis. Briefly, after antigen exposure, certain types of soluble antigen-antibody complexes that are formed in antigen excess freely circulate and, if not cleared by the reticuloendothelial system, are deposited in blood vessel walls. An increase in vascular permeability is an important factor in the deposition of immune complexes and this results, at least in part, from the action of vasoactive amines derived from platelets and IgE-triggered basophils (12, 13). After complexes are deposited in vessel walls, complement components are activated, with some serving as chemotactic factors for polymorphonuclear leukocytes. These cells respond by infiltrating the vessel wall, then releasing their intracytoplasmic lysosomal enzymes, particularly collagenase and elastase, causing damage and necrosis of the vessel wall. This may be accompanied by thrombosis, occlusion, and hemorrhage, and ischemic changes in the surrounding tissue ensues.

In addition to the localized increase in vascular permeability, other factors, such as blood flow turbulence at vessel bifurcations and hydrostatic forces in the lower extremities, predispose to the preferential localization of immune complexes in certain sites of the vascular tree. Furthermore, the concentration of immune complexes in the circulation, the duration of their circulating half-life, and, in particular, the physical characteristics of the antibody molecules forming the complexes (14-17) influence the nature of the disease activity.

Often, investigators fail to identify circulating immune complexes or immune-complex deposition in clinical situations in which it is probable that the disease is immune complex mediated. This may be due to several factors including the fact that complexes are often rapidly cleared from the circulation. Moreover, failure to appreciate immune complexes in involved tissues may be a function of the age of the lesion, because it has been shown in animals that 24 to 48 h after injection of antigen-antibody complexes, immune reactants are undetectable (18).

Besides classic immune complex-mediated vasculitis, other types of immunopathogenic mechanisms may be involved in vascular damage. One of these is cell-mediated immune reactivity. This is not a common or well-studied mechanism of vasculitis, as is the immune complex type. However, in many ways, its mechanisms of vascular damage resemble immune-complex disease and may be reflected in the histopathologic features of certain types of vasculitis.

Theoretical mechanisms of this type of vascular injury

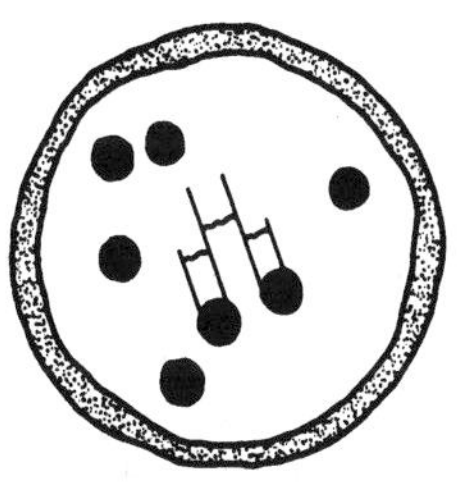

1) Circulating soluble immune complexes in antigen excess.

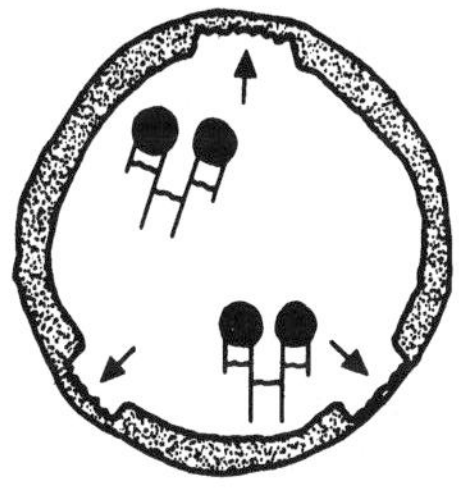

2) Increased vascular permeability via platelet derived vasoactive amines and IgE mediated reactions.

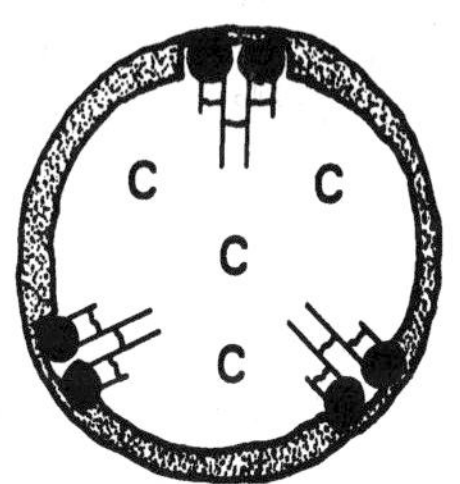

3) Trapping of immune complexes along basement membrane of vessel wall and activation of complement components (C).

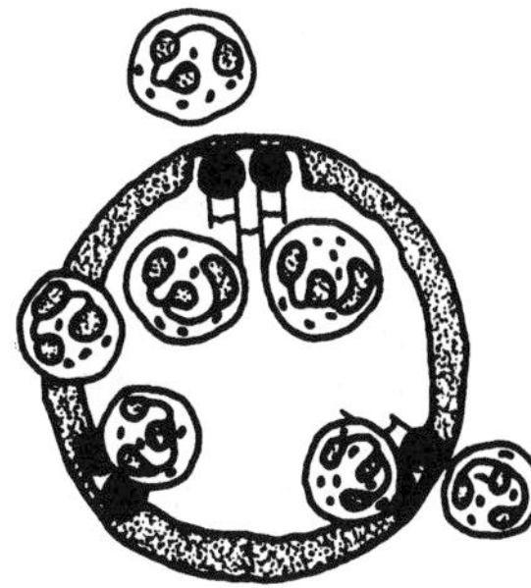

4) Complement derived chemotactic factors (C3a, C5a, C567) cause accumulation of PMNs.

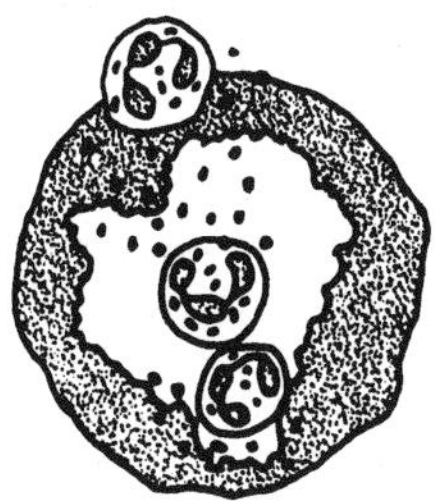

5) PMNs release lysosomal enzymes (collagenase, elastase)

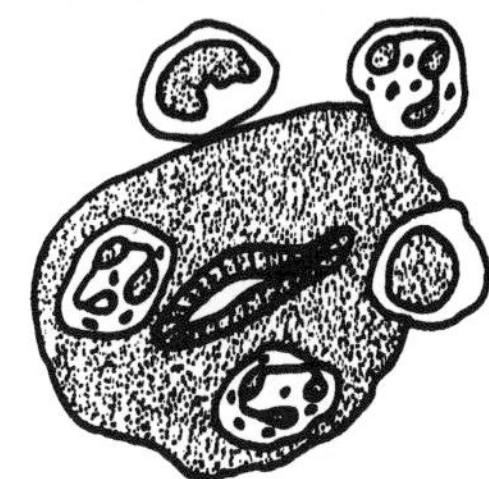

6) Damage and necrosis of vessel wall, thrombosis, occlusion, hemorrhage.

Figure 1. Mechanisms of immune complex vasculitis. Soluble immune complexes formed in antigen excess circulate and are ultimately deposited in blood vessel walls related to increased vascular permeability at the site of deposition. The increased vascular permeability results from the action of vasoactive amines that are derived from platelets and IgE-triggered reactions. The immune complexes are trapped and complement components are activated, some of which are chemotactic for polymorphonuclear leukocytes (*PMNs*) that then migrate in and around the vessel wall. These cells then release their lysosomal enzymes that damage the blood vessel wall.

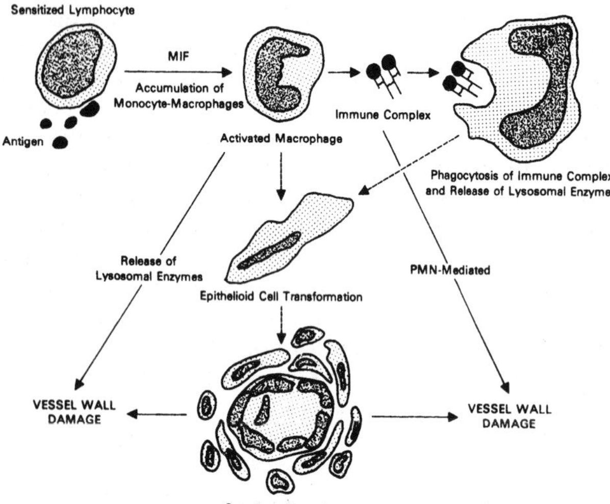

Figure 2. Cell-mediated immune mechanisms of vasculitis. Sensitized lymphocytes react with antigen and most likely release lymphokines. Some of these soluble products, such as macrophage migration inhibitory factor (*MIF*), result in the recruitment of monocytes to the immune reaction site. These cells may transform into activated macrophages that can release lysosomal enzymes capable of damaging blood vessel walls. In addition, these cells may further transform to epithelioid cells and ultimately participate in granuloma formation. When this takes place in and around blood vessels, granulomatous vasculitis occurs. Furthermore, it is possible that macrophages, under certain circumstances, phagocytose or are triggered by immune complexes. This process may then lead to transformation to epithelioid cells, granuloma formation, or release of lysosomal enzymes.

are outlined in Figure 2. Probably, sensitized lymphocytes are triggered by circulating antigen to release a variety of lymphokines, such as macrophage migration inhibitory factor, causing influx and accumulation in and around vessels of monocytes that transform into activated macrophages (19). These cells release their lysosomal enzymes, causing effects similar to neutrophil-mediated vascular damage. Additionally, true granulomatous reactions can develop by transforming monocytes to activated macrophages and, subsequently, to epithelioid cells and multinucleated giant cells of classic granulomata (20).

These mechanisms may, in part, be responsible for the mononuclear cell infiltration seen in certain types of cutaneous vasculitis (21), in addition to the intravascular and extravascular granulomata characteristically seen in the spectrum of granulomatous vasculitides (22). Furthermore, phagocytosis of certain types of immune complexes by macrophages may initiate the chain of events leading to granuloma formation and may explain the presence of granulomatous reactions in diseases that also show strong evidence of immune complex mediation (22).

Although other mechanisms, such as tissue injury, mediated directly by an antibody with specificity against the vessel itself, or via cytotoxic effector cells in antibody-dependent cellular cytotoxicity, can potentially play a role in vascular damage, there is little evidence to support their contribution to the pathogenesis of any of the recognized vasculitides.

The Clinical and Pathologic Spectrum of Vasculitis

Difficulties and confusion have plagued efforts to classify and reclassify the various clinical entities in the broad spectrum of vasculitides. The original prototype of systemic vasculitis (classic polyarteritis nodosa of Kussmaul and Maier [1]), had distinctive clinicopathologic characteristics (discussed later). As other reports of vasculitis appeared, the initial tendency was to group them into one category. However, as it became clear that several of these disorders were obviously different from classic polyarteritis nodosa, attempts were made to strictly classify them according to certain features such as blood vessel size, type, and location, involvement or lack of involvement of the pulmonary vasculature, presence or absence of skin involvement or granulomatous reactions, and association with other entities such as collagen vascular or connective tissue diseases (3, 23-25).

Although several of these classifications lend a useful order and structure to this spectrum of disorders, often they are oversimplified and fail to consider the big overlap that exists. Also, the same disease entities are often called different names by different authors.

In recent years, as discussed later, significant advances have been made in the chemotherapeutic approach to various distinct entities, and groups of diseases highly responsive to various therapeutic regimens have been identified. Under these circumstances, the correct and appropriate classification of these diseases assumes more relevance. Little or no advantage would be gained from completely reclassifying the vasculitic syndromes. However, it may be helpful to extract from previous classifications and outline an updated categorization that more clearly reflects recent clinicopathologic studies, advances in understanding of immunopathogenesis, and distinctions based on differential responses to various therapeutic regimens.

In classifying diseases in the spectrum of vasculitis, certain points should be emphasized. First, and perhaps most important, most, if not all, of these are systemic necrotizing vasculitides, and this term itself connotes little specificity. Within this broad category of systemic vasculitis certain syndromes, such as Wegener's granulomatosis and temporal or cranial arteritis, emerge as well-de-

Table 1. The Spectrum of Vasculitides

Polyarteritis nodosa group of systemic necrotizing vasculitis
Classic polyarteritis nodosa
Allergic granulomatosis
Systemic necrotizing vasculitis—"overlap syndrome"
Hypersensitivity vasculitis
Subgroups of hypersensitivity vasculitis
Serum sickness and serum-sicknesslike reactions
Henoch-Schönlein purpura
Essential mixed cryoglobulinemia with vasculitis
Vasculitis associated with malignancies
Vasculitis associated with other primary disorders
Wegener's granulomatosis
Lymphomatoid granulomatosis
Giant-cell arteritides
Temporal arteritis
Takayasu's arteritis
Thromboangiitis obliterans (Buerger's disease)
Mucocutaneous lymph node syndrome
Miscellaneous vasculitides

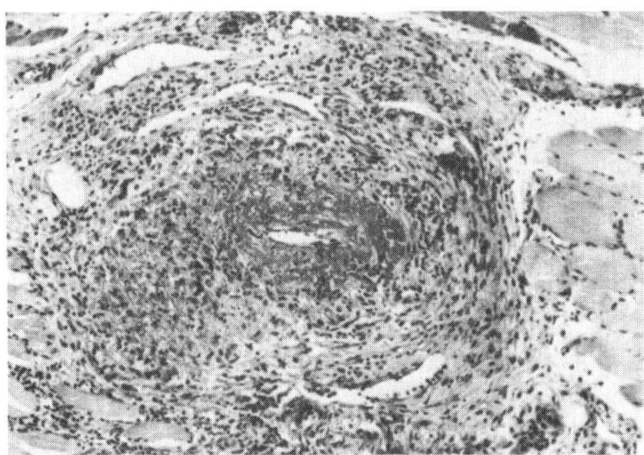

Figure 3. Necrotizing vasculitis in classic polyarteritis nodosa. Muscle biopsy shows fibrinoid necrosis of the wall of a small artery. The lumen of the blood vessel is markedly compromised. (Hematoxylin and eosin; original magnification, × 130.)

fined entities because of the presence of rather well-characterized clinicopathologic features. These disorders, although systemic necrotizing vasculitides in the broad sense, are usually referred to separately because of their distinctive characteristics. Other disorders, however, may not have such distinctive characteristics, but manifest systemic necrotizing vasculitis that may involve vessels of different sizes and locations with variable propensities towards different organs. It is in this group that most of the difficulties and confusion in classification occur because of considerable overlap of clinical and pathologic characteristics. Also, in this group the term polyarteritis nodosa is loosely and, in certain respects, inappropriately used. This is because some people take the term to mean the classic polyarteritis nodosa of Kussmaul and Maier (1), whereas others take it to mean any systemic necrotizing vasculitis that does not fit into any of the other well-defined vasculitic syndromes. Table 1 is a general outline of the vasculitides.

Polyarteritis Nodosa Group of Systemic Necrotizing Vasculitis

The first of these is the group referred to above that should be thought of in terms of the broader category of the polyarteritis nodosa group of systemic necrotizing vasculitides. This takes into account the original classic polyarteritis nodosa, the closely related allergic granulomatosis, and that difficult and most important syndrome that overlaps the other two and does not exclusively have the distinguishing characteristics of either of the other two, but shares features of both, "overlap syndrome."

Because the first two of these three subgroups have been firmly entrenched in the vasculitis literature, it may be helpful to describe briefly the features of the three and to point out that this entire group greatly overlaps and that it is justifiable to consider them together in the broader category already mentioned.

Classic polyarteritis nodosa, as it was originally described (1) and later categorized (23, 24), is a necrotizing vasculitis of small- and medium-sized muscular arteries (Figure 3). The lesions tend to be segmental with a predeliction for bifurcations and branchings of arteries with distal spread involving arterioles and, in some cases, circumferentially involving adjacent veins. Histopathologically, in the acute stages, polymorphonuclear leukocytes infiltrate all layers of the vessel wall and perivascular areas. Mononuclear cell infiltration follows as the lesions become subacute and chronic. Intimal proliferation, vessel wall degeneration with fibrinoid necrosis, thrombosis, ischemia, and infarction are seen in varying degrees. Generally, the simultaneous presence of vascular lesions is found in all stages of development. Multiple organ systems are involved and the clinicopathologic findings reflect the degree and location of vessel involvement with the resulting ischemic changes.

Table 2 outlines the salient clinicopathologic features of classic polyarteritis nodosa (22-24). Certain points should be emphasized with regard to the classic syndrome and its distinction from, and overlap with, other disorders in this subgroup. Allergic histories are uncommon, as are eosinophilia and eosinophilic tissue involvement. Also, granulomata are not characteristically found, and lung and spleen are not characteristically involved. These are important distinguishing features and have been sources of confusion, since Rose and Spencer (24) divided polyarteritis nodosa according to the presence or absence of lung involvement and granulomata. However, as discussed later, the disease that these authors were labeling polyarteritis nodosa with lung involvement and granulomata was, in essence, indistinguishable from the allergic granulomatosis of Churg and Strauss (26).

A characteristic feature of this polyarteritis nodosa group of necrotizing vasculitis is the finding of aneurysmal dilatations up to 1 cm in size in medium-sized arteries seen by angiogram in the renal, hepatic, and visceral vasculature (Figure 4). It is believed that this finding is virtually pathognomonic of classic polyarteritis nodosa (27-29). However, multiple aneurysms of this type are seen in overlap syndromes (discussed later) in which vessels of various sizes are involved (30, 31) as well as in other disorders such as systemic lupus erythematosus (32) and fibromuscular dysplasia (33).

Table 2. Typical Clinicopathologic Features of Classic Polyarteritis Nodosa

Necrotizing vasculitis of small- and medium-sized muscular arteries
Eosinophilia and granulomata not characteristic
Allergic history uncommon
Renal involvement
Related to vasculitis (70%)
Glomerulitis (30%)
Hypertension
Gastrointestinal—infarction of viscera
Hepatic—subclinical disease to chronic active hepatitis in patients with hepatitis B antigenemia; liver disease related to vasculitis (up to 50%)
Coronary arteritis—particularly in children
Neurological—mononeuritis multiplex
Lung and spleen characteristically not involved
Cutaneous—uncommon, usually subcutaneous nodules, livido reticularis
Genitourinary—testes, bladder, epididymis, ovary
Arthralgias common; arthritis rare

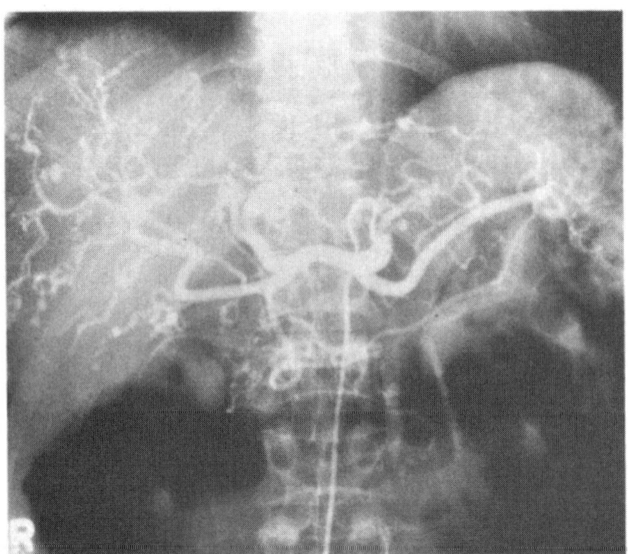

Figure 4. Celiac axis arteriogram in a patient with necrotizing vasculitis of the polyarteritis nodosa group. Arteriogram shows multiple 3-mm to 7-mm aneurysms along the hepatic artery. This patient responded to cyclophosphamide therapy with a complete remission, and, 1 year later, repeat arteriogram showed complete resolution of aneurysms (138).

As previously mentioned, allergic granulomatosis strongly resembles classic polyarteritis nodosa with some obvious distinguishing features and is almost invariably associated with an allergic diathesis, particularly severe asthma (26). Unlike classic polyarteritis nodosa, lung involvement is a sine qua non of this syndrome. Also, it is characterized by high levels of peripheral eosinophilia (usually higher than 1500 per mm^3), eosinophilic tissue infiltration, and granulomatous reactivity. Histopathologically, this disorder manifests, in addition to the fibrinoid necrosis of small- and medium-sized muscular arteries that is the hallmark of classic polyarteritis nodosa, a substantial degree of involvement of small vessels such as capillaries and venules. Apart from these differences, the presentation, clinicopathologic manifestations, organ system involvement, and clinical course of these two syndromes are similar.

The third disorder in this group of systemic necrotizing vasculitides is the overlap syndrome. It manifests in the same patient features that would be considered characteristic, or even pathognomonic, of either classic polyarteritis nodosa or allergic granulomatosis. It is a multisystem disease with the associated protean clinical manifestations. Small-vessel (arterioles, capillaries, and venules), together with the classic small- and medium-sized muscular artery involvement with characteristic angiographically demonstrable small aneurysms, can be seen in the same patient. Allergic history, peripheral eosinophilia, eosinophilic tissue infiltration, granulomatous reactions, and lung involvement may all be seen in the same patient, or one or more of these may be seen to the exclusion of the others.

It is this syndrome that has caused the most difficulty in classification and has appeared under various designations in the literature. The typical perplexing case is that of a young person who presents with a multisystem necrotizing vasculitis with hypertension, renal involvement, and mononeuritis multiplex. Visceral and renal angiography may or may not show multiple aneurysms of medium-sized arteries. By most accepted criteria, this would be called classic polyarteritis nodosa (1, 22-24). Yet, this same patient may have lung involvement, a predominance of small-vessel involvement, and an allergic history with or without eosinophilia and granuloma, all of which should not be seen in classic polyarteritis nodosa.

The difficulties and dilemmas with classification and the obvious overlap of the above disorders have been firmly established by the careful clinicopathologic observations in a group of patients with hepatitis B-associated necrotizing vasculitis (7) and the vasculitis reported after bouts of acute serous otitis media (34). Although it is often maintained that the ultimate precise classification of the vasculitides will depend on identification of the various offending antigens, it is obvious that identification of the antigen in hepatitis B-associated vasculitis has confirmed that the type of vasculitic response, even to the same sensitizing antigen, can completely overlap established categories. Even though the majority of patients with hepatitis B antigen-associated vasculitis in that series manifested the classic form of polyarteritis nodosa, several developed syndromes indistinguishable from small-vessel hypersensitivity vasculitis (discussed below), whereas others manifested vasculitic syndromes that defied any strict classification (7). The same held true for those patients who developed necrotizing vasculitis after acute serous otitis media (34). Furthermore, a substantial portion of patients with otherwise typical essential mixed cryoglobulinemic vasculitis (discussed below) were shown to have hepatitis B antigen in serum-derived cryoprecipitates (35), illustrating even a broader range of overlap among vasculitic syndromes.

It is possible that the involvement of small or large vessels, or both, as well as the presence or absence of granulomatous responses, or lung involvement, or any organ involvement in a situation where the same sentitizing antigen is involved, may be a reflection of the degree and chronicity of antigen exposure, the variability genetically, or otherwise, among patients in immunoregulatory mechanisms, as well as various other, as yet unidentified factors.

An appreciation of this overlap is an important reason to consider all three disorders in this polyarteritis nodosa group as mutually overlapping and, hence, refer to them collectively as systemic necrotizing vasculitis of the polyarteritis nodosa group. It is hoped this will obviate unnecessary confusion in the diagnostic and therapeutic approach to these disorders. Regarding the latter, recent advances in therapy of this group of disorders will be considered in more detail later.

Hypersensitivity Vasculitis

Hypersensitivity vasculitis refers to a large and heterogenous group of clinical syndromes that have in common the predominant involvement of small vessels in contradistinction to the involvement of medium-sized muscular arteries in classic polyarteritis nodosa and larger arteries in other vasculitic syndromes (2, 3, 10, 36, 37). Also, the term originally stemmed from the observation that in many patients the inflammatory and immunologic reactivity, that now has been shown to be mediated in most cases by immune complex deposition, could be directly traced to a precipitating antigen, most often a drug or chemical such as sulfa, or a microorganism such as beta-hemolytic *Streptococcus* (2, 3, 10, 37). Recently, it has been appreciated that endogenous antigens, such as tumor antigens or serum proteins, can serve as the sensitizing antigen and elicit syndromes identical to the more classic hypersensitivity vasculitides (3).

However, it must be emphasized that virtually all of the vasculitides are now recognized as resulting from hypersensitivity reactions to various antigens. In fact, a variable but significant proportion of the systemic necrotizing vasculitides have been directly associated with antigen exposure and subsequent abnormal immunologic reactivity, as with the hepatitis B antigen-associated immune complex vasculitis (7). Hence, this group could also be termed hypersensitivity vasculitis, again illustrating the obvious overlap among these vasculitic syndromes. However, the terminology, hypersensitivity vasculitis, continues to be specifically applied to those vasculitides with predominantly small-vessel involvement, usually in the skin and associated with a recognizable precipitating event or exposure. This syndrome has been variously referred to as allergic vasculitis, leukocytoclastic vasculitis (based on the usual histopathologic appearance of the vascular lesions), microscopic polyarteritis nodosa, and several other terms (2, 3, 10, 23, 24, 39). The salient clinicopathologic features characteristic of this syndrome are outlined in Table 3.

A few points deserve emphasis. The skin is the most common organ involved with the characteristic leukocytoclastic vasculitis involving postcapillary venules. This is the classic palpable purpura that is probably due to a combination of endothelial swelling, infiltration by leukocytes, and extravasation of erythrocytes (Figure 5). The lesions may, however, manifest a wide range of appearances, ranging in size from pinpoint to several centimeters, assuming the form of papules, nodules, vesicles, bullae, or ulcers. Furthermore, it has been reported that episodes of recurrent or chronic urticaria, with or without the characteristic purpura, may be a manifestation of an underlying hypersensitivity cutaneous vasculitis (21). The association of immune complex deposition with this type of small-vessel cutaneous vasculitis is well established (40).

Table 3. Clinicopathologic Features of Hypersensitivity Vasculitis

Leukocytoclastic vasculitis—usually involving postcapillary venules; infiltration of polymorphonuclear leukocytes with leukocytoclasis (presence of nuclear debris), fibrinoid necrosis, and extravasation of erythrocytes
Skin—predominant organ involved (palpable purpura); can involve any organ
Usually traced to a precipitating antigen such as a drug, microorganism, heterologous protein, autologous antigen
Usually occurs 1 week to 10 days after antigen exposure
Strong evidence for immune-complex deposition
Lesions usually at the same stage, suggesting episodic, rather than continuous, exposure to immune complexes
Usually self-limiting, but can recur or become chronic
Usually, treatment of various types is unsatisfactory and of little proven efficacy; withdrawal of agent, treat infection, corticosteroid therapy

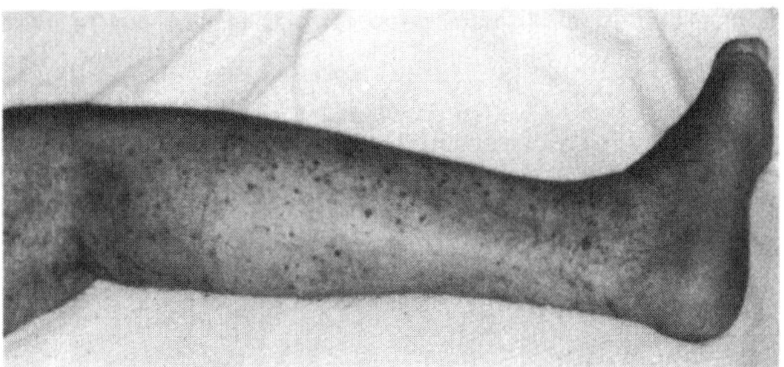

Figure 5. Hypersensitivity vasculitis with primary skin manifestations. This 41-year-old man presented with palpable purpura of the lower extremities. Skin biopsy showed typical leukocytoclastic vasculitis involving the venules.

In addition to the skin involvement, that may be the only manifestation of the disease and can cause significant symptoms and morbidity in and of itself, any organ can be involved with its associated specific clinical and pathologic manifestations. Also, particular constellations of organ system involvement have led to the designations of separate identifiable syndromes within the broader classification of hypersensitivity vasculitis (discussed later). Treatment of this group has been particularly frustrating, because there is little evidence that any of the known modalities, including corticosteroids, significantly alter the course of the disease (10). Fortunately, in many cases the disease is self-limited and confined to the skin. However, when it persists or involves multiple organs, various treatment regimens have not been satisfactory. Moreover, an organized evaluation of treatment protocols has been difficult, because of this group's great heterogeneity.

Another group of syndromes are, in essence, identical to the hypersensitivity vasculitis group, but are usually considered separately because of a characteristic and distinctive constellation of clinicopathologic features or the clinical setting in which they occur. The salient features of several of these syndromes are outlined in Table 4. However, certain points should be emphasized.

For instance, serum sickness in its classic form results from injection of foreign or heterologous serum into a person and is the human counterpart of the classic immune complex-mediated experimental serum sickness that has been elegantly delineated in animal models (11). Recently, it has become rare because of infrequent use of heterologous antisera. However, serum-sicknesslike reactions that are essentially indistinguishable from classic serum sickness can often occur after administration of nonprotein drugs. Often the offender is penicillin (41), although other drugs have been clearly implicated (42).

Usually, typical and obvious immune complex vasculitis does not dominate the clinicopathologic picture of serum sickness and serum-sicknesslike reactions, and fever,

Table 4. Distinct Syndromes Within the Broader Group of Hypersensitivity Vasculitis

Serum sickness and serum-sicknesslike reactions
  Fever, urticiaria, arthralgias, lymphadenopathy 7 to 10 days after primary exposure or 2 to 4 days after secondary exposure (accelerated); heterologous antisera or nonprotein drug (penicillin, sulfa)
Henoch-Schönlein purpura
  Nonthrombocytopenic purpura, joint, gastrointestinal, renal; postinfection or food allergy; tendency to recur several times and resolve; IgA antibody in immune complexes
Essential mixed cryoglobulinemia
  Purpura, arthralgias, anemia, hypergammaglobulinemia, glomerulonephritis; usually IgM rheumatoid factor against IgG; solid evidence for immune complex deposition
Vasculitis associated with connective tissue disease
  Usually rheumatoid arthritis and systemic lupus erythematosus; in rheumatoid arthritis associated with severe erosive and nodular disease; not caused by corticosteroids; combinations of small venule and small- and medium-sized arteries
Vasculitis associated with malignancies
  Chronic lymphocytic leukemia, lymphoma, Hodgkin's disease, multiple myeloma; typical leukocytoclastic vasculitis, seldom a peculiar granulomatous vasculitis of central nervous sytem

urticaria, arthralgias, and lymphadenopathy are the classic findings. However, in a small percentage of cases usually associated with a large amount of antigen exposure, fulminant disseminated vasculitis can occur (43-45).

Mostly, the disease is self-limited, requiring only discontinuation of the offending antigen. In patients with more severe symptoms, antihistamines and brief courses of corticosteroids (prednisone, 40 mg to 60 mg/day for a few days) may be helpful.

Henoch-Schönlein purpura, also called anaphylactoid purpura, is a typical leukocytoclastic vasculitis with a characteristic clinicopathologic picture. There are several points of interest in this syndrome (46-50). For instance, it has a remarkable tendency to resolve and recur several times during a period of weeks or months, usually ending in spontaneous resolution. Also, it is interesting that IgA is the most often seen antibody class in the immune complexes (51-53). Probably, for example, at least one of the mechanisms of disease activity is deposition of IgA immune complexes in blood vessel walls with activation of the alternative complement pathway and subsequent generation of chemotactic factors with influx of neutrophils. The fact that this disease can occur in the absence of the early components of the classic complement pathway has been illustrated by reports of Henoch-Schönlein purpura occurring in patients with congenital absence of C2 (54, 55). Generally, the prognosis of this disorder is good, and treatment usually consists of supportive and symptomatic therapy until resolution. However, some authors have recommended brief courses of corticosteroid therapy in certain patients, usually for abdominal and joint involvement (56).

Cryoglobulinemia may be found in a number of disorders, with or without vasculitis, and is present to a variable degree in many of the vasculitides under discussion. Indeed, there are several categories of cryoglobulinopathies, and vasculitis can be found to a variable degree in a number of them (57, 58). However, a distinct clinical syndrome, essential mixed cryoglobulinemia, has been described in which, for the most part, there is no identifiable underlying disease (59, 60). The histopathology of the purpuric skin lesions shows typical leukocytoclastic small-vessel vasculitis with the immune complexes principally made up of IgM rheumatoid factor directed against IgG molecule, hence the term, mixed cryoglobulinemia. In effect, it is a hypersensitivity reaction against an endogenous protein. As previously mentioned, the recently described finding of hepatitis B antigen in serum-derived cryoprecipitates from patients with essential mixed cryoglobulinemia (35) points out the overlap between the polyarteritis nodosa group of systemic necrotizing vasculitides and other categories of vasculitis. In patients who develop severe glomerulonephritis the prognosis is poor, and the disease has been reported to progress despite corticosteroids and cytotoxic agents (60, 61).

Necrotizing vasculitis may be associated, to various degrees, with the entire spectrum of connective tissue disorders (3, 4, 23, 38). However, systemic lupus erythematosus and rheumatoid arthritis are the two connective tissue diseases in which vasculitis is most commonly seen (4).

Vasculitis associated with rheumatoid arthritis most commonly appears as a typical leukocytoclastic vasculitis of small venules, predominantly involving the skin (62), as is characteristic of classic hypersensitivity vasculitides. Additionally, synovium and early rheumatoid nodules can manifest vasculitis (6). Less often, patients with rheumatoid arthritis, usually those with severe erosive and nodular disease and seropositivity for rheumatoid factor (63), may develop a fulminant disseminated vasculitis involving arterioles, medium-sized muscular arteries, and

Table 5. Characteristic Features of Organ System Involvement in Wegener's Granulomatosis*

Organ System	Approximate Frequency	Typical Features
	%	
Nasopharynx	75	Necrotizing granuloma with mucosal ulceration; saddle nose deformity
Paranasal sinuses	90	Pansinusitis; necrotizing granuloma; secondary bacterial infection
Eyes	60	Keratoconjunctivitis; granulomatous sclerouveitis
Ears	35	Serous otitis media; secondary bacterial infection
Lungs	95	Multiple nodular cavitary infiltrates; necrotizing granulomatous vasculitis
Kidneys	85	Focal and segmental glomerulitis; necrotizing glomerulonephritis later in course
Heart	15	Coronary vasculitis; pericarditis
Nervous system	20	Mononeuritis multiplex; cranial neuritis
Skin	40	Dermal vasculitis with secondary ulcerations
Joints	50	Polyarthralgias

* Adapted from Reference 22.

larger veins (64) similar to the polyarteritis nodosa group of systemic necrotizing vasculitis. Although it was previously believed that administration of corticosteroids either precipitated the development of, or worsened, the systemic vasculitis of rheumatoid arthritis (65, 66), it is now generally thought that this is not the case and that systemic vasculitis in this disease merely reflects very severe rheumatoid arthritis, a condition that probably would evoke corticosteroid therapy (4). The mechanism of vasculitis is probably immune complex deposition, as circulating immune complexes have been clearly shown in the serum of patients with this disease (67), and immune deposits have been seen in walls of involved vessels (68).

As many as 20% of patients with systemic lupus erythematosus develop dermal vasculitis during the course of their disease (69). This is predominantly a small-vessel vasculitis. However, diffuse central nervous system vasculitis and systemic vasculitis, similar to the polyarteritis nodosa group, may also occur, although less commonly (69-71). The mechanism of vasculitis is similar to that described above, as the evidence of immune complex-mediated tissue injury is ample in this disease (38, 68). Treatment of vasculitis in the connective tissue disorders should be directed at the underlying disease. Mostly, this would be with corticosteroids or cytotoxic agents, or both.

Although uncommon, it is nonetheless clear that vasculitis may be seen in association with certain malignancies, usually lymphoid or reticuloendothelial neoplasms such as chronic lymphocytic leukemia, lymphosarcoma, Hodgkin's disease, and multiple myeloma (25, 72, 73). Usually, it is a dermal vasculitis resulting in a clinicopathologic picture similar to the cutaneous necrotizing vasculitis typical of the hypersensitivity vasculitides. Visceral vasculitis occurs even less often. Additionally, there is an interesting syndrome of granulomatous vasculitis of the central nervous system that is associated with lymphoproliferative disorders in which the vasculitis is found in areas not invaded by tumor (74). Although the cause of this type of vasculitis is uncertain, probably it is associated with a hypersensitivity reaction to tumor or tumor-related antigen. Treatment of this condition should be directed at the underlying neoplasm.

In addition to the syndromes of hypersensitivity vasculitis listed in Table 4, there are a number of diseases in which hypersensitivitylike vasculitis can occur but is not a typical feature of the disease, including ulcerative colitis, retroperitoneal fibrosis, primary biliary cirrhosis, and Goodpasture's syndrome (38).

Wegener's Granulomatosis

Wegener's granulomatosis is a disease that has a distinctive clinicopathologic complex of necrotizing granulomatous vasculitis of the upper and lower respiratory tracts, glomerulonephritis, and variable degrees of disseminated small-vessel vasculitis (75-77). Unlike some of the other vasculitides under discussion, its characteristic features cause it to be more easily recognized as a distinct entity. The immunopathogenic, histopathologic, and clin-

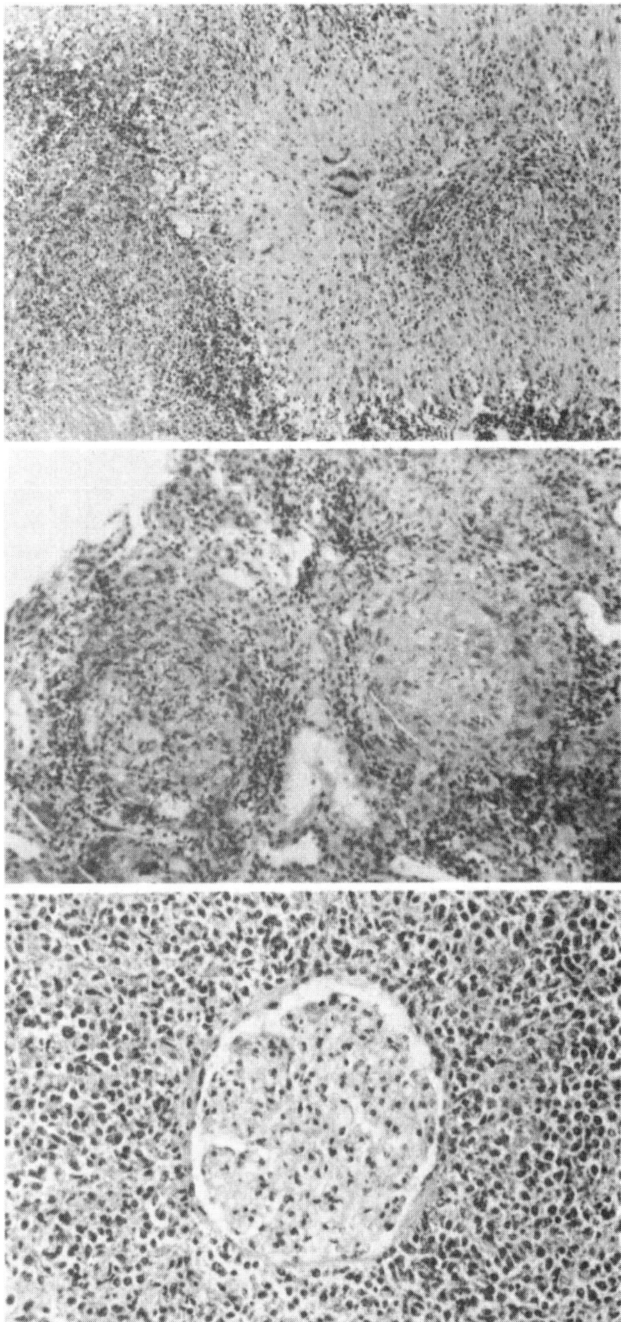

Figure 6 Top. Lung biopsy in a patient with Wegener's granulomatosis. Biopsy of a left upper lobe nodule showed dense infiltration with necrotizing granuloma containing many multinucleated giant cells. Blood vessels in other sections showed typical necrotizing vasculitis. The patient also had severe necrotizing glomerulonephritis as well as granulomatous sinus disease. (Hematoxylin and eosin; original magnification, × 140.) **Middle.** Kidney biopsy in a patient with Wegener's granulomatosis. Biopsy shows severe involvement of glomeruli with a necrotizing glomerulitis. There is extensive involvement of both glomeruli together with copious crescent formation around Bowman's capsule. (Hematoxylin and eosin; original magnification, × 140.) **Bottom.** Renal biopsy in a patient with lymphomatoid granulomatosis. Biopsy shows extensive infiltration of kidney with atypical lymphocytoid and plasmacytoid cells. In contradistinction to Wegener's granulomatosis involving glomeruli with a necrotizing glomerulitis, this biopsy shows the typical pattern of the renal involvement in lymphomatoid granulomatosis in which glomeruli are relatively spared and there is a nodular or even diffuse infiltration of renal parenchyma with atypical cells.

ical features of this disorder have been the subject of recent reviews (22, 77, 78). The characteristic features of the organ system involvement in Wegener's granulomatosis are outlined in Table 5.

The characteristic involvement of upper and lower respiratory tracts with granulomatosis vasculitis (Figure 6, *top*), together with necrotizing glomerulonephritis (Figure 6, *middle*), is quite distinctive. The fact that Wegener's granulomatosis is a distinct entity, clearly separable from allergic granulomatosis and midline granuloma, has been delineated and discussed in detail elsewhere (22, 77-80). The differences between Wegener's granulomatosis and lymphomatoid granulomatosis will be discussed later.

The etiology of this disease is unclear, although a hypersensitivity reaction to an as yet unidentified antigen is highly suspect. Circulating immune complexes have been seen in patients with active disease (81) (Fauci AS, Lawley T, Frank MM: unpublished observations, 1978), and immune reactants and complexlike deposits have been seen in some, but not all, renal biopsies of a group of patients with Wegener's granulomatosis with active glomerulonephritis (77, 82). The exact role of immune complexes in the pathogenesis of Wegener's granulomatosis is not clear, and it is uncertain whether they play a primary role in tissue damage or are only associated or secondarily involved. The demonstration of circulating immune complexes in a vasculitic syndrome with copious granulomatous reactivity promotes an interesting example of overlap of potentially dissociated immunopathogenic mechanisms. For instance, it is possible that the type or properties of immune complexes in Wegener's granulomatosis are partly responsible for triggering the granulomatosis reactivity seen in this disease. In contrast, a delayed hypersensitivitylike response to the hypothetical antigen itself may elicit the granulomatous responses characteristic of the upper and lower airways, with immune complex formation being a secondary phenomenon that may or may not contribute to the pathogensis of disease in organs such as the kidney.

During the past several years, one important aspect in the study of this disease has been the clear-cut demonstration of its exquisite sensitivity to cyclophosphamide therapy. Dramatic responses to this therapy have altered the prognosis from one of almost uniform fatality to that of virtual curability (77, 78, 83, 84). Precise details of the therapeutic approach to Wegener's granulomatosis will be discussed later. This approach in Wegener's granulomatosis has served as a model for using cytotoxic agents, particularly cyclophosphamide, in necrotizing vascilitides of several types. Actual results from using these agents in various vasculitides will be outlined later and are the subject of previous (30) and forthcoming reports.

Lymphomatoid Granulomatosis

Lymphomatoid granulomatosis is an interesting and unusual form of vasculitis, with a granulomatous reaction characterized by an angiotrophic and angiodestructive infiltration of various tissues, particularly lung, with atypical lymphocytoid and plasmacytoid cells (85). The cellular infiltrates are polymorphic and made up of normal-appearing lymphoid cells and atypical lymphocytoid, plasmacytoid, and reticuloendothelial-like cells with varying numbers of mitotic figures, giving it characteristics of a lymphoproliferative disease.

Because this disorder is generally considered as a granulomatous vasculitis, it is often confused with Wegener's granulomatosis. However, granulomata are less copious and less distinct than in Wegener's granulomatosis, and the vasculitis is remarkable in that it is not the characteristic leukocytoclastic or fibrinoid necrotic type of vasculitis seen in Wegener's granulomatosis and other systemic necrotizing vasculitides. In contrast, there is an angiotrophic invasion of blood vessels of various sizes with this bizarre cellular infiltrate. Blood supply through the involved vessels is compromised, and infarction and necrosis occur as with other vasculitides.

Lung involvement is a sine qua non and is usually manifest as multiple nodular infiltrates of various sizes that tend to cavitate. Skin (45%), kidney (45%), and central nervous system (20%) are also often involved (85). Although any organ system can be involved, it is remarkable that the spleen, lymph nodes, and bone marrow are usually spared. This is of interest, given the lymphoproliferative characteristics of the disease and the fact that clear-cut lymphomas evolve in at least 13% of patients (85).

In addition to the characteristic histopathologic features of lymphomatoid granulomatosis, it can be distinguished from Wegener's granulomatosis in several other ways. In contradistinction to Wegener's granulomatosis, sinus and upper-airway involvement are unusual. Furthermore, the renal involvement in lymphomatoid granulomatosis is almost never a necrotizing glomerulonephritis, a hallmark of generalized Wegener's granulomatosis, but is a nodular infiltration of renal parenchyma with the characteristic cellular infiltrate (Figure 6, *bottom*). Additionally, leukopenia, rare in untreated Wegener's granulomatosis, may be seen in some patients with lymphomatoid granulomatosis (84). Also, contrary to the condition of patients with Wegener's granulomatosis (77, 86, 87), the erythrocyte sedimentation rate may be normal in some patients during disease activity, and most patients are anergic before therapy (84).

There is a more benign condition, benign lymphocytic angiitis and granulomatosis (84), that probably is an earlier form of lymphomatoid granulomatosis, because patients' diseases have evolved from this more benign form into fulminant lymphomatoid granulomatosis (80, 84). Hence, it probably should be looked upon as the same disease in different stages of evolution.

Untreated, lymphomatoid granulomatosis is usually rapidly progressive, leading to death. The cause of death is often related to pulmonary complications as well as being commonly related to central nervous system disease (85).

Various treatment regimens, including corticosteroids alone or in combination with various cytotoxic agents, have proved ineffective (84, 85). However, many of these were started late in the course of the disease, and prelimi-

Table 6. Characteristics of the Giant-Cell Arteritides

	Temporal Arteritis	Takayasu's Arteritis
Patients	Disease of the elderly; women more than men	More prevalent in young women; more common in Orient, but neither racially nor geographically restricted
Blood vessels	Characteristically involves branches of carotid artery (temporal artery) but is a systemic arteritis and may involve any medium-sized or large artery	Large- and medium-sized arteries with predeliction for aortic arch and its branches; may involve pulmonary artery
Histopathology	Panarteritis; inflammatory mononuclear cell infiltrates; frequent giant cell formation within vessel wall; fragmentation of internal elastic lamina; proliferation of intima	Panarteritis; inflammatory mononuclear cell infiltrates; intimal proliferation and fibrosis; scarring and vascularization of media; disruption and degeneration of elastic lamina
Manifestations	Classic complex of fever, anemia, high erythrocyte sedimentation rate, muscle aches in an elderly person; headache may be present; strongly associated with polymyalgia rheumatica syndrome	Generalized systemic symptoms; local signs and symptoms related to involved vessels; occlusive phase
Complications	Ocular (sudden blindness)	Related to distribution of involved vessels; death usually occurs from congestive heart failure or cerebrovascular accidents
Diagnosis	Temporal artery biopsy; lesions may be segmental, multiple sections, arteriography, and bilateral biopsy may aid in diagnosis	Arteriography; biopsy of involved vessel
Treatment	Corticosteroids highly effective	Corticosteroids not of proven efficacy; cytotoxic agents untried

nary reports indicate that a relatively high rate of long-term remissions can be achieved if the disease is treated initially and, most importantly, early in the course with cyclophosphamide and corticosteroids in the same regimen as that used for Wegener's granulomatosis (80).

Giant-Cell Arteritides

Two disorders included in the broader category of the giant-cell arteritides are temporal arteritis and Takayasu's arteritis.

The salient features of temporal arteritis and Takayasu's arteritis are juxtaposed in Table 6 (88-105). Although these two disorders are similar, both are panarteritides characterized by inflammation of medium-sized and large arteries, and there are clear-cut differences between the two in age range, distribution of involved vessels, associated syndromes, and response to therapy. The following points are worth emphasizing. Although temporal or cranial arteritis characteristically involves one or more branches of the carotid artery, particularly the temporal artery (hence the name), patients with obvious temporal artery involvement may have concomitant systemic vasculitis of multiple medium-sized and large arteries that goes undetected (88). In fact, the disease may be widespread and virtually any medium-sized or large artery can be involved (92, 96).

Polymyalgia rheumatica syndrome is characterized by stiffness, aching, and pain in the muscles of the neck, shoulders, lower back, hips, and thighs (106). This syndrome has been so closely associated with temporal arteritis at one time or another during the disease in certain series that some authors have found it difficult to practically separate the two, so they consider them part of the same general syndrome (91, 96).

Temporal arteritis has become well recognized by its classic clinical picture of fever, anemia, high erythrocyte sedimentation rate, and associated symptoms in a person more than 55 years old. Often, the diagnosis can be made clinically and confirmed by biopsy of the temporal arteries. Because vessel involvement may be segmental and potentially missed on routine biopsy, some authors have recommended local arteriography (97) and examination of multiple sections from bilateral biopsies (100) to improve the yield of diagnostic biopsies.

A well-recognized and serious complication of temporal arteritis, particularly in untreated patients, is ocular involvement, leading to sudden blindness in some patients (89). Even though the dramatic manifestations of ocular involvement may appear suddenly, most patients have various complaints relating to the head or eyes for months before objective involvement. This emphasizes the need for careful attention to symptomatology and expeditious institution of appropriate therapy. It is of particular relevance, because temporal arteritis and its associated manifestations are generally exquisitely sensitive to corticosteroid therapy (93, 95, 98). Treatment should begin with 40 mg to 60 mg/day of prednisone followed by gradual tapering to a maintenance dose of 7.5 mg to 10 mg/day, with careful attention to readjustment of dosage if symptoms recur. Although there is some debate on this issue, the need for prolonged courses of corticosteroid therapy because of early relapses has been emphasized, and it is now believed that therapy should be continued for at least 1 to 2 years (93, 95, 98). In general, the prognosis is quite good with corticosteroid therapy, and most patients achieve complete remission that is often maintained after withdrawal of therapy.

Takayasu's arteritis is much less common than temporal arteritis (its similar and differing characteristics are listed in Table 6). Although both diseases are true panarteritides and are considered in the broader group of giant-cell arteritides, the finding of clear-cut giant cells in the involved vessels of Takayasu's arteritis is less common than in temporal arteritis.

Pulseless disease is another name given to Takayasu's arteritis because of the ultimate vessel occlusion, although it is a disease of complex manifestations ranging from generalized symptoms characteristic of inflammatory diseases, to local signs and symptoms associated with the involved vessels themselves, to the most characteristic manifestations related to compromise of blood flow to the extremities or other organs (101-105). This leads to a wide variety of changes related to the organ system involved. However, the most common and obvious findings are absent pulses in the involved vessels. Instead, bruits are commonly heard. The clinical course is variable, and, although it usually deteriorates gradually, it may spontaneously remit, stabilize temporarily, insidiously progress, or abruptly decompensate. This variability makes the evaluation of therapeutic regimens difficult. Death usually occurs from congestive heart failure or cerebrovascular accidents (103). Although corticosteroid therapy has been attempted (104, 105) in this disorder with differing results, no good evidence exists that it substantially improved life expectancy. It is quite clear, however, that compared with temporal arteritis, Takayasu's arteritis is quite resistant to corticosteroid therapy.

The etiologies of both these disorders are unclear, and even though immunologic mechanisms have been postulated for both temporal arteritis (107-112) and Takayasu's vasculitis (103, 104), precise pathogenic mechanisms have not been delineated.

Thromboangiitis Obliterans (Buerger's Disease)

Thromboangiitis obliterans is an uncommon inflammatory occlusive peripheral vascular disease involving arteries and veins. The disease is seen predominantly in male patients, usually between the ages of 20 and 40 years (113). There has been considerable disagreement over whether Buerger's disease is really separable from severe arteriosclerosis in young adults. However, now it is generally accepted that the disease is a distinct entity of an inflammatory nature, qualifying as a true vasculitis (113-115). It predominantly involves intermediate- and small-sized arteries, as well as veins in a segmental fashion. The inflammatory process is almost always associated with a thrombus, evolving through several stages. In the acute stage, the vessel wall and thrombus are infiltrated by polymorphonuclear leukocytes. Also, microabscesses may be found within the thrombi (114). This progresses through a subacute stage, in which mononuclear cells and giant cells may be seen and, ultimately, to the chronic stage, characterized by chronic inflammatory infiltrates, fibrosis, and recanalization of the vessel lumen. The entire process may be associated with migratory superficial thrombophlebitis.

Although the cause is unknown, it is well recognized and quite striking that tobacco makes the disease much worse. Almost without exception, the disease is seen in heavy smokers (113). There is no good evidence that immunologic phenomena play a role in the pathogenesis of the disease.

The clinical presentation is variable and may be insidious or abrupt. Coldness of the distal extremities, color changes, dysesthesias, intense hyperemia, excruciating pain, ulceration, gangrene, and pulp atrophy are commonly observed features (113-116). Usually, acute attacks last 1 to 4 weeks, and the disease runs an indolent and recurrent course. Ultimately, collateral circulation can no longer compensate for the progressive ischemia, and amputation of the involved distal extremities is common. Various treatment regimens such as anticoagulation, thromboendarterectomy, bypass operations, and sympathectomy have not been convincingly shown to be associated with an improved prognosis for the involved extremity (116, 117). The most effective approach to this disease seems to be meticulous local care of the involved area, together with complete abstinence from tobacco use.

Mucocutaneous Lymph Node Syndrome

Mucocutaneous lymph node syndrome is an extraordinary and interesting disease that only recently has been recognized as a distinct entity (118, 119). It is an acute febrile illness of infants and children, characterized by unresponsiveness to antibiotics, nonsuppurative cervical adenitis, and changes in the skin and mucous membranes such as edema, congested conjunctivae, erythema of the oral cavity, lips, and palms, and desquamation of the skin of the fingertips. The disease is usually self-limited, and most patients recover uneventfully. However, 1% to 2% of cases end in fatalities, usually sudden death from coronary arteritis similar to infantile polyarteritis nodosa (120). Often, this sudden complication occurs during the convalescent period of the underlying syndrome. Myocarditis, pericarditis, myocardial infarctions, and cardiomegaly are also seen. The syndrome seems to have reached almost epidemic proportions in Japan, where thousands of cases have been reported since 1970 (120). It was first thought to be limited to Japan but has now been reported in several other countries, with at least 100 cases documented in the United States (121).

Histopathologic studies have shown that in nearly all of the reported fatal cases, changes of arteritis were seen along the main trunk and branches of the coronary artery (120). There was intimal thickening and proliferation, infiltration of mononuclear cells, fragmentation of the elastic laminae, and aneurysm formation with thrombosis. Although other vessels may manifest vasculitis, the coronary artery is the most prominent vessel involved.

Some authors have suggested that fatal mucocutaneous lymph node syndrome with coronary artery involvement, and infantile polyarteritis nodosa with involvement of the coronary arteries, are clinically and pathologically indistinguishable, leading to the hypothesis that many of the previously recognized cases of infantile polyarteritis nodosa were really the mucocutaneous lymph node syndrome (120, 122).

A clinical approach to this disease is frustrating. The prognosis in 98% of the patients who do not go on to sudden death seems to be excellent. However, the condition of those who develop obvious coronary arteritis usually goes undetected until the catastrophic event. Additionally, it is uncertain what percent of patients develop subclinical arteritis that will manifest itself as cardiac disease later in life.

What causes the disease is unknown. Although there have been reports of rickettsialike organisms seen through electron microscopy in pathologic specimens, these data remain inconclusive. Given the clinicopathologic pattern of the disease, a reasonable hypothesis is that the underlying disease is caused by an unidentified infectious agent that, in a small percentage of patients, results in a hypersensitivity phenomenon manifested by vasculitis.

Miscellaneous Vasculitides

There are also a number of other syndromes in which vasculitis is either the primary manifestation or a minor component of a broader disease entity. Classic erythema nodosa is a common disease that is well recognized as being a hypersensitivity manifestation of a number of disorders (123). Generally, it is thought of as a painful nodular inflammatory process of the dermis and subcutaneous tissues. However, its histopathology is that of a true vasculitis, predominantly of small venules (124).

Other less common vasculitides that deserve mention are Behçet's syndrome (125), Cogan's syndrome (126), Eale's disease (127), hypocomplementemic vasculitis (128), and erythema elevatum diutinum (129).

Treatment of the Granulomatous Vasculitides

Dr. Barton F. Haynes (Clinical Associate, Clinical Physiology Section, Laboratory of Clinical Investigation, National Institute of Allergy and Infectious Diseases): Perhaps the most dramatic breakthrough in the therapeutic approach to the vasculitides has been clinical experience with cyclophosphamide in treating Wegener's granulomatosis. Although this disease is a granulomatous vasculitis with distinctive and easily recognizable clinicopathologic features, it is a true systemic necrotizing vasculitis. Because of the favorable experience with cyclophosphamide therapy in this disorder, we will discuss it here as the prototype in consideration of specific guidelines for the use of cytotoxic therapy in the necrotizing vasculitides.

Untreated, Wegener's granulomatosis usually pursues a rapidly fatal course represented by a mean survival of 5 months, with 82% of the patients dying within 1 year and more than 90% within 2 years (130). Although corticosteroids have been reported to improve the mean survival to 12.5 months (131), it is clear that the long-term prognosis of the disease is not significantly altered by this therapy, especially in the face of clinically apparent renal disease.

The first recorded use of cytotoxic chemotherapy in Wegener's granulomatosis was by Fahey and associates in 1954 (76). They used nitrogen mustard in a patient with this disorder and noted marked clinical improvement, although detailed follow-up was not provided. Since that time, reports of remissions in patients using various classes of cytotoxic agents have appeared (77, 78). However, it has become clear during the past few years that cyclophosphamide is the treatment of choice in Wegener's granulomatosis (77, 78, 83, 84). This agent, used for an extended period of time in doses of 1 mg to 2 mg/kg body weight per day, has resulted in dramatic long-term remissions in large numbers of patients followed closely for several years (77, 78, 83).

Previously reported was the favorable experience at NIH using cyclophosphamide in 21 patients with Wegener's granulomatosis (77, 78). Since that time this experience has been extended to 47 patients, with a greater than 90% remission rate. On the basis of this experience, it has been possible to delineate certain principles in the therapeutic approach to patients with this disease and, as will be discussed later, to patients with other forms of systemic necrotizing vasculitis.

Two groups of patients with Wegener's granulomatosis, in whom the treatment regimen may vary, can be clinically identified. The first includes those with active multisystem involvement, who manifest a relatively stable clinical course. Usually, they have an abnormal urine sediment, and renal involvement is seen on kidney biopsy. Renal function may be normal or slightly abnormal, but fulminant renal failure is not present. These patients should start on oral cyclophosphamide in a dose of 1 mg to 2 mg/kg body weight per day. The initial dose is maintained for 2 weeks. If evidence of a favorable clinical response is seen, the dose is kept at this level with readjustments to maintain the total leukocyte count above 3000 per mm^3 with a total neutrophil count of 1000 to 1500 mm^3. However, if there is no evidence of a favorable clinical response, the daily dose should be increased by 25 mg and kept at this level for an additional 2 weeks. This rate of increment should be continued until evidence of clinical response is seen or until drug toxicity, such as leukopenia, occurs.

The second category, those patients with fulminant vasculitis, is life threatening and can lead to irreversible organ damage. This includes patients with cerebral vasculitis, severe pulmonary involvement with hypoxemia, rapidly progressive peripheral neuropathy, or rapidly progressive renal failure. Renal failure is the most common and, once recognized, constitutes a medical emergency. Delay in the initiation of therapy for just a few days can lead to irreversible renal failure, whereas early treatment can prevent serious renal damage as well as reverse existing renal functional impairment. The protocol for cyclophosphamide administration in patients with fulminant Wegener's granulomatosis, in contrast to the standard approach just described, is as follows: cyclophosphamide, 4 mg/kg body weight per day either orally or intravenously, is administered daily for 3 days, followed by rapid dose reduction during the subsequent 3-day period until a dose of 1 mg to 2 mg/kg body weight per day is reached. This dose is maintained in the same manner as for nonfulminant disease until evidence of therapeutic response or leukopenia occurs, necessitating dose reduction. In patients with fulminant pulmonary or renal disease, high daily, divided-dose corticosteroid therapy (usually prednisone, 60 mg/day) should be started, together with cyclophosphamide, to initially decrease the acute inflammatory reactions until the effects of cyclophosphamide are seen, usually within 14 days. After 5 to 7 days of daily divided-dose corticosteroid therapy, the

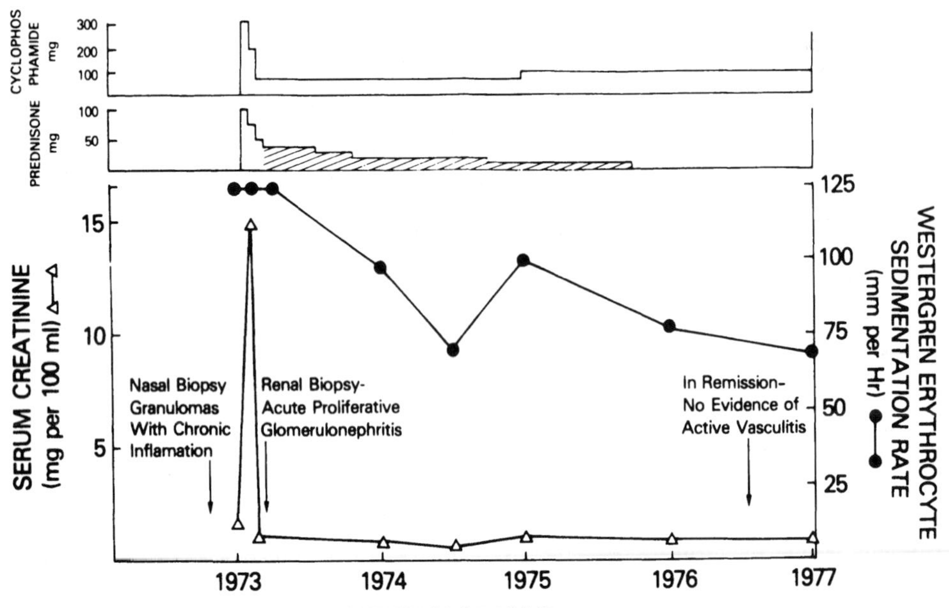

Figure 7. Therapeutic response to cyclophosphamide and corticosteroid therapy in a patient with Wegener's granulomatosis. This patient had severe acute necrotizing glomerulonephritis, together with typical sinus disease. He developed acute renal failure upon admission. Initially, he was treated with cyclophosphamide and prednisone. Shaded area represents alternate-day prednisone therapy. This therapeutic approach resulted in a dramatic reversal of his renal failure. A slight flare in nonrenal manifestations of his disease in 1975 was successfully treated with a small increase in his cyclophosphamide dosage. Prednisone was withdrawn in 1975, and he is currently maintained on cyclophosphamide alone. As with other patients with Wegener's granulomatosis, his cyclophosphamide is being tapered with the intention of ultimately withdrawing the drug.

dose should be rapidly tapered to a single daily dose and then to alternate-day therapy. After a few weeks, corticosteroids can be withdrawn, depending on the individual clinical response. An example of a typical response of fulminant Wegener's granulomatosis to such a therapeutic regimen is depicted in Figure 7.

Corticosteroid therapy is not necessary in every patient with Wegener's granulomatosis (77, 78), and complete remissions can occur rapidly in many patients receiving cyclophosphamide alone. However, there are several specific indications for corticosteroid therapy when treating the disease, in addition to fulminant renal and pulmonary disease. Patients who have severe skin vasculitis, eye involvement of any type (132), or evidence of severe serosal inflammation, such as pericarditis, often benefit from short courses of daily, followed by alternate-day, oral corticosteroids.

In patients who cannot tolerate cyclophosphamide because of severe leukopenia or hemorrhagic cystitis, or in young women who are not willing to accept the ovarian damage associated with cyclophosphamide, azathioprine can be used as an alternative cytotoxic agent. However, experience at NIH has shown that azathioprine is not as effective as cyclophosphamide. Several patients with Wegener's granulomatosis, in whom azathioprine failed to induce remissions, achieved complete remission upon subsequent treatment with cyclophosphamide (77, 78). Although cyclophosphamide is far more effective in inducing remissions in Wegener's granulomatosis, in certain patients azathioprine can adequately maintain these cyclophosphamide-induced remissions (77, 78).

As previously reported (77, 78), NIH continues cyclophosphamide therapy for 1 year after the disappearance of all traces of active disease. In this regard, the erythrocyte sedimentation rate is an excellent monitor of disease activity and, even with the lack of specific organ system disease, the therapy is continued, where feasible, until this variable returns to normal.

With this therapeutic regimen, Wegener's granulomatosis can now be considered a curable disease, if treated early and appropriately with the therapeutic regimen described (77, 78). Of 47 patients, only two can be considered treatment failures, because they died with active disease despite what was considered an adequate therapeutic trial consisting of at least 2 weeks of cyclophosphamide therapy. One of these patients refused consistently to take his medications, so he died with smouldering disease activity.

Two other patients achieved complete remission on cyclophosphamide therapy. They were followed elsewhere and, while in complete remission, developed severe leukopenia that initially went unnoticed and subsequently led to fatal infectious disease complications. This serves to emphasize the extremely important point mentioned above. Apart from rare exceptions, remissions in Wegener's granulomatosis can almost inevitably be achieved with cyclophosphamide without lowering the total leukocyte count below 3000 per mm^3 and the neutrophil count below 1000 to 1500 per mm^3. In general, the experience has been (133) that infectious disease complications related to neutropenia seldom occur when the neutrophil count is kept at, or above, this level. Hence, it is essential to carefully monitor the leukocyte count and adjust the cyclophosphamide dosage, even after complete remission has been achieved. Using this therapeutic approach, complete remissions can be induced and safely maintained in more than 90% of patients with Wegener's granulomatosis.

Because of the dramatic successes in Wegener's granulomatosis using this regimen, the same therapeutic protocol was instituted in lymphomatoid granulomatosis, a disease with certain similarities to Wegener's granulomatosis (80). This disease has characteristics of both a granulomatous vasculitis and a lymphoproliferative disease and carries an extremely poor prognosis (80, 85, 86). Previous reports have indicated that, in most patients, lymphomatoid granulomatosis follows a fulminant and fatal course despite various combined chemotherapeutic regimens including corticosteroids and cytotoxic agents (85, 86). However, at NIH it has been found that if the therapeutic regimen described above for Wegener's granulomatosis is instituted early in the course of lymphomatoid granulomatosis, a substantial portion of long-term remissions can be achieved (80). Indeed, during the past 7 years, eight patients with lymphomatoid granulomatosis have been followed. Initially, two were seen when their disease was fulminant, involving multiple systems including the central nervous system. Both courses were rapidly fatal, despite combined chemotherapeutic regimens including corticosteroids and multiple cytotoxic agents. In contrast, six patients in whom diagnosis was made early were all treated with the cyclophosphamide and corticosteroid regimen described above. All six are now in complete remission with an average follow-up of 3.5 years after onset of disease.

Thus, it is now clear that cyclophosphamide and prednisone therapy, followed by cyclophosphamide maintenance alone, is a highly effective therapeutic approach to the granulomatous vasculitides, particularly Wegener's granulomatosis (77, 78). In addition, lymphomatoid granulomatosis, if treated early, appears to be quite responsive to this therapeutic regimen (80).

Treatment of the Polyarteritis Nodosa Group of Systemic Necrotizing Vasculitis

Dr. Paul Katz (Clinical Associate, Clinical Physiology Section, Laboratory of Clinical Investigation, National Institute of Allergy and Infectious Diseases): Before corticosteroids were used in the systemic necrotizing vasculitides of the polyarteritis nodosa type, the disease almost always progressed with variable degrees of fulminance, usually leading to death (134). The use of corticosteroids improved the 5-year survival from 13% in untreated cases, to 48% in persons receiving corticosteroids (134). In those patients who presented with hypertension or renal disease, the prognosis was even worse. Recently, isolated reports have indicated that the use of cytotoxic agents can induce favorable clinical responses in this disorder (135-138). In fact, it was recently reported that dramatic, long-term remissions were induced with cyclophosphamide in two patients with far-advanced systemic necrotizing vasculitis of the polyarteritis nodosa group (139). Because of experience with Wegener's granulomatosis (77, 78), patients with this disease at NIH are treated with cyclophosphamide immediately upon diagnosis, rather than waiting until corticosteroids alone fail to induce remissions. The results have been favorable.

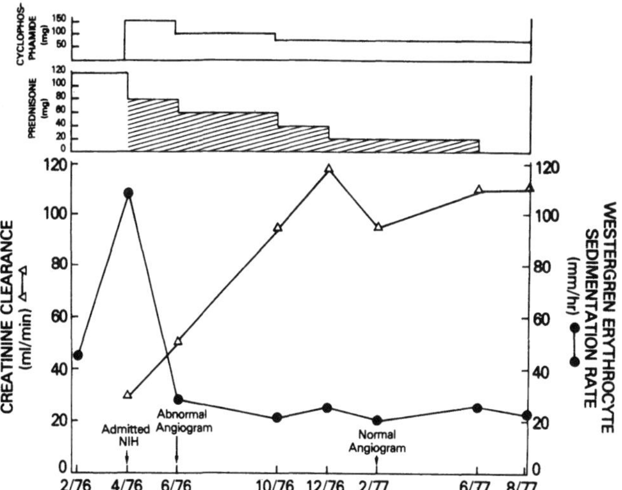

Figure 8. Therapeutic response to cyclophosphamide and corticosteroid therapy in a patient with necrotizing vasculitis of the polyarteritis nodosa group. This patient had multisystem involvement including kidney, lung, central nervous system with seizures, skin, and multiple viscera. He was admitted on prednisone therapy, and his clinical course rapidly deteriorated. Celiac axis arteriogram showed multiple aneurysms. Cyclophosphamide therapy was initiated, and the patient experienced a dramatic remission. Shaded area represents alternate-day prednisone therapy. Repeat arteriogram 1 year later was entirely normal, and the patient was in complete remission. Prednisone was gradually tapered and withdrawn, and the patient is being maintained in remission on tapering doses of cyclophosphamide.

Table 7. Therapeutic Approach to Patients with Systemic Necrotizing Vasculitis

Identification and removal of offending antigen
Treatment of underlying primary disease, such as connective tissue disease, neoplasms
Use of appropriate agents where efficacy has been proved, such as corticosteroids in temporal arteritis; cyclophosphamide in Wegener's granulomatosis
Corticosteroids alone in syndromes without indication of severe disseminated or systemic disease or in apparently self-limiting processes that might benefit from brief courses of therapy, such as resolving hypersensitivity reactions like severe drug reactions
Continual attempts at tapering corticosteroids
Low-dose cytotoxic agents (cyclophosphamide), with or without corticosteroids in severe disseminated necrotizing vasculitis or in corticosteroid failures
Clear-cut understanding of the place of several cytotoxic agents such as cyclophosphamide in systemic necrotizing vasculitis

Figure 8 illustrates the clinical course of a representative patient, admitted with biopsy-proven, well-documented systemic necrotizing vasculitis with multiple-system involvement including central nervous system, hepatic, and renal disease with severe hypertension and seizures. A celiac axis angiogram showed multiple aneurysms of the hepatic and splenic vasculature. At the time of admission, his disease was poorly controlled on high-dose daily prednisone. Within 2 weeks after cyclophosphamide was added, there was an obvious improvement in his clinical course. His disease activity continued to resolve and, within 1 year, he had achieved a complete remission by clinical, angiographic, and laboratory measures. His course has become typical of those patients with systemic necrotizing vasculitis, who are treated early in their disease with cyclophosphamide and prednisone and subsequently maintained on cyclophosphamide.

During the past several years, 11 patients with systemic necrotizing vasculitis have been treated at NIH. The majority displayed a prompt and uniform improvement in their clinical status with gradual amelioration of previously abnormal laboratory findings, functional disturbances, and vasculitic lesions. Patients with the poorest prognosis, those with hypertension and renal disease, showed similar dramatic results with control of their blood pressure and improvement in creatinine clearance and erythrocyte sedimentation rate. As already reported (139), two patients with previous angiographic involvement of multiple viscera had complete resolution of all aneurysms on repeat angiography 1 year after institution of cyclophosphamide therapy. Not surprisingly, mononeuritis multiplex was the symptom complex most recalcitrant to therapy because of previous irreversible nerve damage. In one patient not previously on corticosteroids, cyclophosphamide was instituted as the sole form of therapy and a prompt clinical response was observed.

There have been four deaths. Two of these occurred in patients who were started on cyclophosphamide late in their course, after failure of a previous therapeutic trial of corticosteroids alone. Their disease had already caused significant damage in multiple organ systems, and they died at a time when their disease was inactive or smouldering from causes related to the ravages of previous disease activity. One other patient with far-advanced rapidly progressing disease died within 1 month of the institution of cytotoxic therapy, but received less than 2 weeks of total therapy because of other complications. He probably did not receive an adequate therapeutic trial. The fourth patient with extensive disease died of an unknown cause after 2 months of therapy and had no evidence of active vasculitis on postmortem examination. Despite this lack of evidence of disease activity, she would obviously have to be considered a treatment failure.

The remaining seven patients are in complete remission and have received cytotoxic therapy for a mean of 41 months, ranging from 12 to 108 months. In all of these patients, the cyclophosphamide therapy is being gradually tapered to the point of being ultimately discontinued.

Thus, it is clear that cyclophosphamide, either alone or in combination with pre-existing corticosteroid therapy, can effect a dramatic response in patients with systemic necrotizing vasculitis of the polyarteritis nodosa group if instituted early in the course of the disease process.

Conclusion

Dr. Fauci: The vasculitic syndromes have been re-examined in light of an updated synthesis of clinical, pathologic, and immunologic observations. Clearly one must fully appreciate the distinctive characteristics that make categorization of various syndromes or disease entities into separate groups a feasible and useful undertaking. Also, it is essential to appreciate the significant degree of overlap of different diseases within a broad category. This is particularly true in the overlap within the polyarteritis nodosa group of the systemic necrotizing vasculitides in which classic polyarteritis nodosa overlaps with the systemic necrotizing vasculitides that do not neatly fall into the originally described classic disease (1). This approach is more than an academic interest, because it is becoming evident that several of these serious systemic vasculitides, previously virtually uniformly fatal, are now proving to be responsive to cytotoxic therapy, particularly chronic low-dose cyclophosphamide. Early and correct diagnosis with regard to the particular category of vasculitis, as well as the early institution of aggressive therapy where appropriate, has significantly and dramatically improved the prognosis of several of the serious systemic vasculitides. A general therapeutic approach to patients with systemic necrotizing vasculitis is outlined in Table 7. As greater insight is gained into the immunopathogenesis and pathophysiologic mechanisms of the broader category of vasculitides, the striking therapeutic successes in diseases such as temporal arteritis, Wegener's granulomatosis, and systemic necrotizing vasculitis of the polyarteritis nodosa group may also be seen in the other categories of serious systemic vasculitides with whatever therapeutic modalities prove most appropriate.

▶ Requests for reprints should be addressed to Anthony S. Fauci, M.D.; Head, Clinical Physiology Section, Laboratory of Clinical Investigation, National Institute of Allergy and Infectious Diseases, National Institutes of Health; Building 10, Room 11B09; Bethesda, MD 20014.

Received 24 July 1978; revision accepted 15 August 1978.

References

1. Kussmaul A, Maier K: Über eine bischer nicht beschreibene eigenthümliche Arterienerkrankung (Periarteritis nodosa), die mit Morbus Brightii und rapid fortschreitender allgemeiner Muskellähmung einhergeht. *Dtsch Arch Klin Med* 1:484-517, 1866
2. Zeek PM: Periarteritis nodosa: critical review. *Am J Clin Pathol* 22:777-790, 1952
3. Alarcón-Segovia D: The necrotizing vasculitides. A new pathogenic classification. *Med Clin North Am* 61:24-260, 1977
4. Christian CL, Sergent JS: Vasculitis syndromes: clinical and experimental models. *Am J Med* 61:385-392, 1976
5. Sokoloff L, Willens SL, Bunim JJ: Arteritis of striated muscle in rheumatoid arthritis. *Am J Pathol* 27:157-173, 1951
6. Glass D, Soter NA, Schur PH: Rheumatoid vasculitis. *Arthritis Rheum* 19:950-952, 1976
7. Sergent JS, Lockshin MD, Christian CL, Gocke DJ: Vasculitis with hepatitis B antigenemia: long-term observations in nine patients. *Medicine (Baltimore)* 55:1-18, 1976
8. Conn DL, McDuffie FC, Holley KE, Schroeter AL: Immunologic mechanisms in systemic vasculitis. *Mayo Clin Proc* 51:511-518, 1976
9. Cream JJ: Clinical and immunological aspects of cutaneous vasculitis. *Q J Med* 45:255-276, 1976
10. Sams WM, Thorne EG, Small P, Mass MF, McIntosh RM, Stanford RE: Leukocytoclastic vasculitis. *Arch Dermatol* 112:219-226, 1976
11. Cochrane CG, Dixon FJ: Antigen-antibody complex induced disease, in *Textbook of Immunopathology,* 2nd ed., vol. 1, edited by Meischer PA, Müller-Eberhard HJ. New York, Grune & Stratton, 1976, p. 137
12. Henson PM: Interaction of cells with immune complexes: adherence, release of constituents and tissue injury. *J Exp Med* 134:114-135, 1971
13. Cochrane CG, Koffler D: Immune complex disease in experimental animals and man, in *Advances in Immunology,* vol. 16, edited by Dixon F, Kunkel HG. New York, Academic Press, 1973, p. 185
14. Johnson GD, Edmons JP, Holborrow EJ: Precipitating antibody to DNA detected by two-stage electroimmuno-diffusion. Study in SLE and in rheumatoid arthritis. *Lancet* 2:883-885, 1973
15. Gershwin ME, Steinberg AD: Qualitative characteristics of anti-DNA antibodies in lupus nephritis. *Arthritis Rheum* 17:947-954, 1974
16. Dorsch C, Barnett EV: The occurrence and nature of precipitating antibodies in anti-DNA sera. *Clin Immunol Immunopathol* 2:310-321, 1974
17. Pennybaker J, Gilliam JN, Ziff M: Significance of anti-nDNA classes in serum and skin in prognosis of SLE. *Arthritis Rheum* 19:815, 1976
18. Cochrane CG, Weigle WO, Dixon FJ: The role of polymorphonuclear leukocytes in the initiation and cessation of the Arthus vasculitis. *J Exp Med* 100:481-494, 1959
19. Waksman BH: Delayed (cellular) hypersensitivity, in *Immunological Diseases,* vol. 1, edited by Samter M. Boston, Little, Brown and Co., 1971, p. 220
20. Epstein WL: Granulomatous hypersensitivity. *Prog Allergy* 11:36-88, 1967
21. Soter NA: Clinical presentations and mechanisms of necrotizing angi-

itis of the skin. *J Invest Dermatol* 67:354-359, 1976
22. Fauci AS, Wolff SM: Wegener's granulomatosis and related diseases, in *Disease-a-Month,* vol. 23, no. 7, edited by Dowling HF. Chicago, Year Book Medical Publishers, Inc., 1977, p. 1
23. Zeek PM: Periarteritis nodosa and other forms of necrotizing angiitis. *N Engl J Med* 18:764-772, 1953
24. Rose GA, Spencer H: Polyarteritis nodosa. *Q J Med* 26:43-81, 1957
25. McCombs RP: Systemic "allergic" vasculitis. *JAMA* 194:157-164, 1965
26. Churg J, Straus L: Allergic granulomatosis, allergic angiitis and periarteritis nodosa. *Am J Pathol* 27:277-301, 1951
27. Bron KM, Stroot CA, Shapiro AP: The diagnostic value of angiographic observations in polyarteritis nodosa. *Arch Intern Med* 116:450-453, 1965
28. Fleming RJ, Stern LZ: Multiple intraparenchymal renal aneurysms in polyarteritis nodosa. *Radiology* 84:100-103, 1965
29. Dornfeld L, Lecky LW, Peter JB: Polyarteritis and intrarenal renal artery aneurysms. *JAMA* 215:1950-1952, 1971
30. Fauci AS, Doppman JL, Wolff SM: Cyclophosphamide-induced remissions in advanced polyarteritis nodosa. *Am J Med,* 64:890-894, 1978
31. DeShazo RD, Levinson AI, Lawless OJ, Weisbaum G: Systemic vasculitis with coexistent large and small vessel involvement. A classification dilemma. *JAMA* 238:1940-1942, 1977
32. Longstreth PL, Lorobkin M, Palubinskas AJ: Renal microaneurysms in a patient with systemic lupus erythematosus. *Radiology* 113:65-66, 1974
33. Meyers DS, Grim CE, Kertzer WF: Fibromuscular dysplasia of the renal artery with medial dissection. A case simulating polyarteritis nodosa. *Am J Med* 56:412-416, 1974
34. Sergent JS, Christian CL: Necrotizing vasculitis after acute serous otitis media. *Ann Intern Med* 56:412-416, 1974
35. Levo Y, Gorevic PD, Kassab HJ, Zucker-Franklin D, Franklin EC: Association between hepatitis B virus and essential mixed cryoglobulinemia. *N Engl J Med* 296:1501-1504, 1977
36. Soter NA, Mihm MC Jr, Gigli I, Dvorak HF, Austen KF: Two distinct cellular patterns in cutaneous necrotizing angiitis. *J Invest Dermatol* 66:344-350, 1976
37. Winkelmann RK, Ditto WB: Cutaneous and visceral syndromes of necrotizing or "allergic" angiitis: a study of 38 cases. *Medicine (Baltimore)* 43:59-89, 1964
38. Gilliam JN, Smiley JD: Cutaneous necrotizing vasculitis and related disorders. *Ann Allergy* 37:328-339, 1976
39. Rich AR: Role of hypersensitivity in periarteritis nodosa as indicated by 7 cases developing during serum sickness and sulfonamide therapy. *Bull Johns Hopkins Hosp* 71:123-140, 1942
40. Braverman IM, Yen A: Demonstration of immune complexes in spontaneous and histamine-induced lesions and in normal skin of patients with leukocytoclastic angiitis. *J Invest Dermatol* 64:105-112, 1975
41. Levine BB: Immunologic mechanisms of penicillin allergy. A haptenic model for the study of allergic diseases in man. *N Engl J Med* 275:1115-1125, 1966
42. Parker CW: Drug allergy. *N Engl J Med* 292:511-514, 732-736, 957-960, 1975
43. MacKenzie GM, Hanger FM: Serum disease and serum accidents. *JAMA* 94:260-265, 1930
44. Clark E, Kaplan BI: Endocardial, arterial, and other mesenchymal alterations associated with serum sickness in man. *Arch Pathol* 24:458-475, 1937
45. De La Pava S, Nigogosyan G, Pickren JW: Fatal glomerulonephritis after receiving horse anti-human-cancer serum. *Arch Intern Med* 109:391-399, 1962
46. Ackroyd JF: Allergic purpura, including purpura due to foods, drugs and infections. *Am J Med* 14:605-632, 1953
47. Lindenauer SM, Tank ES: Surgical aspects of Henoch-Schönlein purpura. *Surgery* 59:982-987, 1966
48. Cream JJ, Cumpel JM, Peachy RDG: Schönlein-Henoch purpura in the adult. *Q J Med* 39:461-484, 1970
49. Ballard HS, Eisinger RP, Gallo G: Renal manifestations of the Henoch-Schönlein syndrome in adults. *Am J Med* 49:328-335, 1970
50. Ansell BM: Henoch-Schönlein purpura with particular reference to the prognosis of the renal lesion. *Br J Dermatol* 82:211-215, 1970
51. Lowance DC, Mullins JD, McPhaul JJ: Immunoglobulin A (IgA) associated glomerulonephritis. *Kidney Int* 3:167-176, 1973
52. Harrington JT: Acute oliguric renal failure with IgA glomerular deposits (Henoch-Schönlein purpura) CPC. *N Engl J Med* 290:1365-1369, 1974
53. De La Faille-Kuyper EH, Kater L, Kooiker CJ, Dorhout Mees EJ: IgA deposits in cutaneous blood-vessel walls and mesangium in Henoch-Schönlein syndrome. *Lancet* 1:892-893, 1973
54. Sussman M, Jones JH, Almedia JD, Lachmann P: Deficiency of the second component of complement associated with anaphylactoid purpura and presence of mycoplasma in the serum. *Clin Exp Immunol* 14:531, 1973
55. Gelfand EW, Clarkson JE, Minta JO: Selective deficiency of the second component of complement in a patient with anaphylactoid purpura. *Clin Immunol Immunopathol* 4:269-276, 1975
56. Borges WH: Anaphylactoid purpura. *Med Clin North Am* 56:201-206, 1972
57. Grey HM, Kohler PF: Cryoimmunoglobulins. *Semin Hematol* 10:87-112, 1973
58. Brouet JC, Clauvel JP, Danon F, Klein M, Seligmann M: Biologic and clinical significance of cryoglobulins: a report of 86 cases. *Am J Med* 57:775-788, 1974
59. Lospalluto J, Dorward B, Miller W Jr, Ziff M: Cryoglobulinemia based on interaction between a gamma macroglobulin and 7S gamma globulin. *Am J Med* 32:142-147, 1962
60. Meltzer M, Franklin EC, Elias K, McCluskey RT, Cooper N: Cryoglobulinemia—a clinical and laboratory study. II. Cryoglobulins with rheumatoid factor activity. *Am J Med* 40:837-856, 1966
61. Golde D, Epstein W: Mixed cryoglobulins and glomerulonephritis. *Ann Intern Med* 69:1221-1227, 1968
62. Soter NA, Austen KF, Gigli I: The complement system in necrotizing angiitis of the skin. Analysis of complement component activities in serum of patients with concomitant collagenvascular diseases. *J Invest Dermatol* 63:219-226, 1974
63. Mongan ES, Cass RM, Jacox RF, Vaughan JH: A study of the relation of seronegative and seropositive rheumatoid arthritis to each other and to necrotizing vasculitis. *Am J Med* 47:23-35, 1969
64. Sokoloff L, Bunim JJ: Vascular lesions in rheumatoid arthritis. *J Chronic Dis* 5:668-687, 1957
65. Kemper JW, Baggenstoss AH, Slocumb CH: The relationship of therapy with cortisone to the incidence of vascular lesions in rheumatoid arthritis. *Ann Intern Med* 46:831-851, 1957
66. Schmid FR, Cooper NS, Ziff M, McEwen C: Arteritis in rheumatoid arteritis. *Am J Med* 30:56-83, 1961
67. Winchester RJ, Kunkel HG, Agnello V: Occurrence of -globulin complexes in serum and joint fluid of rheumatoid arthritis patients: use of monoclonal rheumatoid factors as reagents for their demonstration. *J Exp Med* 134:286s-295s, 1971
68. Conn DL, McDuffie FC, Dyck PJ: Immunopathologic study of sural nerves in rheumatoid arthritis. *Arthritis Rheum* 15:135-143, 1972
69. Estes D, Christian CL: The natural history of systemic lupus erythematosus by prospective analysis. *Medicine (Baltimore)* 50:85-95, 1971
70. Klemperer P, Pollack AD, Baehr G: Pathology of disseminated lupus erythematosus. *Arch Pathol* 32:569-631, 1941
71. Mintz G, Fraga A: Arteritis in systemic lupus erythematosus. *Arch Intern Med* 116:55-66, 1965
72. Sams WM Jr, Harville DD, Winkelmann RK: Necrotizing vasculitis associated with lethal reticuloendothelial diseases. *Br J Dermatol* 80:555-560, 1968
73. Copeman PWM, Ryan TJ: The problems of classification of cutaneous angiitis with reference to histopathology and pathogenesis. *Br J Dermatol* 82:2-14, 1970
74. Rewcastle NB, Tom MI: Non-infectious granulomatous angiitis of the nervous system associated with Hodgkin's disease. *J Neurol Neurosurg Psychiatry* 25:51-58, 1962
75. Wegener F: Über generalisierte, septische Gefässerkrankungen. *Verh Dtsch Ges Pathol* 29:202-210, 1936
76. Fahey J, Leonard E, Churg J, Godman G: Wegener's granulomatosis. *Am J Med* 17:168-179, 1954
77. Fauci AS, Wolff SM: Wegener's granulomatosis: studies in eighteen patients and a review of the literature. *Medicine* 52:535-561, 1973
78. Wolff SM, Fauci AS, Horn RG, Dale DC: Wegener's granulomatosis. *Ann Intern Med* 81:513-525, 1974
79. Fauci AS, Johnson RE, Wolff SM: Radiation therapy of midline granuloma. *Ann Intern Med* 84:140-147, 1976
80. Fauci AS: Granulomatous vasculitides: distinct but related (editorial). *Ann Intern Med* 87:782-783, 1977
81. Howell SB, Epstein WV: Circulating immunoglobulin complexes in Wegener's granulomatosis. *Am J Med* 60:259-268, 1976
82. Horn RH, Fauci AS, Rosenthal AS, Wolff SM: Renal biopsy pathology in Wegener's granulomatosis. *Am J Pathol* 74:423-434, 1974
83. Reza MJ, Dornfeld L, Goldberg LS, Bluestone P, Pearson CM: Wegener's granulomatosis. Long-term follow-up of patients treated with cyclophosphamide. *Arthritis Rheum* 18:501-506, 1975
84. Israel HL, Patchefsky AS, Saldana MJ: Wegener's granulomatosis, lymphomatoid granulomatosis, and benign lymphocytic angiitis and granulomatosis of lung. Recognition and treatment. *Ann Intern Med* 87:691-699, 1977
85. Liebow AA, Carrington CRB, Friedman PJ: Lymphomatoid granulomatosis. *Hum Pathol* 3:457-558, 1972
86. Fauci AS, Wolff SM, Johnson JS: Effect of cyclophosphamide upon the immune response in Wegener's granulomatosis. *N Engl J Med* 285:1493-1496, 1971

87. Fauci AS, Wolff SM: Immunological features of Wegener's granulomatosis. *Lancet* 1:688-689, 1974
88. Cooke WT, Choake PCP, Govan ADT, Colbeck JC: Temporal arteritis. A generalized vascular disease. *Q J Med* 15:47-75, 1946
89. Wagener HP, Hollenhorst RW: The ocular lesions of temporal arteritis. *Am J Ophthalmol* 45:617-630, 1958
90. Paulley JW, Hughes JP: Giant-cell arteritis or arthritis of the aged. *Br Med J* 2:1562-1567, 1960
91. Kogstad OA: Polymyalgia rheumatica and its relation to arteritis temporalis. *Acta Med Scand* 178:591-598, 1965
92. Hamrin B, Jonsson N, Landberg T: Involvement of large vessels in polymyalgia arteritica. *Lancet* 1:1193-1196, 1965
93. Healey LA, Parker F, Wilske KR: Polymyalgia rheumatica and giant cell arteritis. *Arthritis Rheum* 14:138-141, 1971
94. Hauser WA, Ferguson RH, Holley KE, Kurland LT: Temporal arteritis in Rochester, Minnesota, 1951-1967. *Mayo Clin Proc* 46:597-602, 1971
95. Hamilton CR Jr, Shelley WM, Tumulty PA: Giant cell arteritis: Including temporal arteritis and polymyalgia rheumatica. *Medicine (Baltimore)* 50:1-27, 1971
96. Fauchald P, Rygvold O, Oystese B: Temporal arteritis and polymyalgia rheumatica. Clinical and biopsy findings. *Ann Intern Med* 77:845-852, 1972
97. Hunder GG, Baker HL Jr, Rhoton AL Jr, Sheps SG, Ward LE: Superficial temporal arteriography in patients suspected of having temporal arteritis. *Arthritis Rheum* 15:561-570, 1972
98. Beevers DG, Harpur JE, Turk KAD: Giant cell arteritis—the need for prolonged treatment. *J Chronic Dis* 26:571-584, 1973
99. Hunder GG, Sheps SG, Allen GL, Joyce JW: Daily and alternate-day corticosteroid regimens in treatment of giant cell arteritis. *Ann Intern Med* 82:613-618, 1975
100. Klein RG, Campbell RJ, Hunder GG, Carney JA: Skip lesions in temporal arteritis. *Mayo Clin Proc* 51:504-510, 1976
101. McKusick VA: A form of vascular disease relatively frequent in the Orient. *Am Heart J* 63:57-64, 1962
102. Vinijchaikul L: Primary arteritis of the aorta and its main branches (Takayasu's arteriopathy). *Am J Med* 43:15-27, 1967
103. Nakao K, Nütani H, Miyahara M, Ishimi ZI, Hashiba K, Takeda Y, Ozawa T, Matsushita S, Kuramochi M: Takayasu's arteritis. Clinical report of eighty-four cases and immunological studies of seven cases. *Circulation* 35:1141-1155, 1967
104. Fraga A, Mintz G, Valle L, Flores-Izquierdo G: Takayasu's arteritis: frequency of systemic manifestations (study of 22 patients) and favorable response to maintenance steroid therapy and adrenocorticosteroids (12 patients). *Arthritis Rheum* 15:617-624, 1972
105. Ishikawa K: Natural history and classification of occlusive thromboaortopathy (Takayasu's disease). *Circulation* 57:27-35, 1978
106. Barber HS: Myalgic syndrome with constitutional effects. Polymyalgia rheumatica. *Ann Rheum Dis* 16:230-237, 1957
107. Esiri MM, MacLennan ICM, Hazleman BL: Lymphocyte sensitivity to skeletal muscle in patients with polymyositis and other disorders. *Clin Exp Immunol* 14:25-35, 1973
108. Liang GC, Simkin PA, Hunder GG, Wilske KR, Healey LA: Familial aggregation of polymyalgia rheumatica and giant cell arteritis. *Arthritis Rheum* 17:19-24, 1974
109. Hazleman BL, MacLennan ICM, Esiri MM: Lymphocyte proliferation to artery antigen as a positive diagnostic test in polymyalgia rheumatica. *Ann Rheum Dis* 34:122-127, 1975
110. Bacon PA, Doherty SM, Zuckerman AJ: Hepatitis-B antibody in polymyalgia rheumatica. *Lancet* 2:476-480, 1975
111. Malmvall BE, Bengtsson BA, Kaijser B, Nelsson LA, Alestig K: Serum levels of immunoglobulin and complement in giant-cell arteritis. *JAMA* 236:1876-1978, 1976
112. Liang GC, Simkin PA, Mannick M: Immunoglobulins in temporal arteries. An immunofluorescent study. *Ann Intern Med* 81:19-24, 1974
113. McKusick VA, Harris WS: The Buerger syndrome in the Orient. *Bull Johns Hopkins Hosp* 109:241-291, 1961
114. McKusick VA, Harris WS, Goodman RM, Shelley WM, Bloodwell RD, Ottesen OE: Buerger's disease: a distinct clinical and pathologic entity. *JAMA* 181:5-12, 1962
115. Williams G: Recent views on Buerger's disease. *J Clin Pathol* 22:573-578, 1969
116. Hill GL: A rational basis for management of patients with the Buerger syndrome. *Br J Surg* 61:476-481, 1974
117. Shionoya S, Ban I, Nakata Y, Matsubara J, Shinjo K, Hirai M, Kawai S, Suzecki S, Tsai WH: Diagnosis, pathology, and treatment of Buerger's disease. *Surgery* 75:695-700, 1974
118. Kawasaki T, Kosaki F, Shigematsu I, Yanagawa H, Okawa S: A new infantile acute febrile mucocutaneous lymph node syndrome (MLNS) prevailing in Japan. *Pediatrics* 54:271-276, 1974
119. Kawasaki T: Acute febrile mucocutaneous syndrome with lymphoid involvement with specific desquamation of the fingers and toes in children. *Jpn J Allergy* 16:178-222, 1967
120. Tanaka N, Sekimoto K, Naoe S: Kawasaki disease. Relationship with infantile periarteritis nodosa. *Arch Pathol Lab Med* 100:81-86, 1976
121. Morens DM, O'Brien RJ: Kawasaki disease in the United States. *J Infect Dis* 137:91-93, 1978
122. Landing BH, Larson EJ: Are infantile periarteritis nodosa with coronary artery involvement and fatal mucocutaneous lymph node syndrome the same? Comparison of 20 patients from North America with patients from Hawaii and Japan. *Pediatrics* 59:651-662, 1977
123. Blomgren SE: Erythema nodosum. *Semin Arthritis Rheum* 4:1-24, 1974
124. Winkelmann RK, Förström L: New observations in the histopathology of erythema nodosum. *J Invest Dermatol* 65:441-446, 1975
125. O'Duffy JD, Carney JA, Deodhar S: Behçet's disease. Report of 10 cases, 3 with new manifestations. *Ann Intern Med* 75:561-570, 1971
126. Cheson BD, Bluming AZ, Alroy J: Cogan's syndrome: a systemic vasculitis. *Am J Med* 60:549-555, 1976
127. Sheie HG, Albert DM: *Textbook of Ophthalmology*, 9th ed. Philadelphia, W. B. Saunders Co., 1977, p. 32
128. McDuffie FC, Sams WM Jr, Maldonado JE, Andreini PH, Conn DL, Samayoa EA: Hypocomplementemia with cutaneous vasculitis and arthritis: Possible immune complex syndrome. *Mayo Clin Proc* 48:340-348, 1973
129. Katz SI, Gallin JI, Hertz KC, Fauci AS, Lawley TJ: Erythema elevatum diutinum: skin and systemic manifestations, immunologic studies, and successful treatment with dapsone. *Medicine (Baltimore)* 56:443-455, 1977
130. Walton EW: Giant-cell granuloma of the respiratory tract (Wegener's granulomatosis). *Br Med J* 2:265-270, 1958
131. Hollander D, Manning RT: The use of alkylating agents in the treatment of Wegener's granulomatosis. *Ann Intern Med* 67:393-398, 1967
132. Haynes BF, Fishman ML, Fauci AS, Wolff SM: The ocular manifestations of Wegener's granulomatosis. Fifteen years' experience and review of the literature. *Am J Med* 63:121-141, 1977
133. Dale DC: Abnormalities of leukocytes, in *Harrison's Principles of Internal Medicine*, 8th ed., edited by Thorn GW, Adams RD, Braunwald E, Isselbacher KJ, Petersdorf RG. New York, McGraw-Hill Book Co., 1977, pp. 304-411
134. Frohnert PP, Sheps SG: Long-term follow-up study of periarteritis nodosa. *Am J Med* 43:8-14, 1967
135. Melam H, Patterson R: Periarteritis nodosa. A remission achieved with combined prednisone and azathioprine therapy. *Am J Dis Child* 121:424-427, 1971
136. Tuma S, Chaimovitz C, Szylman P, Gellei B, Better OS: Periarteritis nodosa in the kidney. Recovery following immunosuppressive therapy. *JAMA* 235:280-281, 1976
137. Glanz S, Bittner SJ, Berman MA, Dolan TF Jr, Talner NS: Regression of coronary-artery aneurysms in infantile polyarteritis nodosa. *N Engl J Med* 294:939-941, 1976
138. Reimold EW, Weinberg AG, Fink CW, Battles ND: Polyarteritis in children. *Am J Dis Child* 130:534-541, 1976
139. Fauci AS, Doppman JL, Wolff SM: Cyclophosphamide-induced remissions in advanced polyarteritis nodosa. *Am J Med* 64:890-894, 1978

REVIEW

Glucocorticoid-Induced Osteoporosis: Pathogenesis and Management

Barbara P. Lukert, MD; and Lawrence G. Raisz, MD

Purpose: To review the clinical picture, pathogenesis, and management of glucocorticoid-induced osteoporosis.

Data Identification: Studies published since 1970 were identified from a MEDLINE search, articles accumulated by the authors, and through bibliographies of identified articles.

Study Selection: Information for review was taken from 160 of the more than 200 articles examined.

Data Extraction: Pertinent studies were selected; the relative strengths and weaknesses of these studies are discussed.

Results of Data Synthesis: Studies in tissue and organ cultures suggest that glucocorticoids have a direct effect on bone, causing inhibition of bone formation and enhancing bone resorption. Glucocorticoids decrease calcium absorption from the intestine and increase renal excretion. Osteoporosis occurs in at least 50% of persons who require long-term glucocorticoid therapy. Long-term trials of therapy for the prevention of glucocorticoid-induced osteoporosis have not been done, but reasonable recommendations include the use of a glucocorticoid with a short half-life in the lowest dose possible, maintenance of physical activity, adequate calcium and vitamin D intake, sodium restriction and use of thiazide diuretics, and gonadal hormone replacement. In refractory cases, the use of calcitonin, bisphosphonates, sodium fluoride, or anabolic steroids should be considered.

Conclusions: Osteoporosis is common in patients requiring long-term treatment with glucocorticoids. Careful attention to preventive management may minimize the severity of this serious complication.

Annals of Internal Medicine. 1990;**112**:352-364.

From the University of Kansas Medical Center, Kansas City, Kansas; and the University of Connecticut Health Center, Farmington, Connecticut. For current author addresses, see end of text.

Glucocorticoid-induced osteoporosis has been recognized since 1932 when Cushing first described skeletal decalcification as a characteristic feature of adrenal hyperplasia secondary to pituitary tumors producing adrenocorticotrophic hormone (ACTH) (1). Because of the rarity of the Cushing syndrome, glucocorticoid-induced bone loss did not become a significant problem until these agents began to be used therapeutically. It soon became apparent that patients receiving prolonged therapy developed vertebral fractures (2). We review the metabolic effects of glucocorticoids on bone and mineral metabolism and the clinical features, pathogenesis, prevention, and treatment of glucocorticoid-induced osteoporosis.

Clinical Features

The anti-inflammatory and immunosuppressive properties of glucocorticoids have prompted their extensive use (3, 4); however, the side effects of these potent drugs are dramatic. The patient receiving large doses of glucocorticoids presents a distinctive clinical picture: centripetal obesity with peripheral subcutaneous fat atrophy, thinning of the skin with increased fragility and ecchymoses, proximal muscle weakness, fluid retention, hyperglycemia, and, frequently, vertebral fractures. Bone loss with resulting fractures is the most incapacitating sequela of steroid therapy. The severity of bone loss appears to parallel that of the other side effects. Synthetic derivatives have been developed in an attempt to reduce the number of detrimental side effects of cortisol, particularly sodium retention, and augment the anti-inflammatory effect of the parent compound. The compounds most frequently prescribed are prednisone, prednisolone, methylprednisolone, betamethasone, dexamethasone, and triamcinolone. The relative anti-inflammatory potencies of these compounds are due largely to differences in half life, but other differences include protein binding, ability to traverse membranes, and intrinsic effectiveness of the molecule at its site of action (3, 4). Patients most prone to adverse side effects of glucocorticoids are those with the slowest clearance rates of the drug (5). Unfortunately, although many of these compounds cause less sodium retention, the severity of other side effects is proportional to their anti-inflammatory potency. Deflazacort, an oxazoline derivative of prednisone, has been used in Europe recently with the hope of reducing the incidence of the catabolic effects of glucocorticoids, including bone loss (6).

The true incidence of osteoporosis in patients receiving glucocorticoid therapy is unknown. Very few

Table 1. *Results from Sixteen Studies of the Effect of Glucocorticoids on Humans**

Study	Reference	Study Design	Number of Patients	Dose of Prednisone (*mg/d*)	Duration of Treatment (*y*)	Method of Bone Measurement†	Bone Measured	Difference from Control (*%*)‡
1	7	Retrospective	128	> 15	> 1	SPA	Lumbar vertebrae 2 to 4	−15.0
2	11	Retrospective	25	9 to 12	3 to 5	SPA	Distal forearm	−14.0
3	12	Retrospective	70	< 15	1 to 5	Histomorphometry	Iliac crest	−33.8
4	13	Longitudinal	13	Average, 7.4	4.4 ± 1.9	SPA	Distal forearm	pre 0
		Longitudinal	17	Average, 7.4	5.4 ± 1.6			post −2.6/y
		Longitudinal	22	Average, 7.4	4.6 ± 0.9			men −1.7/y
5	14	Retrospective	23	11.3 ± 4.2	7.3 ± 1.6	SPA	Distal forearm	−28.0
6	15	Retrospective	21	5.3 ± 36.7	9.7	MCT	Second metacarpal	−5 to −10
7	16	Retrospective	17	Average, 17.3	4.2 ± 1	SPA	Distal forearm	−33
8	17	Prospective	5	20 to 80	1.7 to 2.8	NAA	Total body calcium	0
9	18	Retrospective	114	NA§	NA	DPA	Proximal forearm	0
10	19	Retrospective	44	Average, 8.0	0.7 ± 1	DPA	Lumbar vertebrae 2 to 4	−9.6
							Femoral neck	−12.2
11	20	Cross-sectional	22	6.8 ± 1.9	12.5 ± 6.4	NAA	Total body calcium	−17.0
12	21	Prospective	15	Average, 24.6	0.4	SPA	Distal forearm	−3.1
13	8	Prospective	20	Average, 25, every other day	1	QCT	Distal tibia and radius	−13.0
14	22	Retrospective	30	22.8 ± 17.9 g cumulated dose	7.34 ± 5.6	DPA	Lumbar vertebrae 2 to 4	−19.5
							Femoral neck	−9.0
							Femoral diaphysis	−5.7
15	23	Retrospective	28	Average 8.9	4.7	DPA	Lumbar vertebrae 2 to 4	−12.3
16	10	Prospective	3	Average 15	2	DPA	Lumbar vertebrae 2 to 4	−10 to −20

* The differences observed in study 10 were not statistically significant; study 12 was of only 24 weeks duration.
† SPA = single-photon absorptiometry, MCT = cortical thickness, NAA = neutron activation, DPA = dual-photon absorptiometry.
‡ Pre = premenopausal women, post = postmenopausal women.
§ NA = not available.

prospective studies have compared bone loss in patients who received glucocorticoid with that in patients with the same disease process who did not receive steroids. Available data suggest that the incidence is 30% to 50% (7, 8). (Incidence is defined as number of patients suffering atraumatic fractures.) These data are consistent with the report of a 50% incidence of osteoporosis in patients with Cushing disease (9). The extent of bone loss is equally difficult to evaluate because so many of the studies are cross-sectional, making it impossible to determine the condition of the subjects' skeletons before glucocorticoid therapy or whether the loss was linear over time. One short longitudinal study suggests that there is rapid early loss and a plateau after approximately 6 months (10). Table 1 lists the results of bone density measurements from 15 studies. Only five studies (4, 8, 12, 13, and 16) contain prospective data, and only three studies (4, 8, and 9) failed to observe significant bone loss in patients receiving glucocorticoids. Study 13 was a prospective study with observations made over a period of 1 year. It showed a close relation between rate of bone loss and glucocorticoid dose. Patients receiving less than 17 mg over 2 days lost an insignificant amount of bone, those receiving 17 to 34 mg over 2 days lost 0% to 8% per year, and those receiving 34 to 51 mg over 2 days lost up to 17.5% per year. Only four studies (10, 14, 15, and 16) included lumbar spine density measurements, and these measurements showed losses from the lumbar spine to be proportionately greater than losses seen in the distal radius. All studies showed significantly greater losses of trabecular bone than of cortical bone. Study 4 suggests that premenopausal women were protected from bone loss while receiving low doses of glucocorticoid, and men were particularly sensitive to low-dose therapy. However, at higher doses, premenopausal women and young people lost significant amounts of bone (Study 13).

In summary, doses of prednisone of 7.5 mg per day or greater appear to cause significant loss of trabecular bone in most patients. Smaller doses have less dramatic effects on premenopausal women, but postmenopausal women and men will lose bone even on low-dose therapy. The limited data available show that approximately 50% of patients taking glucocorticoids will experience fractures. Comparisons of longitudinal and cross-sectional data suggest that bone loss must be more rapid in the early weeks of glucocorticoid therapy with subsequent slowing.

The usual risk factors for osteoporosis (age, race, sex, menopausal state, and parity) do not apply to the same extent to glucocorticoid-induced bone loss (23-26). A study by Ruegsegger and colleagues (8) suggests that young people receiving glucocorticoids lose bone more rapidly than do older patients and premenopausal women; however, postmenopausal women receiving equivalent doses of steroids are more at risk for fractures, presumably because they also have age- and menopause-related bone loss (24). Men are equally susceptible to the skeletal effects of glucocorticoids (8), and blacks lose bone to the same extent as whites. In diseases such as rheumatoid arthritis, the inflammatory process and immobilization contribute to bone loss. Even so, glucocorticoids clearly play a significant role (24-26). Steroid-induced bone loss occurs primarily in trabecular bone (26, 27). Histologically, there is reduction of mean wall thickness of trabecular bone packets, with a consequent decrease in total bone volume (12, 28). Parameters of bone resorption are elevated with increases in eroded surface (12, 28), osteoclast-covered surface, and a suggestion of increased osteoclast number (16). Calcium kinetic studies also suggest that bone resorption is increased (29, 30). We will discuss the mechanisms responsible for these findings.

Pathogenesis

Glucocorticoid-induced osteoporosis is the result of a number of factors that adversely affect calcium homeostasis. Abnormalities in gonadal hormone secretion, calcium absorption and renal handling of calcium, and direct effects of glucocorticoids on bone all contribute to bone loss.

Glucocorticoid Effect on Secretion of Sex Hormones

Glucocorticoids alter gonadal function by two mechanisms: inhibition of pituitary gonadotrophin secretion and direct effects on ovary or testes. Glucocorticoids blunt secretion of luteinizing hormone in response to luteinizing-hormone-releasing hormone (LHRH) in both men and women (31, 32). Glucocorticoids inhibit follicle-stimulating-hormone (FSH)-induced estrogen production by cultured rat granulosa cells and decrease testosterone production by the testes (33-36). Circulating levels of androstenedione and estrone are further suppressed by reduced adrenal production of androstenedione due to suppression of ACTH and the resultant adrenal atrophy (37). These aberrations in the production of gonadal hormones may play an important role in glucocorticoid-induced osteoporosis. Recent studies (38) in rats showed that estrogen deficiency and glucocorticoids were additive in increasing the rate of bone loss, and postmenopausal women receiving glucocorticoids are particularly susceptible to bone loss (25).

Effect on Intestinal Calcium Absorption

It is generally accepted that glucocorticoids decrease net intestinal calcium absorption in both humans (39-47) and animals (48-54), but the mechanism is not known. Balance studies in patients with the Cushing syndrome have shown increased fecal calcium, although net calcium absorption was not depressed in the presence of an adequate dietary intake of calcium. Radioisotope techniques have shown calcium absorption to decrease (56-58), increase (59), or remain unchanged (60). There are several possible explanations for these divergent results. First, animal and in-vitro studies demonstrate that glucocorticoids may influence individual intestinal segments differently. Duodenal absorption is depressed (48-51), whereas absorption in the colon may be stimulated by glucocorticoids (61, 62). Thus, studies looking at the early time points may see decreased absorption that reflects only the effect of glucocorticoids on the upper bowel; whereas, studies looking at a more prolonged period may see greater rates of absorption because of the increase in absorption occurring in the colon. This concept is supported by studies showing decreased calcium absorption in the first hour, absorption similar to that in normal controls in the second hour, and greater absorption than in controls thereafter (59, 63).

Second, studies in the rat duodenum have shown that, with low doses of cortisol, calcium absorption increases but, with high doses, although transcellular transport increases, intestinal secretion rises exponentially as a function of the dose (64). Thus, at high doses, net calcium absorption is reduced secondary to a marked increase in calcium secretion into the intestinal lumen. In this case, divergent results could depend on differences in the dose of glucocorticoid administered in the study.

Despite discrepancies seen in isolated studies, most patients receiving the usual pharmacologic doses of glucocorticoids apparently have impaired intestinal absorption of calcium. The mechanisms responsible for glucocorticoid-induced inhibition of the active transcellular transport of calcium in the duodenum are poorly understood. Table 2 lists the mechanisms proposed in the literature. Glucocorticoids do not alter the initial uptake of calcium by brush border membrane vesicles (65). Synthesis of calcium binding protein is decreased (66) and release of calcium from mitochondria appears to be inhibited because of depletion of mitochondrial adenosine triphosphate (ATP) (67). Paracellular back flux of calcium has been reported to be increased; this increase may be secondary to stimulation of the sodium-potassium-ATPase pump (68) by glucocorticoids, causing an increase in the flow of sodium and water through the cell into the serosal space and then through the paracellular pathway to the lumen carrying calcium with it by a solvent drag effect (69). The relative role of each of these aberrations in producing impairment of the calcium transport mechanism is unknown.

Effect on Vitamin D Metabolism

The possible contribution of alterations in vitamin D metabolism to glucocorticoid-induced changes in calcium absorption have been extensively studied, with divergent findings. Glucocorticoid-induced vitamin D deficiency has been suggested, and both low (41, 70) and normal (16, 71) serum levels of 25-OHD have been reported. This discrepancy may be due to differences in the dietary intake and absorption of vitamin D and differences in sunlight exposure imposed by the underlying disease process and the debility of the subjects.

Circulating levels of 1,25-$(OH)_2D$ have been reported as low (70), normal (71), or increased (51, 72). Synthesis and clearance rates of 1,25-$(OH)_2D$ have been shown to be normal in humans receiving glucocorticoids (73), and subcellular localization is normal in the intestinal mucosa of glucocorticoid-treated rats (49). Intestinal receptors for 1,25-$(OH)_2D$ have been reported to be increased in the rat and decreased in the mouse (74). It has been suggested that glucocorticoids accelerate the breakdown of 1,25-$(OH)_2D$ at the mucosal receptor site (75). 1,25-$(OH)_2D$ improves calcium transport but does not return it to normal in either humans (40) or animals (49). 1,25-$(OH)_2D$ may improve the transcellular transport but not diminish the paracellular back flux of calcium. The defect in calcium transport induced by glucocorticoids is made worse by a high sodium intake (46) and by a low calcium intake (49-55). In summary, the mechanisms responsible for the inhibition of the gastrointestinal absorption of calcium induced by glucocorticoids are unknown, but appear to be independent of an interaction with vitamin D.

Effects on Renal Excretion of Calcium and Phosphorus

The renal loss of calcium has not been studied as extensively, but is thought to play an important role in the development of secondary hyperparathyroidism (76). Fasting urinary calcium excretion is elevated in normal subjects receiving glucocorticoids for only 5 days before immunoreactive parathyroid hormone (iPTH) levels rise (77). This may be due to an abrupt rise in filtered load of calcium because of a rapid decrease in bone formation that results in a lower uptake of calcium by newly formed bone or because of more direct effects of glucocorticoids on the kidney. In patients on long-term glucocorticoid therapy, hypercalciuria is most likely due to increased skeletal mobilization of calcium and decreased renal tubular reabsorption that occurs in spite of elevated levels of PTH. Renal loss of calcium is accentuated by a high sodium intake and is decreased by sodium restriction and thiazide diuretics (46).

Table 2. *Studies on Mechanisms for Effects of Glucocorticoids on Calcium Transport in the Intestine*

Effect	Reference
Decrease active transcellular transport.	48 to 51
Decrease transport with normal brush border vesicle uptake.	65
Decrease synthesis of calcium-binding protein.	66
Decrease release of calcium from mitochondria.	67
Stimulate basolateral membrane sodium-potassium-ATPase.	68
Increase back flux through paracellular pathway.	69
Decrease binding of 1,25-$(OH)_2D$ to intestinal mucosal cell (mouse).	74
Increase rate of degradation of 1,25-$(OH)_2D$ at mucosal binding site.	75
Induce vitamin D deficiency.	42, 70

Regardless of the mechanisms responsible for the transport defect, the net effect of glucocorticoids is to decrease the gastrointestinal absorption of calcium and to increase urinary excretion, resulting in a negative calcium balance. This negative balance leads to secondary hyperparathyroidism as evidenced by elevated iPTH levels in patients receiving glucocorticoids (16, 76, 78, 79). The observations that glucocorticoids stimulate release of PTH by rat parathyroid glands in organ culture (80) and cause an abrupt rise (within 15 minutes) in serum iPTH levels after the intravenous infusion of cortisol (79) suggest a direct stimulating effect on PTH secretion. The elevated iPTH levels can be suppressed by calcium infusion, suggesting that the elevation is more likely to be related to negative calcium balance than to direct stimulating effect of glucocorticoids (78). Tissue response to PTH may also be augmented by glucocorticoids. The rise in serum cyclic adenosine monophosphate (cAMP) stimulated by PTH infusion is doubled by pretreatment with prednisone for 3 days (10).

Glucocorticoids induce phosphaturia, and decreased tubular reabsorption of phosphate has been reported (81). These effects can be attributed in large part to secondary hyperparathyroidism; however, glucocorticoids also have direct effects on the kidney. Glucocorticoids increase the amiloride-sensitive Na^+-H^+ exchange activity in rat proximal tubule brush border vesicles and decrease the Na^+ gradient-dependent phosphate uptake, resulting in increased acid secretion and phosphaturia (80).

Effects on Bone

Bone Resorption

Histomorphometric and calcium kinetic studies (82, 83) suggest that bone resorption is enhanced by glucocorticoids. This enhanced bone resorption may be attributed in large part to secondary hyperparathyroidism. In vivo, the enhanced resorption is prevented by parathyroidectomy (84, 85). Nevertheless, it seems unlikely that glucocorticoid-induced osteoporosis is due solely to secondary hyperparathyroidism, because formation and resorption are usually coupled in the presence of PTH excess, and trabecular bone loss is not prominent in primary hyperparathyroidism yet is characteristic of glucocorticoid-induced osteoporosis (82, 86). Inhibition of bone formation, therefore, must play a role.

Studies of the direct effect of glucocorticoids on bone resorption in organ culture have yielded confusing results. One study (87) using mouse calvaria showed a direct stimulating effect on osteoclasts, and studies (88) using fetal rat calvaria showed a transient increase in the release of previously incorporated ^{45}Ca. Glucocorticoids can enhance the attachment of macrophages to bone by altering cell surface oligosaccharides (89). However, glucocorticoids can inhibit bone resorption in vitro (90), particularly in unstimulated bone organ cultures and cultures stimulated by osteoclast activating factors (interleukin-1 and tumor necrosis factor) (91). The effect of glucocorticoids on osteoclasts may be biphasic with physiologic concentrations being required for the late stages of differentiation and function of osteoclasts, whereas the generation of new osteoclasts that involves cell replication is inhibited by high doses and prolonged exposure (92).

Effect on Bone Formation

The hypothesis that glucocorticoids decrease bone formation is supported by histomorphometric studies (12, 28, 93) that show a marked decrease in the number of osteoid seams, a low mineral apposition rate measured by tetracycline labeling, and reduced mean wall thickness. The total amount of bone replaced in each remodeling cycle has been shown to be reduced by 30% (28). The reduction in mean wall thickness is thought to be due to a shortening of the life span of the active osteoblast population in each basic multicellular unit (12, 28). Osteoblast-like cells have glucocorticoid receptors, and glucocorticoids appear to have a direct inhibitory effect on osteoblast replication and differentiation. In addition, glucocorticoids act on osteoblasts by modulating their responses to PTH, $1,25\text{-}(OH)_2D$, prostaglandins, and growth factors.

Glucocorticoids and PTH

The sensitivity of osteoblasts to PTH is enhanced by glucocorticoids. It has been suggested that glucocorticoids act on or near the stimulatory guanine nucleotide binding regulatory protein complex (94). The potentiation of PTH-induced increases in cAMP response appears to be due to increases in cAMP activity and inhibition of phosphodiesterase (95-98). PTH-mediated inhibition of alkaline phosphatase activity, collagen synthesis, and citrate decarboxylation are all potentiated by glucocorticoids (99). These findings have implications for resorption as well as formation, because osteoblastic control of the initiation of the resorption process may be altered.

Glucocorticoids and $1,25\text{-}(OH)_2D$

The effect of glucocorticoids on calcitriol receptors is complex with variations seen depending on species and growth phase. Glucocorticoids downregulate the $1,25\text{-}(OH)_2D$ receptor in mouse osteoblasts, but upregulate the receptor in rats (100, 101). Recent studies (102) have shown increased nuclear uptake of $1,25\text{-}(OH)_2D$ in human monocytes exposed to prednisone. We do not know if this information can be applied to human bone cells.

Glucocorticoids and Prostaglandins

Prostaglandin E_2 at concentrations of 10^{-8} to 10^{-7}M stimulates collagen and noncollagen protein synthesis in bone (103, 104). Prostaglandin E_2 is produced by bone in organ culture, and glucocorticoids inhibit prostaglandin E_2 production (105). When prostaglandin E_2 is added to bones treated with glucocorticoids, the glucocorticoid-induced decrease in DNA and collagen synthesis is reversed (106). This reversal suggests that part of the inhibitory effects of glucocorticoids may be mediated by inhibition of prostaglandin production. However, the effect of glucocorticoids cannot be explained solely on the basis of low prostaglandin levels, because the effect cannot be reproduced by inhibition of prostaglandin synthesis with nonsteroidal drugs such as indomethacin.

Glucocorticoids and Cytokines

Interleukin-1 is known to induce bone resorption and inhibit bone formation. However, it is unlikely that interleukin-1 plays a role in glucocorticoid-induced osteoporosis, because production of cytokines by T-lymphocyte clones is inhibited in vitro by glucocorticoids in concentrations of 10^{-8} to 10^{-6} M (107), and the bone resorbing activity of interleukin-1 is partially inhibited by hydrocortisone (108).

Effects of Glucocorticoids on Growth Hormone and Growth Factors

Insulin-like growth factor-1 or somatomedin-C is a growth-hormone-dependent polypeptide known to stimulate skeletal growth. Growth hormone and somatomedin-C (insulin-like growth factor-1) concentrations are normal in patients receiving glucocorticoids (109, 110), and insulin-like growth factor-1 receptor binding by rat osteoblast-like cells in tissue culture is increased by glucocorticoids (111). Despite this, somatomedin activity measured by bioassay is decreased in the serum of patients with glucocorticoid excess (112). This discrepancy might be explained by a somatomedin inhibitor that has been found in the serum of children receiving glucocorticoids (112). It has been shown recently that fetal rat calvariae synthesize growth factors (113) and glucocorticoids decrease the local production of insulin-like growth factor-1 (McCarthy TL, Canalis E. Personal communication). A better understanding of the interactions between glucocorticoids and growth factors may shed light on the genesis of glucocorticoid-induced bone loss.

Direct Effects on Osteoblasts

Glucocorticoids have a biphasic effect in organ culture systems. Physiologic concentrations of glucocorticoids appear to enhance the function of differentiated osteoblasts (92, 114); however, prolonged exposure and supraphysiologic concentrations inhibit synthetic processes. During the first 24 hours of exposure to cortisol, collagen synthesis is increased; whereas, after 48 to 96 hours in culture, collagen synthesis is markedly inhibited (115, 116). When periosteum and osteoblast-rich central bone are examined separately, glucocorticoids stimulate collagen synthesis in central bone but not in the periosteum (117). At 48 hours, cortisol causes a decrease in DNA synthesis, and histologic sections confirm decreased mitoses (115, 116). Osteoblasts in central bone must be replaced from periosteal precursor cells. The late inhibitory effects on collagen synthesis seen in central bone may be the result of a decrease in the proliferation of periosteal precursor cells (117, 118). An additional direct inhibitory effect on differentiation of osteoblasts for collagen synthesis is quite likely, because we have found that collagen synthesis is slowly inhibited by glucocorticoids in the presence of inhibitors of cell replication such as hydroxyurea and aphidicolin (Figure 1) (Lukert BP, Kream BE, Raisz LG. Unpublished results).

Collagenase production has been shown to be increased by cortisol in mouse calvaria (119). High collagenase concentrations could also decrease the collagen content of bone. Synthesis of other components of matrix, such as mucopolysaccharides and sulfated glucosaminoglycans, is decreased in bone cultures and mouse dermal fibroblasts exposed to cortisol (120, 121).

The combination of secondary hyperparathyroidism and inhibition of matrix synthesis in bone leads to a rapid rate of bone loss. Secondary hyperparathyroidism increases the birth rate of bone remodeling units and probably also increases the amount of bone resorbed, but glucocorticoids reduce the quantity of bone formed at each remodeling site. The result is an increase in resorption and an inability of osteoblasts to replace the bone that is removed (28).

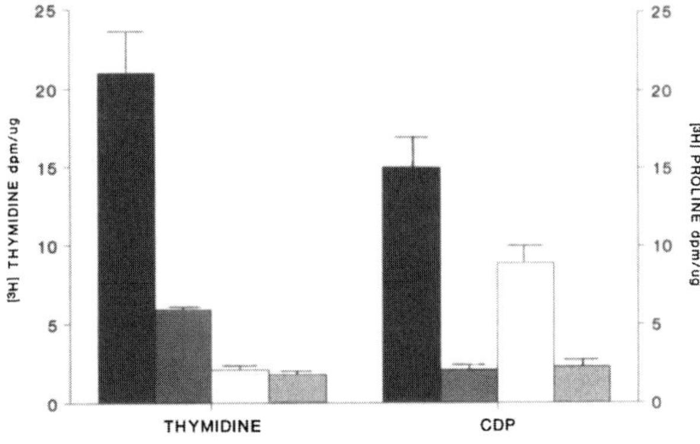

Figure 1. The effect of aphidocolin and cortisol on DNA and collagen synthesis in fetal rat calvariae after 96 hours of incubation. Closed bars indicate control; dark gray bars indicate treatment with cortisol 10^{-6} M; open bars indicate treatment with aphidocolin, 30 μM; light gray bars indicate treatment with aphidocolin, 30 μM, plus cortisol, 10^{-6} M. DNA synthesis, measured by ^{3}H-thymidine incorporation, is more than 95% inhibited by aphidocolin within 24 hours and remains so. Collagen synthesis, measured by ^{3}H-proline incorporation, is significantly inhibited by cortisol in the presence of aphidocolin, suggesting that cortisol affects osteoblast differentiation and function as well as replication (Lukert BP, Kream BE, Raisz LG. Unpublished results).

Table 3. *Major Mechanisms in the Pathogenesis of Glucocorticoid-Induced Osteoporosis*

Systemic Effects	Skeletal Effects
Decrease gastrointestinal calcium absorption and increase renal excretion (?) leading to 2° HPT.	Directly inhibit osteoblast function: decrease replication, differentiation, and life span.
Decrease gonadal hormone secretion (ovarian, testicular, and adrenal).	Decrease production of prostaglandin E_2 and insulin-like growth factor-1.
Inhibit insulin-like growth factor-1 production and action.	Increase sensitivity to parathyroid hormone and 1,25-$(OH)_2$D.
Cause muscle wasting.	Directly stimulate osteoclastic activity?

Mechanisms that may play an important role in the pathogenesis of glucocorticoid-induced osteoporosis are summarized in Table 3. Factors that are affected by glucocorticoids but do not fit logically into a scheme of pathogenesis are not included in Table 3. Glucocorticoid-induced increases in osteoblast sensitivity to insulin-like growth factor-1 and increases in differentiation of osteoblasts would not be expected to result in loss of bone. Likewise, the decrease in bone resorption observed in some in-vitro systems does not fit into the pathogenesis of bone loss but may be either a direct effect on osteoclast function or mediated through a decrease in prostaglandin E_2.

Osteonecrosis

Osteonecrosis (also known as aseptic necrosis) is a serious complication of steroid therapy that can occur in patients who are otherwise asymptomatic from bone loss. Glucocorticoid-induced osteonecrosis was recognized in 1957 and usually involves the femoral and humeral heads (122-124). Several theories about cause include a vascular theory that attributes glucocorticoid-osteonecrosis to bone ischemia caused by microscopic fat emboli (124, 125); a mechanical theory that attributes ischemic bone collapse of the epiphysis to osteoporosis and the accumulation of unhealed trabecular microcracks, resulting in fatigue fractures through the epiphysis (125-127); and the theory that increased intraosseous pressure due to fat accumulation as part of the Cushing syndrome leads to mechanical impingement on the sinusoidal vascular bed and decreased blood flow within bone (128). The pain and impaired mobility caused by glucocorticoid-osteonecrosis could increase the rate of bone loss.

Effect of Glucocorticoids on Muscle

Steroid-induced myopathy deserves further discussion, because it appears to be closely associated with bone loss. Reports of muscle weakness occurring with glucocorticoid administration began appearing in the literature soon after the introduction of corticosteroids to clinical medicine (129-131). Symptoms of myopathy can begin with myalgias or unusual sudden weakness. Weakness is always most severe in the pelvic girdle muscles, with lesser involvement of shoulder girdle and, later, distal muscles (132). Myopathy can develop after brief exposure to glucocorticoids and is not always dose dependent. Glucocorticoid-induced myopathy can be difficult to distinguish from muscle weakness resulting from the disease process in such entities as rheumatoid arthritis or polymyositis (132). The distinguishing feature is creatinuria in the presence of normal concentrations of muscle enzymes, aspartate aminotransferase, creatine kinase, and aldolase (132). Biopsies of the vastus lateralis have shown selective atrophy of type II (fast twitch, high glycolytic) muscle fibers in the Cushing syndrome (133, 134). Recent studies (135) have shown a relative increase in the number of type IIb fibers and a decrease in type I fibers, although there was severe atrophy of type IIb fibers. The glycolytic enzyme, lactate dehydrogenase, is normal, but glycogen synthase is low, suggesting insulin resistance (135). The enzymes of fatty acid oxidation, β-hydroxyacyl-CoA dehydrogenase and citric acid synthase, are lower in muscle from glucocorticoid-treated patients than in muscle from disease-matched controls (134). These metabolic changes result in significant loss of muscle strength. There is a striking association between the presence of steroid myopathy and osteoporosis (132). Preliminary studies have suggested that exercise can reverse the negative nitrogen balance but not the negative calcium balance induced by glucocorticoids; further investigation is needed in this important area. Significant myopathy and the resulting muscle weakness may contribute to bone loss by removing the normal forces on bone produced by strong muscle contraction and by the relative immobility imposed by weakness.

Assessment

Bone loss is most rapid in areas of the skeleton containing the greatest proportion of trabecular bone: the spine, hip, distal radius, pelvis, and ribs. However, recent animal studies (136) have also shown increased fragility of cortical bone. Earliest changes can be detected in the spine and femoral neck using dual-energy photon or x-ray absorptiometry or computed tomography (26). Because some patients who are on glucocorticoid therapy do not develop osteoporosis, it is important to identify persons at risk for closer follow-up of the effectiveness of preventive measures.

Patients who are most likely to develop osteoporosis have the lowest initial bone mass and strength, the most serious impairment of calcium absorption, the highest urinary loss of calcium, the greatest degree of secondary hyperparathyroidism, and respond most dramatically to the direct inhibitory effect of glucocorticoids on osteoblastic function. Measurement of urine calcium concentrations is helpful in assessing calcium balance and susceptibility to secondary hyperparathyroidism (78, 79). Serum osteocalcin (bone gamacarboxyglutamic acid) levels are low in most patients receiving glucocorticoids and are useful in assessing the degree of inhibition of osteoblastic activity (137-141). Recent studies (77, 141) have shown that doses of prednisone as small as 2.5 mg will suppress serum osteocalcin levels. Total urinary hydroxyproline excretion is an indicator of the rate of bone resorption. Because vitamin D deficiency augments the adverse effects of glucocorticoids, serum 25-OHD should be measured to assess the state of vitamin D nutriture. Assessment of calcium absorption would be valuable, if an inexpensive, convenient method were developed. The clinical usefulness of these measurements of mineral metabolism in patient management has not been studied prospectively; however, a retrospective study (142) has shown that patients who have developed glucocorticoid-induced osteoporosis had lower radiocalcium absorption and higher fasting urinary calcium and hydroxyproline than patients who did not have roentgenogram evidence of osteoporosis while receiving glucocorticoids.

Radiologic Assessment

Distinctive features of glucocorticoid-induced bone disease can be seen on a roentgenogram (143). In postmenopausal osteoporosis, horizontal trabeculae are lost out of proportion to vertical trabeculae, leading to a "corduroy stripe" appearance of the vertebra. In glucocorticoid-induced osteoporosis, vertical and horizontal trabeculae tend to be equally thin, thus producing a uniformly translucent appearance of the vertebrae, ribs, and pelvis. Abundant pseudocallus formation at the site of stress fractures is another hallmark of glucocorticoid-induced osteoporosis. This formation is most frequently seen just at the end plates of collapsed vertebrae or around stress fractures in the pelvis or ribs. Microscopic examination shows grossly diminished osteoblastic activity with production of a cartilaginous callus that becomes highly mineralized in an amorphous fashion. The presence of pseudocallus is regarded as a highly specific sign for glucocorticoid-induced osteoporosis. It has been observed in only one other situation, osteogenesis imperfecta, another entity in which collagen production is abnormal.

Any patient receiving steroids who suddenly has pain or weakness in a joint, particularly the hip or shoulder, may have osteonecrosis. The essential radiologic finding is an isolated epiphyseal compression or subchondral fracture of the symptomatic epiphysis (143). Early diagnosis is frequently difficult and may require bone scan or magnetic resonance imaging for confirmation. Ischemic vertebral collapse can occur in patients receiving glucocorticoids. In such cases, there is a transverse radiolucent cleft running under one of the end plates, similar in appearance to the subchondral fractures seen in glucocorticoid-induced osteonecrosis.

Evaluation of Bone Density

Bone loss is most rapid in areas of the skeleton containing the greatest proportion of trabecular bone: the spine, hip, distal radius, pelvis, and ribs. Early changes

Table 4. *Studies Using Vitamin D in Treatment of Glucocorticoid-Induced Osteopenia**

Study	Reference	Subjects (*n*)	Type of Treatment	Duration	Response†‡	Complications (number of patients)
1	145	11	Dihydrotachysterol, 4000 IU every other day	2 y	L2-4, + 3.7	Hypercalciuria (7), hypercalcemia (3)
		10	Calcium, 500 mg/d	2 y	L2-4, + 1.7	Hypercalciuria (4), hypercalcemia (3)
2	16	9	Calcidiol, 40 μg/d; calcium, 500 mg/d	2 y	DR, + 13.0	Hypercalciuria
3	146	5	Vitamin D, 0.5 to 1 mg/d	1 to 3 mo	Calcium balance, + in 3	Hypercalcemia (2)
4	21	16	Sodium fluoride, 50 mg/d; $CaPO_4$, 4.5 g/d; vitamin D, 45 000 IU 2x/w	6 mo	DR, −3.6 PR, −2.9	Urine calcium not measured
5	147	7	1-OH vitamin D, 2 μg/d	3 mo	Bone biopsy: decrease in osteoclast number	Urine calcium not measured
6	14	13	Calcitriol, 0.4 μg/d; calcium, 500 mg/d	18 mo	DR: no change. Bone biopsy: decrease in clast and blast activity	Hypercalciuria or hypercalcemia (12)

* All studies were prospective. These studies are flawed by a small number of subjects, and studies 3 to 5 are of short duration. *See* text for discussion.
† Percent change from baseline.
‡ L2-4 = density measured in lumbar vertebrae 2 to 4, DR = density measured in distal forearm, PR = density measured in proximal forearm.

can be detected in the spine and femoral neck using dual-photon or dual-energy x-ray absorptiometry or quantitative computed tomography (26). However, recent studies (136) have also shown increased fragility of cortical bone. It may also be useful to measure bone density in the forearm. Evaluation at 6-month intervals should be used to identify patients who are losing bone rapidly.

Assessment of Effects on Muscle

Since steroid-induced myopathy contributes so much to the general debility of the patient, a careful evaluation of muscle strength should be done with particular attention to proximal muscle groups, and appropriate exercise programs should be developed. A well-trained physical therapist can be helpful.

Prevention and Treatment

First, sufficient data do not exist to allow recommendation of any definite treatment protocol. Long-term, prospective, controlled studies on the effect of any treatment on glucocorticoid-induced trabecular bone loss in the axial skeleton are limited. Most studies have looked at bone density in the distal radius, although, in other situations, bone loss in the distal radius correlates only poorly with changes in the spine (144); consequently, measurements in the arm may be misleading as an indicator of what is occurring in the rest of the skeleton.

Prevention

Bone loss in patients receiving glucocorticoids is dose related; therefore, it is prudent to prescribe the lowest effective dose and to use topical preparations when possible. Although alternate-day therapy preserves normal function of the pituitary-adrenal axis, it does not prevent bone loss (11). As previously mentioned, deflazacort may have less inhibitory effect on calcium absorption and produce less bone loss than prednisone while maintaining its anti-inflammatory effect (5). If long-term prospective trials confirm this, it will be a useful compound. Most attempts to prevent bone loss associated with glucocorticoids have tried to improve calcium retention by increasing calcium absorption and decreasing urinary excretion, thus reversing secondary hyperparathyroidism. Vitamin D and its metabolites, calcium supplements, and thiazide diuretics have been used.

Pharmacologic doses of vitamin D are widely used to prevent and treat glucocorticoid-induced osteoporosis, although this action is not justified by reported study results. Table 4 shows six studies of the response of glucocorticoid-treated patients to various doses and preparations of vitamin D. Study 2, using calcidiol and calcium over a period of 2 years, was the only study to show a significant response. In study 2, the increase in bone density in the distal radius was rapid over the first 6 months, then it plateaued. Because the study reports only mean values and standard deviations, it is impossible to know how many patients responded. The changes in lumbar spine density reported for study 1 are not significantly different from the precision error of the test. Study 4 produced negative results even though sodium fluoride was added to the program; however, the study was relatively short, making results less reliable. Evidence of vitamin D toxicity (hypercalciuria and hypercalcemia) was reported in a high percentage of patients in all of the studies. The investigators reporting study 6 results recommend that 1,25-$(OH)_2D$ not be used in the treatment of glucocorticoid-induced osteoporosis because of the frequency of hypercalciuria and hypercalcemia and the potential for inhibiting osteoblastic activity. Calcium supplements alone have been reported to reduce urinary hydroxyproline excretion in patients receiving glucocorticoids, suggesting that calcium supplementation decreases bone turnover (148). Current knowledge does not justify the widespread use of large doses of vitamin D or its metabolites for the prevention or treatment of glucocorticoid-induced bone loss. Patients with low 25-OHD certainly should be considered to be vitamin D deficient and should receive small supplements of vitamin D or 25-OHD. Because treatment of patients with high normal serum 25-OHD levels with large doses of vitamin D can be hazardous (149), we reserve pharmacologic vitamin D therapy for patients with low bone mass or clinical osteoporosis who will receive close follow-up care.

Sodium restriction and thiazide diuretics have been shown to improve gastrointestinal absorption of calcium and decrease urinary excretion of calcium (46, 76). This treatment would be expected to reverse secondary hyperparathyroidism, but the long-term effect on bone loss has not been reported. Complete inhibition of PTH secretion may be undesirable, because physiologic concentrations may have an anabolic effect. In fact, intermittent low dose PTH therapy has been shown to increase trabecular bone mass in osteoporosis (150). Thiazide diuretics may aggravate hypokalemia in glucocorticoid-treated patients, and a combination of thiazide and amiloride, a potassium-sparing diuretic that also diminishes hypercalciuria, may be useful. Even with this combination, serum potassium levels must be closely monitored. Serum calcium should also be checked in patients receiving both vitamin D and thiazides, because these patients are more prone to hypercalcemia (146, 149).

Treatment

The use of gonadal hormones to prevent and treat glucocorticoid-induced osteoporosis has not been adequately studied. Balance studies from the 1940s suggest a positive effect of estrogens (151) and androgens (152) in patients with Cushing disease. The studies (37) do not include measurement of estradiol levels in women receiving glucocorticoids, but they report low levels of estrone and androstenedione. Glucocorticoids have been shown to blunt the secretion of luteinizing hormone in response to LHRH (31) and to inhibit FSH-induced estrogen production in cultured rat granulosa cells (33). Previously cited studies (38) show that bone loss is more rapid in oophorectomized rats receiving glucocorticoids than in those with intact ovaries. These data support the administration of estrogen to women receiving glucocorticoids. Not only postmenopausal but also premenopausal women who become amenorrheic while receiving glucocorticoids could benefit from estrogen therapy. Men receiving glucocorticoids should also be evaluated for hypogonadism. Serum testosterone levels are reduced in men during chronic glucocorticoid therapy (35, 36), and testosterone deficiency can cause osteoporosis (153). It seems reasonable to assume that low testosterone levels would adversely affect the skeleton in men receiving glucocorticoids and, therefore, that testosterone replacement is in order.

The anabolic steroid, nandrolone decanoate, in doses of 50 mg intramuscularly every 3 weeks, has been shown to increase forearm bone density in glucocorticoid-treated patients (154). Only about 10% of women were reported to develop virilizing signs or symtoms after 6 months of therapy. Long-term follow-up studies, including studies of effects on serum lipids, are needed before this drug is used routinely.

Agents that stimulate the replication, differentiation, and function of osteoblasts should be useful in treating glucocorticoid-induced osteoporosis. Sodium fluoride is such an agent, but the response to treatment is variable. Subjects in a 6-month study of 13 patients with a wide variety of disease states were given sodium fluoride, 50 mg/d, and calcium phosphate, 4.5 g/d. Their rate of bone loss did not differ from that of a matched group receiving equivalent doses of glucocorticoids (21). However, more prolonged studies of the effect of fluoride on bone histology in glucocorticoid-treated patients showed a dramatic increase in bone formation and trabecular bone mass (155).

Agents that reduce bone resorption independent of any effects on secondary hyperparathyroidism include calcitonin and bisphosphonates. Short-term studies on 18 patients given salmon calcitonin, 100 MRC units every other day for 6 months, showed an increase in mean forearm bone mass in patients on glucocorticoids (156). However, in this study, 4 of 16 patients receiving glucocorticoids alone did not lose bone; in fact, 3 of them showed small increases in bone mass. In the calcitonin group, 11 patients gained bone, 4 remained unchanged, and 3 showed a decrease. Sixteen patients receiving continuous glucocorticoid and aminohydroxypropylidene bisphosphonate for 12 months had a 19% increase in bone density, whereas controls on glucocorticoids had an 8.8% decrease (not statistically significant). Iliac crest bone biopsies showed a marked decrease in osteoclastic bone resorption, but osteoblastic surfaces were also decreased (157). Nevertheless, bone mass in patients treated with aminohydroxypropylidene bisphosphonate was significantly higher than in controls, and a 2-year follow-up of 5 of these patients showed relatively stable bone density (158). Aminohydroxypropylidene bisphosphonate does not cause impairment of mineralization; therefore, it is safer than etidronate, the only bisphosphonate currently available in the United States. More studies are needed to assess the usefulness of these agents.

It is important to keep an optimistic view when treating bone disease in patients receiving glucocorticoids; a study (159) has shown that bone loss in patients with the Cushing syndrome is partially reversible. An informative review of pathogenesis and treatment (160) has recently been reported. Specific recommendations for management of glucocorticoid-treated patients are given in the Appendix. These recommendations are based on theoretical considerations, as results of long-term clinical trials are not available. Although glucocorticoid-induced osteoporosis is a serious disorder, fear of this side effect does not justify withholding glucocorticoid therapy from patients whose disease cannot be adequately managed with other forms of treatment. Diligence in early assessment and management of glucocorticoid-related bone loss will minimize its severity.

Acknowledgments: The authors thank Dr. Barbara Kream for reviewing the manuscript and Charlotte Johnson for secretarial assistance.

Requests for Reprints: Barbara P. Lukert, MD, University of Kansas Medical Center, Room 4023C, 39th Street and Rainbow Boulevard, Kansas City, KS 66103.

Current Author Addresses: Dr. Lukert: University of Kansas Medical Center, Room 4023C, 39th Street and Rainbow Boulevard, Kansas City, KS 66103.

Dr. Raisz: University of Connecticut Health Center, Farmington, CT 06032.

Appendix. *Specific Recommendations for Patient Management*

1. Use the lowest effective dose of glucocorticoid.
2. Use a glucocorticoid with a short half life.
3. Use topical steriods when possible.
4. Maintain as much physical activity as possible.
5. Maintain a good nutritional status and restrict sodium intake to 2 to 3 g/d.
6. Replace gonadal hormones in postmenopausal women or women with glucocorticoid-induced amenorrhea and testosterone in men with low serum testosterone levels, unless contraindicated.
7. Give a thiazide- and potassium-sparing diuretic, if hypercalciuria is present.
8. Maintain serum 25-OHD concentrations within normal range with either calcidiol or vitamin D.
9. Follow bone density of spine at 6-month intervals for the first 2 years.
10. Consider giving sodium fluoride, 50 mg/d, calcitonin, bisphosphonates,* or anabolic hormones, if the patient continues to have crush fractures with conservative management or has marked bone loss.

* The efficacy of the only bisphosphonate available in the United States, etidronate, in the treatment of glucocorticoid-induced osteoporosis has not been studied. (3-amino-1-hydroxypropylidene)-1, 1-bisphosphonate was used in studies showing efficacy.

References

1. **Cushing H.** Basophile adenomas. *J Nerv Ment Dis.* 1932;**76**:50.
2. **Curtiss PH, Clark WS, Herndon CH.** Vertebral fractures resulting from prolonged cortisone and corticotrophin therapy. *JAMA.* 1954;**156**:467-9.
3. **Swartz SL, Dluhy RG.** Corticosteroids: clinical pharmacology and therapeutic use. *Drugs.* 1978;**16**:238-55.
4. **Ballard PL, Carter JP, Graham BS, Baxter JD.** A radioreceptor assay for evaluation of the plasma glucocorticoid activity of natural and synthetic steroids in man. *J Clin Endocrinol Metab.* 1975;**41**:290-304.
5. **Kozower M, Veatch L, Kaplan MM.** Decreased clearance of prednisolone, a factor in the development of corticosteroid side effects. *J Clin Endocrinol Metab.* 1974;**38**:407-12.
6. **Gennari C, Imbimbo B, Montagnani M, Bernini M, Nardi P, Avioli LV.** Effects of prednisone and deflazacort on mineral metabolism and parathyroid hormone activity in humans. *Calcif Tissue Int.* 1984;**36**:245-52.
7. **Adinoff AD, Hollister JR.** Steroid-induced fractures and bone loss in patients with asthma. *N Engl J Med.* 1983;**309**:265-8.
8. **Ruegsegger P, Medici TC, Anliker M.** Corticosteroid-induced bone loss. A longitudinal study of alternate day therapy in patients with bronchial asthma using quantitative computed tomography. *Eur J Clin Pharmacol.* 1983;**25**:615-20.
9. **Ross EJ, Linch DC.** Cushing's syndrome–killing disease: discriminatory value of signs and symptoms aiding early diagnosis. *Lancet.* 1982;**2**:646-9.
10. **Gennari C.** Glucocorticoids and bone. In: Peck WA, ed. *Bone and Mineral Research/3.* Amsterdam: Elsevier Publishers B.V.; 1985:213-32.
11. **Gluck OS, Murphy WA, Hahn TJ, Hahn B.** Bone loss in adults receiving alternate day glucocorticoid therapy. A comparison with daily therapy. *Arthritis Rheum.* 1985;**24**:892-8.
12. **Bressot C, Meunier PJ, Chapuy MC, Lejeune E, Edourd C, Darby AJ.** Histomorphometric profile, pathophysiology and reversibility of corticosteroid-induced osteoporosis. *Metab Bone Dis Rel Res.* 1979;**1**:303-19.
13. **de Deuxchaisnes CN, Devogelaer JP, Esselinckx W, et al.** The effect of low dosage glucocorticoids on bone mass in rheumatoid arthritis: a cross-sectional and a longitudinal study using single photon absorptiometry. *Adv Exp Med Biol.* 1984;**171**:210-39.
14. **Dykman TR, Haralson KM, Gluck OS, et al.** Effect of oral 1,25-dihydroxyvitamin D and calcium on glucocorticoid-induced osteopenia in patients with rheumatic diseases. *Arthritis Rheum.* 1984;**27**:1336-43.
15. **Greenberger PA, Hendrix RW, Patterson R, Chmiel JS.** Bone studies in patients on prolonged systemic corticosteroid therapy for asthma. *Clin Allergy.* 1982;**12**:363-8.
16. **Hahn TJ, Halstead LR, Teitelbaum SL, Hahn BH.** Altered mineral metabolism in glucocorticoid-induced osteopenia. Effect of 25-hydroxyvitamin D administration. *J Clin Invest.* 1979;**64**:655-65.
17. **Hosking DJ, Chamberlain MJ.** Osteoporosis and long-term corticoid therapy. *Br Med J.* 1973;**3**:125-7.
18. **Meuller MN.** Effects of corticosteroids on bone mineral in rheumatoid arthritis and asthma. *Am J Roentgenol.* 1976;**126**:1300.
19. **Sambrook PN, Eisman JA, Yeates MG, Pocock NA, Eberl S, Champion GD.** Osteoporosis in rheumatoid arthritis: safety of low dose corticosteroids. *Ann Rheum Dis.* 1986;**45**:950-3.
20. **Reid DM, Nicoll JJ, Smith MA, Higgins B, Tothill P, Nuki G.** Corticosteroids and bone mass in asthma: comparisons with rheumatoid arthritis and polymyalgia rheumatica. *Br Med J [Clin Res].* 1986;**293**:1463-6.
21. **Rickers H, Deding A, Christiansen C, Rodbro P.** Mineral loss in cortical and trabecular bone during high-dose prednisone treatment. *Calcif Tissue Int.* 1984;**36**:269-73.
22. **Schaadt O, Bohr H.** Loss of bone mineral in axial and peripheral skeleton in aging, prednisone treatment and osteoporosis. In: Dequeker JV, Johnston CC Jr, eds. *Non-Invasive Bone Measurements: Methodological Problems.* Oxford: IRL Press; 1982:207-14.
23. **Verstraeten A, Dequeker J.** Vertebral and peripheral bone mineral content and fracture incidence in postmenopausal patients with rheumatoid arthritis: effect of low dose corticosteroids. *Ann Rheum Dis.* 1986;**45**:852-7.
24. **Dykman TR, Gluck OS, Murphy WA, Hahn TJ, Hahn BH.** Evaluation of factors associated with glucocorticoid-induced osteopenia in patients with rheumatic diseases. *Arthritis Rheum.* 1985;**28**:361-8.
25. **Als OS, Gotfredsen A, Christiansen C.** The effect of glucocorticoids on bone mass in rheumatoid arthritis patients. *Arthritis Rheum.* 1985;**28**:369-75.
26. **Seeman E, Wagner HW, Offord KP, Kumar R, Johnson WJ, Riggs BL.** Differential effects of endocrine dysfunction on the axial and appendicular skeleton. *J Clin Invest.* 1982;**69**:1302-9.
27. **Gallagher JC, Aaron J, Horsman A, Wilkinson R, Nordin BE.** Corticosteroid osteoporosis. *Clin Endocrinol Metab.* 1973;**2**:355-68.
28. **Dempster DW, Arlot MA, Meunier PJ.** Mean wall thickness and formation periods of trabecular bone packets in corticosteroid-induced osteoporosis. *Calcif Tissue Int.* 1983;**35**:410-7.
29. **Wajchenberg BL, Pereira VG, Kieffer J, Ursic S.** Effect of dexamethasone on calcium metabolism and ^{47}Ca kinetics in normal subjects. *Acta Endocrinol (Copenh).* 1983;**61**:173-92.
30. **Caniggia A, Nuti R, Lore F, Vattimo A.** Pathophysiology of the adverse effects of glucoactive corticosteroids on calcium metabolism in man. *J Steroid Biochem.* 1981;**15**:153-61.
31. **Sakakura M, Takebe K, Nakagawa S.** Inhibition of luteinizing hormone secretion induced by synthetic LRH by long-term treatment with glucocorticoids in human subjects. *J Clin Endocrinol Metab.* 1975;**40**:774-9.
32. **Luton JP, Thieblot P, Valcke JC, Mahoudeau JA, Bricaire H.** Reversible gonadotropin deficiency in male Cushing's disease.

J Clin Endocrinol Metab. 1977;**45:**488-95.
33. **Hsueh AJ, Erickson GF.** Glucocorticoid inhibition of FSH-induced estrogen production in cultured rat granulosa cells. *Steroids.* 1978;**32:**639-48.
34. **Doerr P, Pirke KM.** Cortisol-induced suppression of plasma testosterone in normal adult males. *J Clin Endocrinol Metab.* 1976;**43:**622-9.
35. **Schaison G, Durand F, Mowszowicz I.** Effect of glucocorticoids on plasma testosterone in men. *Acta Endocrinol (Copenh).* 1978;**89:**126-31.
36. **MacAdams MR, White RH, Chipps BE.** Reduction of serum testosterone levels during chronic glucocorticoid therapy. *Ann Intern Med.* 1986;**104:**648-51.
37. **Crilly RG, Cawood M, Marshall DH, Nordin BE.** Hormonal status in normal, osteoporotic and corticosteroid-treated postmenopausal women. *J R Soc Med.* 1978;**71:**733-6.
38. **Goulding A, Gold E.** Effects of chronic prednisolone treatment on bone resorption and bone composition in intact and ovariectomized rats and in ovariectomized rats receiving B-estradiol. *Endocrinology.* 1988;**122:**482-7.
39. **Caniggia A, Gennari C.** Effect of 25-hydroxycholecalciferol (25-OHCC) on intestinal absorption of ^{47}Ca in four cases of iatrogenic Cushing's syndrome. *Helv Med Acta.* 1973;**37:**221-5.
40. **Colette C, Monnier L, Pares Herbute N, Blotman F, Mirouze J.** Calcium absorption in corticoid treated subjects effects of a single oral dose of calcitriol. *Horm Metabol Res.* 1987;**19:**335-8.
41. **Klein RG, Arnaud SB, Gallagher JC, DeLuca HF, Riggs BL.** Intestinal calcium absorption in exogenous hypercortisonism. Role of 25-hydroxyvitamin D and corticosteroid dose. *J Clin Invest.* 1977;**60:**253-9.
42. **Gallagher JC, Aaron J, Horsman A, Wilkinson R, Nordin BE.** Corticosteroid osteoporosis. *Clin Endocrinol Metab.* 1973;**2:**355-68.
43. **Wajchenberg BL, Pereira VG, Kieffer J, Ursic S.** Effect of dexamethasone on calcium and ^{47}Ca kinetics in normal subjects. *Acta Endrocrinol (Copenh).* 1969;**61:**173-92.
44. **Harrison HE, Harrison HC.** Transfer of ^{45}Ca across intestinal wall in vitro in relation to action of vitamin D and cortisol. *Am J Physiol.* 1960;**199:**265-71.
45. **Lindgren U, Lindholm S, Sarby B.** Short-term effects of 1-alpha-hydroxy-vitamin D_3 in patients on corticosteroid treatment and in patients with senile osteoporosis. *Acta Med Scand.* 1978;**204:**89-92.
46. **Adams JS, Wahl TO, Lukert BP.** Effects of hydrochlorothiazide and dietary sodium restriction on calcium metabolism in corticosteroid treated patients. *Metabolism.* 1981;**30:**217-21.
47. **Findling JW, Adams ND, Lemann J, Gray RW, Thomas CJ, Tyrrell JB.** Vitamin D metabolites and parathyroid hormone in Cushing's syndrome: relationship to calcium and phosphorus homeostasis. *J Clin Endocrinol Metab.* 1982;**54:**1039-44.
48. **Kimberg DV, Baerg RD, Gershon E, Graudusius RT.** Effect of cortisone treatment on the active transport of calcium by the small intestine. *J Clin Invest.* 1971;**50:**1309-21.
49. **Favus MJ, Walling MW, Kimberg DV.** Effects of 1,25-dihydroxycholecalciferol on intestinal calcium transport in cortisone-treated rats. *J Clin Invest.* 1973;**52:**1680-5.
50. **Aloia JF, Semla HM, Yeh JK.** Discordant effects of glucocorticoids on active and passive transport of calcium in the rat duodenum. *Calcif Tissue Int.* 1984;**36:**327-31.
51. **Lukert BP, Stanbury SW, Mawer EB.** Vitamin D and intestinal transport of calcium: effects of prednisolone. *Endocrinology.* 1973;**93:**718-22.
52. **Collins EJ, Garrett ER, Johnston RL.** Effect of adrenal steroids on radiocalcium metabolism in dogs. *Metabolism.* 1962;**11:**716-26.
53. **Fox J, Care AD, Blahos J.** Effects of low calcium and low phosphorus diets on the duodenal absorption of calcium in betamethasone-treated chicks. *J Endocrinol.* 1978;**78:**255-60.
54. **Glade MJ, Krook L, Schryver HF, Hintz HF.** Calcium metabolism in glucocorticoid-treated pony foals. *J Nutr.* 1982;**112:**77-86.
55. **Liddle GW.** Effect of antiinflammatory steroids on electrolyte metabolism. *Ann N Y Acad Sci.* 1959;**82:**854-67.
56. **Williams GA, Bowser EN, Henderson WJ, Uzgiries V.** Calcium absorption in the rat in relation to excessive vitamin D and cortisone. *Proc Soc Exp Biol Med.* 1962;**110:**889-92.
57. **Hahn TJ, Halstead LR, Strates B, Imbimbo B, Baran DT.** Comparison of subacute effects of oxazacort and prednisone on mineral metabolism in man. *Calcif Tissue Int.* 1980;**31:**109-15.
58. **Milhaud G, Remagen W, deMatos G, Aubert JP.** Etude du metabolisme du calcium chez le rat a l'aide du calcium 45. II. Action de la cortisone. *Rev Fr Etud Clin Biol.* 1960;**5:**354-8.
59. **Lekkerkerker JF, Van Woudenberg F, Doorenbos HD.** Influence of low dose of sterol therapy on calcium absorption. *Acta Endocrinol (Copenh).* 1972;**69:**488-96.
60. **Sjoberg HE.** Retention of orally administered 47-calcium in man under normal and diseased conditions studied with a whole-body counter technique. *Acta Med Scand.* 1970;**509**(Suppl):1-28.
61. **Lee DB.** Unanticipated stimulatory action of glucocorticoids on epithelial calcium absorption. Effect of dexamethasone on rat distal colon. *J Clin Invest.* 1983;**71:**322-8.
62. **Binder HJ.** Effect of dexamethasone on electrolyte transport in the large intestine of the rat. *Gastroenterology.* 1978;**75:**212-7.
63. **Nordin BE, Young MM, Oxby C, Bulusu L.** Calculation of calcium absorption rate from plasma radioactivity. *Clin Sci.* 1968;**35:**177-82.
64. **Ferretti JL, Bazan JL, Alloatti D, Puche RC.** The intestinal handling of calcium by the rat in vivo, as affected by cortisol. Effect of dietary calcium supplements. *Calcif Tissue Res.* 1978;**25:**1-6.
65. **Shultz TD, Bollman S, Kumar R.** Decreased intestinal calcium absorption in vivo and normal brush border membrane vesicle calcium uptake in cortisol-treated chickens: evidence for dissociation of calcium absorption from brush border vesicle uptake. *Proc Natl Acad Sci USA.* 1982;**79:**3542-6.
66. **Feher JJ, Wasserman RH.** Intestinal calcium binding protein and calcium absorption in cortisol treated chicks: effects of vitamin D_3 and 1,25-dyhydroxyvitamin D_3. *Endocrinology.* 1979;**104:**547-51.
67. **Kimura S, Rasmussen H.** Adrenal glucocorticoids, adenine nucleotide translocation, and mitochondrial calcium accumulation. *J Biol Chem.* 1977;**252:**1217-25.
68. **Charney AN, Kinsey MD, Myers L, Giannella RA, Gots RE.** Na^+-K^+-activated adenosine triphosphatase and intestinal electrolyte transport. Effect of adrenal steroids. *J Clin Invest.* 1975;**56:**653-60.
69. **Adams JS, Lukert BP.** Effects of sodium restriction on ^{45}Ca and ^{22}Na transduodenal flux in corticosteroid-treated rats. *Miner Electrolyte Metab.* 1980;**4:**216-26.
70. **Chesney RW, Mazess RB, Hamstra AJ, DeLuca HF, O'Reagan S.** Reduction of serum-1, 25-dihydroxyvitamin D_3 in children receiving glucocorticoids. *Lancet.* 1978;**2:**1123-5.
71. **Zerwekh JE, Emkey RD, Harris ED Jr.** Low-dose prednisone therapy in rheumatoid arthritis: effect on vitamin D metabolism. *Arthritis Rheum.* 1984;**27:**1050-2.
72. **Hahn TJ, Halstead LR, Baran DT.** Effects of short term glucocorticoid administration on intestinal calcium absorption and circulating vitamin D metabolite concentrations in man. *J Clin Endocrinol Metab.* 1981;**52:**111-5.
73. **Seeman E, Kumar R, Hunder GG, Scott M, Heath H III, Riggs BL.** Production, degradation, and circulating levels of 1,25-dihydroxyvitamin D in health and in chronic glucocorticoid excess. *J Clin Invest.* 1980;**66:**664-9.
74. **Hirst M, Feldman D.** Glucocorticoid regulation of 1,25(OH)2-vitamin D_3 receptors: divergent effects on mouse and rat intestine. *Endocrinology.* 1982;**111:**1400-2.
75. **Carre M, Ayigbede O, Miravet L, Rasmussen H.** The effect of prednisolone upon the metabolism and action of 25-hydroxy- and 1,25-dihydroxyvitamin D_3. *Proc Natl Acad Sci USA.* 1974;**1:**2996-3000.
76. **Suzuki Y, Ichikawa Y, Saito E, Homma M.** Importance of increased urinary calcium excretion in the development of secondary hyperparathyroidism of patients under glucocorticoid therapy. *Metabolism.* 1983;**32:**151-6.
77. **Nielsen HK, Thomsen K, Eriksen EF, Charles P, Storm T, Mosekilde L.** The effect of high-dose glucocorticoid administration on serum bone gamma carboxyglutamic acid-containing protein, serum alkaline phosphatase and vitamin D metabolites in normal subjects. *Bone Miner.* 1988;**4:**105-13.
78. **Lukert BP, Adams JS.** Calcium and phosphorus homeostatis in man. Effect of corticosteroids. *Arch Intern Med.* 1976;**136:**1249-53.
79. **Fucik RF, Kukreja SC, Hargis GK, Bowser EN, Henderson WJ, Williams GA.** Effect of glucocorticoids on function of the parathyroid glands in man. *J Clin Endocrinol Metab.* 1975;**40:**152-5.
80. **Au WY.** Cortisol stimulation of parathyroid hormone secretion by rat parathyroid glands in organ culture. *Science.* 1976;**193:**1015-7.
81. **Frieberg JM, Kinsella J, Sacktor B.** Glucocorticoids increase the Na^+-H^+ exchange and decrease the Na^+ gradient-dependent phosphate-uptake systems in renal brush border membrane vesicles. *Proc Natl Acad Sci USA.* 1982;**79:**4932-6.
82. **Meunier PJ, Bressot C.** Endocrine influences on bone cells and bone remodeling evaluated by clinical histomorphometry. In: Parsons JA, ed. *Endocrinology of Calcium Metabolism.* New York: Raven Press; 1982:445-65.
83. **Lund B, Storm TL, Lund B, et al.** Bone mineral loss, bone histomorphometry and vitamin D metabolism in patients with rheumatoid arthritis on long-term glucocorticoid treatment. *Clin Rheumatol.* 1985;**4:**143-9.
84. **Kukreja SC, Bowser EN, Hargis GK, Henderson WJ, Williams GA.** Mechanisms of glucocorticoid-induced osteopenia: role of parathyroid glands. *Proc Soc Exp Biol Med.* 1976;**152:**358-61.
85. **Stern PH.** Inhibition by steroids of parathyroid hormone-induced ^{45}Ca release from embryonic rat bone in vitro. *J Pharmacol Exp Ther.* 1969;**168:**211-7.
86. **Baron R, Magee S, Silverglate A, Broadus A, Lang R.** Estimation

of trabecular bone resorption by histomorphometry: evidence for prolonged reversal phase with normal resorption in post-menopausal osteoporosis and coupled increased resorption in primary hyperparathyroidism. In: Frame B, Potts JT, eds. *Clinical Disorders of Bone and Mineral Metabolism.* Princeton, NJ: Excerpta Medica; 1983:191-5.

87. **Reid IR, Katz JM, Ibbertson HK, Gray DH.** The effects of hydrocortisone, parathyroid hormone, and the bisphosphonate, APD, on bone resorption in neonatal mouse calvaria. *Calcif Tissue Int.* 1986;**38:**38-43.
88. **Gronowicz G, McCarthy MB, Woodiel F, Raisz LG.** Effects of corticosterone and parathyroid hormone on formation and resorption in cultured fetal rat parietal bones [Abstract]. *Amer Soc Bone Mineral Research.* 1988;**3**(Suppl 1):5114.
89. **Bar-Shavit Z, Kahn AJ, Pegg LE, Stone KR, Teitelbaum SL.** Glucocorticoids modulate macrophage surface oligosaccharides and their bone binding activity. *J Clin Invest.* 1984;**73:**1277-83.
90. **Raisz LG, Trummel CL, Wener JA, Simmons H.** Effect of glucocorticoids on bone resorption in tissue culture. *Endocrinology.* 1972;**90:**961-7.
91. **Knudsen PJ, Dinarello CA, Strom TB.** Glucocorticoids inhibit transcriptional and post-transcriptional expression of interleukin-1 in U937 cells. *J Immunol.* 1987;**139:**4129-34.
92. **Wong GL.** Basal activities and hormone responsiveness of osteoclast-like and osteoblast-like bone cells are regulated by glucocorticoids. *J Biol Chem.* 1979;**254:**6337-40.
93. **Frost HM, Villanueva AR.** The effect of cortisone on lamellar osteoblastic activity. *Henry Ford Hosp Med J.* 1961;**9:**97-9.
94. **Catherwood BD.** 1,25-Dihydrocholecalciferol and glucocorticoid regulation of adenylate cyclase in an osteoblast-like cell line. *J Biol Chem.* 1985;**160:**736-43.
95. **Chen TL, Feldman D.** Glucocorticoid receptors and actions in subpopulations of cultured rat bone cells. Mechanism of dexamethasone potentiation of parathyroid hormone-stimulated cyclic AMP production. *J Clin Invest.* 1979;**63:**750-8.
96. **Ng B, Hekkelman JW, Heersche JN.** The effect of cortisol on the adenosine 3',5'-monophosphate response to parathyroid hormone in cultured rat bone cells. *Endocrinology.* 1979;**102:**589-96.
97. **Hahn TJ, Halstead LR.** Cortisol enhancement of PTH-stimulated cyclic AMP accumulation in cultured fetal rat long bone rudiments. *Calcif Tissue Int.* 1979;**29:**173-5.
98. **Chen TL, Feldman D.** Glucocorticoid potentiation of the adenosine 3',5'-monophosphate response to parathyroid hormone in cultured rat bone cells, *Endocrinology.* 1978;**102:**589-96.
99. **Heersche JN, Jez DH, Aubin J, Sodek J.** Regulation of hormone responsiveness of bone in vitro by corticosteroids, PTH, PGE2 and calcitonin. In: Talmage RV, Cohn DV, Matthews JL, eds. *Hormonal Control of Calcium Metabolism.* Amsterdam: Excerpta Medica; 1981: 157-62. (International Congress Series no. 511.)
100. **Chen TL, Cone CM, Morey-Holton E, Feldman D.** Glucocorticoid regulation of 1,25(OH)2-vitamin D_3 receptors in cultured mouse bone cells. *J Biol Chem.* 1982;**257:**13564-9.
101. **Chen TL, Cone CM, Morey-Holton E, Feldman D.** 1 alpha,25-dihydroxyvitamin D_3 receptors in cultured rat osteoblast-like cells. Glucocorticoid treatment increases receptor content. *J Biol Chem.* 1983;**258:**4350-5.
102. **Nielsen HK, Eriksen EF, Storm T, Mosekilde L.** The effects of short-term, high-dose treatment with prednisone on the nuclear uptake of 1,25-dihydroxyvitamin D_3 in monocytes from normal human subjects. *Metabolism.* 1988;**37:**109-14.
103. **Blumenkrantz N, Sondergaard J.** Effect of prostaglandins E1 and F1 on biosynthesis of collagen. *Nature New Biol.* 1972;**239:**246.
104. **Chyun YS, Raisz LG.** Stimulation of bone formation by prostaglandin E2. *Prostaglandins.* 1984;**27:**97-103.
105. **Raisz LG, Simmons HA.** Effects of parathyroid hormone and cortisol on prostaglandin production by neonatal rat calvaria in vitro. *Endocr Res.* 1985;**11:**59-74.
106. **Chyun YS, Raisz LG.** Opposing effects of prostaglandin E2 and cortisol in bone growth in organ culture. *Clin Res.* 1982;**30:**387A.
107. **Kelso A, Munck A.** Glucocorticoid inhibition of lymphokine secretion by alloreactive T lymphocyte clones. *J Immunol.* 1984;**133:**784-91.
108. **Sato K, Fujii Y, Kasono K, Saji M, Tsushima T, Shizume K.** Stimulation of prostaglandin E2 and bone resorption by recombinant human interleukin 1-alpha in fetal mouse bones. *Biochem Biophys Res Commun.* 1986;**138:**618-24.
109. **Morris HG, Jorgensen JR, Jenkins SA.** Plasma growth hormone concentrations in corticosteroid-treated children. *J Clin Invest.* 1968;**47:**427-35.
110. **Gourmelen M, Girard F, Binoux M.** Serum somatomedin/insulin-like growth factor (IGF) and IGF carrier levels in patients with Cushing's syndrome or receiving glucocorticoid therapy. *J Clin Endocrinol Metab.* 1982;**54:**885-92.
111. **Bennett A, Chen T, Feldman D, Hintz RL, Rosenfeld DG.** Characterization of insulin-like growth factor I receptors on rat bone cells: regulation of receptor concentration by glucocorticoids. *Endocrinology.* 1984;**115:**1577-83.
112. **Unterman TG, Phillips LS.** Glucocorticoid effects on somatomedins and somatomedin inhibitors. *J Clin Endocrinol Metab.* 1985;**61:**618-26.
113. **Canalis E, McCarthy T, Centrella M.** Isolation of growth factors from adult bovine bone. *Calcif Tissue Int.* 1988;**43:**346-51.
114. **Hahn TJ, Westbrook SL, Halstead LR.** Cortisol modulation of osteoblast metabolic activity in cultured neonatal rat bone. *Endocrinology.* 1984;**114:**1864-70.
115. **Dietrich JW, Canalis EM, Maina DM, Raisz LG.** Effect of glucocorticoids on fetal rat bone collagen synthesis in vitro. *Endocrinology.* 1979;**104:**715-21.
116. **Canalis EM.** Effect of glucocorticoids on type I collagen synthesis, alkaline phosphatase activity, and deoxyribonucleic acid content in cultured rat calvariae. *Endocrinology.* 1983;**112:**931-9.
117. **Canalis EM.** Effect of corticol on periosteal and nonperiosteal collagen and DNA synthesis in cultured rat calvariae. *Calcif Tissue Int.* 1984;**36:**158-66.
118. **Chyun YS, Kream BE, Raisz LG.** Cortisol decreases bone formation by inhibiting periosteal cell proliferation. *Endocrinology.* 1984;**114:**477-80.
119. **Uphill PF, Daniel MR.** A comparison of the effects of tixocortol pivalate (JO 1016), hydrocortisone acetate and beclomethasone dipropionate on collagen synthesis and degradation. *Arzneimittelforschung.* 1981;**31:**467-9.
120. **Verbruggen LA, Salomon DS, Greene RM.** Inhibition of collagen and sulfated glycosaminoglycan synthesis in neonatal mouse dermal fibroblasts by corticosterone. *Biochem Pharmacol.* 1981;**30:**3285-9.
121. **Saarni H, Jalkanen M, Hopsu-Havu VK.** Effect of five anti-inflammatory steroids on collagen and glycoaminoglycan synthesis in vitro. *Br J Dermatol.* 1980;**103:**167-73.
122. **Pietrogrande V, Mastromarino R.** Osteopatia da prolungato trattamento cortisonico. *Orthop Traum Appar Mot.* 1957;**25:**791-3.
123. **Bloch-Michel H, Benoist M, Peyron J.** Osteonecroses aseptiques au cours de la corticotherapie du pemphigus. *Rev Rhum Mal Osteoartic.* 1959;**26:**648-50.
124. **Fisher DE, Bickel WH.** Corticosteroid-induced avascular necrosis. A clinical study of seventy-seven patients. *J Bone Joint Surg [Am].* 1971;**53:**859-73.
125. **Cruess RL, Ross D, Crawshaw E.** The etiology of steroid-induced avascular necrosis of bone. A laboratory and clinical study. *Clin Orthop.* 1975;**113:**178-83.
126. **Frost HM.** Presence of microscopic cracks in vivo in bone. *Henry Ford Hosp Med J.* 1960;**8:**25.
127. **Frost HM.** *Orthopaedic Biomechanics.* Springfield: C.C. Thomas; 1973:185-90.
128. **Laurent J, Meunier P, Vignon PJ Jr.** Etude anatomique et pathogenique de l'osteonecrose de la tete femorale chez l'adult. *Lyon Med.* 1973;**230:**163.
129. **Afifi AK, Bergman RA, Harvey JC.** Steroid myopathy. Clinical, histologic and cytologic observations. *Johns Hopkins Med J.* 1968;**123:**158-73.
130. **William RS.** Triamcinolone myopathy. *Lancet.* 1959;**1:**698-701.
131. **Harman JB.** Muscular wasting and corticosteroids therapy. *Lancet.* 1959;**1:**887.
132. **Askari A, Vignos PJ Jr, Moskowitz RW.** Steroid myopathy in connective tissue disease. *Am J Med.* 1976;**61:**485-92.
133. **Pleasure DE, Walsh GO, Engel WK.** Atrophy of skeletal muscle in patients with Cushing's syndrome. *Arch Neurol.* 1970;**22:**118-25.
134. **Rebuffe-Scrive M, Krotkiewski M, Elfverson J, Bjorntorp P.** Muscle and adipose tissue morphology and metabolism in Cushing's syndrome. *J Clin Endocrinol Metab.* 1988;**67:**1122-8.
135. **Danneskiold-Samsoe B, Grimby G.** The influence of prednisolone on the muscle morphology and muscle enzymes in patients with rheumatoid arthritis. *Clin Sci.* 1986;**71:**693-701.
136. **Ortoft G, Oxlund H.** Reduced strength of rat cortical bone after glucocorticoid treatment. *Calcif Tissue Int.* 1988;**43:**376-82.
137. **Lukert BP, Higgins JC, Stoskopf MM.** Serum osteocalcin is increased in patients with hyperthyroidism and decreased in patients receiving glucocorticoids. *J Clin Endocrinol Metab.* 1986;**62:**1056-8.
138. **Nielsen HK, Thomsen K, Eriksen EF, Storm T, Mosekilde L.** The effect of high-dose glucocorticoid administration on serum bone gamma carboxyglutamic acid containing protein, serum alkaline phosphatase and vitamin D metabolites in normal subjects. *Bone Miner.* 1987;**4:**105-8.
139. **Reid IR, Chapman GE, Fraser TR, et al.** Low serum osteocalcin levels in glucocorticoids-treated asthmatics. *J Clin Endocrinol Metab.* 1986;**62:**379-83.
140. **Ekenstam E, Stalenheim G, Hallgren R.** The acute effect of high dose corticosteroid treatment on serum osteocalcin. *Metabolism.* 1988;**37:**141-4.
141. **Nielsen HK, Charles P, Mosekilde L.** The effect of single oral

doses of prednisone on the circadian rhythm of serum osteocalcin in normal subjects. *J Clin Endocrinol Metab.* 1988;**67:**1025-30.

142. **Need AG, Philcox JC, Hartley TF, Nordin BE.** Calcium metabolism and osteoporosis in corticosteroid-treated postmenopausal women. *Aust N Z J Med.* 1986;**16:**341-6.
143. **Maldague B, Malghem J, de Deuxchaisnes C.** Radiologic aspects of glucocorticoid-induced bone disease. *Adv Exp Med Biol.* 1984;**171:**155-90.
144. **Riggs BL, Wahner HW, Dunn WL, Mazess RB, Offord KP, Melton LJ III.** Differential changes in bone mineral density of appendicular and axial skeleton with aging: relationship to spinal osteoporosis. *J Clin Invest.* 1981;**67:**328-35.
145. **Bijlsma JW, Raymakers JA, Mosch C, et al.** Effect of oral calcium and vitamin D on glucocorticoid-induced osteopenia. *Clin Exp Rheumatol.* 1988;**6:**113-9.
146. **Condon JR, Nassim JR, Dent CE, Hilb A, Stainthorpe EM.** Possible prevention and treatment of steroid-induced osteoporosis. *Postgrad Med J.* 1978;**54:**249-52.
147. **Braun JJ, Birkenhager-Frenkel DH, Rietveld AH, Juttman JR, Vissen TJ, Birkenhager JC.** Influence of 1 α-(OH)D_3 administration on bone and bone mineral metabolism in patients on chronic glucocorticoid treatment; a double-blind controlled study. *Clin Endocrinol (Oxf).* 1983;**19:**265-73.
148. **Reid IR, Ibbertson HK.** Calcium supplements in the prevention of steroid-induced osteoporosis. *Am J Clin Nutr.* 1986;**44:**287-90.
149. **Schwartzman MS, Franck WA.** Vitamin D toxicity complicating the treatment of senile, postmenopausal, and glucocorticoid-induced osteoporosis. Four case reports and a critical commentary on the use of vitamin D in these disorders. *Am J Med.* 1987;**82:**224-30.
150. **Slovik DM, Rosenthal DI, Doppelt SH, et al.** Restoration of spinal bone in osteoporotic men by treatment with human parathyroid hormone (1-34) and 1,25-dihydroxyvitamin D. *J Bone Miner Res.* 1986;**1:**377-81.
151. **Dunn CW.** The Cushing's syndrome. *Endocrinology.* 1938;**22:**375-85.
152. **Keutmann EH, Friedman HA, Bassett SH, Kochakian CD, Russ EM.** Metabolic studies in Cushing's syndrome: treatment with various androgens and a six-year follow-up. *Am J Med.* 1948;**5:**518-31.
153. **Foresta C, Ruzza G, Mioni R, Meneghello A, Baccichetti C.** Testosterone and bone loss in Klinefelter syndrome. *Horm Metab Res.* 1983;**15:**56-7.
154. **Need AG.** Corticosteroids and osteoporosis. *Aust N Z J Med.* 1987;**17:**267-72.
155. **Meunier PJ, Birancon D, Chavassieux P, et al.** Treatment with fluoride: bone histomorphometric findings. In: Christiansen C, Johansen JS, Riis BJ, eds. *Osteoporosis 1987.* Copenhagen: Osteopress; 1987:824-8.
156. **Ringe JD, Welzel D.** Salmon calcitonin in the therapy of corticoid-induced osteoporosis. *Eur J Clin Pharmacol.* 1987;**33:**35-9.
157. **Reid IR, King AR, Alexander CJ, Ibbertson HK.** Prevention of steroid-induced osteoporosis with (3-amino-1-hydroxypropylidene)-1,1-bisphosphonate (APD). *Lancet.* 1988;**1:**143-6.
158. **Reid IR, Heap SW, King AR, Ibbertson HK.** Two-year follow-up of biphosphonate (APD) treatment in steroid osteoporosis [Letter]. *Lancet.* 1988;**2:**1144.
159. **Pocock NA, Eisman JA, Dunstan CR, Evans RA, Thomas DH, Huq NL.** Recovery from steroid-induced osteoporosis. *Ann Intern Med.* 1987;**107:**319-23.
160. **Reid IR.** Pathogenesis and treatment of steroid osteoporosis. *Clin Endocrinol (Oxf).* 1989;**30:**83-103.

Wegener Granulomatosis: An Analysis of 158 Patients

Gary S. Hoffman, MD; Gail S. Kerr, MD; Randi Y. Leavitt, MD, PhD; Claire W. Hallahan, MS;
Robert S. Lebovics, MD; William D. Travis, MD; Menachem Rottem, MD;
and Anthony S. Fauci, MD

■ *Objective:* To prospectively study the clinical features, pathophysiology, treatment, and prognosis of Wegener granulomatosis.

■ *Design:* Of the 180 patients with Wegener granulomatosis referred to the National Institute of Allergy and Infectious Diseases during the past 24 years, 158 have been followed for 6 months to 24 years (a total of 1229 patient-years).

■ *Measurements:* Characteristics of clinical presentation, surgical pathology, course of illness, laboratory and radiographic findings, and the results of medical and surgical treatment have been recorded in a computer-based information retrieval system.

■ *Setting:* The Warren Magnuson Clinical Center of the National Institutes of Health.

■ *Main Results:* Men and women were equally represented; 97% of patients were white, and 85% were more than 19 years of age. The mean period of follow-up was 8 years. One hundred and thirty-three patients (84%) received "standard" therapy with daily low-dose cyclophosphamide and glucocorticoids. Eight (5.0%) received only low-dose cyclophosphamide. Six (4.0%) never received cyclophosphamide and were treated with other cytotoxic agents and glucocorticoids. Ten patients (6.0%) were treated with only glucocorticoids. Ninety-one percent of patients experienced marked improvement, and 75% achieved complete remission. Fifty percent of remissions were associated with one or more relapses. Of 99 patients followed for > 5 years, 44% had remissions of > 5 years duration. Thirteen percent of patients died of Wegener granulomatosis, treatment-related causes, or both. Almost all patients had serious morbidity from irreversible features of their disease (86%) or side effects of treatment (42%).

■ *Conclusions:* The course of Wegener granulomatosis has been dramatically improved by daily treatment with cyclophosphamide and glucocorticoids. Nonetheless, disease- and treatment-related morbidity is often profound. Alternative forms of therapy have not yet achieved the high rates of remission induction and successful maintenance that have been reported with daily cyclophosphamide treatment. Despite continued therapeutic success with cyclophosphamide, our long-term follow-up of patients with Wegener granulomatosis has led to increasing concerns about toxicity resulting from prolonged cyclophosphamide therapy and has encouraged investigation of other therapeutic regimens.

Annals of Internal Medicine. 1992;**116:**488-498.

From the National Institutes of Health, Bethesda, Maryland. For current author addresses, see end of text.

Wegener granulomatosis is distinguished from other necrotizing vasculitides by its predilection to affect the upper and lower respiratory tracts and, in most cases, the kidneys. Inflammatory lesions typically include necrosis, granulomatous changes, and vasculitis (1-7). Relatively mild forms of disease without renal involvement have been previously described. The course of illness in such patients may vary from indolence to rapid progression. However, most patients with untreated or ineffectively treated generalized disease (including glomerulonephritis) experience a rapidly progressive, fatal illness (7, 8). In prospective studies (5, 6) we have shown that Wegener granulomatosis could be effectively treated using low-dose daily cyclophosphamide and glucocorticoids. These observations have been confirmed by other investigators (9). The National Institutes of Health (NIH) experience has grown to include 180 patients with Wegener granulomatosis. Adequate follow-up to characterize disease and treatment was available for 158 of these patients. Although treatment has been life-saving, extended follow-up has led to recognition of a greater frequency of disease relapse, morbidity, and drug toxicity than had been previously recognized.

Methods

Enrollment of patients in the NIH protocol required a clinical history that was compatible with Wegener granulomatosis and histopathologic evidence of either vasculitis or granulomatous changes in a typical organ system. Cultures and special stains for bacteria, fungi, and mycobacteria were obtained from all nonrenal biopsy samples and appropriate body fluids to rule out infectious granulomatous processes.

Treatment Protocol

The protocol treatment regimen has been previously described (6). In brief, the regimen consisted of daily, oral therapy with cyclophosphamide, 2 mg/kg body weight, and prednisone, 1 mg/kg body weight. Several patients with fulminant and rapidly progressive disease received 3 to 5 mg/kg of cyclophosphamide daily. We used the leukocyte count to guide subsequent dosage adjustments in these patients. Under these circumstances, prednisone (or a soluble parenteral equivalent) was usually given for the first few days at a daily dose that varied from 2 to 15 mg/kg. Daily prednisone therapy was continued for approximately 4 weeks and then changed over 1 to 3 months to 60 mg on alternate days. The dose was tapered gradually until the patient no longer received prednisone and was maintained solely on cyclophosphamide. The duration of alternate-day prednisone therapy varied according to individual responses to therapy. Cyclophosphamide was continued for at least 1 year after the patient achieved complete remission. Cyclophosphamide was then tapered by 25-mg decrements every 2 to 3 months until discontinuation or until disease recurrence required a dose increase.

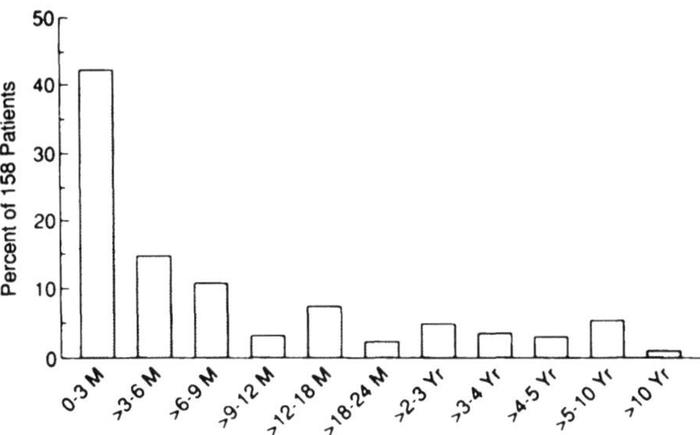

Figure 1. Time from onset of Wegener granulomatosis to diagnosis. Patients with limited disease, without renal involvement or severe lung disease, may have an indolent course. Such atypical presentations may result in marked delay in diagnosis.

Criteria for Remission

Partial remission was defined as clear-cut suppression of disease with stabilization of renal function and at least partial resolution of pulmonary infiltrates. Further, other organ system disease was required to show signs of improvement to be classified as a partial remission. Criteria for complete remission included the absence of evidence of active disease, complete resolution of pulmonary infiltrates or evidence of stable scarring without signs of active inflammation, absence of systemic inflammatory disease such as serositis and fever, and stabilization or improvement in renal function with no further evidence of active renal sediment. Minor abnormalities of urine sediment, compatible with previous glomerular damage, were present in some patients who achieved a complete remission.

Results

Patient Sample

Although our previously reported experience suggested a slight male predominance (6), our larger sample of 158 patients included equal numbers of men and women. Of these patients, 97% were white, 2% were black, and 1% were of other racial backgrounds. The mean age was 41 years (range, 9 to 78 years), and 15% of patients were less than 19 years of age.

Presenting Features of Disease

The median and mean periods from the onset of symptoms to a diagnosis of Wegener granulomatosis were 4.7 and 15 months, respectively. In some cases, the correct diagnosis was apparent at the first physician visit. The diagnosis of Wegener granulomatosis was made within 3 months of symptom onset in 42% of patients, but in 8% of patients the diagnosis was not made until 5 to 16 years later. Patients in this latter group had indolent progression of mild disease that led to delays in diagnosis. Inclusion of these patients accounts for the large variation between the mean and the median (Figure 1).

The signs and symptoms of Wegener granulomatosis that were present at disease onset and during the course of illness are shown in Figures 2 and 3. Most patients first sought medical care because of upper or lower airway symptoms or both (90%). Nasal, sinus, tracheal (upper airway), or ear abnormalities were initially responsible for symptoms in 73% of patients and occurred in 92% of patients overall (Figure 2 and Figure 3, *top left*). In the absence of systemic illness, these problems were often considered to be secondary to allergy or infection. Symptomatic treatment, followed by persistent symptoms and complications, especially recurrent epistaxis, mucosal ulcerations, nasal septal perforation, or nasal deformity, led in some cases to more extensive evaluation. The findings of an active urine sediment, pulmonary infiltrates or nodules, elevated erythrocyte sedimentation rates, unexplained anemia, and, in recent years, antineutrophil cytoplasmic antibodies (ANCA) prompted some referring physicians to pursue definitive diagnosis by biopsy of the involved organs. In 30% of cases, the absence of rigorous pursuit of diagnosis, the lack of symptomatic pulmonary and renal findings, or the indolent course of illness led to delays in diagnosis greater than 1 year.

Pulmonary infiltrates, nodules, or both were initially present in 45% of patients (Figure 3, *top right*, and Figure 4). Symptoms included cough (19%), hemoptysis (12%), and pleuritis (10%). During the entire course of illness, 66% of all episodes (241) of Wegener granulomatosis were associated with either cough (46%), hemoptysis (30%), and/or pleuritis (28%). In about 34% of cases radiographs showed infiltrates or nodules that were asymptomatic. Eighty-five percent of patients eventually developed lung disease related to Wegener granulomatosis.

As previously reported (6), several patients (18%) presented with features of glomerulonephritis (*see* Figure 2); in all such cases renal disease was asymptomatic. Seventy-seven percent of patients later developed glomerulonephritis, usually within the first 2 years of disease onset.

Ocular abnormalities were noted in 15% of patients (*see* Figure 2 and Figure 3, *bottom left*) during the early phases of Wegener granulomatosis and in most cases produced significant symptoms. Fifty-two percent of patients eventually developed one or more features of eye disease, which, in general, were nonspecific. The most diagnostically helpful ocular finding was proptosis, which, when present in the setting of upper or lower airway disease or glomerulonephritis, was strongly suggestive of Wegener granulomatosis. Proptosis was present in 2% of patients at disease onset and in 15% at

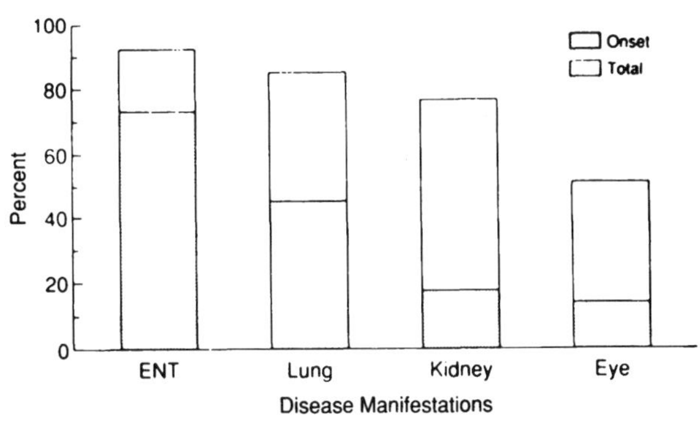

Figure 2. Major organ systems affected by Wegener granulomatosis. ENT = ear, nose, and throat involvement.

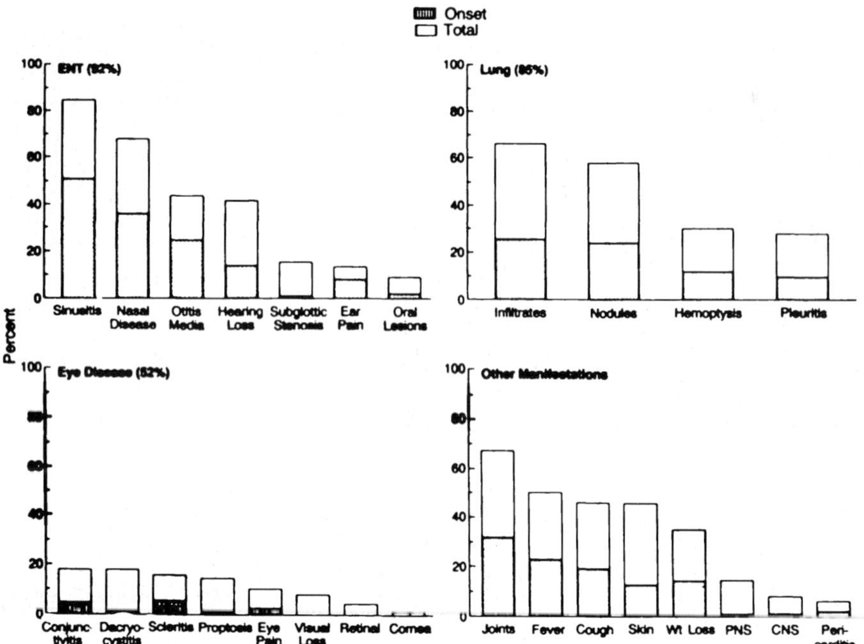

Figure 3. Type and frequency of disease manifestations are represented at the time of presentation and as they may have occurred during the course of illness. ENT = ear, nose, and throat involvement.

some time during the course of illness. Proptosis was usually painful (Figure 5). About half of the patients with retro-orbital pseudotumors lost vision due to optic nerve ischemia. Entrapment of extraocular muscles also led to loss of conjugate gaze that caused diplopia.

Other Manifestations

Musculoskeletal symptoms were a prominent feature of disease in 67% of patients. Most patients experienced only arthralgias or myalgias. In patients with persistent or recurrent musculoskeletal symptoms, the differential diagnosis was perplexing. In several cases symmetrical involvement of small and large joints, in conjunction with false-positive test results for rheumatoid factor (60%), led to the incorrect diagnosis of rheumatoid arthritis. In several patients monarticular disease needed to be distinguished from microcrystalline and septic arthritis. Other patients had pauciarticular or migratory polyarthritis. In no instance did deformity occur. For some patients in whom musculoskeletal symptoms were the main initial feature of disease, the diagnosis of Wegener granulomatosis was not made until other, more classic features of illness were present.

Fever due to Wegener granulomatosis was initially present in 23% of patients and occurred in 50% during the course of illness. In all cases, the presence of fever led to an evaluation for secondary infection. Significant weight loss, defined as a loss greater than 10% of usual body weight, occurred in 15% of patients at disease onset and in 35% of patients overall. When weight loss was present initially in conjunction with persistent fever, patients had frequently been evaluated by referring physicians for occult malignancy before a diagnosis of Wegener granulomatosis was made.

Skin disease occurred in 13% of patients initially and in 46% of patients overall. Lesions included palpable purpura, ulcers, vesicles, papules, and subcutaneous nodules.

Nervous system involvement was rare at initial presentation, but mononeuritis multiplex developed eventually in 15% of patients, and central nervous system abnormalities occurred in 8% of patients. The latter included stroke, cranial nerve abnormalities, and one case of diabetes insipidus.

Ten (6%) patients developed pericarditis. In eight patients, pericarditis was symptomatic. In one patient, hemodynamic compromise required pericardiocentesis and pericardiectomy. Cardiac muscle or vessel involvement unequivocally due to Wegener granulomatosis was uncommon (< 2% of patients).

Biopsy-proven Wegener granulomatosis was noted rarely (< 1% of patients) in the parotid gland, pulmonary artery, breast, urethra, cervix, and vagina.

Laboratory Data

Sera from 106 patients with Wegener granulomatosis, 40 healthy controls, and 70 patients with disease other

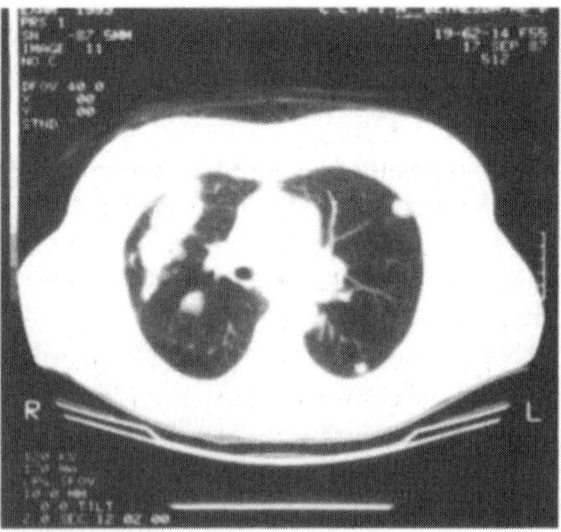

Figure 4. Wegener granulomatosis lung disease may be unilateral or bilateral and may consist of infiltrates, nodules, hemorrhage, or a combination of abnormalities. The right lung field (*left*) seen in the computed axial tomographic scan in this patient includes an example of coalescent nodules.

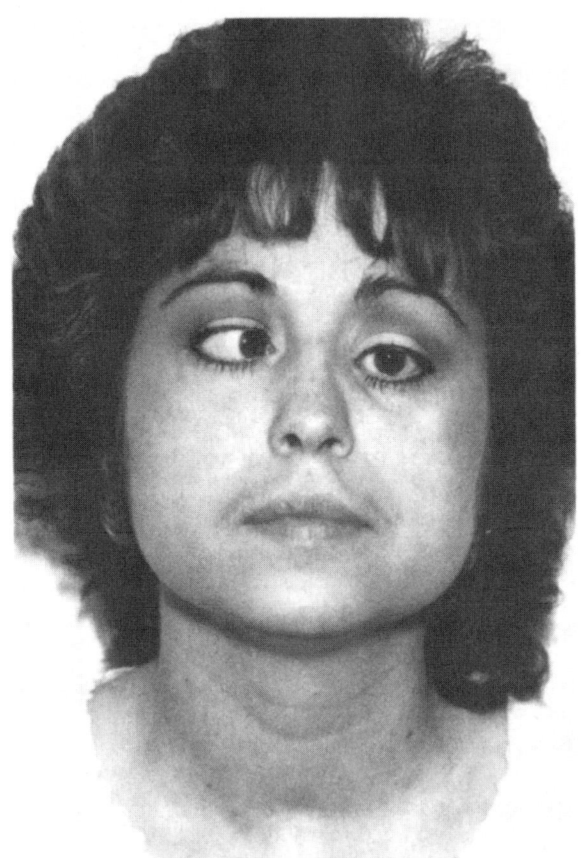

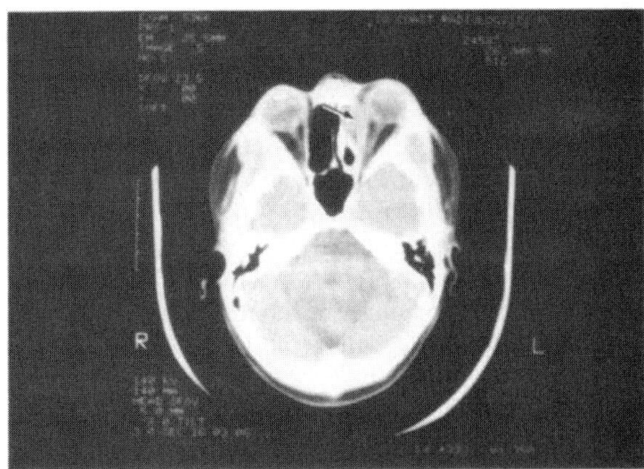

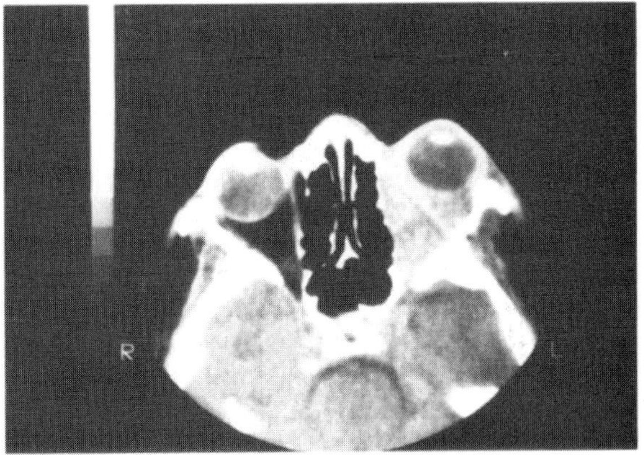

Figure 5. Optic and retro-orbital manifestations of Wegener granulomatosis. Left. Retro-orbital pseudotumor has resulted in proptosis; the position of the left eye is fixed and unable to deviate in conjunction with the right eye. **Right, top.** A computed axial tomographic scan of the orbits shows entrapment (*arrow*) of the medial and inferior rectus muscles, as well as impingement on the optic nerve. **Right, bottom.** In a similar patient, a computed axial tomographic scan shows complete filling of the retro-orbital space with inflammatory-fibrotic tissue that caused blindness. The extent to which fibrous tissue has filled the retro-orbital space is a major determinant of visual outcome after immunosuppressive treatment.

than Wegener granulomatosis were tested using indirect immunofluorescence (10) for the presence of ANCA. Leukocytes from normal volunteers were placed on glass slides and fixed in 95% ethanol. Sera from 88% of patients with active Wegener granulomatosis and 43% of patients in remission produced diffuse granular cytoplasmic (C-ANCA) immunofluorescent staining of neutrophils. The difference in positive results between patients with active disease and those in remission was significant (P = 0.008, Fisher exact test). Among patients with active disease, however, no significant differences in test results were noted between treated and untreated patients. Sera from five patients (5%) produced perinuclear (P-ANCA) immunofluorescent staining, which is not a useful diagnostic tool for Wegener granulomatosis. The C-ANCA findings are similar to those previously reported (11-13), in which about 40% of patients in remission and > 90% of patients with active Wegener granulomatosis had positive test results. None of the ANCA studies in the 40 normal controls, 13 patients with polyarteritis nodosa, 21 with idiopathic inflammatory lung disease, 12 with uveitis, 2 with systemic lupus erythematosis, or 2 with polymyositis showed granular cytoplasmic staining. One of 12 patients with Takayasu disease, 1 of 3 with lymphomatoid granulomatosis, and 1 patient with isolated cutaneous vasculitis had positive C-ANCA results at a low titer (≤ 1:80). Sera from one patient each with polyarteritis nodosa, uveitis, and polymyositis produced a P-ANCA pattern.

In a previous study, Cohen Tervaert and colleagues (14) suggested that in stable patients with Wegener granulomatosis, a rise in C-ANCA titer usually portends a clinical exacerbation. Although some investigators feel that this association justifies increased immunosuppressive therapy, we feel that such measures may be premature. The sample in this study was small (20 patients), and about half of the patients who had an asymptomatic rise in C-ANCA experienced delays in clinical exacerbation of 1 to 2 years. Currently, it seems more prudent to simply follow more closely those patients with such isolated serologic changes.

Before initiation of therapy, patients with active Wegener granulomatosis often had leukocytosis (mean leukocyte count, 10.5 × 10^9/L; range, 4.3 to 19.4 × 10^9/L). Leukopenia (leukocyte count, < 3.5 × 10^9/L) was not observed. Anemia (hematocrit, < 0.35 [<35]; hemoglobin, < 125 g/L) occurred in 73% of patients and was usually normocytic or normochromic. The mean hematocrit was 0.327 [32.7], and the mean hemoglobin was 111 g/L (ranges, 0.13 to 0.45 [13 to 45] and 50 to 151 g/L, respectively). Thrombocytosis (platelets, ≥ 400 × 10^9/L) occurred in 65% of patients with active disease. The mean platelet count was 481 × 10^9/L (range, 113 to 1017 × 10^9/L). Thrombocytopenia (platelets, 113 × 10^9/L) was noted in only one patient before therapy. Response to treatment was associated with a parallel resolution of thrombocytosis in all cases. These findings are similar to our previous observations (5, 6).

Before treatment, the erythrocyte sedimentation rate (ESR, Westergren method) correlated with disease activity in 80% of patients (mean, 71 mm/h; range, 17 to 140 mm/h). Serum immunoglobulin levels before treatment were generally within the normal range. The use of prednisone and daily cyclophosphamide therapy occasionally resulted in persistent hypogammaglobulinemia, which did not correlate with clinical response to therapy.

Pathology

The pathologic manifestations of Wegener granulomatosis in the upper and lower airway of our patients are summarized in Table 1 and have been reported in detail elsewhere (15-17). Eighty-two open lung biopsies were done. Combined vasculitis and necrosis were found in 89% of biopsy samples; granulomas and necrosis were found in 90%; and the combinations of granulomas and vasculitis as well as vasculitis, necrosis, and granulomatous inflammation were found in 91% of biopsy specimens (16) (Figure 6). Fifty-nine transbronchial biopsies were done in 48 patients. In only four specimens (7%) was vasculitis identified, and granuloma were present in three of those four.

The small amount of tissue available in biopsy specimens from the head and neck may make it difficult or impossible to identify pathologic features of Wegener granulomatosis. Both vasculitis and necrosis were found in 23% of upper-airway biopsy specimens; vasculitis and granulomatous inflammation were present in 21%; and in only 16% were vasculitis, necrosis, and granulomatous inflammation all present (15). Diagnostically useful tissue in the upper airway was obtained in decreasing order of frequency from the paranasal sinuses, nose, and the subglottic region (*see* Table 1). This order may reflect the quantity of tissue usually obtained by each procedure.

The characteristic finding from renal biopsy in patients with Wegener granulomatosis was segmental necrotizing glomerulonephritis, which was usually focal (Figure 7, *left*) (18-20). One hundred and forty-four renal biopsies were done in 103 patients in our study. Varying degrees of segmental necrotizing glomerulonephritis were noted in 80%. Vasculitis unrelated to glomerular vessels occurred in 8% of specimens (Figure 7, *right*), and vasculitis and granulomatous changes were both present in 3% of specimens. In one patient, large necrotizing granulomas presented as a renal mass lesion. Skin specimens most commonly showed small vessel leukocytoclastic vasculitis and, less commonly, dermal necrotizing granulomas or necrotizing vasculitis involving larger dermal arteries or veins.

Seventy-nine percent of patients had at least one biopsy specimen with evidence of vasculitis. Eighty-nine percent of patients had vasculitis, granulomatous changes, or both in these specimens. The remainder of patients in whom biopsy findings were less diagnostic had evidence of glomerulonephritis shown by renal biopsy.

Table 1. Pathologic Findings from Open-Lung and Upper-Airway Biopsy Samples in Patients with Wegener Granulomatosis*

Variable	Type of Inflammation				
	Nasal (n = 60)	Paranasal Sinuses (n = 27)	Larynx (n = 17)	Lung (n = 82)	
	← n (%) →				
Parenchymal changes†					
Geographic necrosis‡	12(20)	15(56)	3(18)	56(68)	
Poorly formed granulomas	28(47)	16(59)	4(23)	48(59)	
Scattered giant cells	28(47)	16(59)	4(23)	64(78)	
Microabscesses	20(33)	10(37)	3(18)	53(65)	
Microabscesses plus granulomas	12(20)	9(33)	3(18)	56(68)	
Vascular changes§					
Granulomatous vasculitis	4(7)	4(15)	0(0)	NG 8(22)¶ NNG 21(26)	NG 6(7)** NNG 8(10)
Acute vasculitis	10(17)	8(30)	0(0)	30 (37)	23 (28)
Chronic vasculitis	14(23)	8(30)	1(6)	71(87)	23 (28)
Fibrinoid necrosis	6(10)	3(11)	0(0)	9 (11)	5 (6)
Cicatricial changes‖	0(0)	1(4)	1(6)	33(40)	13 (16)

* Data combined from references 25 and 26. NG = necrotizing granulomas; NNG = non-necrotizing granulomas.
† Sarcoid-like granulomas were not seen in any biopsy samples from the upper airway and were found in only 3 (4%) from the lung.
‡ Geographic necrosis was defined as parenchymal necrosis characterized by a basophilic, granular center with a serpentine border often lined by a peripheral rim of palisading histocytes and multinucleated giant cells.
§ Capillaritis was observed in 31% of open-lung biopsy specimens and was characterized primarily by acute inflammation.
‖ Cicatricial changes are nonspecific and should not be used as diagnostic criteria.
¶ Data in this column (six entries) refer to the arteries.
** Data in this column (six entries) refer to the veins.

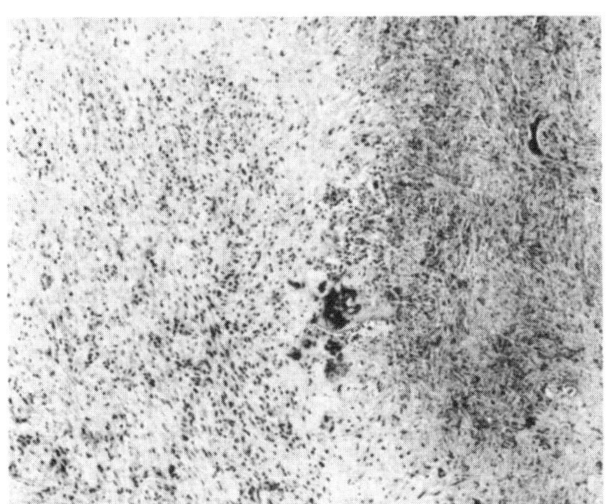

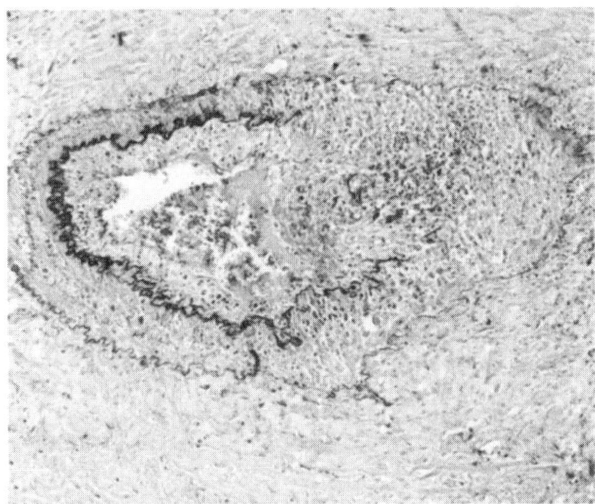

Figure 6. Lung biopsy showing a necrotizing granuloma characteristic of Wegener granulomatosis. Left. An area of necrosis (seen at right) is surrounded by a fibroinflammatory infiltrate that contains multinucleated giant cells. (Hematoxylin and eosin stain, 100 × original magnification). **Right.** Another site in this biopsy sample shows necrotizing vasculitis that involves a pulmonary arteriole. The destructive inflammatory infiltrate is eccentric, transmural, and has destroyed the inner and outer elastic laminae. (Verhoeff elastic stain, 200 × original magnification).

Clinical Outcome

One hundred and thirty-three patients (84%) were treated with standard therapy (daily cyclophosphamide and glucocorticoids). Eight (5.0%) received only low-dose cyclophosphamide therapy. Ten patients (6.0%) were treated with only glucocorticoids, and 6 patients (4.0%) who never received cyclophosphamide were treated with other cytotoxic agents and glucocorticoids. Standard treatment resulted in marked improvement or partial remission in 91% of patients and complete remission in 75% of patients. Among those patients who achieved remission while receiving standard therapy, conversion from daily to alternate-day prednisone occurred within a median of 3.2 months. The median time to complete discontinuation of glucocorticoids was 12 months. Although some patients achieved complete remission within a few months, the median time for all patients receiving standard therapy to achieve remission was 12 months (Figure 8). Some patients (8.3%) with seemingly intractable disease eventually did achieve remission up to 4 to 6 years after initiation of therapy. Fifty percent of complete remissions were followed by one or more relapses. Relapses occurred from 3 months to 16 years after achieving remission. If outcome, as measured by remission, were expressed in terms of total patient years of follow-up (1229 patient years), 46% of all patients' time during the study was spent in remission. When remission analysis focused only on the 98 patients with at least 5 years of follow-up, several other important observations emerged. Remission was

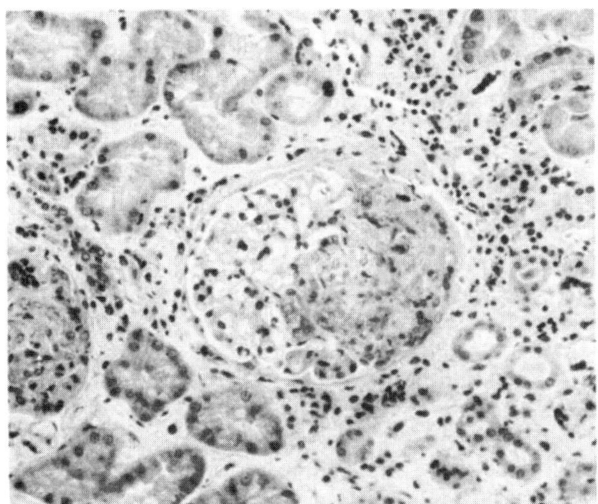

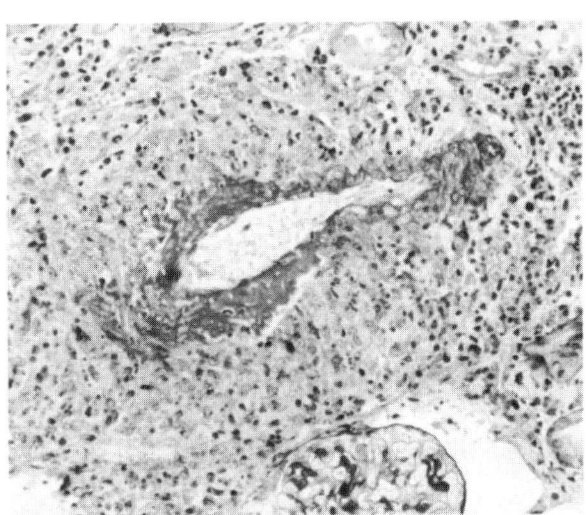

Figure 7. Renal abnormalities in Wegener granulomatosis. Left. A segmental necrotizing glomerular lesion (Hematoxylin and eosin stain, × 250 original magnification). **Right.** Necrotizing vasculitis with fibrinoid necrosis is present in the extraglomerular tissue of this renal biopsy specimen (Hematoxylin and eosin stain, × 250 original magnification).

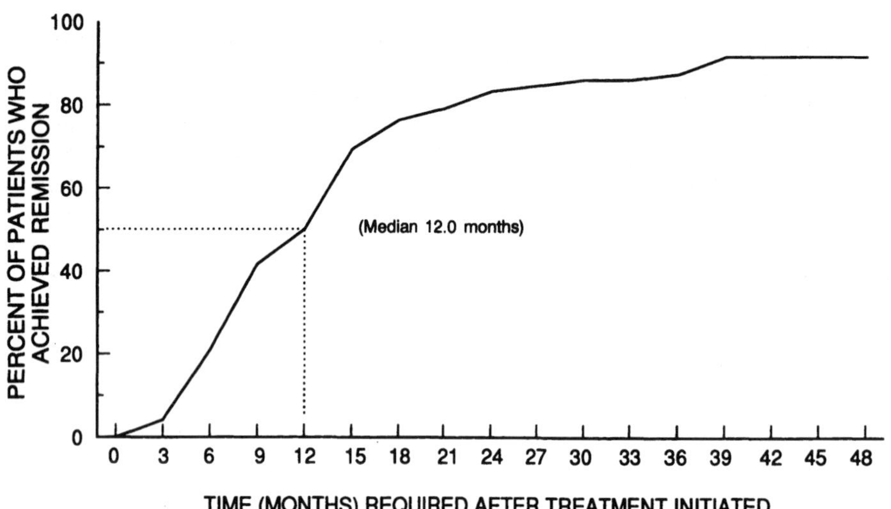

Figure 8. Graphic representation of the cumulative remission rate from the beginning of standard treatment. The cumulative rate is illustrated only for those patients (75% of total) in whom complete remission occurred. Although 50% of all individuals who achieved remission did so within 12 months, 20% required treatment for over 2 years before all features of disease had resolved. The remaining 8.3% of patients achieved remission after 48 months.

achieved at least once in 96% of patients. However, 49% later experienced at least one relapse. Forty-four percent of patients had remissions of more than 5 consecutive years duration. Thirteen percent of patients in this group experienced subsequent relapse. Similarly, 10 of 54 patients (18.5%) with over 10 years of follow-up experienced remissions of at least 10 consecutive years; two (20%) of these patients later relapsed.

Ten patients (6.0%) were treated with only glucocorticoids during the course of our study. Six patients had limited (no evidence of renal disease) and four had generalized disease. Only two of six patients with limited Wegener granulomatosis achieved sustained remission. One of four patients with limited disease improved while receiving glucocorticoid therapy but did not achieve remission and later died of active Wegener granulomatosis. All four patients with generalized disease who received only glucocorticoid therapy died of active Wegener granulomatosis. Deaths among patients treated with only glucocorticoids occurred before recognition of the efficacy of cyclophosphamide therapy (5, 6).

Eight patients (5.0%) were treated exclusively with low-dose daily cyclophosphamide. Four patients had limited disease, and four had generalized disease. Two of the four patients with glomerulonephritis had significant renal failure (serum creatinine, 389 μmol/L [4.4 mg/dL] and 592 μmol/L [6.7 mg/dL], respectively) when cyclophosphamide treatment was initiated. Both patients died within 1.5 years due to active Wegener granulomatosis and end-stage renal disease. Two patients with glomerulonephritis had normal serum creatinine values at the start of cyclophosphamide therapy and achieved remission after about 2 years. These patients remained in remission without medication for 2 and 6 years, respectively, and were then lost to follow-up. All four patients with limited Wegener granulomatosis who were treated with only cyclophosphamide achieved remission after 1 to 2.5 years of therapy and have remained in remission without cyclophosphamide therapy for 1 to 11 years.

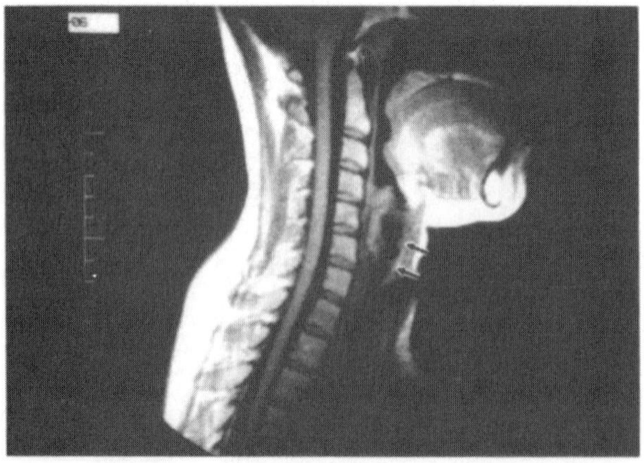

Figure 9. Subglottic (tracheal) stenosis. Magnetic resonance imaging (Picker, 0.5 Tesla magnet, T1 weighted image). Arrows show two foci of subglottic stenosis above the tracheostomy site. Failure of dilatations to restore normal tracheal patency led to tracheal reconstructive surgery that was only partially successful.

Morbidity

We divided morbidity into three categories: that which resulted from disease only, from disease plus treatment, and from treatment only. Permanent disease-related morbidity occurred in 86% of patients and included chronic renal insufficiency (42%), hearing loss (35%), cosmetic and functional nasal deformities (28%), tracheal stenosis (13%), and visual loss (8%). Many patients experienced more than one permanent type of morbidity.

Renal insufficiency was often severe; the median creatinine level was 225.4 μmol/L (2.55 mg/dL). Although the most common histopathologic renal abnormality was focal segmental glomerulonephritis, most patients with irreversible renal impairment had developed varying degrees of diffuse proliferative, crescentic, necrotic, and sclerotic lesions. Of our 158 patients, 17 (11%) eventually required dialysis, and 5% (about half of the patients needing dialysis) had renal transplantation. All eight renal transplant recipients were in remission and were not receiving immunosuppressive medications at the time of surgical engraftment. Follow-up after transplantation varied from 6 months to 13 years (mean, 5 years). Only one patient experienced recurrence of active Wegener granulomatosis that contributed to renal failure. This observation has reinforced our belief in the feasibility of renal transplantation in patients with Wegener granulomatosis who are in remission.

Hearing loss was related to recurrent serous or suppurative otitis media, sensorineural impairment, or to a combination of these factors. Most affected patients had partial unilateral or bilateral hearing loss (33%) that required hearing aids. Rarely, complete unilateral (1%) or bilateral (1%) deafness occurred. Five patients (3%) required mastoid sinus exenterations for secondary chronic infection or Wegener granulomatosis that was unresponsive to medical therapy.

Nasal deformity occurred only rarely in patients without concurrent chronic sinus disease. The emotional impact of this deformity is usually substantial. Most affected patients were eager to have nasal cosmetic surgery. Concern about relapsing disease, however, led to restraint in carrying out such procedures.

Of our 158 patients, 25 (16%) had tracheal stenosis (Figures 9 and 10). The most common symptom was shortness of breath. Symptoms and findings in five patients were modest and resolved during the course of treatment. In 20 patients, subglottic tracheal stenosis was irreversible. In 12 patients with severe tracheal stenosis the presentation included stridor and required emergency tracheostomy. Three patients had moderate degrees of stenosis that permitted manual or laser dilatation without a preceding tracheostomy. In four patients, mild fixed stenosis was followed but not treated during serial examinations. Five patients failed to achieve adequate subglottic patency after multiple attempts at dilatation and required open tracheal reconstruction procedures.

Visual loss (8%) occurred primarily as the result of retro-orbital Wegener granulomatosis, taking the form of a pseudotumor or mass lesion (*see* Figure 5, *bottom right*). The histopathologic features of pseudotumors varied within and between specimens with regard to the extent of inflammatory disease and fibrosis. Extensive fibrotic changes in chronic lesions may explain the relative resistance of this problem to treatment.

Permanent morbidity attributed to disease plus medical or surgical treatment or both included chronic sinus dysfunction (47%) and pulmonary insufficiency (17%). The combined effects of disease activity, upper airway surgery to provide drainage of impacted sinuses or to obtain diagnostic material, and medical therapy probably all contributed to atrophic rhinitis and sinusitis, chronic mucosal crusting, impaired mucosal immunity, and recurrent infections. *Staphylococcus aureus* was the most common cause of purulent sinusitis and was treated using antibiotics and sinus irrigation. Persistent or recurrent infections also required surgical drainage. Clinical distinction between worsening sinus disease due to Wegener granulomatosis, infection, or both, was often difficult. In the absence of purulent drainage and a prompt response to antibiotics, surgical drainage and biopsy were often required for a more definitive diagnosis. Most patients, regardless of disease activity, had mucosal glandular atrophy. They required daily (one to three times per day) saline irrigations to minimize accumulation of sinus and nasal secretions and crusts associated with an increased risk for impaction and infection.

Serial pulmonary function studies documented moderate to severe degrees of progressive pulmonary insufficiency in at least 17% of patients. We could not distinguish to what degree restrictive changes were caused by fibrosis that followed active Wegener granulomatosis, by cyclophosphamide-induced pneumonitis, or by a combination of these factors. Endobronchial lesions and scarring due to Wegener granulomatosis caused obstructive lung disease and recurrent postobstructive pneumonias in several patients.

Some forms of morbidity were attributed solely to treatment toxicity, when complications were well known medication side effects and were not known to be manifestations of untreated Wegener granulomatosis. Transient, mild to moderate cyclophosphamide-induced hair loss occurred in 17% of patients, and glucocorticoid-induced diabetes mellitis occurred in 8%, of whom 3% required insulin. All glucocorticoid-treated patients

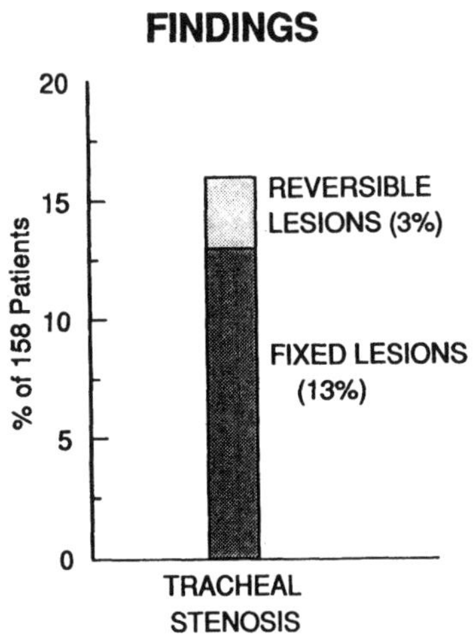

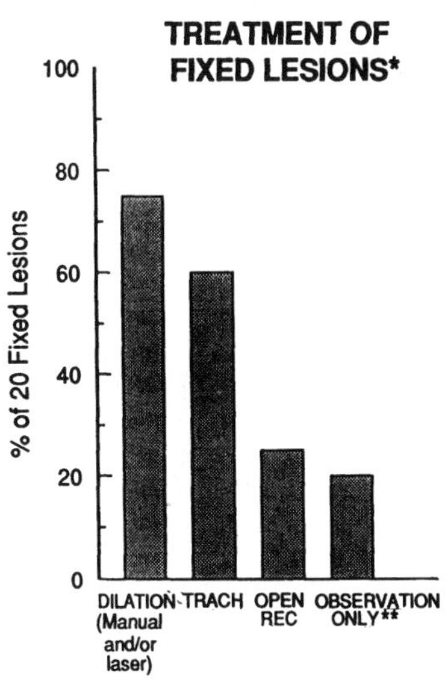

Figure 10. Tracheal stenosis in patients with Wegener granulomatosis. Sixteen percent of all patients had tracheal stenosis. In a minority, lesions were reversible with immunosuppressive therapy. However, most patients required surgical intervention to restore adequate ventilation. * Totals exceed 100% because some patients required more than one surgical intervention. ** Indicates mild stenosis. Open rec = tracheal reconstructive surgery; Trach = tracheostomy.

experienced transient Cushingoid features. Examples of persistent or more permanent treatment-associated morbidity included cyclophosphamide-cystitis (43%), bladder cancer (2.8%), myelodysplasia (2%) and glucocorticoid-related cataracts (21%), fractures (11%), and aseptic necrosis (3%).

In 28 women, ranging in age from 18 to 35 years, adequate information was available to estimate fertility status after at least 1 year of therapy with daily low-dose cyclophosphamide. Sixteen patients (57%) had stopped having menses for more than 1 year, were unable to become pregnant, or had hormonal studies that supported the impression of ovarian failure. Data regarding fertility and hormonal status in men were not available.

To determine whether cyclophosphamide could be implicated in the genesis of malignancies, the malignancy rate among patients with Wegener granulomatosis (791 per 100 000 persons annually) was compared with that in the National Cancer Institute Registry (1982 to 1986) for adult men and women in the general population (335 per 100 000 persons annually). The results indicate a 2.4-fold overall increase in malignancies, a 33-fold increase in bladder cancers (ratio of cases observed to those expected, 4 to 0.12), and an 11-fold increase in lymphomas (ratio of cases observed to those expected, 2 to 0.18). The latency period from the start of cyclophosphamide therapy to detection of transitional cell carcinoma of the bladder varied from 7 months in one patient who was receiving daily cyclophosphamide, to 12 years in a patient who had not received cyclophosphamide for 10 years. Cyclophosphamide-treated patients who have experienced hematuria unrelated to glomerulonephritis have been evaluated using cystoscopy and bladder biopsy. All cyclophosphamide-treated patients, even after treatment has been stopped, have continued to have urinary cytologic examinations.

All four patients (two men and two women) with bladder cancer developed hematuria (microscopic hematuria in three, gross hematuria in one) in the absence of red blood cell casts, which led to cystoscopic evaluation and a subsequent diagnosis of malignancy. One patient also had atypical cells observed during urinary cytologic screening before the diagnosis of bladder cancer. Features that might enhance the risk for cyclophosphamide-induced bladder cancer, such as obstructive uropathy and neurogenic bladder, were not present in any of these patients.

Two patients developed lymphomas after 1.5 and 8.6 years of cyclophosphamide treatment, respectively. Myelodysplasia followed 1.6, 9.6, and 13 years of similar therapy in three patients, respectively.

Infectious Complications

Because the degree to which tissue damage (such as that leading to impaired mucosal immunity) or immunosuppressive therapies led to infections was unclear, these complications are reported separately. Seventy-three patients (46%) experienced 140 serious infections over 1229 patient years (0.11 infections per patient year). Serious infection was defined as that which required hospitalization and intravenous antibiotics. Examples of serious infections included pneumonias (57 episodes, 39% of serious infections) due to *Pseudomonas aerugenosa* (8 episodes), *Staphylococcus aureus* (8 episodes), and fungal organisms such as *Coccidioides immitis*, *Aspergillus fumigatus*, and *Candida albicans* (8 episodes), *Hemophilus influenza* (7 episodes), *Pneumocystis carinii* (6 episodes), *Streptococcus pneumonia* (3 episodes), *Mycobacterium tuberculosis* (1 episode), *Mycobacterium avium-intracellulare* (1 episode); skin infections (38 episodes, 26% of serious infections) that were most often due to herpes zoster (34 episodes); and bacterial or fungal sepsis (13 episodes, 9% of serious infections). Although sinus infections of bacterial origin were common, most patients were treated by their personal referring physicians on an outpatient basis using oral antibiotics. The precise frequency of such therapy is unclear, but 9% of all serious hospital-treated infections involved the sinuses. When medical therapy, including sinus irrigation, superficial debridement, and antibiotics was unsuccessful, surgical sinus drainage was done. Fifty percent of all serious bacterial, pneumocystis, and fungal infections (0.208 infections per patient year) occurred during periods of daily glucocorticoid therapy. A significantly smaller proportion of serious infections occurred during alternate-day therapy with glucocorticoids (21%), single agent cytotoxic therapy (16%), and periods without therapy (12%). This observation underscores the rationale behind the change from daily to alternate-day glucocorticoid therapy as quickly as was clinically feasible. The incidence of cutaneous herpes zoster was 0.004 infections per patient year during periods of no treatment and was about 10-fold increased in patients receiving daily or alternate-day glucocorticoids or only daily cyclophosphamide therapy. Compared with periods of no treatment, the frequency of herpes zoster infection was increased 20-fold when glucocorticoids and cyclophosphamide were used concurrently. Thus, glucocorticoids and cyclophosphamide independently and in combination enhanced the risk for herpes zoster infections.

Mortality

Twenty percent of all patients in our study died. In 13% of patients, death could be completely or partially attributed to active Wegener granulomatosis, chronic morbidity from previously active disease, complications of treatment, or a combination of these factors. Factors contributing to death included renal disease (3%), pulmonary disease (3%), concomitant renal and pulmonary disease (1%), infection (3%), and malignancy (2.5%). No significant differences in morbidity and mortality were noted between men and women.

Discussion

In 1973 Fauci and Wolff (5) reported the initial prospective NIH experience with Wegener granulomatosis. Our studies, which now extend over 24 years, have enhanced our understanding of the broad spectrum of organ system involvement, the atypical and indolent forms of disease, the efficacy of standard therapy to induce remission, and the tendency of patients to relapse and accrue additive morbidity from both disease and treatment. Our 158 patients (followed for up to 24 years) were remarkably similar to the 18 patients in our earlier study cohort with regard to the frequency and quality of clinical abnormalities. An important observation that has been repeatedly confirmed since the early reports by Klinger (1) and Wegener (2, 3) is that the airway is almost always initially involved in Wegener granulomatosis. Although upper or lower respiratory symptoms (or both) are usually present, about 34% of patients with radiographic, biopsy-proven, pulmonary abnormalities may be asymptomatic. We have recently shown that some persons with active Wegener granulomatosis, who lack airway symptoms and who have normal chest radiographs and computerized axial tomographic results, may have neutrophilic alveolitis and pulmonary production of ANCA as determined by bronchoalveolar lavage analysis (21, 22). Although it is not known whether similar findings occur in sinus lavage specimens, we have observed significant abnormalities of the nasal mucosa and sinus radiographs in asymptomatic patients. These findings have practical application in the evaluation of patients in whom Wegener granulomatosis is suspected. The upper airway and lungs of such patients should be studied by direct inspection or imaging techniques, even when these sites are not the source of symptoms.

Our current experience has confirmed the life-saving potential of daily therapy with cyclophosphamide and glucocorticoids for this once usually fatal disease (7). However, long-term follow-up has also produced greater awareness of disease relapse in about half of our patients and serious morbidity resulting from the disease and its treatment. Our standard protocol was designed to minimize daily glucocorticoid therapy. In those patients experiencing partial or complete remission within 4 to 8 weeks of starting daily therapy with cyclophosphamide and glucocorticoids, prednisone was gradually tapered over the next 4 to 8 weeks to an alternate-day schedule. Among the 75% of patients who achieved remission, a median of 3.2 months was required to taper daily glucocorticoid therapy to an alternate-day schedule, and a median of 12 months was required to discontinue glucocorticoids entirely. Patients who did not achieve or sustain remission received longer courses of glucocorticoid therapy. Despite efforts to minimize the use of glucocorticoids, such therapy ultimately contributed to opportunistic infections, (especially during the period of daily glucocorticoid use), osteoporosis, fractures, cataracts, and Cushingoid features.

The frequencies of cyclophosphamide-induced cystitis (43%), bladder cancer (2.8%), and myelodysplasia (2%) among our patients were higher than those previously recognized (6). The known extended latency period for expression of malignancy, even after discontinuation of treatment with alkylating agents, is of great concern.

Treatment-related morbidity has led us to search for safer and effective alternative therapies. We have evaluated the potential efficacy of intermittent high-dose intravenous ("pulse") cyclophosphamide (23), trimethoprim-sulfamethoxazole, and low-dose weekly methotrexate therapies. Our interest in pulse cyclophosphamide stemmed from its successful application in the treatment of systemic lupus erythematosus with nephritis (24-27). After 4 months of pulse cyclophosphamide therapy, 13 of 14 patients (93%) with Wegener granulomatosis markedly improved, and half had achieved remission. Despite further treatment over 6 to 24 months, however, 72% of patients were unable to sustain remission. Our patients received monthly high-dose intravenous cyclophosphamide and daily prednisone that was later tapered to alternate-day therapy after clinical improvement. Steppat and Gross (28) also used a monthly pulse cyclophosphamide protocol and reported results similar to ours. Their protocol differed in that monthly high-dose glucocorticoid therapy was given as well. Other, as yet untried, pulse cyclophosphamide regimens may prove more beneficial.

Several reports have suggested that trimethoprim-sulfamethoxazole therapy may be useful in the treatment of Wegener granulomatosis (29-33). The anecdotal nature of these reports, the tenuous nature of the diagnosis in some cases, the use of concurrent immunosuppressive therapies, and failure to rule out infection for which trimethoprim-sulfamethoxazole may be an effective antimicrobial, all cast some doubt on purported efficacy (34). We studied this agent in an ongoing prospective open study. Patients were required to have active biopsy-proven disease, no evidence of infection, and to have not initiated or increased immunosuppressive therapies for at least 3 months. Thus far, only one of nine patients has had prolonged improvement while receiving trimethoprim-sulfamethoxazole therapy (one double-strength tablet, twice daily). This experience has reinforced our skepticism regarding the role of trimethoprim-sulfamethoxazole in the treatment of Wegener granulomatosis.

The benefits of methotrexate in the treatment of rheumatoid arthritis (35-41) and rheumatoid vasculitis (42) led to initiation of a trial of low-dose weekly methotrexate (0.15 to 0.30 mg/kg) in patients with systemic vasculitides, including Wegener granulomatosis. Although remissions have occurred in 14 of 18 patients (unpublished observations), our impressions remain guarded because of the brief (1 year) follow-up period. Further study is necessary to determine what role methotrexate will play in the treatment of Wegener granulomatosis.

Without a better understanding of the events that trigger and perpetuate expression of Wegener granulomatosis, nonspecific immunosuppressive therapies are not likely to provide uniform long-term remissions without relapse. The heterogeneity of our patient sample with regard to age, geographic origins, previous illness, environmental inhalant exposure (data not shown), and the inability to identify microorganisms in lung tissue or bronchoalveolar lavage fluid (21) casts doubt on whether Wegener granulomatosis is triggered by any single agent. Stimulation of the upper or lower airway by various airborne substances may, in a predisposed person, lead to systemic illnesses, such as Wegener granulomatosis. Whether proteinase-3 antibodies play a role in an airway-mediated systemic illness being expressed as Wegener granulomatosis is unclear (43-45).

Our imperfect understanding of Wegener granulomatosis leaves us to apply broadly immunosuppressive therapies in the hope of producing remission and minimizing disease and treatment-associated morbidity. Standard therapy with daily cyclophosphamide and glucocorticoids is currently the best known means of achieving these ends. However, drug toxicity associated with such treatment is substantial and requires continued efforts to better understand disease pathophysiology and to identify effective alternative less toxic therapy.

Acknowledgments: The authors thank the National Institute of Allergy and Infectious Diseases Clinical Fellows and Clinical Center nursing staff for the care of our patients and Mary Rust for preparation of the manuscript.

Requests for Reprints: Gary S. Hoffman, MD, National Institutes of Health, Building 10, Room 11B12, Bethesda, MD 20892.

Current Author Addresses: Drs. Hoffman, Kerr, Leavitt, Lebovics, Travis, Rottem, and Fauci and Ms. Hallahan: National Institutes of Health, 9000 Rockville Pike, Building 10, Room 11B12, Bethesda, MD 20892.

References

1. **Klinger H.** Grenzformen der periarteritis nodosa. Frankf Z Pathol. 1931;42:455-80.
2. **Wegener F.** Über generalisierte, septische efäberkrankungen. Verh Dtsch Pathol Ges. 1936;29:202-10.
3. **Wegener F.** Über eine eigenartige rhinogene granulomatose mit besonderer beteiligung des arterien systems und der nieren. Beitr Pathol Anat Allg Pathol. 1939;36-68.
4. **Pinching AJ, Lockwood CM, Pussell BA, Rees AJ, Sweny P, Evans DJ.** Wegener's granulomatosis: observations on 18 patients with severe renal disease. Q J Med. 1983;208:435-60.
5. **Fauci AS, Wolff SM.** Wegener's granulomatosis: studies in eighteen patients and a review of the literature. Medicine. 1973;52:535-61.
6. **Fauci AS, Haynes BF, Katz P, Wolff SM.** Wegener's granulomatosis: prospective clinical and therapeutic experience with 85 patients for 21 years. Ann Intern Med 1983;98:76-85.
7. **Walton EW.** Giant cell granuloma of the respiratory tract (Wegener's granulomatosis). Br Med J. 1958;2:265-70.
8. **Hollander D, Manning RT.** The use of alkylating agents in the treatment of Wegener's granulomatosis. Ann Intern Med. 1967;67:393-8.
9. **Reza MJ, Dornfeld L, Goldberg LS, Bluestone R, Pearson CM.** Wegener's granulomatosis. Long-term followup of patients treated with cyclophosphamide. Arthritis Rheum. 1975;18:501-6.
10. **Van Der Woude FJ, Lobatto S, Permin H, van der Giessen M, Rasmussen N, Wiik A.** Autoantibodies against neutrophils and monocytes: Tool for diagnosis and marker of disease activity in Wegener's granulomatosis. Lancet. 1985;1:425-9.
11. **Specks U, Wheatley CL, McDonald TJ, Rohrbach MS, DeRemee RA.** Anticytoplasmic autoantibodies in the diagnosis and follow-up of Wegener's granulomatosis. Mayo Clin Proc. 1989;64:28-36.
12. **Nölle B, Specks U, Lüdemann J, Rohrback MS, DeRemee RA, Gross WL.** Anticytoplasmic autoantibodies: their immunodiagnostic value in Wegener's granulomatosis. Ann Intern Med. 1989;111:28-40.
13. **Lüdemann J, Csernok E, Ulmer M, Lemke H, Utecht B, Rautmann A.** Anti-neutrophil cytoplasm antibodies in Wegener's granulomatosis: immunodiagnostic value, monoclonal antibodies and characterization of the target antigen. Neth J Med. 1990;36:157-62.
14. **Cohen Tervaert JW, Huitem MG, Hene RJ, Sluiter WJ.** Prevention of relapses in Wegener's granulomatosis by treatment based on anti-neutrophil cytoplasmic antibody titer. Lancet. 1990;336:709-11.
15. **Devaney KO, Travis WD, Hoffman GS, Leavitt RY, Lebovics R, Fauci AS.** Interpretation of head and neck biopsies in Wegener's granulomatosis. A pathologic study of 126 biopsies in 70 patients. Am J Surg Pathol. 1990;14:555-64.
16. **Travis WD, Hoffman GS, Leavitt RY, Pass HI, Fauci AS.** Surgical pathology of the lung in Wegener's granulomatosis. Review of 87 open lung biopsies from 67 patients. Am J Surg Pathol. 1991;15:315-33.
17. **Travis WD, Colby TV, Lombard C, Carpenter HA.** A clinicopathologic study of 34 cases of diffuse pulmonary hemorrhage with lung biopsy confirmation. Am J Surg Pathol. 1990;14:112-25.
18. **Antonovych TT, Sabnis SG, Tuur SM, Sesterhenn IA, Balow JE.** Morphologic differences between polyarteritis and Wegener's granulomatosis using light, electron and immunohistochemical techniques. Mod Pathol. 1989;2:349-59.
19. **Watanabe T, Yoshikawa Y, Toyoshima H.** Morphological and clinical features of the kidney in Wegener's granulomatosis. A survey of 28 autopies in Japan. Jap J Nephrol. 1981;23:921-30.
20. **Weiss MA, Crissman JD.** Renal biopsy findings in Wegener's granulomatosis: Segmental necrotizing glomerulonephritis with glomerular thrombosis. Hum Pathol. 1984;15:943-56.
21. **Hoffman GS, Sechler JM, Gallin JI, Shelhamer JH, Suffredini A, Ognibene FP, et al.** Bronchoalveolar lavage analysis in Wegener's granulomatosis. Am Rev Respir Dis. 1991;143:401-7.
22. **Baltaro RJ, Hoffman GS, Sechler JM, Suffredini AF, Shelhamer JH, Fauci AS, et al.** Immunoglobulin G antineutrophil cytoplasmic antibodies are produced in the respiratory tract of patients with Wegener's granulomatosis. Am Rev Respir Dis. 1991;143:275-8.
23. **Hoffman GS, Leavitt RY, Fleisher TA, Minor JR, Fauci AS.** Treatment of Wegener's granulomatosis with intermittent high-dose intravenous cyclophosphamide. Am J Med. 1990;89:403-10.
24. **Balow JE, Austin HA, Muenz LR, Joyce KM, Antonovych TT, Klippel JH, et al.** Effect of treatment on the evolution of renal abnormalities in lupus nephritis. N Engl J Med. 1984;311:491-5.
25. **Balow JE, Austin HA, Tsokos GC, Antonovych TT, Steinberg AD, Klippel JH.** Lupus nephritis. Ann Intern Med. 1987;106:79-94.
26. **Austin HA, Klippel JH, Balow JE, LeRiche NG, Steinberg AD, Plotz PH, et al.** Therapy of lupus nephritis. Controlled trial of prednisone and cytotoxic drugs. N Engl J Med. 1986;314:614-9.
27. **Sessoms SL, Kovarsky J.** Monthly intravenous cyclophosphamide in the treatment of severe systemic lupus erythematosus. Clin Exp Rheumatol. 1984;2:247-51.
28. **Steppat D, Gross WL.** Stage adapted treatment of Wegener's granulomatosis. Klin Wochenschr. 1989;67:666-71.
29. **De Remee RA, McDonald TJ, Weiland LH.** Wegener's granulomatosis: observations on treatment with antimicrobial agents. Mayo Clin Proc. 1985;60:27-32.
30. **West BC, Todd JR, King JW.** Wegener's granulomatosis and trimethoprim-sulfamethoxazole: complete remission after a twenty-year course. Ann Intern Med. 1987;106:840-2.
31. **Yuasa K, Tokitsu M, Goto H, Kato H, Shimada K.** Wegener's granulomatosis: diagnosis by transbronchial lung biopsy, evaluation by gallium scintigraphy and treatment with sulfamethoxazole/trimethoprim. Am J Med. 1988;84:371-2.
32. **De Remee RA.** The treatment of Wegener's granulomatosis with trimethoprim/sulfamethoxazole: illusion or vision? Arthritis Rheum. 1988;31:1068-72.
33. **Israel HL.** Sulfamethoxazole-trimethoprim therapy for Wegener's granulomatosis. Arch Intern Med. 1988;148:2293-5.
34. **Leavitt RY, Hoffman GS, Fauci AS.** Response: the role of trimethoprim/sulfamethoxazole in the treatment of Wegener's granulomatosis. Arthritis Rheum. 1988;31:1073-4.
35. **Anderson PA, West SG, O'Dell JR, Via CS, Claypool RG, Kotzin BL.** Weekly pulse methotrexate in rheumatoid arthritis. Ann Intern Med. 1985;103:489-96.
36. **Weinstein A, Marlowe S, Korn J, Farouhar F.** Low dose methotrexate treatment of rheumatoid arthritis. Am J Med. 1985;79:331-7.
37. **Kremer JM, Lee JK.** The safety and efficacy of the use of methotrexate in long-term therapy for rheumatoid arthritis. Arthritis Rheum. 1986;29:822-31.
38. **Williams HJ, Wilkens RF, Samuelson CO, Alarcon GS, Guttadauria M, et al.** Comparison of low dose oral pulse methotrexate and placebo in the treatment of rheumatoid arthritis. Arthritis Rheum. 1985;28:721-30.
39. **Hamdy H, McKendry RJ, Mierins E, Liver JA.** Low dose methotrexate compared to azathioprine in the treatment of rheumatoid arthritis. Arthritis Rheum. 1987;30:361-8.
40. **Tugwell P, Bennett K, Gent M.** Methotrexate in rheumatoid arthritis. Indications, contraindications, efficacy and safety. Ann Intern Med. 1987;107:358-66.
41. **Weinblatt ME, Kaplan H, Germain BF, Merriman RC, Solomon SD, Wall B, et al.** Low dose methotrexate compared with auranofin in adult rheumatoid arthritis. A thirty-six week, double blind trial. Arthritis Rheum. 1990;33:330-8.
42. **Espinoza LR, Espinoza CG, Vasey FB, Germain BF.** Oral methotrexate for chronic rheumatoid arthritis ulcerations. J Am Acad Dermatol. 1986;15:508-12.
43. **Falk RJ, Terrell RS, Charles LA, Jennette JC.** Anti-neutrophil cytoplasmic autoantibodies induce neutrophils to degranulate and produce oxygen radicals in vitro. Proc Natl Acad Sci USA. 1990;87:4115-9.
44. **Van der Woude FJ, Van Es LA, Daha MR.** The role of the C-ANCA antigen in the pathogenesis of Wegener's granulomatosis. A hypothesis based on both humoral and cellular mechanisms. Neth J Med. 1990;36:169-71.
45. **Kallenberg CG.** Antineutrophil cytoplasmic antibodies (ANCA) and vasculitis. Clin Rheumatol 9. (suppl) 1990;132-5.

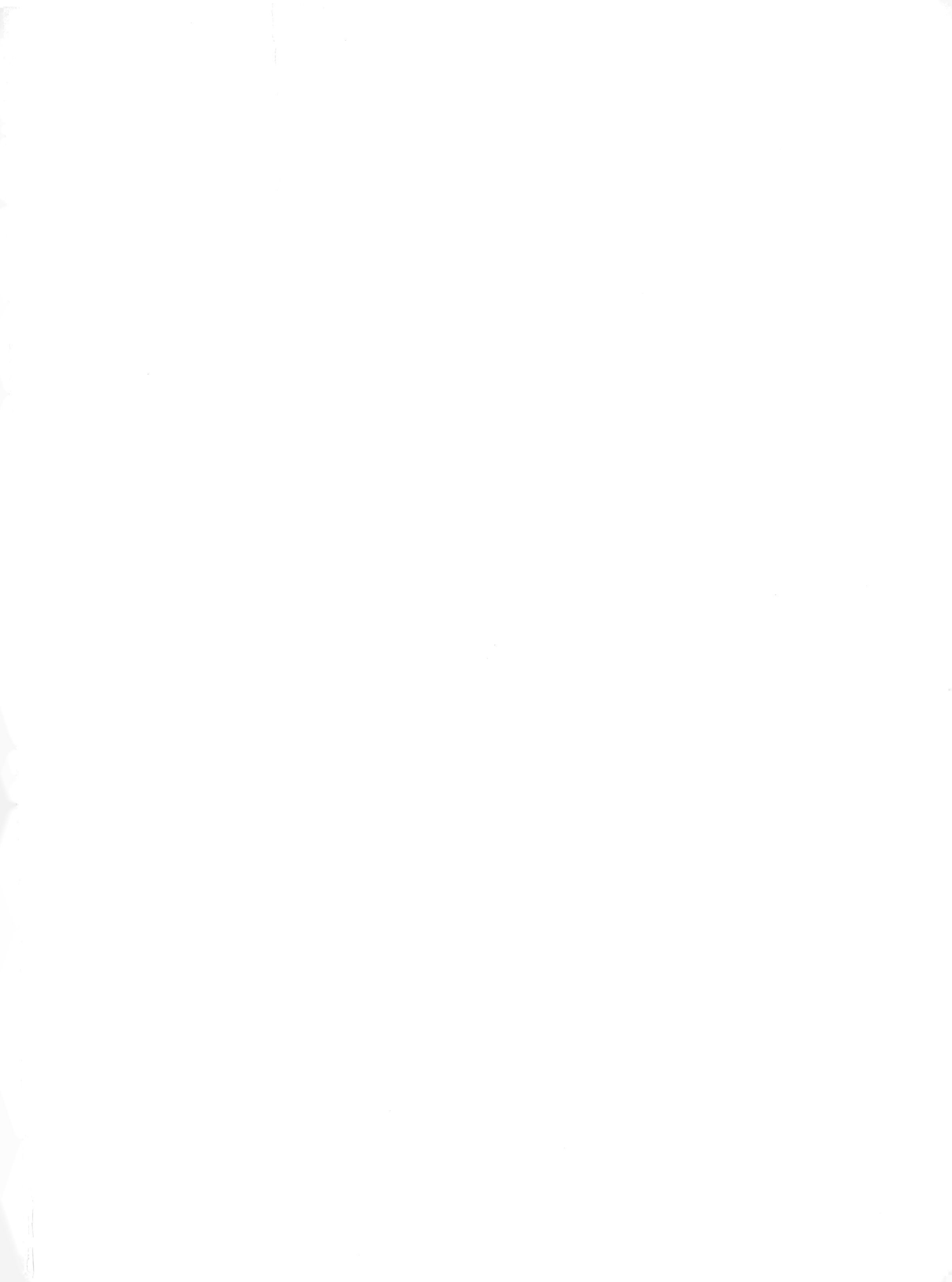